AF778739

Anglo-Saxon Prognostics, 900-1100

Brill's Studies in Intellectual History

General Editor

A.J. Vanderjagt, University of Groningen

Editorial Board

C.S. Celenza, Johns Hopkins University, Baltimore
M. Colish, Oberlin College
J.I. Israel, Institute for Advanced Study, Princeton
J.D. North, University of Groningen
W. Otten, Utrecht University

VOLUME 153

Brill's Texts and Sources in Intellectual History

General Editor

Han van Ruler, Erasmus University Rotterdam

Editorial Board

A. Fix, Lafayette College, Easton
J. Lagrée, Université de Rennes-1
U. Renz, Swiss Federal Institute of Technology Zurich
A. Uhlmann, University of Western Sydney

VOLUME 3

Anglo-Saxon Prognostics, 900-1100

Study and Texts

By

László Sándor Chardonnens

BRILL

LEIDEN • BOSTON
2007

Cover illustration: Oxford, St. John's College, MS 17, fol. 8r (detail), by permission of the President and Scholars of Saint John Baptist College in the University of Oxford.

Brill has done its best to establish rights to use of the materials printed herein. Should any other party feel that its rights have been infringed we would be glad to take up contact with them.

This book is printed on acid-free paper.

Library of Congress Cataloging-in-Publication data

A C.I.P. record for this book is available from the Library of Congress.

ISSN 0920-8607
ISBN 978-90-04-15829-0

© Copyright 2007 by Koninklijke Brill NV, Leiden, The Netherlands.
Koninklijke Brill NV incorporates the imprints Brill, Hotei Publishing, IDC Publishers, Martinus Nijhoff Publishers and VSP.

All rights reserved. No part of this publication may be reproduced, translated, stored in a retrieval system, or transmitted in any form or by any means, electronic, mechanical, photocopying, recording or otherwise, without prior written permission from the publisher.

Authorization to photocopy items for internal or personal use is granted by Koninklijke Brill NV provided that the appropriate fees are paid directly to The Copyright Clearance Center, 222 Rosewood Drive, Suite 910, Danvers, MA 01923, USA.
Fees are subject to change.

PRINTED IN THE NETHERLANDS

For Max Förster, Ditta and Femke
For learning, life and love

CONTENTS

FIGURES, PLATES, TABLES

ACKNOWLEDGMENTS

This book is a complete revision of my Ph.D. thesis, *Anglo-Saxon Prognostics: a Study of the Genre with a Text Edition*, which was written between 1998 and 2005 with financial aid from the Netherlands Organization for Scientific Research (NWO) and the research institute of the Faculty of Arts and Letters of Leiden University (Pallas). The thesis was supervised by Rolf H. Bremmer, Jr., and Bart Westerweel, reviewed by Elaine Treharne (University of Leicester), and defended with honours at Leiden University in 2006.

There are many people who have contributed in some way to my Ph.D. thesis and therefore also to the present book. Foremost are Rolf Bremmer and Bart Westerweel, who have, in addition to their supervision and guidance, maintained confidence and repeatedly managed to steer me clear of the dangers of Ph.D. research combined with the rough edges of my mind. Elaine Treharne has been very helpful in reviewing my thesis critically and meticulously from cover to cover before it went to the manuscript committee. I extend my gratitude to the manuscript committee: Wim van Anrooij (University of Leiden), Kees Dekker (University of Groningen), and Onno Kneepkens (University of Groningen); to the opposition committee: Manfred Horstmanshoff (University of Leiden), and Sophie van Romburgh (University of Leiden); and to the external examiners: Alasdair MacDonald (University of Groningen), and John North (University of Groningen). My dear friends Frederik Maes and Johan Oldenziel have been a great support in assisting me during the Ph.D. ceremony.

Furthermore, I should like to thank Marianne Elsakkers, Concetta Giliberto, Alan Griffiths, John C. Hirsh, Patrizia Lendinara, Roy Liuzza and Linda Voigts for their food for thought, Femke Prinsen for her help in the graphical field, Tom Hall, Erik Kooper, and Patrizia Lendinara, Rolf Bremmer and Kees Dekker for providing me with an opportunity to test my ideas at the International Congress on Medieval Studies at WMU, Kalamazoo (2000, 2002), the English Medievalists' Research Symposium in Utrecht (1998), and the Palermo and Leiden workshops of the Storehouses of Wholesome Learning project (2004, 2005). I owe my gratitude to Onno Kneepkens, whose advice and insight have proved truly invaluable in revising the text edition in the present book.

Needless to say, any mistakes in the text edition are my own or the scribes'.

My thanks go to Boris van Gool, Assistant Editor History of Brill Academic Publishers, and to the editors of Brill's Studies in Intellectual History and Brill's Texts and Sources in Intellectual History for accepting this volume in their series.

In preparing the text edition I have made use of microfilms, photographs and facsimiles. For a collation with the manuscripts, I visited libraries in Cambridge, London and Oxford in December 2002 and April 2006. These visits would not have been possible without the help of Gill Cannell, the Parker Library of Corpus Christi College, Cambridge; Joanna Ball, the Wren Library of Trinity College, Cambridge; Jayne Ringrose, the University Library, Cambridge; Joe Maldonado and Justin Clegg, the British Library, London; Richard Palmer, the Lambeth Palace Library, London; Bruce Barker-Benfield, the Bodleian Library, Oxford; and Catherine Hilliard, the Library of St. John's College, Oxford. I should like to thank the trustees and librarians of the libraries, and the masters and fellows of the colleges for granting me access to their manuscript collections.

The cover image (St. John's College, MS 17, fol. 8r, detail) is reproduced by permission of the President and Scholars of Saint John Baptist College in the University of Oxford. Plates are reproduced by permission of the Master and Fellows of Trinity College, Cambridge (Trinity College, O. 7. 41, fol. 1r), the British Library, London (Cotton Caligula A. xv, fol. 125v; Cotton Tiberius C. i, fol. 7v; Cotton Tiberius C. vi, fol. 6v; Cotton Vitellius E. xviii, fols 14v, 16r; Harley 3667, fols 4v, 5r), the Bodleian Library, University of Oxford (Bodley 579, fols 49v, 50r), the President and Scholars of Saint John Baptist College in the University of Oxford (St. John's College, MS 17, fols 8r, 41r).

My (continued) existence would be impossible, perhaps even inconceivable, without the support, love and friendship of my partner Femke Prinsen, and our mutual parents Ditta Huigen, and Harm and Harma Prinsen.

ABBREVIATIONS

Add.	Additional
Archiv	*Archiv für das Studium der neueren Sprachen und Literaturen*
ASE	*Anglo-Saxon England*
ASMMF	Anglo-Saxon Manuscripts in Microfiche Facsimile
CCCC	Cambridge, Corpus Christi College
CCSL	Corpus Christianorum, Series Latina
cont	continental
CPC	Cambridge, Pembroke College
CSASE	Cambridge Studies in Anglo-Saxon England
CTC	Cambridge, Trinity College
CUL	Cambridge, University Library
CUP	Cambridge University Press
ed.	editor(s)
EEMF	Early English Manuscripts in Facsimile
EETS	Early English Text Society
fig.	figure(s)
fol./fols, f./ff.	folio/folios
HBS	Henry Bradshaw Society
ill.	illustration(s)
L	Latin
ns	new series
OE	Old English
os	original series
OUP	Oxford University Press
pl.	plate(s)
rpt.	reprinted
ser.	series
ss	supplementary series
Sudhoff	*Sudhoffs Archiv für Geschichte der Medizin und der Naturwissenschaften, der Pharmazie und der Mathematik*
transl.	translator(s)
Univ.	University
UP	University Press
ZfdA	*Zeitschrift für deutsches Altertum und deutsche Litteratur*

INTRODUCTION

Prognostics foretell the future with the help of natural phenomena, dreams, and divinatory instruments such as the alphabet or dice. The everlasting relevance of such texts lies in the fascination people which display towards knowing their own future. Foreknowledge of the future places that which has yet to happen on the same level of certainty and interpretability as the present and the past, thereby lending comfort to and providing justification for events in the future. Human inquisitiveness ensured that, at various times in history, prognostics were considered important enough to be committed to clay tablets and papyri, vellum and paper.

The Anglo-Saxon prognostics represent but a brief phase in the long history of prognostication, which spans a period of over four thousand years and which extends into the present. Even though methods of prognostication hail from different cultures, from Assyrian to Egyptian, and from Greek to Roman, the practice of prognostication can be regarded as a continuum through time and space, because each culture built upon, expanded and modified its own prognostic knowledge and assimilated that of other cultures. Thus, a dream of being blind may be encountered in Assyrian, Greek and Anglo-Saxon dreambooks and an early twentieth-century *Dictionary of Dreams*:

> Assyrian: "If the eyes of a man do not see: for an important person [this means: more] importance, for a poor person: [more] poverty, [also] and an important person will be removed [i.e. die]".
> Greek: "If you dream of being blind, this signifies a matter of hindrance".
> Anglo-Saxon: "If anyone sees himself blind, it signifies hindrance".
> *Dictionary of Dreams*: "To dream of being blind, denotes a sudden change from affluence to almost abject poverty".[1]

At the same time, a dream about electricity will have been inconceivable to an Anglo-Saxon reader, but is not exceptional to us,[2] while a dream

[1] Oppenheim (1956: 258), Oberhelman (1981: I.81), translation of text 7/4, ll. 87-88, Miller (1909: 97, s.v. *Blind*), respectively.

[2] "To dream of electricity, denotes there will be sudden changes about you, which will not afford you either advancement or pleasure" (Miller 1909: 215, s.v. *Electricity*).

about kissing a dead person is not included in the modern dreambook, but features in many (pre-)medieval dreambooks.[3]

The age of some prognostic genres is considerable, especially that of the alphabetical dreambooks. Other genres, such as the Egyptian Days, the Dog Days and Apuleian Spheres, may have emerged in classical times, but the majority cannot be traced further back than the earliest witnesses in eighth- and ninth-century continental manuscripts. None of the prognostic genres known in England can be ascribed to a Germanic tradition of superstition: these prognostics are composed either in Latin or are translated directly from continental, Latin sources. Nevertheless, nowhere in Western Europe has the vernacularisation of prognostics enjoyed such an early start as in England. The Old English text on the Dog Days in Royal 12. D. xvii is the earliest prognostic in the vernacular ever encountered, to my knowledge. In addition, a number of prognostic genres is first attested in the Old English language, or in Anglo-Saxon and early post-Conquest manuscripts.

In this book the Anglo-Saxon prognostics will be analysed, a fraction of the medieval prognostic material available. My aim is twofold: to study the genre and its place in Anglo-Saxon culture and to provide an edition of all prognostics in Old English and a representative range in Latin.

The book is structured as follows: chapter one provides a definition of the genre and a history of the study of Anglo-Saxon prognostics. Chapter two delves into the manuscript contexts of the prognostics and offers a method to analyse the attestation of particular prognostic genres in relation to the manuscript context. Chapter three deals with the language of the texts and the date and place of origin of the manuscripts. Chapter four places prognostics within a framework of superstition in order to facilitate an investigation of opinions on prognostication in late Anglo-Saxon England. Chapter five, finally, addresses the issue of the intended use of Anglo-Saxon prognostics. It will become apparent that the corpus of prognostics does not constitute a modern effort at grouping an arbitrary range of texts together under one guise. Rather, the various types of prognostics were already organised into larger units and collected for different purposes in the Anglo-Saxon period.

The text edition features all prognostics which are discussed in the study, introduced and grouped by genre. The introductions to the

[3] See Oppenheim (1956: 259), Oberhelman (1981: I.81), Fischer (1982a: 55-57).

editions describe the working principle behind the genres and focus on their history and text transmission.

The appendices provide additional, mostly tabular information in the form of reference lists and concordances. Of these, appendix one is the most important because it offers a handlist of manuscripts and texts. It is the first place to look for information on the date, place of origin and contents of the manuscripts containing prognostics, and contains exhaustive descriptions of each prognostic in the corpus. Appendix two is a reference list based on appendix one, compounded by data analysed in chapters two and three. Appendix three is a concordance to the indexation of prognostics in catalogues and reference works on Anglo-Saxon texts. Appendix four features tables of numbers used in several prognostic genres. These tables can be consulted by those who actually wish to rely on prognostics in times of need, and by those who are, like me, appreciative of tables in general.

A number of interesting discoveries will be presented in this book: (1) a fivefold division of manuscript contexts which proves essential in understanding why some Anglo-Saxon prognostics are encountered more often than others and why certain prognostic genres appear in some contexts but not in others; (2) a correlation between language and manuscript context, and language and prognostic genre; (3) an analysis of a vogue in prognostics, specifically in the vernacular, in the period of the Benedictine Reform; (4) evidence that the status of prognostics changed in the course of time: though prognostics have usually been regarded as static expressions of superstition, medicine or arithmetic, they are not necessarily for that reason always superstitious, medical, or arithmetical texts; (5) ample indication that prognostics were not always held in strong opposition to orthodox Christianity, as some contemporaries, such as Ælfric, would have us believe, and that prognostics were probably not used in a pastoral capacity either.

The prognostic corpus collected here survives in thirty-seven manuscripts or fragments thereof. Most of the texts were copied in New Minster, Winchester, Christ Church, Canterbury, Worcester Cathedral and Ramsey Abbey. I have collected 174 texts: forty-nine in Old English, eleven in Latin with running glosses in Old English, and 114 in Latin. This collection comprises all glossed prognostics and those in Old English, from the earliest text on the Dog Days in Royal 12. D. xvii (s. x^{med}) to the prognostics in the twelfth-century booklet 5 of Hatton 115.[4] The 114 Latin texts in the corpus do not form a closed collection, but they do constitute a fair sample of English prognostics from the earliest witnesses in Digby 63 (867-92) to texts copied in the twelfth century. [5]

I have focussed on Anglo-Saxon prognostics, but many post-Conquest eleventh- and twelfth-century texts are included for two reasons. First, most of these early post-Conquest prognostics were copied from older, Anglo-Saxon exemplars, e.g. those in the eleventh-century manuscript Caligula A. xv + Egerton 3314, and the twelfth-century manuscripts Tiberius C. i + Harley 3667 and St. John's College 17. A negligible number of late eleventh- and twelfth-century prognostics are representative of genres or redactions unknown in England before the Norman Conquest. Second, an important collection of Old English prognostics was copied in the twelfth century in booklet 5 of Hatton 115, from Canterbury(?). The exemplar of this booklet was probably also used for some of the vernacular prognostics in the eleventh-century manuscript Tiberius A. iii. The testimony of Hatton 115 is, therefore, illustrative of a continued tradition of text transmission in the vernacular in the twelfth century. Moreover, the booklet also testifies to the uniquely English phenomenon of gathering prognostics into separate sections, first attested in the eleventh century. Such sections are of prime importance in preserving prognostics in the vernacular. For these reasons, the scope of this book is somewhat wider than Anglo-Saxon prognostics 900-1100.

[4] In Chardonnens (2006, 2007c) I have included the thirteenth-century copy of a vernacular prognostic by the Tremulous Worcester hand in CCCC 391, p. 721. In the present book, however, this prognostic is excluded from the corpus since a solitary witness from the thirteenth century is unrepresentative of the large number of texts from this period that have not been taken into account (see also p. 505, n. 20).

[5] Prognostics identified after I had compiled the prognostic corpus are not included in the study or the edition, but they are listed in a supplement (see pp. 545-48).

CHAPTER ONE

PROGNOSTICS DEFINED

Anglo-Saxon prognostics were first published, translated and studied on an appreciable scale by the Rev. Thomas Oswald Cockayne, Max Förster and Heinrich Henel, from the second half of the nineteenth to the first half of the twentieth century.[1] Remarkably, these scholars did not give a definition of the genre,[2] nor do present-day studies of prognostics. At most, the genre is described in terms of status: Förster saw prognostics as a exponent of 'Volkskunde' (folklore), whereas Henel identified them as 'Mönchsaberglaube' (monkish superstition).[3] The index to Neil Ker's *Catalogue of Manuscripts Containing Anglo-Saxon*, significantly, reads: "Prognostics. See Folklore".[4] 'Folklore', judging by Ker's classification, comprises a heterogeneous group of writings ranging from charms to (the majority of) prognostic genres.[5] Förster, Henel and Ker were not ignorant of what prognostics are, but still they preferred to describe the genre in terms of status. These scholars were preoccupied with the position of prognostics in low and high culture, rather than with the textual structure of prognostics or their intended purpose.

This one-sided approach is by no means restricted to any particular period. Ælfric had first-hand experience of prognostics,[6] and though he used the Old English verb "cepan" (to observe, to regulate by) in connection with prognostication, there is no comprehensive reference to prog-

[1] Cockayne (1861, 1864-66), Förster (1903, 1908a-c, 1910, 1911, 1912a-c, 1916, 1921, 1925-26, 1929, 1936, 1944), Henel (1934-35). See also pp. 16-23.

[2] In this entire book, I use the word 'genre' to refer both to prognostics as a whole, viz. the genre of prognostics, and to individual types of prognostic texts, i.e. alphabetical dreambooks are a prognostic genre rather than a subgenre of prognostics.

[3] Förster (1908a: 43-44), Henel (1934-35: 329-30).

[4] Ker (1957: 545).

[5] Ker (1957: 523). In Quinn and Quinn (1990) and in Cameron's list of Old English texts for the *Old English Corpus* and the *Dictionary of Old English* (Cameron 1973, Healy and Venezky 1980, 2000), prognostics and charms are gathered under the header "folklore" as well. Greenfield and Robinson's *Bibliography* (1980: 355-56) reads "folklore and prognostics", giving equal status to both categories. Scragg (2001: 275) wrote that prognostics are "texts that straddle the boundary between medicine and folklore".

[6] See pp. 98-101, 117-21.

nostics in Anglo-Saxon times.[7] At the other end of the time-line, Roy Liuzza, in the most recent study of Anglo-Saxon prognostics, noted that to regard prognostics in view of their status may lead to misrepresentations of the genre, yet Liuzza did not transcend the level of description to offer a definition.[8] Other recent studies in which prognostics play a major role similarly avoid a denotation of the genre.[9]

The only recent definition I have come across is from Treharne and Pulsiano's introduction to their outstanding *Companion to Anglo-Saxon Literature*, which relates that "prognostications attempt to pre-empt particular bad fates or unfortunate outcomes, by warning, among other things, of the probable occurrence of events on specific days or in specific periods".[10] This definition can be improved upon in three ways. First, prognostication does not necessarily deal with "bad fates or unfortunate outcomes". Therefore, prognostics do not so much warn as inform their users. Second, there can be no question of a "probable occurrence of events", because prognostication does not allow for probability: it offers certainty. Third, it is true that most prognostic genres are temporal, i.e. structured by time sequences,[11] but there are also genres which are non-temporal, e.g. alphabetical dreambooks. An example which illustrates my first two objections is a prognostic on the miraculous birthdays:

> There are three days and three nights in twelve months on which no girl is born, and the body of a boy that is born on these days will not decompose or rot before Judgement Day. Now one of these days is at the end of December, and the other two at the beginning of the month January, and there are few who have heard of or know this secret.[12]

This text shows that not all prognostics predict adverse events. It is a good thing that the body of a boy born on these days stays intact until Judgement Day at least. In addition, the text discloses a secret which not many people are aware of: not a "probable occurrence of events" but a fact. This knowledge is presented as a certainty; to question whether the outcome of the prediction pertains to reality will not detract from the conviction that is apparent in the text. The idea of relating prognostic

[7] Toller (1908-21: 122, s.v. *cepan* Ia, II), Cameron *et al.* (1980-: fiche C 1.2, s.v. *cepan* B.1.c). For Anglo-Saxon opinions towards prognostication, see chapter four.

[8] Liuzza (2001: 182-83).

[9] Cf. Hollis and Wright (1992: 257-70), Wallis (1995), Hollis (2001).

[10] Treharne and Pulsiano (2001: 7).

[11] See p. 11.

[12] Translation of text 3.1.2/2.

knowledge to reality is not new, as the following text on the twenty-four Egyptian Days illustrates:

> The doctors of old wrote in Latin books that there are always two days in each month on which it is very hurtful to drink any [medicinal] potion or to let blood, because there is a time on each of these days that if one opens a vein on this time, it will cause death or protracted pain. A doctor knew this and bled his horse on such a time, and it lay dead immediately.[13]

This quotation shows that there is no reason to doubt the dangers of Egyptian Days, because here knowledge is backed by reported medical experiment and experience. In fact, any second thoughts on the risks involved vanish in view of the evidence presented in the text. To regard prognostication in the light of probability rather than certainty is, therefore, inappropriate. Before I offer my own definition of prognostics, let me turn to a lexicographical source.

The *Oxford English Dictionary* defines the term 'prognostic' in a non-medical sense as follows:

> 1. that which foreshows or gives warning of something to come, or from which the future may be foreknown; a pre-indication, token, omen.
> 2. a prediction or judgement of the future drawn from such an indication; a forecast, prophecy, anticipation.[14]

These definitions may suffice for lexicographical purposes, but they cover too much ground with reference to the text corpus at hand. The type of prognostics under discussion is to be distinguished from other prognostics (in the sense of the *OED*), such as biblical prophecies or animal omens, because these belong to wholly different methods of prediction. With the help of an Old English prognostic, I list the three constituents of a proper definition of the genre. The prognostic known as the agenda lunary purports to list various tasks that can be carried out on particular days of the moon. One of the predictions is:

> On the sixth night of the moon, put [fresh] hay in your bed; then you will have none of the customary pain in it, but you will be glad thereof. It is also a good moon to build a church or to begin the construction of a ship.[15]

First, prognostics are codified. These texts can be traced from Assyrian clay tablets and Egyptian papyri to modern publications, including in

[13] Translation of text 8.3/1, ll. 1-5 .
[14] Simpson and Weiner (1992: s.v. *prognostic* n1).
[15] Translation of text 9.2.1/2, ll. 15-17.

their long history early medieval, Western-European branches, such as the Anglo-Saxon texts of which the agenda lunary is but one representative.[16] Codification is one means by which our prognostics distinguish themselves from animal omens, which were not usually committed to vellum.[17] There is no foundation for a belief in the oral transmission of prognostics in Anglo-Saxon England, despite a recent claim to the contrary.[18] Second, the forecast must have a direct relevance for the life or life-time of an individual, or for the immediate surroundings of the questioner. Refreshing the hay on one's bed with its subsequent beneficial effects, is an example of the personal approach of prognostics. The prediction does not carry over into the afterlife, nor does it apply to unidentifiable groups of people, which effectively rules out biblical prophecies and predictions based on the appearance of comets, for instance. Third, the majority of prognostics deals with observation of signs, such as dreams, or times, such as the days of the moon in the agenda lunary. A few instances of non-observatory prognostics can be found, but these are limited to mantic divination, usually by dice or letters of the alphabet.[19] I am not aware of prognostics relating to other forms of divination or to magic.[20]

With these three criteria in hand, I define the genre of prognostics as "a codified means of predicting events in the life-time of an individual or identifiable group of individuals, using observation of signs and times, or mantic divination".

The Nature of Prognostics

Prognostics predict the immediate future in a variety of ways. Moreover, they are found in a number of different manuscript contexts. A corpus of prognostics does, therefore, not exist as such: it is a group of writings

[16] Alphabetical dreambooks, for instance, have enjoyed continuous attention over a period of about four thousand years.

[17] NB the use of animal omens may be reported in historical sources, but the working principle behind these omens and the range of interpretations open to the user were not committed to writing.

[18] Wilcox (2001: 51) opined that prognostics were orally transmitted as well, but evidence for this claim is lacking.

[19] The *Sortes Sanctorum* and the alphabet prognostic are representative of this kind of divinatory prognostication.

[20] On the distinction between observation, divination and magic, see pp. 104-07.

which exists as a coherent unit in our minds only. Nevertheless, these predictive texts can be brought together loosely under the heading 'prognostics' because they share the features outlined above.

The subjects to be queried in prognostics are legion, ranging from questions on health, illness, birth and death (by far the most popular subjects), to the recovery of stolen goods or the gender of an unborn child. These subjects pertain to the personal—an individual's recovery from illness—, or have an indirect bearing on the questioner—the size of next year's harvest or the death of a bishop. Despite their unspecific nature (they are not tailored to any one particular user), all prognostics are specialist tools that give insight into the prospective life of the person consulting the text. The influence of the predictions may extend to the death of this person, but the prediction has no influence in the afterlife. In this sense, prognostics are patently in a class of their own as compared to long-term prophecies, such as those concerning the end of times.[21]

The excerpt from the agenda lunary may shed light on the working principle behind prognostics. The text exhibits a link between the day of the moon and something which can be undertaken with good results. All prognostics operate in this manner, i.e. they rely on a trigger or sign that points to something signified. The link between sign and signified can be regarded in terms of synchronicity or causality. In the agenda lunary, the sixth day of the moon does not cause a refreshed bed to be particularly beneficial. Rather, the sixth day of the moon and the benefits of a refreshed bed coincide synchronically, and this coincidence (in the etymological sense of 'falling together') is the link between sign and signified. Such a relationship does not apply to the Dog Days, a period of roughly fifty days, ending in Anglo-Saxon England on 5 September, in which the Dog-star is visible and bloodletting proves fatal. The Dog-star causes bloodletting to be fatal, either through its direct influence or through secondary causes, such as a rise in temperature and subsequent lowered hygiene. Both the link through synchronicity and through causality between sign and signified have subjected prognostics to misinterpretation and ridicule in modern scholarship, which does not acknowledge any links between prognostic signs and actual events.[22]

The structure of prognostics is threefold and consists of (1) the thing to be observed; (2) the (sometimes implicit) subject of the query; and (3) the

[21] Occasionally, however, prognostics are found near texts dealing with the fifteen signs of Judgement Day.

[22] Cf. Singer (1917, 1928, 1961), Grattan and Singer (1952).

outcome of the query. An entry from a sunshine prognostic, for instance, runs as follows: "If the sun shines brightly on the seventh day [of Christmas], the Lord will send many fruits on the trees this coming year".[23] The structure of this entry is as follows: (1) sunshine is to be observed on the twelve days of Christmas; (2) events in the coming year are the subject of the query; (3) plenty of fruit on the trees is the outcome. Alphabetical dreambooks query the outcome of a dream based on the contents of the dream: "If it seems to him that he sees a dragon, it is [a] good [sign]".[24] Again, the structure is threefold: (1) a dream is to be observed; (2) the content of the dream is the subject of the query; (3) the propitious sign is the outcome. For each individual prognostic, the thing to be observed and the subject of the query remain identical throughout the text, whereas the outcome differs per entry.

The examples I have adduced so far mainly concern descriptive prognostics: texts that simply describe what will happen in the future. Proscriptive prognostics are quite another type: they foretell the course of events if one does not follow the advice provided. This type is represented by the Dog Days; the various genres of Egyptian Days, on which bloodletting, medication and the consumption of gooseflesh are lethal; and the unlucky days, on which a task newly begun will never be completed. I know of only one prescriptive genre, that of the regimen, a list of dietary and hygienic rules based on the seasons or the months.[25] The number of proscriptive genres is not as large as that of descriptive ones, but the number of proscriptive texts by token makes up a considerable part of the prognostic corpus under discussion:[26]

	descriptive	proscriptive	prescriptive
by type	81.3%	15.6%	3.1%
by token	55.7%	43.7%	0.6%

table 1: descriptive, pro- and prescriptive prognostics

This table illustrates the large share of proscriptive prognostics, even though there are not that many proscriptive genres to begin with. The main reason for this phenomenon is that proscriptive genres often feat-

[23] Translation of text 14/1, ll. 7-8.

[24] Translation of text 7/1, l. 59.

[25] The role of prescriptive prognostics can be largely ignored for Anglo-Saxon England (see pp. 31-33, 44-45).

[26] The exact number of prognostics in the corpus is 174 (see pp. 3-4, 503-44); the total number of prognostic genres is thirty-two (see pp. 14-15).

ure in calendars and computi, contexts which are encountered frequently in late Anglo-Saxon manuscripts.[27]

A second way to categorise types of prognostics is to see whether or not they are structured by time. Alphabetical dreambooks are non-temporal, whereas agenda lunaries are temporal. The sunshine prognostic occupies a position in between, because it forecasts the future by using sunshine (non-temporal) on the twelve days of Christmas (temporal). Temporal prognostics may employ various time units, e.g. hours (unspecified, canonical, night and day office), days (weekdays, New Year's Day, Days of Christmas, miraculous days), weeks, months, and days of the moon.[28] Non-temporal categories are: alphabets and dice, numbers, human behaviour, dreams, compass directions and natural phenomena, such as wind, the moon, sunshine and thunder.[29]

Some prognostic genres make use of more than one structuring component. Apuleian Spheres, for instance, predict the outcome of an illness, based on a combination of the letters in one's name, the day of the moon and the weekday on which one fell ill, and an arbitrary system of numbers.[30] Care should be taken to distinguish between a structural component, and the subject and/or outcome. In the sunshine prognostic, sunshine is part of the structure of the prognostic, but it does not pertain to the subject or outcome of the prediction, that is, the text does not foretell the amount of sunshine. A weekday bloodletting prognostic, in contrast, assigns appropriate times for bloodletting based on the days of the week. In this case, weekdays are the structural component, but bloodletting relates to the outcome of the prognostic. Hence, bloodletting is not a non-temporal component in this example, whereas sunshine is in the previous example. The relevance of this distinction becomes apparent when the names of prognostic genres are considered. The structure of a dream lunary, for example, consists of days of the moon, but the outcome of the prognostic deals with dreams.

---

[27] The influence of the manuscript context on the type of prognostics contained therein is exhaustively dealt with in chapter two.

[28] The temporal element can be differentiated further, see pp. 31-33.

[29] There are many more non-temporal prognostic structures, but that these seem not to have been employed for prognostication in Anglo-Saxon England, e.g. zodiacal signs, geomancy, palmistry. Moreover, the range of natural phenomena is limited to the categories mentioned. Earthquakes, volcanoes, comets and planets are not commonly used as prognostic devices, but these may be used as predictive devices.

[30] The letters of the alphabet, the weekday, and sometimes the days of the moon, are represented by numerical values on which calculations are based.

Yet another approach to grouping prognostics is by inspecting the content or the method by which the structure of a particular genre is realised. Förster was the first to group prognostics in this way. At first, he recognised eleven genres: 'Bauernpraktiken' (year prognoses), wind prognostics, sunshine prognostics, brontologies, unlucky days, three Egyptian Days, three miraculous birthdays, weekday birth prognostics, illness lunaries, dream lunaries and alphabetical dreambooks.[31] Later on, Förster distinguished five brontological genres, and added six more genres: birth, bloodletting and agenda lunaries (the last of which he confused with collective lunaries), Apuleian Spheres, twenty-four Egyptian Days and collective lunaries.[32] Overall, Förster's method was based upon genre divisions solely, and since he made no systematic attempt to distinguish broader categories, this makes his approach highly effective.[33]

Ker tried to find a larger perspective: (1) texts dealing with "lucky and unlucky days", (2) "prognostics from dreams, thunder, the moon, &c.", (3) a "prohibition against blood-letting in the Dog-Days"; glosses to the (4) Egyptian Days, and (5) the Apuleian Sphere.[34] This crude division gives the impression that prognostics may be too eclectic a kind of texts to be gathered into one corpus.[35] Ker's system has found a ready audience,[36] even though the groupings are arbitrary and show either overlap or are too inclusive.[37] All prognostic genres that existed in Anglo-Saxon England are filed under (2), except Ker's (1, 3-5). This means that Ker thought groups (1, 3-5) did not really belong to a core of prognostic texts, otherwise his division is senseless. The same would seem to apply to the system in Gneuss's *Handlist of Anglo-Saxon Manuscripts*, in which prognos-

[31] Förster (1903).

[32] Förster (1908a: 45-52; 1912c: 16-30, 36-37, 37-45, 45-49; 1929: 265-70; 1944).

[33] I have adopted Förster's classification with some modifications, see pp. 14-15.

[34] Ker (1957: 523, 524, 525). This categorisation excludes certain unusual prognostics, such as the text on the development of the foetus.

[35] Indeed, Jorge Luis Borges's list of animals in his essay "El idioma analítico de John Wilkins" is more comprehensive than Ker's classification of Old English prognostics.

[36] Ker's division seems to have been retained in the Cameron numbers: "folklore" (B23) is divided into "prose charms and charm headings" (B23.1), and "tables of lucky and unlucky days" (B23.2), "prognostics" (B23.3), a "prohibition against blood-letting" (B23.4), while glosses to the Egyptian Days (C67), prognostics (C16), and the Apuleian Sphere (C37) are included as well (Healey and Venezky 1980: 73-75, 95, 158-60, 161, 151, 160-61, 148, respectively).

[37] Overlap is shown by the fact that Egyptian Days and Dog Days are unlucky, while one of Ker's genres of unlucky days is that of the three Egyptian Days.

tics are grouped together against isolated instances of the Egyptian Days, lunaries, and alphabetical dreambooks.[38]

Hollis and Wright's *Old English Prose of Secular Learning* has largely followed Ker's grouping: (1) prognostics; (2) the alphabet prognostic; (3) "tables of lucky and unlucky days"; and (4) a "prohibition against bloodletting".[39] They transferred the Egyptian Days but not the Dog Days (i.e. 4) to the lucky and unlucky days, separated the alphabet prognostic from the larger group of prognostics, and omitted the Apuleian Sphere included in Ker's classification. In their discussion of the individual genres, however, Hollis and Wright seem to prefer Förster's system, reduced to a fourfold group of "divination by natural phenomena", "nativity prognostics and propitious days", "dream interpretation", and "medical prognostics".[40] Again, the inclusiveness of the categories is open to discussion.

Liuzza isolated six main groups: "predictions of the *if* ... *then* type based on the calendar"; "predictions based on some natural occurrence"; "lists of lucky and unlucky days in the year"; lunaries; alphabetical dreambooks; and "devices for divination".[41] Liuzza's categories are partly based on structure and partly on content. This practice leads to strange distinctions. For instance, alphabetical dreambooks are "predictions of the *if*... *then* type", but not "based on the calendar", which begs the question: why not distinguish between temporal and non-temporal "predictions of the *if*... *then* type"?

Scholars of the Middle English prognostics have made more headway in devising a classification than Anglo-Saxonists have. The works of Braswell, Keiser, Means, Mooney, Taavitsainen and Voigts should not be disregarded by those interested in the earlier medieval prognostics.[42] A fourfold classification has been advanced by Means for Middle English prognostics. She grouped prognostics into: (1) electionary or horary, i.e. "a guide for choosing... activities according to the most favourable astrological conditions"; (2) lunary, i.e. "a set of prognostications based upon the position of the moon at specific times"; (3) destinary, i.e. "a horoscope; a group of prognostications based upon time of birth, deter-

[38] Gneuss (2001: 177, 162, 172, 180).

[39] Hollis and Wright (1992: 257-58).

[40] Hollis and Wright (1992: 263). A similar system is used by Epe (1995: 56-64).

[41] Liuzza (2001: 183-90).

[42] Braswell (1978, 1984), Keiser (1998, 2004), Means (1992, 1993), Mooney (1994, 1998), Taavitsainen (1987, 1988, 1994), Taavitsainen and Pahta (2004), Voigts (1984, 1986, 1994, 1995), Voigts and Kurtz (2000).

mining destiny... decided by the position of the sun or moon at the time of nativity"; and finally (4) questionary, which is "only concerned with specific questions, who and how they are asked, and the means by which they may be answered".[43] The system devised by Means is practicable if one is not content simply to list the prognostic genres individually, and it is a pity that this classification has not been acknowledged more often in recent scholarship on the prognostics.

Hollis and Wright stated that "the possibilities for grouping and classification are numerous", to which one might add that such groupings are, moreover, a matter of individual preference.[44] I propose a classification of prognostics that unites this diverse group of texts and still acknowledges the variety in subject matter and structure. This grouping is, therefore, not based on any of the somewhat random or indeterminate systems outlined above, because these are either too inclusive, too broad or too arbitrary. Instead, I have adopted Förster's method of referencing individual genres, and improved it through: (1) a distinction between temporal and non-temporal texts;[45] and (2) an incremental approach, i.e. prognostics are listed in alphabetical order, in temporal order (from hours to months), in range (from general to specific). The result is a list of seventeen genres, some of which are further differentiated on the basis of their temporal structure or the subject of the query:[46]

Prognostic genres	
1	Alphabet prognostic
2	Apuleian Sphere
3.1.1	Birth prognostic, temporal, development of the foetus
3.1.2	Birth prognostic, temporal, three miraculous days
3.1.3	Birth prognostic, temporal, day of the week
3.2	Birth prognostic, non-temporal, gender prediction
4	Bloodletting prognostic, day of the week
5.1.1.1	Brontology, temporal, canonical hours (night office)
5.1.1.2	Brontology, temporal, canonical hours (day office)
5.1.2	Brontology, temporal, hours
5.1.3	Brontology, temporal, day of the week
5.1.4	Brontology, temporal, month of the year
5.2	Brontology, non-temporal, compass directions
6	Dog Days

[43] Means (1992: 370, 376, 386, 395).
[44] Hollis and Wright (1992: 263).
[45] This is of use in discussing prognostics in the manuscript context (see chapter two).
[46] On the numbering in my system, see p. 502.

Prognostic genres	
7	Dreambook
8.1	Egyptian Days, three days per year
8.2	Egyptian Days, twelve days per year
8.3	Egyptian Days, twenty-four days per year
9.1	Lunary, collective
9.2.1	Lunary, specific, agenda
9.2.2	Lunary, specific, birth
9.2.3	Lunary, specific, bloodletting
9.2.4	Lunary, specific, dreams
9.2.5	Lunary, specific, illness
10	Month prognosis
11	Moon colour
12	Regimen
13	*Sortes Sanctorum*
14	Sunshine prognostic
15	Unlucky days
16	Wind prognostic
17	Year prognosis

table 2: classification of prognostic genres

The Study of Prognostics

History of the Subject

In the publication history of Old English texts, prognostics have enjoyed a relatively brief vogue. Up to the nineteenth century, Old English texts were infrequently edited or transcribed, but from then on they attracted growing attention.[47] From the earliest editions to those of the present, the collecting and editing of prognostics spans roughly one century, from 1841 to 1944. Within this period, all known Old English prognostics had been published, but despite these efforts a collective edition has never appeared.[48] Below, I trace the publication history of the prognostics in chronological order. In doing so, I concentrate on the pioneers. Authoritative re-editions will be mentioned but are not discussed separately.

[47] See Graham (2001), Hall (2001), and Sauer (2001).

[48] With respect to Förster's publications on prognostics, Sauer (1998: 344) wrote: "the preparation of a clear, comprehensive, critical edition of these texts is a difficult task, and it is not surprising that a complete edition has not yet been achieved".

Franciscus Junius the Younger

The Dutch scholar Franciscus Junius the Younger (1591-1677) never published a single prognostic, but he is included here for his great interest in the Anglo-Saxon vernacular.[49] Two manuscripts which were in his keeping, Hatton 113 (formerly Junius 99) and Hatton 115 (formerly Junius 23) contain prognostics. Of these, Hatton 115 is of considerable importance for its large collection of prognostics in a separate booklet. Junius also had access to Tiberius A. iii, a remarkable miscellany of post-Benedictine Reform England which features many prognostics in Old English and Latin. Junius's interest in prognostics is evident from his copies of prognostic texts in the manuscripts Junius 41, 43 and 44.[50] He did not copy these texts at random, but organised them from different manuscripts by structural or thematic unity, which shows that he was aware of the genre divisions of prognostics and of the common features of these different prognostic genres. Junius 41 features the two odd birth prognostics from Tiberius A. iii: the texts on the development of the foetus and gender prediction. Junius 43 has dream prognostics in the form of dreambooks and dream lunaries from Tiberius A. iii and Hatton 115. Junius 44, finally, includes lunaries (both collective and specific ones), brontologies and year prognoses, again from Tiberius A. iii and Hatton 115.

Robert Thomas Hampson

The first edition ever of some Anglo-Saxon prognostics is found in the monumental two-volume *Medii aevi kalendarium: Dates, Charters, and Customs of the Middle Ages*, by Robert Thomas Hampson (1793-1858).[51] This work is unique in that it provides an unparalleled, in-depth analysis of medieval folkloric customs and all manner of medieval feast days. To my knowledge, no later study on this topic has been carried out in such a comprehensive way.[52] Consequently, *Medii aevi kalendarium* remains an indispensable tool for those interested in the medieval calendar and the uses connected with it. In the glossary of *Medii aevi kalendarium* (volume 2,

[49] The life and scholarship of Junius are studied in Bremmer (1998).

[50] Wanley (1705: II.87-90) listed the contents of these manuscripts. Stanley (1998: 164) only mentioned the prognostics in Junius 44.

[51] Hampson (1841).

[52] Although the reliability of Hampson's work is diminished in the light of modern scholarship, there is no single work that can replace *Medii aevi kalendarium*.

which matches the study in length), three prognostics have been edited and translated to exemplify several types of dangerous days.[53] In addition, Hampson's study (volume 1) contains a translation of a year prognosis in connection with popular customs on New Year's Day.[54] The publication of these four Old English prognostics has been superseded by Förster's more authoritative editions.[55] At several points in *Medii aevi kalendarium*, Hampson refers to Wanley's catalogue of Anglo-Saxon manuscripts,[56] which must have served as his source of information on the prognostics.

Thomas Oswald Cockayne

Twenty years elapsed after the publication of Hampson's work, before Thomas Oswald Cockayne (1807-73),[57] author of several historical, philological and grammatical works, edited a slim volume of Old English texts entitled *Narratiunculæ anglice conscriptæ*, which includes the text on the development of the foetus.[58] A few years later, Cockayne published an edition and translation of Anglo-Saxon scientific texts in three volumes, Teutonically entitled *Leechdoms, Wortcunning, and Starcraft of Early England*.[59] This publication contains an almost complete collection of Anglo-Saxon medical texts, herbal remedies and prognostics.

Cockayne published roughly two-fifths of all Old English and glossed prognostics.[60] He used three manuscripts as his main source. From Caligula A. xv and Hatton 115 (booklet 5), all Old English prognostics are represented. A Latin Apuleian Sphere was reproduced from Caligula A. xv. The prognostics in Tiberius A. iii were used as variants to those in the former two manuscripts. The running Old English glosses of the two longest Latin prognostics (a collective lunary and an alphabetical dreambook) in Tiberius A. iii were edited as well, though without the

[53] Hampson (1841: II.76-77, s.v. *Dies Malæ*, II.107, s.v. *Egyptian Days*).

[54] Hampson (1841: I.133-34).

[55] See pp. 22-23.

[56] Hickes (1703-05: II).

[57] For biographical information, see Stephen and Lee (1885-1900: XI.176), Singer (1961: I.xi-xviii), Hall (2001: 441).

[58] Cockayne (1861: 49-50).

[59] Cockayne (1864-66).

[60] This number does not take into account the variant texts in Cockayne's collated editions because his collations are far from accurate. Prognostics can be found in Cockayne (1864-66: II.14-17, 146-49, III.76-77, 82-85, 144-47, 150-215, 224-25).

Latin texts themselves. Skipping several prognostics in Tiberius A. iii, Cockayne presented the two curious birth prognostics and the same number of minor prognostics, viz. a brontology and a lunary. At first sight, it may seem strange that Cockayne favoured the weekday brontology and the illness lunary over the other prognostics in Tiberius A. iii. It is likely, however, that the latter were omitted because they are all Latin prognostics with Old English glosses, in contrast to the Old English brontology and illness lunary.[61]

One peculiar incident regarding the reprint of the *Leechdoms* deserves mention. When Singer published a partly stripped reprint of the *Leechdoms* with a new introduction, he left out the greater portion of the prognostics. Moreover, in introducing the revamped third volume, Singer mentioned the manuscripts Caligula A. xv and Tiberius A. iii explicitly, but he did not once refer to Hatton 115, the texts of which are somehow not included in the reprint.[62] Singer further noted:

> There follows in Vol. III a *mass of senseless prognostications from dreams* (p. 198), *no source for which has been traced*.... Next come (p. 231-p. 283) translations from the works of Bede [= Ælfric's *De temporibus anni*]. These may be linguistically important but Bede's scientific works are now available in modern critical editions and *they are here omitted because of the special limitation of their interest.*[63]

The "mass of senseless prognostications from dreams, ... no source for which has been traced" is a particularly uninformed statement in view of the fact that many prognostics have been traced back to Greek and Latin texts, but the alphabetical dreambook to which Singer referred ultimately derives from Assyrian clay tablets and Egyptian papyri,[64] as Singer must undoubtedly have known in view of publications on the dreambooks by Förster and Oppenheim, among others.[65] Aside from my objection to Singer's careless dismissal of dreambooks, his statement is

[61] This is, of course, true for the collective lunary and alphabetical dreambook, as well as for several other Latin prognostics with Old English glosses in Tiberius A. iii, but the lunary and dreambook certainly commanded some interest as substantial texts in their own right. The Old English glosses of the other Latin prognostics were used solely as variant readings to Cockayne's edition of the prognostics from Caligula A. xv and Hatton 115.

[62] Singer (1961: I.xxv).

[63] Singer (1961: I.xxvi); emphasis is mine. Singer's references to page numbers in this citation are to Cockayne's edition (1864-66: III).

[64] See pp. 290-96.

[65] Förster (1908c, 1910, 1916, 1921, 1925-26), Oppenheim (1956).

rather ambiguous. His remark that "they are here omitted" seems to refer to Ælfric's *De temporibus anni*. Nevertheless, this text, which had found a place in Cockayne's collection, is retained in Singer's edition of the *Leechdoms*, whereas most of the prognostics are not. A mistake on the part of either editor or publisher is unlikely because the prognostics excluded, from Hatton 115, should have started halfway down pages 158/159 (i.e. directly following those from Caligula A. xv and Tiberius A. iii), while the bottom halves of these pages are blank in Singer's edition. Furthermore, the pages following are renumbered consecutively from page 160 onwards. Finally, Singer does not mention the prognostics from Hatton 115, the edition of which was to start where Singer started cutting in the *Leechdoms*. It would seem, therefore, that the exclusion of the prognostics from Hatton 115 was deliberate, perhaps "because of the special limitation of their interest". Did Singer refer to *De temporibus anni* or to the prognostics? On account of *De temporibus anni* being "now available in modern critical editions",[66] one would think Singer would have wanted to exclude Ælfric's work rather than the prognostics.[67]

Cockayne's publication was groundbreaking in providing the first comprehensive edition of the prognostics; yet his editorial methods left much to be desired. Of course, Cockayne's shortcomings exist only in the mind of the modern editor. Placed in its original cultural climate, the *Leechdoms* was neither exceptionally Germanic in tone, nor overly folkloric in character.[68] Even so, there are some flaws which diminish the reliability of the *Leechdoms* as an authoritative text edition.

Cockayne's first shortcoming is his carelessness in the transcriptions.[69] In the large enterprise which the *Leechdoms* is, mistakes and faulty emendations are to be expected, but they are almost ubiquitous. Second, his collated editions of prognostics of the same type are inaccurate in that he tends to mark variant readings haphazardly. In a collated edition of an

[66] I.e. Henel (1942).

[67] One other reason springs to mind: Singer was quite keen on ridiculing English prognostics and medicine, judging by his analysis of magical and pagan elements therein, which would make him more inclined to omit *De temporibus anni* than prognostics (cf. Grattan and Singer 1952: 3-94; Singer 1917, 1928: 133-67; 1961: I.xxvi-xxxviii).

[68] Cf. Stanley (1975). The language of Cockayne's translation is deliberately Germanic (neologistic Germanic words were preferred above the existing Romance vocabulary), which gives the subject an undeservedly quaint air of Germanic folklore.

[69] Cf. Chardonnens (2000).

Old English dreambook,[70] for instance, Cockayne recorded just a fraction of the variant readings. He must have sensed a certain inadequacy, because he added an apologetic note stating that a "minute collation seemed unsuitable in this piece",[71] yet why this is so never transpires. In another instance, Cockayne proved even more obtuse: he presented a collated edition of two Latin illness lunaries with Old English glosses and prefixed the text with the diagram of an Apuleian Sphere, Apuleian Spheres being an altogether different prognostic genre.[72] Additionally, he did not mention that there is no Apuleian Sphere in one of the two manuscripts presented, and he omitted the explanatory text that is an essential part of this prognostic genre. The third and final objection I would raise against Cockayne's edition is that it omitted the Latin text whenever the Old English glosses a Latin prognostic.[73] The edition of the Old English glosses of the longest extant Latin alphabetical dreambook from Anglo-Saxon England, for example, is preceded by the comment "the Saxon glosses some Latin", which is quite an understatement.[74] My critical remarks on Cockayne's edition do not deny the fact that the *Leechdoms* is invaluable in that it formed the first publication of a wide range of Old English non-literary and non-historical texts, including prognostics.

Eduard Sievers

In response to a series of articles which presented alphabetical lists of letters with a clause attached to each letter in Latin and the vernacular,[75] Eduard Sievers (1850-1932)[76] published the text that is now known as the Old English alphabet prognostic.[77] The conclusion of this text, viz.

[70] Cockayne (1864-66: III.168-76).

[71] Cockayne (1864-66: III.169 n. a).

[72] Cockayne (1864-66: III.150-51).

[73] The aforementioned glossed illness lunary, which lacks a translation probably because of the Latin, is an exception.

[74] Cockayne (1864-66: III.199). This is probably not what Singer had in mind when he remarked that Cockayne was "over-scrupulous in excluding material" (1961: I.xx).

[75] Martin (1867: 368), Steinmeyer (1874), Schönbach (1875), Sievers (1875).

[76] Although an enumeration of Sievers' pioneering work in the manifold disciplines of philology is beyond my scope and purpose, his extensive scholarship is hereby acknowledged. For biographical information, see Frings (1933), Ganz (1978), Pope (1998), Sauer (2001: 457-60).

[77] Sievers (1877).

the three metrical lines following the letter Z, have become known as the poem "The Gloria II".[78]

Walter de Gray Birch

Walter de Gray Birch (1842-1924) was senior assistant of the manuscript department in the British Museum (now British Library).[79] His interests ranged from charters and seals to methods of bookbinding. Birch published a partial edition of the contents of one of the more important prognostic collections: that in the manuscripts Titus D. xxvi and xxvii.[80] Despite the fact that he was mainly interested in the religious and codicological aspects of these manuscripts, Birch did not desist from editing and analysing the prognostics. In addition to the one Old English prognostic (the aforementioned alphabet prognostic), Titus D. xxvi, xxvii contain no less than twenty Latin prognostics, sixteen of which were edited by Birch (sometimes in part). Beate Günzel has recently published a critical edition of the entire contents of Titus D. xxvi, xxvii.[81] For a better understanding of the transmission of prognostics into the vernacular, the Latin texts in these manuscripts prove invaluable.

Bruno Assmann

The next scholar who edited some prognostics was Bruno Assmann.[82] For his *Angelsächsische Homilien und Heiligenleben*,[83] Assmann used Vespasian D. xiv, consisting almost entirely of homilies to which two prognostics were added at a later date.[84] In his study of this manuscript, Assmann must have noticed the year prognosis and the month brontology, which he subsequently published.[85] Rubie Warner published a critical edition of the entire manuscript.[86]

[78] Dobbie (1942: lxxxiii-lxxxiv, 94).

[79] For biographical information, see *Who was Who, 1916-1928* (1947: 93), Keynes (1992: 61), Hall (2001: 444).

[80] Birch (1878). The article was reprinted in a condensed and slightly modified in his *Liber Vitae: Register and Martyrology of New Minster and Hyde Abbey, Winchester* (1892).

[81] Günzel (1993).

[82] I have not been able to find any biographical information except for a brief mention in Sauer's account of nineteenth-century Anglo-Saxon scholarship (2001: 462).

[83] Assmann (1889b: 246, 266).

[84] See p. 46.

[85] Assmann (1888, 1889a: 369).

[86] Warner (1917).

Max Förster

The scholar to subject the Old English prognostics to an exhaustive analysis, both as compared to analogues in other vernaculars and Latin, and in a wide cultural context, was Max Förster (1869-1954).[87] His bibliography contains hundreds of titles on a great variety of subjects. A minute, though invaluable, fraction of his writings concerned prognostics, which he first analysed in an article entitled "Die Kleinliteratur des Aberglaubens im Altenglischen" ("The Non-Literary Canon of Superstition in Old English").[88] Förster explored the sources of Old English prognostics and was able to supply Latin analogues for many of the texts edited by Cockayne and Assmann. The article proved to be the start of a programme, for in a long series of articles called "Beiträge zur mittelalterlichen Volkskunde" ("Contributions to Medieval Folklore"), Förster edited many more prognostics.[89] Several years after the "Beiträge", the article "Die altenglischen Traumlunare" ("The Old English Dream Lunaries") appeared, closely followed by "Die altenglischen Verzeichnisse von Glücks- und Unglückstagen" ("The Old English Lists of Lucky and Unlucky Days").[90] His last article on the Anglo-Saxon prognostics appeared in 1944, entitled "Vom Fortleben antiker Sammellunare im englischen und in anderen Sprachen" ("On the Continuation of Antique Collective Lunaries in English and in other Languages").[91]

Förster's training in comparative, Germanic, Celtic and Romance philology is evident from his choice of sources and analogues in these articles: from early Latin prognostics to modern almanacs, from classical and Byzantine Greek to a wide range of sources in European vernaculars. Förster edited most of the Old English prognostics. His endea-

[87] For biographical information, see Stolberg-Wernigerode (1953-: V.279-80), Sauer (1998; 2001: 460-62), Killy and Vierhaus (1995-2000: III.364).

[88] Förster (1903).

[89] Förster (1908a-c, 1910, 1911, 1912a-c, 1916). The following is a checklist of the contents of the "Beiträge" series: I (1908a) introduction, 1. brontologies; II (1908b) 2. year prognoses, 3. alphabetical dreambook; III (1908c) 4. contents of Tiberius A. iii; IV (1910) 5. alphabetical dreambook; V (1911) 6. alphabetical dreambook in verse, 7. alphabetical dreambook in prose; VI (1912a) 8. wind prognostics, 9. sunshine prognostics; VII (1912b) 10. brontologies, 11. year prognoses, 12. (non-prognostic) calendar verses, 13. weekday birth prognostics; VIII (1912c) 14. birth lunaries, 15. illness lunaries, 16. bloodletting lunaries, 17. agenda lunaries, 18. Apuleian Spheres; IX (1916) 19. alphabetical dreambook.

[90] Förster (1925-26, 1929).

[91] Förster (1944). He also edited a Welsh dreambook, and two Welsh redactions of the *Sortes Sanctorum* (Förster 1921, 1936).

vours in the field of the Anglo-Saxon prognostics testify to his pioneering interest in a comparative study of the genre. Furthermore, his editions are annotated exhaustively and are invariably accompanied by an introduction on the transmission and history of each particular prognostic genre. Some of Förster's analyses are now outdated, and sometimes more and closer Latin analogues have been discovered. Yet for many prognostic genres his editions and studies are still the standard against which new insights must be measured. If it is true that Cockayne prepared the ground for the study of the Anglo-Saxon prognostics, it is equally true that the study of the genre matured with Förster.

Heinrich Henel

Heinrich Henel (1905-81) is a scholar whose interest ranged "von Beowulf bis Kafka".[92] Henel wrote his article "Altenglischer Mönchsaberglaube" ("Old English Monkish Superstition") well after Förster had published the greater part of his work on the prognostics,[93] but its importance should not be underestimated because Henel contributed valuable Latin analogues to prognostics already edited by Förster. Moreover, Henel was more successful than Förster in deciphering the prognostics in those parts of Vitellius E. xviii which had been badly damaged in the Cottonian Fire of 1731, as he had actually seen the manuscript, whereas Förster worked from photographs.[94] Henel published collated editions of six prognostic genres.

Emanuel Svenberg

Eight years before Förster published the only Latin collective lunary with Old English glosses, Emanuel Svenberg[95] published a slim volume containing collated editions of collective lunaries, among which a number of texts from England.[96] Svenberg edited the collective lunaries in Titus D. xxvii, Sloane 475, and the Latin part of the text in Tiberius A. iii, the Old English glosses of which had been published by Cockayne.

[92] Seidlin (1981: 290). For biographical information, see Sammons and Schürer (1970), Seidlin (1981).

[93] Henel (1934-35).

[94] Henel (1934-35: 336, n. 1).

[95] I have not been able to find any biographical information.

[96] Svenberg (1936).

State of Affairs

The scholars introduced above have published between them all the extant Old English prognostics, and many of the Latin ones from Anglo-Saxon manuscripts. Some, such as Assmann and Sievers, contributed a few texts only; others, like Cockayne, Henel and Förster, discovered and published between them almost the entire corpus of Old English prognostics. Despite the relative antiquity of these editions, they still are the touchstone for modern research on the prognostics.

For some reason, the study of Anglo-Saxon prognostics became unfashionable after Förster had published his "Antiker Sammellunare" in 1944. In fact, no new authoritative editions of Anglo-Saxon prognostics have appeared since that time.[97] This does not mean that the prognostics were neglected, as recent articles by Liuzza attest.[98] Moreover, a fair number of studies of medieval continental and Middle English prognostics have been carried out after the 1940s.[99]

In the past decade, several publications have focussed on Anglo-Saxon prognostics from an iatromathematical perspective. Most noteworthy are the following articles: Wallis's "Medicine in Medieval Calendar Manuscripts", Hollis's "Scientific and Medical Writings", and Liuzza's "Anglo-Saxon Prognostics in Context".[100] Useful reference works are Hollis and Wright's *Old English Prose of Secular Learning*, and Voigts and Kurtz's *Scientific and Medical Writings in Old and Middle English: an Electronic Reference*.[101] The manuscript descriptions of the series *Anglo-Saxon Manuscripts in Microfiche Facsimile* may prove helpful,[102] though judging by the volumes published thus far not always in equal measure with regard to prognostics.[103]

---

[97] Granted that Löweneck (1896) published the *Peri didaxeon*, Leonhardi (1905) Bald's *Leechbook*, Grattan and Singer (1952) the *Lacnunga*, Günzel (1993) re-edited Titus D. xxvi, xxvii, not one book has appeared which focusses on the Anglo-Saxon prognostics in particular, except for Epe's edition of the English dreambooks (1995).

[98] Liuzza (2001, 2004, 2005).

[99] For instance, Svenberg (1963), Wickersheimer (1966), Martin (1981), Weißer (1982), Taavitsainen (1988), Means (1993), Matheson (1994).

[100] Wallis (1995), Hollis (2001), Liuzza (2001). A short characterisation of these articles is provided on p. 146.

[101] Hollis and Wright (1992), Voigts and Kurtz (2000).

[102] Pulsiano and Doane (1994-).

[103] See p. 501.

CHAPTER TWO

THE MANUSCRIPT CONTEXT

The extant English prognostics are found in manuscripts known principally for the various other genres they contain. Prognostics have thus been discovered in computi, in volumes on science or medicine, and in miscellanies which present a host of different text genres. I am not aware of any medieval manuscript containing prognostics only. Despite the large number of contexts possible, I argue that there are in fact just five contexts in which prognostics have been found:[1] (1) in calendars; (2) in computi; (3) in medical sections;[2] (4) as guest texts; and (5) collected in prognostic sections.[3] Moreover, prognostics are sometimes transmitted in fixed series. I present three such sequences for analysis.

This chapter is the first of four contextual studies of the prognostics: the others pertain to the language, date and place of origin (chapter three), superstition and prognostication (chapter four), and the intended use of the Anglo-Saxon prognostics (chapter five). A footnote at the head of each section lists the manuscripts under discussion. Descriptions of the date, origin and contents of each manuscript discussed in this chapter, as well as a detailed survey of the prognostics, have been provided in appendix one. A condensed reference list to the prognostic corpus is provided in appendix two.

---

[1] I acknowledge the risk of simplification by fitting prognostics into particular contexts, but I have yet to meet a situation where my method causes inconsistencies.

[2] I am indebted to the following scholars, whose works have been very helpful in shaping my thoughts for the sections on calendars, computus and medicine: Henel (1934a), Hollis and Wright (1992), Cameron (1993), Borst (1993), Baker and Lapidge (1995), Stevens (1995), Wallis (1995; 1999), Hollis (2001), D'Aronco (2005; 2007).

[3] The word 'section' is here not used in a codicological sense. A section should be understood as a grouping of texts which bear a thematic relationship. Thus, a prognostic section is a unit predominantly composed of prognostics, while a medical section is a unit of medical texts. I call these sections because more often than not they reflect thematic divisions of manuscripts containing several units of thematically linked texts, i.e. consisting of more than one section. A psalter, for instance, may be preceded by a computus, e.g. CCCC 391. Likewise, St. John's College 17 consists of a medical section (fols 1-2), a computus (fols 3-174), and yet another medical section (fols 175-177). By 'section', then, I refer to thematic units, not to the entire contents of a manuscript.

Manuscript Contexts

Calendars[4]

Of the thirty-seven manuscripts which compose the prognostic corpus, twenty-three feature calendars with prognostic material.[5] By prognostic material is understood the incorporation of prognostic data in calendars, in contrast to stand-alone prognostics. Egyptian Days, for instance, have been attested as independent texts but also feature as entries in the calendar, where they are mentioned as "dies egyptiacus", "dies mala", "dies", "d eg", "d m", "d", etc. Prognostic material is of a more hermetic nature than stand-alone prognostics because the prospective user will have to be able to recognise the somewhat cryptic references and to interpret their meaning without the help of the explanatory notes often present in stand-alone texts. The scope of prognostic material is of necessity limited to those genres that use fixed dates: the Dog Days and the twenty-four Egyptian Days.[6]

Easter tables, often accompanied by a calendar, form the core of the computus.[7] The computus concerns itself with time reckoning, which is important for liturgical purposes.[8] It is not surprising, then, that many of the calendars under discussion can be found in manuscripts of a religious nature. Twelve out of twenty-three manuscripts incorporate prognostic material in the calendar only, the remaining eleven have stand-alone prognostics in addition to prognostic material. Prognostic material in

[4] This section pertains to the calendars in CCCC 9, CCCC 422, CTC O. 7. 41, CTC R. 15. 32, CUL Kk. 5. 32, Add. 37517, Arundel 60, Arundel 155, Nero A. ii, Titus D. xxvii, Vitellius A. xii, Vitellius A. xviii, Vitellius E. xviii, Egerton 3314, Harley 863, Bodley 579, Digby 63, Douce 296, Hatton 113, St. John's College 17, Reg. lat. 12, Rouen 274, Salisbury 150.

[5] Many of the Anglo-Saxon calendars have been published in their entirety, see Hampson (1841: I.389-472), Wilson (1896: 9-20), Wildhagen (1921), Atkins (1928), Wormald (1934), Muir (1988: 3-14), Günzel (1993: 91-102), and the facsimiles available on microfiche (Pulsiano and Doane 1994-).

[6] The only other genres which assign fixed dates are the twelve Egyptian Days and the three miraculous birthdays. I do not know of any medieval calendars which incorporate the dates assigned in these prognostics, however. The unlucky days, a genre which shows some affinity with the twenty-four Egyptian Days though is not to be confused with the latter, uses dating by the age of the moon.

[7] Wallis (1995: 106). The importance of the calendar and the Easter tables as two different ways of measuring time is discussed below.

[8] See pp. 29-39 for more information on prognostics in the computus.

calendars makes up a large proportion of the entire prognostic corpus, but calendars have hitherto been neglected in the study of prognostics.[9] In this section I limit myself to an overview of prognostic material to illustrate the relevance of this context for the study of prognostics. In the next section, the wider, computistical context will be addressed.

Wallis studied the development of ecclesiastical calendars from Roman civil and agricultural calendars in the fifth century. She has argued that early church calendars had no use for Roman festivals, and that the number of Christian feasts was small at the time. This would leave considerable gaps in the calendar, whereas "a calendar was fundamentally a list of *named* days".[10] Because early ecclesiastical calendars would have been rather empty, "meteorological and seasonal indicators, as well as other paraphernalia such as Egyptian Days" were incorporated.[11] This scenario would account for the inclusion of Dog Days and Egyptian Days in early medieval calendars, but I have some reservations with regard to Anglo-Saxon calendars.

First, incorporation of prognostic material is not always the rule in English calendars, which in sporadic cases lack entries for the Dog Days and Egyptian Days altogether. One manuscript, CCCC 391, which boasts a large prognostic section towards the end of the volume and a computus at the beginning, does not have any prognostic material in the calendar.[12] Five calendars have entries for the Dog Days only, and six feature Egyptian Days solely.[13] Second, early calendars do not invariably include prognostic material, the calendar of St. Willibrord (658-739) being a case in point.[14] Moreover, some early Anglo-Saxon calendars show impaired transmission of the Dog Days and Egyptian Days. Of the four Anglo-Saxon calendars antedating the eleventh century, two contain an incomplete and haphazard selection of Egyptian Days; the other two mention the beginning of the Dog Days but not the end. In comparison, of the nineteen calendars from the eleventh century and after, three have selected entries on the Egyptian Days, and another four

[9] Prognostic material in calendars is rarely mentioned by scholars. Exceptions are: Camus (1891: 254-55), James (1900-04: III.379 [1369.2]), Wildhagen (1921: 77, n. 2), Thorndike (1923-58: I.686).

[10] Wallis (1995: 106-07). Emphasis is Wallis's.

[11] Wallis (1995: 107).

[12] See pp. 51-53.

[13] The entries for Dog Days and Egyptian Days in Vitellius A. xii are in two separate calendars.

[14] Wilson (1918).

do not mention the end of the Dog Days.[15] My third and final observation is that some calendars originally lacking Egyptian Days had these entries added at a post-Conquest date, which indicates a deliberate reintroduction of prognostic material into the calendar.[16] The later addition of prognostic material is the more significant as it demonstrates that, in late Anglo-Saxon calendars, Egyptian Days were not included for reasons of filling up blank space, something which may have applied to the early (non-Anglo-Saxon) ecclesiastical calendars.

The three reservations mentioned seem to indicate that the Dog Days and Egyptian Days in Anglo-Saxon calendars were incorporated for a different reason compared to early ecclesiastical calendars. Wallis mentioned that in early calendars, Egyptian Days filled awkward gaps. In contrast, Anglo-Saxon calendars do not exhibit a lack of entries and are not in need of "paraphernalia such as Egyptian Days" for this reason. This is substantiated by the relative scarcity or impaired transmission of entries on the Egyptian Days and Dog Days in early Anglo-Saxon calendars, and the addition of the same in some Anglo-Saxon calendars at a later point in time. If the scribes of Anglo-Saxon calendars did not suffer from *horror vacui*, there must be another reason why prognostic material was in demand. As I pointed out in the second reservation, we should distinguish between calendars from before the eleventh century, and those that have come into existence in the eleventh century and after. None of the pre-eleventh-century calendars has a complete set of dates for either the Egyptian Days or the Dog Days, whereas a large majority of the later calendars does. This would suggest that, by the eleventh century, the Egyptian Days and Dog Days were becoming a standard ingredient of Anglo-Saxon calendars, which is confirmed by the addition of Egyptian Days in calendars originally lacking these entries. Additional evidence for this claim is found in the dates for the twenty-four Egyptian Days. These dates display greater variation in early English calendars but seem to have become regularised in late Anglo-Saxon and early post-Conquest calendars. Therefore, the incorporation and introduction of prognostic material in English calendars from the eleventh cen-

[15] Calendars from the twelfth century and after almost invariably include Egyptian Days and Dog Days as standard ingredients, cf. Wormald (1939-46).

[16] On pp. 45-49, I discuss prognostics as guest texts, i.e. texts that fill space originally left blank. I do not think, however, that insertion of Egyptian Days in the calendar is an example of guest material since there is no blank space to speak of in late Anglo-Saxon calendars.

tury and after testifies to the making of a tradition, rather than the display of a fear of, by that time non-existent, blank spaces in the calendar.

Computi[17]

In addition to prognostic material embedded in calendars, several computi contain stand-alone redactions of prognostics. Computus, 'gerim' in Old English, is defined by the *Oxford English Dictionary* as "the mediæval name for a set of tables for practically calculating astronomical occurrences and the movable dates of the calendar; a calendar".[18] However, the computus is not strictly a matter of tabular material, nor is it just a calendar. Baker and Lapidge established that "the computus was a collection of letters, instructions and tables relating to the calendar".[19] The term 'computus' is used by Bede to denote both calculation in general, and time reckoning in particular, while the specific use is more usual among later Anglo-Saxon writers such as Ælfric.[20] At the heart of the computus are the Easter tables accompanied by a series of commentaries, and, later, the calendar, all designed to monitor correctly time and its progress. A proper understanding of time, after all, meant a correct observation of the liturgy.[21]

Accretion of Prognostics in the Computus

Wallis explained succinctly how non-computistical texts found their way into the computus:

---

[17] This section pertains to CCCC 422, CTC O. 7. 41, CTC R. 15. 32, Arundel 60, Caligula A. xv + Egerton 3314, Tiberius C. i + Harley 3667, Tiberius C. vi, Titus D. xxvii, Vitellius A. xii, Vitellius C. viii, Vitellius E. xviii, Harley 3271, Lambeth Palace 427, Bodley 579, St. John's College 17. The following limitations apply: (a) the prognostics in CCCC 422, p. 49, Tiberius C. vi, fol. 114r, and Titus D. xxvii, fols 55v-56v, are excluded since they are later additions (see p. 47); (b) by Titus D. xxvii I do not mean D. xxvii and xxvi, for which see pp. 57-59.

[18] Simpson and Weiner (1992: s.v. *computus*).

[19] Baker and Lapidge (1995: xl). Cf. Henel (1934a: 1-4). Wallis (1995: 105) asserted that the computus was "for the most part, and certainly in its most formative period, not built around texts at all, but rather around tables".

[20] Wallis (1999: 425-26).

[21] I realise that the way in which I represent the computus here is somewhat simplistic, yet the scope of my argument does not allow a more exhaustive discussion. For a lucid introduction to medieval computus, see Wallis (1999: xv-lxxxv).

> as these tables [viz. the calendar and the Easter tables] crossed North Africa and Italy in the sixth and seventh centuries, they also took on board additional tables and formulae, as well as useful supplementary materials such as notes on astronomy and mathematics, and even peripheral elements (texts on medicine, music, grammar, and tables of weights and measures) that attached themselves to the computus by a kind of associative attraction. Some of the earliest surviving Western computus manuscripts already contain a halo of noncomputistical materials, some of which can be described as propaedeutic to the computus (e.g., astronomy, cosmology, and mathematics), but much of which is simply analogous to the computus, the common element being time and its measurement.[22]

The accretive process which Wallis called "associative attraction" accounted for a large body of non-computistical texts being drawn into the computus, including prognostics.[23] The majority of prognostic genres known in Anglo-Saxon England has a temporal structure, i.e. is ordered by time sequences. The emphasis on time, the essence of the computus, is, therefore, patently visible in the Anglo-Saxon prognostics as well. Indeed, the prognostics hitherto encountered in computi are without exception temporal.[24] There are two noteworthy examples of associative attraction.

First, Apuleian Spheres are frequently included in computi, and it is likely that this genre made its entry on account of its scientific appearance (diagrams and tables of letters and numbers), which makes the genre fit in very well with computistical tables and diagrams. In fact, all Anglo-Saxon Apuleian Spheres are found in computi; some manuscripts even contain more than one Apuleian Sphere.[25] A typical example of associative attraction is found in St. John's College 17, fols 3-12.[26] These pages contain a series of tables and diagrams, including a diagram of an Apuleian Sphere on folio 8rb. It is likely that this Apuleian Sphere was

[22] Wallis (1995: 107-08).

[23] Cf. Thorndike (1923-58: I.676). Martin (1977: 24-26) tried to explain the presence of dreambooks in computus manuscripts. This, however, does not pertain to English manuscripts, which do not have dreambooks in the computus. Taavitsainen (1988: 133-51) studied the manuscript context of Middle English lunar prognostics.

[24] The (non-temporal) alphabet prognostic in Titus D. xxvii is excluded from consideration since it is a later addition to the original computus (see p. 47).

[25] Vitellius E. xviii has two Apuleian Spheres. Tiberius C. i + Harley 3667 and St. John's College 17 have three each. The Sphere in the medical volume Sloane 475 is an exception, but that may have to do with the origin of the texts (see pp. 42-43).

[26] Wallis (1985; 1995: 122-27) made an outstanding analysis of the contents of this manuscript and the position of the texts.

copied because of its similarity to scientific diagrams: the Apuleian Sphere lacks both the explanatory text and the lists of letter and weekday values that usually accompany the diagram. The diagram itself is placed next to a similar looking tidal diagram.[27] Moreover, the former contains Greek labels and a form of cryptographic writing, which contribute to its scientific appeal.[28] These indications seem to illustrate that there was, at this point in the manuscript, an interest in the Apuleian Sphere for the scientific guise of the diagram, rather than for its value as a prognostic.

Second, associative attraction is present in the nature of the temporal structure of prognostics in the computus. The calendar and the Easter tables can be considered a twofold system of absolute and relative time, realigned in a lunar Easter cycle of nineteen solar years.[29] The solar calendar is concerned with fixed dates, while lunar time shifts with reference to the solar calendar.[30] This twofold mechanism of time reckoning has attracted prognostics which follow the same division, as is evident from those genres most frequently attested in the computus: the Egyptian Days, the Dog Days, lunaries and Apuleian Spheres. The solar component is exemplified by the Dog Days, the twelve and twenty-four Egyptian Days, and the three miraculous birthdays, which are on fixed dates in the year. Lunar time, which shifts with reference to the solar cycle, is represented by all other temporal genres, notably by lunaries and Apuleian Spheres. Of the fifteen computi under discussion, eleven contain prognostics that follow both the solar and lunar cycle.

Wallis discussed a system of time reckoning in the computus which is largely identical to the one I have just outlined: a division of seasonal, astronomical and calendric time.[31] Seasonal time is manifested by regimens, texts which prescribe dietary and hygienic rules appropriate to the seasons. These texts, according to Wallis, were usually, though not always, adapted to fit the solar calendar, i.e. they were changed from

---

[27] See p. 222, pl. 12.

[28] Although the diagrams and the structure of Apuleian Spheres vary considerably, a diagram bearing resemblance to the one under discussion is found in Caligula A. xv.

[29] On Easter cycles and ways of measuring time in Anglo-Saxon England, see Harrison (1978), Stevens (1981, 1985, 1992, 1993).

[30] This is comparable to—but not to be identified with—the liturgical sanctorale and temporale cycles. The temporale is, after all, linked to lunar time through the determination of the Easter date. However, the temporale cycle also includes Christmas, which is not a movable feast. Therefore, solar and lunar time had better be equated to the system of movable and immovable feasts.

[31] Wallis (1995: 112-18).

seasonal to monthly, since seasons are not a central part of the computus whereas months are.[32] In essence then, the seasonal-turned-monthly regimen had become an application of calendric time. Wallis described astronomical time as follows:

> *Lunare* time is astronomical time, and the medical effects of changes in heavenly bodies like the Moon can only be inferred or deduced on the basis of a theory of celestial influence; they cannot be experienced directly and somatically, as can seasonal changes.[33]

The Egyptian Days, finally, are representative of calendric time: "their character is determined not by the natural seasons, nor yet by the visible movements of the heavens, but by the arbitrary artifice of the Roman calendar".[34]

This threefold system may be required for the continental computus, but it is cumbersome for Anglo-Saxon computi, which, to my knowledge, do not feature regimens. This makes seasonal time a highly marginal issue for Anglo-Saxon computi. In fact, the few Anglo-Saxon regimens in existence are not incorporated into the computus at all.[35] In comparison, the continental part of the composite manuscript Sloane 475 has no less than five regimens, which goes to show that prognostics in Anglo-Saxon manuscripts should be treated differently from ones in continental manuscripts.[36] Works on the seasons and the humours were known in Anglo-Saxon England,[37] but it has been argued that "an emphasis on diet" and hygiene, as manifested in regimens, was somehow related to the emergence of the medical school of Salerno.[38] This is a rather misguided view in the light of the many pre-eleventh-century regimens and writings on hygiene and the humours in Western European

[32] Wallis (1995: 114).

[33] Wallis (1995: 116). Italics are Wallis's.

[34] Wallis (1995: 117).

[35] In Harley 3271 (see pp. 38-39) and CUL Gg. 5. 35; in prognostic and medical sections, respectively.

[36] I address the difference between the treatment of Anglo-Saxon and continental prognostics on pp. 44-45.

[37] Cameron (1993: 28, 53) referred to Bede quoting from the *Epistula Vindiciani ad Pentadium nepotem*, a tract on the humours, health, and the seasons of the year (printed Rose 1894: 484-92).

[38] Singer (1917: 116). On what has traditionally been considered Salernitan medicine (but is not necessarily so), see Payne (1904: 143-57), Singer (1917: 115-17; 1928: 148; 1961: I.xxiv, I.xxxix-xl), Thorndike (1923-58: I.731-41), Grattan and Singer (1952: 74-79), Bonser (1963: 47), Talbot (1967: 38-55), Rubin (1974: 190).

manuscripts.[39] Cameron remarked that the Anglo-Saxons were familiar with the theory of the humours, but that their understanding of the system was limited.[40] Whether the Anglo-Saxons had a limited understanding of diet and hygiene or not, it is a fact that pre-Conquest English science hardly dealt with the topic in the form of regimens.

I agree with Wallis that the Egyptian Days are dates arbitrarily appointed throughout the year, but it is possible to find another prognostic genre which also assigned fixed dates, yet the dates of which were not determined arbitrarily: the Dog Days. These days are connected with the period in which the Dog-star, Sirius in Canis Major, is visible. Granted that the latitude of the observer and the precession of the equinoxes influence the period on which the Dog Days fall, these days are entered into the calendar because they are on fixed dates.[41] Although I would class the Dog Days under solar time, it is unclear where Wallis would accommodate them, either as seasonal, astronomical or calendric time: the Dog Days fall in a specific season, they are determined "by the visible movements of the heavens", and they appear in the calendar. The advantage of the twofold system of solar and lunar time is its adequacy for Anglo-Saxon computi and the temporal prognostics.[42]

Types of Computi

Sixty-two computi have survived in forty-five English manuscripts from before the thirteenth century.[43] These computi are not all identical to one another because they reflect knowledge acquired at various points in time, from various sources and drawing on various scientific traditions. Computus manuscripts are usually studied in the light of their computistical contents solely. It may prove worthwhile, however, to study the transmission of prognostics in these manuscripts in correlation to the transmission of types of computi.

---

[39] One only needs to consult a few pages of the catalogue of medical manuscripts compiled by Beccaria (1956) to realise how extensive learning was on this point.

[40] Cameron (1993: 161, 168). On bloodletting , hygiene and the humours, see Bonser (1963: 34-37, 294-99), Rubin (1974: 140-44), Cameron (1993: 28, 159-68).

[41] The precession of the equinoxes is negligible unless one considers a period of hundreds of years, which generally exceeds the life span and validity of computi.

[42] Please note that I do not question Wallis's threefold division in a wider perspective.

[43] Hollis (2001: 189). Stevens (1992: 143, n. 1) mentioned "sixty-two independent *computi*" from Anglo-Saxon England, probably referring to individual computi rather than discrete versions of the computus.

Baker and Lapidge distinguished a number of computus types, starting with the earliest: Bede's and the Canterbury computus.[44] These made use of Irish computi which ultimately derived from Spain and North Africa. The next development that influenced English time reckoning was the continental Abbonian computus, which came into being in the tenth century under the influence of Abbo of Fleury.[45] The Abbonian computus was to shape the computistical work of Byrhtferth, Abbo's pupil at Ramsey. The so-called Leofric-Tiberius computus was developed around 970 and is named after the two manuscripts containing relatively independent representatives of this type of computus.[46] The Winchester computus, which came into being around 978, is next and may have been the work of one person. It is partly indebted to the Leofric-Tiberius computus. A number of manuscripts have derived their versions of the computus from the Winchester type. Finally, Byrhtferth compiled a computus of his own, based on an Abbonian computus probably in his possession, while also taking material from the Leofric-Tiberius and Winchester computi, and from an unidentified pre-Abbonian computus. Byrhtferth also added new material of his own design.

From the text edition it appears that within the same genre, individual prognostics are sometimes related. This relationship is borne out by similarities in phrasing, idiom and grammar, and in the case of Apuleian Spheres by correspondences in the diagrams. Texts which share these similarities can be grouped as one redaction of a prognostic genre, while texts within the same genre which do not share these features form separate redactions. In order to discover how prognostics were transmitted from one computus to the next, we can trace redactions of these prognostics from one type of computus to the next.[47] An example will illustrate how this works.

The diagrams of a specific redaction of Apuleian Spheres may serve as indicators of how these Spheres are related.[48] This redaction repre-

[44] The following sketch of developments in the English computus is based on Baker and Lapidge's study of the computus (1995: xl-lx). Any mistakes are mine.

[45] On the writings and career of Abbo, see van de Vyver (1935) and the outstanding biography by Riché (2004).

[46] The manuscripts are Tiberius B. v and Bodley 579.

[47] Henel (1934a: 40-70) did the same for Old English computistical texts in CCCC 422, Caligula A. xv, Titus D. xxvii, Vitellius E. xviii, and Harley 3271. He noted strong links between, for instance, Canterbury and Winchester computi.

[48] The number of redactions distinguished for Apuleian Spheres depends heavily upon the criteria used, however (see pp. 181-95).

sents the two main subdivisions of the diagram as figures of Life and Death and is attested in three manuscripts, the earliest and most ornate rendering of which is in Bodley 579; the other two are in Tiberius C. vi and Harley 3667.[49] These manuscripts represent Leofric-Tiberius, Winchester and Byrhtferth's computi, respectively. Of both Winchester and Byrhtferth's computi there are more manuscripts containing Apuleian Spheres, none of which have the figures of Life and Death other than Tiberius C. vi and Harley 3667. In this case, vertical text transmission took place, whereas lateral transmission did not occur.

The example illustrates that prognostics moved from one type of computus to the next but were not necessarily copied into other manuscripts of the same type of computus. It is conceivable that there are prognostics which show lateral transmission. Some of the prognostics in Tiberius C. i + Harley 3667 and St. John's College 17, both Byrhtferth's computi, are related, for instance, as are the calendars containing Dog Days in Vitellius A. xii, Bodley 579 and Add. 37517. This, however, is the result of the material having been copied from the same exemplar. When a common exemplar has been used, lateral transmission is to be expected. In conclusion, the accretion and transmission of prognostics in the computus is far from systematic. Having found a redaction of a prognostic in one type of computus does not mean it will be encountered in other manuscripts of the same type of computus, nor does it imply that other types of computi will incorporate this prognostic. Vertical transmission between different types of computi is just as likely to take place as lateral transmission in the case of several copies from one exemplar. In the development of a certain type of computus a scribe copying computistical material at hand added a temporal prognostic which merited inclusion in the computus. Other scribes working on the same type of computus may have added other (redactions of) prognostics to the manuscripts they were working on. One of these manuscripts is then used as a source of information for another type of computus, and the scribe using this manuscript would copy the prognostic he encountered and would perhaps even add some of his own liking. This scenario demonstrates how prognostics were copied from one type of computus to the next, an effective but haphazard mechanism which aided the preservation and transmission of prognostics.

[49] See pp. 200, 202, 204, 206, pl. 3-6.

Four Computi containing Old English Prognostics

Most of the findings pertaining to prognostics in computi were gathered from computi containing Latin prognostics. Without this Latin material, our perspective would have been distorted since relatively few vernacular prognostics have survived from the Anglo-Saxon period. There is, for instance, only one Latin Apuleian Sphere with a partial Old English gloss,[50] which, if limited to this attestation, would have discouraged an analysis of Apuleian Spheres in Anglo-Saxon manuscripts. Moreover, Old English prognostics, or Latin ones with Old English glosses for that matter, are infrequently encountered in computi. Four manuscripts deserve mention since they are the only ones to contain Old English and/or glossed prognostics in the computus, to wit Vitellius C. viii, Caligula A. xv + Egerton 3314, Vitellius E. xviii and Harley 3271.

Vitellius C. viii

Folios 22-25 of this manuscript constitute no more than a fragment of a Winchester computus. Two of the computistical texts in this fragment are related to corresponding ones in Vitellius E. xviii, though said texts in the former might be slightly later than the others in this fragment and are written in another hand than the other texts in Vitellius C. viii. The prognostic in Vitellius C. viii, in the main hand, is one of five extant Old English texts on the three Egyptian Days. Unlike the two computistical texts in this fragment, the prognostic is not related to the Old English text on the three Egyptian Days in Vitellius E. xviii. In fact, the prognostic in Vitellius C. viii is nearly identical to the one in the medical manuscript Harley 585.[51] The other three manuscripts discussed below have more extensive prognostic collections in the computus. One cannot help but wonder what the original computus to which Vitellius C. viii once belonged might have contained in the way of prognostics.

Caligula A. xv + Egerton 3314

Caligula A. xv, fols 120-153, formed one manuscript with Egerton 3314, fols 1-78. This manuscript contains a Canterbury computus with miscellaneous notes, charms, prognostics, annals of Christ Church, Canterbury, and excerpts from Ælfric's *De temporibus anni*. The prognostics do not appear in consecutive order because other texts intervene. Seven

[50] Vitellius E. xviii, fol. 16r.

[51] See p. 41 for this manuscript.

prognostics are in Latin, one of which is an illness lunary glossed in Old English; five are in Old English. The prognostics are not ordered by language, grouped together, or separates from the immediate context, which suggests that material was copied as it came to hand or aroused the scribe's interest. Some similarities can be observed between Caligula A. xv + Egerton 3314 and Tiberius A. iii, a manuscript composed around the same time and also from Christ Church, Canterbury.[52] Some of the prognostics in these manuscripts are closely related, to wit the glossed illness lunary and the Old English dream and birth lunaries. The other prognostics in Caligula A. xv + Egerton 3314 are not found in Tiberius A. iii, and although Tiberius A. iii antedates the former, it cannot have been used as an exemplar on the basis of text-internal evidence. One or more exemplars can be posited from which both manuscripts drew some prognostics. The link between Caligula A. xv + Egerton 3314 and St. John's College 17, through the Apuleian Sphere, has been remarked upon above.[53]

Vitellius E. xviii

This manuscript is a psalter prefaced by a Winchester computus with miscellaneous notes, charms, medical texts and prognostics, on folios 1-17.[54] As with Caligula A. xv + Egerton 3314, the computistical texts, so not just the prognostics, are both in Latin and in Old English, and no attempt has been made on the part of the scribe to put texts together on the basis of language or genre, though there is an agglomeration of prognostics on folios 14v-15v. In addition to prognostic material in the calendar, the computus of Vitellius E. xviii hosts seven prognostics: one in Latin and one glossed (both Apuleian Spheres), and five in Old English. Furthermore, there are indications that the calendar on folios 2-7 was preceded by a bloodletting lunary (*fol. 1**, now lost), as is customary with Winchester calendars related to the one in Vitellius E. xviii.[55]

The collection of prognostics in Vitellius E. xviii is invaluable as it presents a series of unique texts as well as texts with links to various other manuscripts. The Old English text on the Dog Days is unique in this

[52] See pp. 53-57 for the latter manuscript.

[53] See p. 31, n. 28.

[54] Pulsiano (1994b: 51-53).

[55] E.g. in CCCC 422, Arundel 60 and Titus D. xxvii. See Henel (1934a: 26, n. 78), Budny (1997: I.647). On the link between Vitellius E. xviii and Titus D. xxvii, see Pulsiano (1998a; 1998b: 99-103).

redaction,[56] as is the glossed Apuleian Sphere. Caligula A. xv + Egerton 3314 and Vitellius E. xviii are the only Anglo-Saxon manuscripts to have an Old English text on the unlucky days, a genre of which I have found only one insular Latin representative, in St. John's College 17. The two Cottonian manuscripts, together with Harley 3271, also have a closely corresponding redaction of an Old English text on the twenty-four Egyptian Days.[57] Additionally, the Old English texts on the three Egyptian Days and the three miraculous birthdays in Vitellius E. xviii are closely related to those in CCCC 391, from Worcester.[58] In short, Vitellius E. xviii contains a series of prognostics with parallels in manuscripts from a number of religious establishments.

Harley 3271

A large part of the contents of this Winchester(?) manuscript is taken up by a copy of Ælfric's *Grammar* preceded by grammatical and encyclopedic notes,[59] and followed by computistical and encyclopedic notes and a prognostic section. The only Old English prognostic, a text on the twenty-four Egyptian Days, is part of the computus.[60] There are nine Latin prognostics in Harley 3271, three of which appear twice. The first prognostic, a guest text,[61] is a bloodletting lunary written in a blank space within the grammatical treatise *Beatus quid est*. The remaining eight prognostics constitute a prognostic section.[62] This section starts out with a β-sequence in Latin: the twenty-four Egyptian Days, the Dog Days and the three Egyptian Days.[63] The first of these prognostics is a severely corrupted copy which has undergone extensive revision at the hands of the scribe. A mass of seventeen lines intervenes between the second and third prognostic, but a line in the margin indicates that the latter should have followed the text on the Dog Days. The same prognostic sequence is

[56] Dog Days in Old English also feature in Royal 12. D. xvii, fols 54v-55v (see pp. 40-41) and the *Peri didaxeon* (see p. 42).

[57] See pp. 366-69.

[58] See pp. 51-53 for CCCC 391. On the sequence of three Egyptian Days and three miraculous birthdays, see pp. 61-62.

[59] On the origin and contents of Harley 3271, see Chardonnens (2007b).

[60] McGowan (2001b: 297) discussed instances of "Anglo-Latin prose curiosities" in Harley 3271, for which he listed the rubrics of a number of short tracts, among which *De diebus malis*. This is quite ironic, however, because the rubric is affixed to the only prognostic in Old English in Harley 3271.

[61] For prognostics as guest texts, see pp. 45-49.

[62] For the other manuscripts containing prognostic sections, see pp. 49-59.

[63] On this sequence, see p. 61.

repeated immediately, but now the copy of the text on the twenty-four Egyptian Days is impeccable and the text on the three Egyptian Days follows the one on the Dog Days. This second series is in a hand different from the first, but does not start on a new quire. It is unlikely that these two sets are simultaneous copies from the exemplar by two scribes who did not check up on each other's progress. Rather, the second scribe probably decided to recopy the series from the exemplar because the first had done a bad job. Directly after the second series of prognostics is a month regimen,[64] and yet another text on the Dog Days, in a different redaction than the other two and related to the one in Titus D. xxvi.

It is interesting to observe that the three Old English texts on the twenty-four Egyptian Days are found in all three of the larger manuscripts discussed above. The Old English redaction of this prognostic is thus limited to transmission within computi and did not circulate outside this context. Furthermore, Caligula A. xv + Egerton 3314 and Vitellius E. xviii, Canterbury and Winchester computi, respectively, share an Old English text on the unlucky days, otherwise unattested. These two instances not only illustrate that some (redactions of) prognostic genres are not found outside a computistical context, but they also give credit to the relevance of vertical transmission in the dissemination of prognostics.

Medical Sections and Manuscripts[65]

Medical writings are a source in which one would expect to find prognostics that deal with illness and health. This expectation, however, is belied: only the *Lacnunga* (Harley 585, fols 130-93), the *Peri didaxeon* (Harley 6258B, fols 51-66) and Bald's *Leechbook* (Royal 12. D. xvii, fols 1-108) contain one Old English prognostic each. The first medical section of St. John's College 17 (fols 1-2) contains tracts on bloodletting and the humours, two of which mention the Dog Days. Finally, Sloane 475, fols 125-231, contains six Latin prognostics in what seem to me to be continental redactions. The scarcity of prognostics in medical writings is awkward in view of the relatively many Anglo-Saxon medical manuscripts and texts that have come down to us. A comparison between continental

[64] On regimens in English manuscripts, see pp. 31-33.

[65] This section pertains to Harley 585, Harley 6258B, Royal 12. D. xvii, Sloane 475, St. John's College 17.

and Anglo-Saxon medical manuscripts will reveal that the Anglo-Saxon medical context is not the vehicle of choice for prognostics.

Manuscripts containing Medical Sections

Medical sections may be included in basically non-medical manuscripts, such as the medical sections in St. John's College 17 (fols 1-2 and 175-77), or they may be found in manuscripts entirely devoted to this subject. These medical manuscripts can be subdivided into volumes containing one or two large medical tracts (Royal 12. D. xvii), or those comprising a collection of various works on medicine (Harley 585, Harley 6258B, Sloane 475).[66] This distinction seems to determine to what extent the prognostics in question are integrated into the text.

Royal 12. D. xvii

In Bald's *Leechbook*, the text on bloodletting and the Dog Days is placed towards the end of book I, "after the organizational format has broken down",[67] yet consolidation is evident from the consecutive numbering of the recipes in book I proper and the table of contents. The Dog Days are embedded in a tract on bloodletting. This tract is in the same hand as the rest of the text, so it can be assumed that it is original to Bald's *Leechbook* as it stands. Since Royal 12. D. xvii is the copy of exemplars now lost, it is difficult to determine how the prognostic got into Bald's *Leechbook* in the first place. Nokes has argued that a number of recipes, including the tract on bloodletting, were added later, after the core of books I and II had come into being.[68] Cameron spoke of Bald's *Leechbook* as a "more consciously ordered piece of work [than *Leechbook 3*, in the same manuscript]", and he praised the "blending into a harmonious whole" of sources from a number of cultures and backgrounds.[69] The prognostic, then, can be said to be an integral part of Bald's *Leechbook*, even if it does not belong to the core of recipes that shaped Bald's *Leechbook* in the first place. Moreover, the lengthy introduction of the Dog Days in the table of contents suggests that the compiler who added the text to the original batch or remedies made note of the prognostic value of the text, i.e. com-

[66] Cameron (1983: 144-45).
[67] Nokes (2004: 60).
[68] Nokes (2004: 58-61, 65-70). See Payne (1904: 40).
[69] Cameron (1993: 42), cf. Meaney (1984a: 237, 251).

pared to the instructions for bloodletting the prognostic content was not of secondary importance to him.

Harley 585

The text on the three Egyptian Days is a different case as it appears in the *Lacnunga*, a medical commonplace book which is not at all homogenous in content: "a compilation made by non-medical collectors" in the words of Cameron.[70] The *Lacnunga* was copied in two parts, though probably not much time elapsed between the copying.[71] The text on the three Egyptian Days is found near the end of the second part. The prognostic in the *Lacnunga* is one of four attestations of the three Egyptian Days outside a computistical context;[72] seven more texts on the three Egyptian Days are found within computi. The text in Harley 585 is not accompanied by a birthday prognostic, in contrast to most other attestations of the three Egyptian Days.[73] The prognostic on the three Egyptian Days does not strike me as fitting in very well with the context —if there ever was a conscious design in the collection of texts contained in the *Lacnunga*.[74] Some scholars have commented upon the *Lacnunga* as "a rambling collection",[75] and Meaney suggested that the scribe "simply put down everything as it came to hand",[76] in contrast to the compiler of Bald's *Leechbook*. We probably owe the survival of the Old English prognostic in the *Lacnunga* more to accident than to intent.[77]

---

[70] Cameron (1993: 34).

[71] Doane (1994: 26).

[72] The other three are in CCCC 391, CCCC 422 and Titus D. xxvi. Despite being found outside a computistical context, the redaction of the three Egyptian Days in Harley 585 is identical to the one in Vitellius C. viii, a fragment of a computus (see p. 36).

[73] See pp. 61-62 on this sequence.

[74] The *Lacnunga* is a construct rather than a volume of unified texts, as Grattan and Singer's analysis of the contents makes clear (1952: 18-22). Grattan and Singer distinguished five strata of texts based on the type of sources used for the "Anglo-Saxon medico-magic" (their phrase) in the *Lacnunga*. Though Grattan and Singer rail against what they considered Anglo-Saxon medicine "deformed by a perverted learning", filled with "monastic stupidity", and "barbarian interpretation and mishandling" (1952: 15, 16, 18), they do have a point in establishing that the texts in the *Lacnunga* are so varied that they cannot possibly form a unified corpus of well-adjusted texts. Talbot's comment that the *Lacnunga* "has been dealt with adequately, if not excessively, by those whose intention has been to denigrate Anglo-Saxon medicine" (1967: 21) seems to be a jibe at Grattan and Singer's study and edition of the treatise.

[75] Talbot (1967: 23). Cf. Cameron (1993: 31, 45).

[76] Meaney (1984a: 245).

[77] Cf. Cameron (1993: 35).

Harley 6258B
This manuscript from the late twelfth century contains a number of medical tracts including the *Peri didaxeon*. This treatise is a translation into late Old English of parts of the *Practica Petrocelli Salernitani*, a non-Salernitan collection of medical treatises.[78] The earliest continental manuscript witness of this compilation that has been identified so far is ninth-century; the *Practica* is thought to have reached England in the eleventh century.[79] The *Peri didaxeon* opens with an adaptation of a letter on the schools of medicine, the *Epistola peri hereseon*, followed by an adaptation of the *Disputatio Platonis et Aristotelis* on the humours.[80] Yellow bile is said to be active on the Dog Days, and the text issues a warning for doctors not to treat a patient on these days. As with the text on the Dog Days in Royal 12. D. xvii, the prognostic component in Harley 6258B is embedded into a larger medical context.

Sloane 475
Reportedly, folios 125-231 of this medical miscellany are the English part of a composite manuscript in Latin.[81] This part dates from the eleventh century and contains a mutilated version of an Apuleian Sphere.[82] In addition, there is a bloodletting prognostic, unattested anywhere else, to my knowledge. Finally, a sequence of a collective lunary, the twenty-four Egyptian Days, a year prognosis and an alphabetical dreambook are found near the end of the English part. The redactions of the prognostics in Sloane 475 are totally unlike those I have encountered in English manuscripts, which raises questions as to the place of origin of Sloane 475, fols125-231, or that of its exemplar. The texts are sloppy copies impaired by numerous errors: they are riddled with grammatical and spelling mistakes; abbreviation marks are often omitted; word division is often such that the last syllable of a word is joined to the first syllable of the next; texts are incomplete or jumbled; transpositions are frequent; minims cause considerable problems. In short, the manuscript "suffers from a severe degree for inherent vice".[83]

---

[78] On the *Practica Petrocelli Salernitani* and its relationship to the *Peri didaxeon*, see Glaze (2007) and Maion (2007).

[79] Glaze (2007), Maion (2007).

[80] On the *Epistola peri hereseon* and an edition of the text, see Glaze (2007); on the *Disputatio*, see Maion (2007).

[81] Gameson (1999: 121 [567]), Gneuss (2001: 85 [498.1]).

[82] The text is severely mangled; the diagram was never drawn.

[83] Derow (1993: 8)

The prognostics in Sloane 475 are poorly executed and some appear in a context unusual for these genres. The Apuleian Sphere shows that this genre is not attested in a computistical context only. But why would an Apuleian Sphere have been incorporated in the first place? Even if the Sphere had been intended for actual use, its utilitarian value is nil as it is not close to being finished. Moreover, the presence of a prognostic like the dreambook is awkward in a medical context. In Anglo-Saxon manuscripts, prognostic sections are the sole context for dreambooks. Sloane 475, fols 125-231, is the only English(?) medical section known to me which contains so many prognostics, included for no immediately apparent reason. If these texts interested the scribe, why did he copy them so carelessly? Folios 125-231 cannot have been a draft for a hypothetical fair copy since the condition of the prognostics is so poor that they cannot possibly serve as a source of information without the help of comparable texts in a better state. Despite the state the texts are in, it is clear from the deliberate inclusion of prognostics in between medical treatises that the compiler saw a medical use for these texts.

A large number of English prognostics are encountered in related redactions more than once, which is not the case for the prognostics in Sloane 475. The repeated attestation of one redaction of a prognostic genre can be said to represent the extent to which the text has become naturalised. The fact that the redactions of the prognostics in Sloane 475 had up to then not been attested in England should give rise to caution, as should the unique attestation of a weekday bloodletting prognostic. The 'Si tenebrae' redaction of the text on the twenty-four Egyptian Days, is, for this period, more common on the continent (this also applies to the one in Egerton 3314). Cameron has argued that the exemplar of the entire English part was written in Anglo-Saxon minuscule on the basis of confusion between 'r' and 'n'.[84] If the exemplar was in an Anglo-Saxon hand, this does not rule out the possibility that the exemplar (or even Sloane 475, folios 125-231, itself) was produced on the continent. In fact, judging from the prognostic redactions—alien compared to Anglo-Saxon prognostics—, an exemplar of continental origin is highly likely. The presence of material from the *Practica Petrocelli Salernitani* would fit in with the introduction of this compendium in England in the late eleventh century.[85] In conclusion, even if Sloane 475, fols 125-231, is an English production, its links with the continent are still very strong.

[84] Cameron (1983: 144).

[85] Maion (2007).

St. John's College 17
This largely computistical manuscript has an extensive collection of Latin prognostics. It contains two prognostics in the first medical section, on folios 1-2. The second medical section, folios 175-77, does not have any prognostics. Cameron pointed out that these sections cannot have been part of the original set-up of Byrhtferth's computus in the exemplar of St. John's College 17.[86] The prognostics are two texts on the Dog Days embedded in medical tracts on the four humours and bloodletting. This is somewhat akin to the inclusion of Dog Day information in the *Peri didaxeon*, some parts of the *Practica Petrocelli Salernitani*, and Bald's *Leechbook*. The redactions of the Dog Days in St. John's College 17 are unlike the ones in Titus D. xxvi, xxvii, and Harley 3271, but as the former do not form independent texts this is hardly surprising.

English versus Continental Medical Manuscripts

With regard to Sloane 475, fols 125-231, I raised the issue of prognostic genres in a context atypical for English manuscripts. The only prognostics which seem to fit into their medical contexts are the ones in Royal 12. D. xvii, Harley 6258B and St. John's College 17, and these are embedded in more extensive medical tracts on bloodletting or the humours. Two other English medical sections contain prognostics, but in Harley 585 the prognostic does not really fit in, and in Sloane 475 the prognostics are in what I conclude are continental redactions.

There is a marked difference between English and continental medical manuscripts in that prognostics are far more common in the latter, and out of context in the former. Careful analysis of two representative manuscript catalogues in this field, Beccaria's *I codici di medicina del periodo presalernitano* and Wickersheimer's *Les manuscrits latins de médecine du haut moyen âge dans les bibliothèques de France*,[87] confirms that not only are prognostics found frequently in continental medical manuscripts, but also that the range of genres attested in continental volumes is more extensive than in English volumes.[88] The size of the Anglo-Saxon prognostic corpus is correlated to contextual embedding, and to a lesser extent to the

[86] Cameron (1993: 54). Cf. Hollis and Wright (1992: 161-62).

[87] Beccaria (1956), Wickersheimer (1966).

[88] In a chapter on Anglo-Saxon and continental medicine in the early Middle Ages, Thorndike (1923-58: I.719-41) did not note this difference between continental and English medical manuscripts.

survival of manuscripts. Granted that there are few prognostics in English medical manuscripts anyhow, the extant number of such manuscripts will hardly exert influence upon the overall number of Anglo-Saxon prognostics. Continental medical manuscripts, on the other hand, contribute extensively to the continental prognostic corpus. Apuleian Spheres, for example, are regularly found in continental medical manuscripts, which is one more reason to posit a continental connection for Sloane 475. Another example are regimens; these texts, too, seem to have been more current in continental manuscripts at the time.[89] whereas there are few English manuscripts containing regimens. The inclusion of five regimens in the continental part of Sloane 475 confirms this notion.

Most of the Anglo-Saxon prognostics are attested in a computistical context and in prognostic sections. The cause for this can be found in the accretive influence of computistical writings, compounded by a renewed interest in the computus in the tenth and eleventh centuries. The first prognostic sections came into being in the eleventh century. These sections usually include a large number of prognostics. The existence of prognostics in Anglo-Saxon England is, therefore, largely dependent upon computi and prognostic sections.

From the above it is evident that the manuscript context exerts influence upon the presence of certain prognostic genres, and that prognostics in English medical manuscripts are treated differently from those in continental manuscripts. Accordingly, this different treatment underlies the near absence of Anglo-Saxon prognostics in a medical context, that is if these prognostics are not integrated properly into larger tracts on bloodletting or the humours.

Prognostics as Guest Texts[90]

Sporadically, prognostics were used as guest material. Guest texts are added at a later date in blank spaces of existing (parts of) manuscripts. This usage has led to the preservation of two unique prognostics. For-

[89] See pp. 31-33. Reiche (1973) published eight different continental regimens, Stuart (1979) four.

[90] This section pertains to CCCC 391, p. 721, CCCC 422, p. 49, Tiberius C. vi, fol. 114r, Titus D. xxvii, fols 55v-56v, Vespasian D. xiv, fols 75v and 103v, Harley 3271, fol. 102v, Royal 2. B. v, fol. 190rv.

tunate though this may be, it is difficult to establish conclusively why prognostics, of all possible types of texts, were chosen as guest texts.[91] I have tried to discover whether the presence of prognostics as guest material could be justified in view of the immediate manuscript context, but I have been unable to find such a justification.[92] Six manuscripts contain eight guest prognostics in all, two of which are in a computus, one following a prognostic section, the other ones in contexts atypical for prognostics. One of these texts, in Harley 3271, has been introduced elsewhere.[93]

Vespasian D. xiv

The first instance of guest texts is from Vespasian D. xiv. Two Old English prognostics found their way into this Old English homiletic collection: a year prognosis and a month brontology. The latter prognostic is uniquely attested in Old English. Both prognostics were added by the main hand in blank spaces at quire endings on folios 75v and 103v.[94] There cannot be any doubt that the prognostics were intended as guest texts since they were added at a later date and their relevance to the immediate context is not directly apparent. It is likely that they did not serve a practical purpose as predictive devices in view of their being atypical for the context in which they are found.

Royal 2. B. v

The second manuscript, the tenth-century Regius Psalter, has the only Latin month brontology from Anglo-Saxon England. The manuscript originally consisted of a glossed psalter, to which a quire containing an Office of the Virgin was prefixed.[95] Several other additions were made in blank spaces in this manuscript and following the psalter text, some in the place of origin, Winchester, and some in Christ Church, Canterbury, where the manuscript had been transferred to in the eleventh cen-

[91] I return to some of the choices underlying guest texts on pp. 69-70, 149-50.

[92] In Chardonnens (2006, 2007c) I have called these filler texts because this is precisely what such texts do. However, since the role and purpose of guest texts is in need of further investigation, I have replaced the prejudicial term 'filler material' with 'guest material' in accordance with current practice (see, for instance, Gumbert 2004).

[93] See pp. 38-39. CCCC 391 contains a guest prognostic added by the Tremulous Worcester hand, but I have excluded this text on account of its late genesis (see p. 4).

[94] For additions at the quire endings of Vespasian D. xiv, see Handley (1974).

[95] Pulsiano (1994b: 57).

tury. Of these additions, the most interesting to me is that of a series of encyclopedic notes concluded by a Latin month brontology, all in the same hand and immediately following the psalter.[96] This entire group of guest texts was added at the end of the tenth century and is of Winchester origin. After the notes and the prognostic, Old English prayers and directions for fasting were added, some of which in Canterbury.[97]

Tiberius C. vi

The third manuscript, the Tiberius Psalter from the third quarter of the eleventh century, contains an Apuleian Sphere in the computus. A Latin text on the twenty-four Egyptian Days and an Anglo-Norman text on the unlucky days were added on folio 114r in the twelfth century. Folios 31r-129v constitute the glossed psalter, interspersed with full-page illuminations and ornamentation.[98] Folio 114v contains a full-page illustration, and the blank space following the original text on folio 114r has been used to add the two prognostics.

Titus D. xxvii

The fourth instance of a guest text is the alphabet prognostic added on folios 55v-56v of Titus D. xxvii.[99] This manuscript, known as Ælfwine's *Prayerbook* together with Titus D. xxvi, has a computus in which several temporal prognostics can be found, followed by a non-computistical section containing offices, prayers and devotions. The alphabet prognostic was added after the computus.[100]

---

[96] In Pulsiano (1994b: 62-63), the notes are listed as item (7) and the month brontology as (8), which does not make it sufficiently clear that these items were copied in one stint. Furthermore, Pulsiano classified item (7) as computistical notes whereas they are not since they deal with the age of Christ, the size of the arc, and various other such matters. Warner and Gilson (1921: I.41) saw items (7) and (8) as one unit of "chronological and other commonplaces", thereby avoiding such complications. See Dekker (2007) for an outstanding treatment of these encyclopedic notes.

[97] Ker (1957: 320 [249]).

[98] Wilcox (2000: 38).

[99] Note that this prognostic is non-temporal and in Old English, whereas all other prognostics in this manuscript and its companion volume Titus D. xxvi are in Latin.

[100] See pp. 57-59 for a more detailed discussion of this text and Titus D. xxvi, xxvii.

CCCC 422

The fifth attestation of guest prognostics, finally, is in CCCC 422, part B. This segment contains a computus with a calendar and prognostics. The first prognostic in CCCC 422 is a glossed bloodletting lunary. This lunary is followed by a calendar with uniquely preserved glossed entries on the Dog Days. These two items are original to the manuscript, which was produced at New Minster, Winchester, and intended for use at Sherborne. In Sherborne, a γ-sequence of two Latin prognostics, the three Egyptian Days and the three miraculous birthdays, was added on page 49.[101] These two prognostics are not out of place in the computus, but they are guest texts nevertheless.

Lambeth Palace 427

One other manuscript deserves mention in this section, viz. Lambeth Palace 427. The original manuscript consisted of psalter prefaces, the psalter itself, and canticles, on folios 1-2, 5-202. Folios 203-08, containing a litany and prayers, were added in the fifteenth century.[102] Folio 209 and a final unnumbered leaf are later binding leaves enveloping folios 210-11, which are leaves from another manuscript and contain an Old English history of Kentish royal saints.[103] O'Neill has argued that the leaves of interest, folios 3-4, are later additions as well.[104] The texts on these leaves are in an eleventh-century hand, and comprise prognostics and computistical tables in Latin. The prognostics, two lunaries, are on folio 3r. O'Neill observed that folios 3-4 do not fit in the psalter context,[105] and the absence of a larger computistical section in the host volume makes their presence even more conspicuous. Folios 3-4 resemble the status of guest material in that they lack contextual justification for their presence in this manuscript. Nevertheless, the prognostics are original to the computus to which they once belonged, so they are not guest texts despite the fact that folios 3-4 were added to Lambeth Palace 427 at a later date.

[101] See pp. 61-62 for this sequence.
[102] Ker (1957: 342 [280]), O'Neill (1991: 144-46).
[103] Ker (1957: 342-43 [280, 281]), O'Neill (1991: 144-46).
[104] O'Neill (1991: 146).
[105] O'Neill (1991: 146).

In these six manuscripts, including Harley 3271 and excluding Lambeth Palace 427, prognostics were added in blank spaces. The computistical context in CCCC 422 lent itself to prognostic additions. The remaining five manuscripts, a homiletic collection, two psalters, a miscellany and a prayerbook, provide contexts in which one does not expect prognostics to be added. There can be no doubt that all eight prognostics were intended as guest material since they were added at a later date, though the reason why prognostics specifically were chosen is obscure. One of the constraints on guest material is the relative brevity of the text in view of the space available. It seems unlikely, however, that prognostics were selected because of their conciseness only, seeing that in some cases other types of guest texts were added alongside prognostics.

Prognostic Sections[106]

There are no Anglo-Saxon manuscripts which contain prognostics only. Nevertheless, a number of manuscripts include substantial prognostic sections, i.e. parts in which one finds prognostics mainly, and in some cases exclusively. Such manuscripts are varied in contents, and they are principally known not for the prognostics, but for the other genres they contain. I have not encountered prognostic sections in continental manuscripts, or in manuscripts antedating the eleventh century.[107] Furthermore, it would appear that no underlying system governs in what type of manuscript prognostic sections are included. The importance of these sections should not be underestimated, because they are the main source of Old English prognostics (in contrast to Latin prognostics, which are most frequently encountered in computi). Furthermore, the range of prognostic genres in computi is more limited than that in prognostic sections, which uniquely feature non-temporal prognostics and a wide range of temporal prognostics. It is noteworthy that prognostics outside a computistical or medical context tend to stick together. Below, four manuscripts will be analysed that contain prognostic sections, valuable both on account of the large number of vernacular prognostics they

[106] This section pertains to CCCC 391, Tiberius A. iii, Titus D. xxvi, xxvii, Harley 3271, Hatton 115.

[107] Arguably, the continental manuscript Harley 3017 contains a prognostic section on fols 58r-60r, but this is an embryonic section at best in view of its limited size and the small number of prognostics included. Moreover, the range of genres and non-temporal prognostics, a characteristic of English sections, is absent in Harley 3017, fols 58r-60r.

have preserved and because they shed light on the placement of such sections in manuscripts. Some (parts) of these volumes have already been referred to before. One of the manuscripts with a prognostic section, Harley 3271, has already been discussed.[108]

Hatton 115

Perhaps the most remarkable manuscript to include a prognostic section is Hatton 115. This volume consists of five separate booklets bound together, the first four booklets of which are linked by their homiletic content.[109] Booklets 1-3 had been kept together for a while, as is evident from the original table of contents and the first layer of glosses by the Tremulous Worcester hand. At a later time booklets 4 and 5 were added, though it is unlikely that they were inserted simultaneously. The Tremulous hand applied a second layer of glosses to booklets 1-4, and a still later text fragment in his hand is found at the end of booklet 5. The place of origin of the eleventh-century booklets 1-4 is unknown, but booklet 5 is probably from Christ Church, Canterbury, and dates to the middle of the twelfth century.[110] Booklet 5 does not fit in with the four homiletic booklets because it contains prognostics and two short non-prognostic texts on the number of masses or psalms that equal a certain period of fasting. The nine prognostics in booklet 5 are in Old English and written in one hand. The wind prognostic is not attested elsewhere. Two texts are incomplete, and a third, the most complete agenda lunary in Old English, ends on the seventeenth day of the moon. The latter prognostic concludes the collection and strong punctuation is used to denote the end, though two blank leaves remained. Strong punctuation and the availability of space indicate that the scribe deliberately terminated his work. As noted before, outside the context of the computus non-temporal prognostics are encountered, in the case of Hatton 115 a dreambook closely resembling one of the dreambooks in Tiberius A. iii.

It is unknown what happened to booklet 5 between the time of its composition and the first half of the thirteenth century, when the manuscript is thought to have taken its present form. How and why it travelled from the south-east to Worcester is likewise not known. Furthermore, if

[108] See pp. 38-39.

[109] On the notion of booklets, see Robinson (1978).

[110] Canterbury was one of the centres which contributed extensively to the prognostic corpus, see pp. 71-77.

booklets 1-5 were bound together before the second layer of glosses, why did the Tremulous hand skip booklet 5 altogether at the time of glossing, only to return to this booklet later to add the text fragment mentioned earlier? A copied fragment of the three Egyptian Days in CCCC 391 illustrates that the Tremulous hand was not averse to prognostics, despite the fact that he may not have been interested in the prognostics in Hatton 115.

A prognostic section bound with four homiletic booklets is awkward, and the underlying purpose of this union is not revealed. The only plausible reason I can think of is that booklet 5 was lying around in the Worcester Cathedral library and to prevent its loss or misplacement (booklet 5 consists of two quires of four leaves each), it was incorporated in a manuscript to be rebound at the time. Anything other than a utilitarian purpose behind the union of booklets 1-5 can be dismissed for the contents of booklets 1-4 have nothing in common with that of booklet 5, except for the language in which the texts are written. Indeed, a "revival of interest in Old English manuscripts in Worcester in the early thirteenth century" may prove to be the main reason why the prognostic section in Hatton 115 has survived.[111]

CCCC 391

CCCC 391 is also known as the *Portiforium Wulfstani* since it may have been made for, or was owned by Wulfstan II, bishop of Worcester (1062-95). This voluminous work consists of a psalter preceded by a computus and followed by a litany, hymnal, collectar and a prognostic section. Many additional texts found their way into the manuscript after completion, but the prognostic section, on pages 713-21, is contemporary with the main part of the manuscript, so there can be no doubt that this section was meant to be included in the manuscript. Ker identified the scribe of the prognostic as "probably identical with the first of the two main hands of the manuscript".[112]

The prognostic section in CCCC 391 bears some similarity to booklet 5 in Hatton 115, not because of the type of prognostics in these volumes, but because the section in CCCC 391 is on a separate quire as well (pages 713-24). The section opens midway in the third entry of a sunshine prognostic (the only other sunshine prognostic from Anglo-Saxon

[111] Franzen (1991: 186). Cf. Franzen (1991: 185, 189-93).

[112] Ker (1957: 115 [67]), cf. James (1912: II.246).

England is in Hatton 115), followed by four brontologies, three of which are unique, to wit one for the canonical hours of the night office, one for the compass direction from which thunder comes, and one for the hours of the day office.[113] The directional brontology is the only non-temporal prognostic in CCCC 391. The manuscript contains thirteen prognostics in all: eleven in Old English, and a unique dream lunary with Psalm readings in Latin. These twelve texts are in one hand. The thirteenth prognostic in CCCC 391 is a guest text on the three Egyptian Days, an incomplete rendering in the early thirteenth century by the Tremulous Worcester hand of the Old English text preceding it on page 718.[114]

As I have mentioned, the sunshine prognostic is incomplete. It would be illogical for a scribe to start his work at an arbitrary point in the text, on the blank recto page of a new quire. Furthermore, the beginning of the sunshine prognostic does not appear on the preceding quire, since pages 711-12 were originally blank until a later hand added collects on these pages.[115] At present the prognostic section is a quire of six leaves (pages 713-24).[116] These considerations make it highly likely for another bifolium (for ease of reference pages *712**, *712†*, *725*, *726*), now lost, to have enclosed the extant quire. Alternatively, the prognostic section may have started with a single half-sheet, so that pages *725* and *726* may not have existed or may have been cancelled. Signs of the use of page 724 as a back pastedown argue against a bifolium: "it has traces of paste, offsets of wood-grain, and brown-colored offsets of unevenly trimmed leather turn-ins with mitered corners".[117] Budny assigns an early (twelfth-century?) binding to the manuscript as we have it, which is further corroborated by rust marks of a binding mechanism on pages 709-24, and wormholes on pages 719-24.[118] The pastedown page 724 seems to indi-

[113] A related hour brontology has the compass directions incorporated in the main text, in Tiberius A. iii and Titus D. xxvi.

[114] Why the scribe chose this particular prognostic is not clear; there are ten other prognostics in Old English in CCCC 391. Franzen (1991: 189) wrote that "somewhere... someone with a trembling hand was glossing Old English manuscripts, for some reason". She adduced various motives for a revived interest in Old English on the part of the Tremulous hand, such as educational or pastoral intentions (Franzen 1991: 183-94; cf. Thomson and Gullick 2001: xxiv). The reason that would underlie the copying of a prognostic, however, may have been an antiquarian interest in the Old English language.

[115] James (1912: II.246).

[116] James (1912: II.242).

[117] Budny (1997: I.633).

[118] *Ibid.*

cate that either the lost leaf is a bifolium which had disappeared before the manuscript was bound, or a singleton. The prognostics end on page 721 with the prognostic fragment in the Tremulous hand, which makes it improbable that pages *725* and *726*, if present at all, contained any prognostics. The blank pages 711-12 indicate that the text on the quire preceding that of the prognostic section had ended, so the lost page before 713, i.e. *712†*, is certain to have contained the beginning of the sunshine prognostic on the last six or so lines of the page. In addition, pages *712** and *712†* will conceivably have contained more prognostics, though it would be impossible to reconstruct the precise contents. Marks of the former binding reveal that the prognostic section was already placed at the end of the manuscript when it was bound for the first time.

Why would CCCC 391 incorporate prognostics, atypical as this genre is for a psalter? Wulfstan II carried a psalter with him when travelling, as William of Malmesbury's *Vita Wulfstani* attests, and Budny suggested that CCCC 391 may have been the volume referred to.[119] If this is so, Wulfstan II, in touring his diocese may have had need of utilitarian texts. Such texts range from exorcisms and ordeals, and might extend to prognostics. This interpretation, however, depends upon the attribution—by no means certain—of this volume to the travelling Wulfstan II. The more plausible part of the hypothesis, i.e. that Wulfstan II owned or commissioned CCCC 391,[120] suggests that the bishop felt the need to have not only a breviary within easy reach, but also a collection of other texts, including prognostics. An interest in prognostics by the higher clergy is not unusual: Ælfwine, when dean of New Minster, Winchester (before 1032), owned Titus D. xxvi, xxvii; Leofric, bishop of Exeter (1046-72), presented Bodley 579 to Exeter Cathedral.

Tiberius A. iii, fols 2-173

The third volume, Tiberius A. iii, is a miscellany containing texts ranging from Ælfrician to Alcuinian material, a *Life of St. Margaret*, a glossed *Regularis concordia*, homilies, prayers and devotions, the *Monasteriales indicia* and the largest extant collection of prognostics in Latin and Old English in a single Anglo-Saxon manuscript. Förster, the first scholar to have provided an extensive analysis of the contents, divisions and hands of the entire(!) manuscript, divided the book into six separate booklets

[119] Budny (1997: I.631-32).
[120] Franzen (1991: 184).

gathered into one by Sir Robert Cotton.[121] It is certain that Förster's booklets 4-6, i.e. folios 174-79, were taken from other manuscripts and bound with folios 2-173.[122] Gneuss, however, has argued convincingly that folios 2-173 do not constitute a manuscript consisting of separate booklets, as Förster once thought.[123]

The prognostics in this volume consist of one section of seven glossed and eleven Old English prognostics on folios 27v-43r, and a second section of four Latin prognostics on folio 65rv. This number is only rivalled by Titus D. xxvi, xxvii, which has twenty-one prognostics. In Tiberius A. iii, the glossed part of the first series of prognostics includes, among others, one of the largest extant alphabetical dreambooks, the only glossed collective lunary and a brontology. Among the Old English prognostics are two alphabetical dreambooks, a unique month prognosis and two unique birth prognostics—on the development of the foetus and the gender of the unborn child. The first of two Old English alphabetical dreambooks is closely related to that in Hatton 115. The link between several prognostics in Tiberius A. iii and Caligula A. xv + Egerton 3314 has already been remarked upon.[124] The second prognostic section in Tiberius A. iii contains a sequence in Latin of a bloodletting lunary, a birth prognostic, and birth and illness lunaries.[125]

In contrast to those in Hatton 115 and CCCC 391, the prognostic sections in Tiberius A. iii do not appear on separate quires, nor are they written in one hand. Ker gave the signature of the pertinent sections as three quires of eight leaves, folios 27-50, and one quire of eight leaves, folios 65-72.[126] The first prognostic section starts on folio 27v, following upon the glossed *Regularis concordia* on folios 3-27, and crosses two quire boundaries: folios 34v-35r and 42v-43r. The second prognostic section opens a quire also containing an excerpt of Ælfric's *De temporibus anni* on folios 65v-73r. The last prognostic in the second section is an incomplete illness lunary; it is possible that the scribe deliberately intended to discontinue copying the prognostics.

[121] Förster (1908c: 30).

[122] Förster (1908c: 44 [V]), Ker (1957: 196-97 [155], 248-49 [187], 249-50 [188]), Gneuss (1997: 16).

[123] Gneuss (1997: 15-17).

[124] See pp. 36-37.

[125] See pp. 60-61 for this sequence.

[126] Ker (1957: 247 [186]).

Among the two Latin and five Old English hands distinguished by Ker,[127] one is responsible for the Latin prognostics on folios 27v-37v, 65rv, one for the Old English glosses on folios 27v-37v, and one for the Old English prognostics on folios 37v-43r/2. These hands also contributed to various other portions of Tiberius A. iii. From the crossing of quire boundaries and the changes of hands, the prognostic sections would seem to be fully integrated into the rest of the miscellaneous material in this manuscript, or, in the words of Gneuss: "the distribution of the work of the several scribes speaks against this assumption [of separate booklets]".[128] Furthermore, the sequence of the glossed *Regularis concordia* is immediately followed by a series of glossed prognostics, which is in turn followed by a series of prognostics in Old English, i.e. a gradual transition from glossed non-prognostic material to prognostics in the vernacular. The crossing of quire boundaries, the variety of hands and the transition from glossed Latin to the vernacular seem to suggest that the prognostics were purposefully included in Tiberius A. iii.

The second prognostic section is twenty-two leaves removed from the first. This distance is remarkable, especially since the same hand was responsible for both the Latin part of the glossed prognostics in the first section, and for the prognostics in the second section. Tiberius A. iii is a miscellany for which a large number of sources may have been used. It is reasonable, then, to assume that different sources were accessed at different times during the production of the manuscript, and that the source used for the second prognostic section may have been another than that of the first section. Similarly, the first prognostic section is divided into glossed prognostics and Old English prognostics, produced by three hands. The coexistence of prognostics in Old English and Latin (with or without glosses) is rare. Two other manuscripts which have this are Caligula A. xv + Egerton 3314 and Vitellius E. xviii.[129]

The two prognostic sections may have been included in Tiberius A. iii for various reasons. The first section follows a glossed Rule of St. Benedict, supplements to the Rule, and the glossed *Regularis concordia*,[130] of

[127] Ker (1957: 248 [186]) assigned one hand to the Old English texts on fols 37v-42v, and one to fols 43r-45r. The two lines completing the birth prognostic on fol. 43r are, however, in the same hand as the rest of the text.

[128] Gneuss (1997: 16).

[129] These volumes are unusual in that they are the only ones to have glossed and Old English prognostics in a computus, see pp. 36-38.

[130] Ker (1957: 241-42 [186]), Gneuss (1997: 14). The material preceding the first prognostic section is on fols 117-73, 2-27, as fols 117-73 originally preceded 2-116.

which Gneuss remarked: "there would be next to no problem if we only had to deal with articles one to seven [the items listed above and the first prognostic section], a compendium of the Benedictine Reform movements in Carolingian Francia and in tenth-century England".[131] With regard to the nature of the text in Tiberius A. iii, Clayton and Magennis observed that the beginning of the manuscript is a collection of monastic writings inspired by the Benedictine Reform, after which the manuscript "takes on a much more miscellaneous character":[132]

> While some of the texts, such as the directions for confessors and the Office of the Virgin, were written for a particular practical purpose, it is difficult to imagine this manuscript as having been intended for direct use in practical contexts, as texts for very different situations are placed side by side. The manuscript perhaps came to be viewed primarily as a type of reference book, preserving texts of interest to the community and serving as a handy repository for such diverse items as the lapidary and the guide to monastic sign language.[133]

It is beyond doubt that the prognostics gained in popularity with the renewed interest in the computus in the final decades of the tenth century and the first decades of the eleventh. This is evident from the concern with time reckoning during and after this period: the furtherance of computistical knowledge by Byrhtferth, Ælfric and Gerland, and the varying types of computi already in existence by that time.[134] An important impulse on a scientific level was the sojourn of Byrhtferth's teacher at Ramsey in 985-87, Abbo of Fleury, the leading figure in science and time reckoning, at the invitation of two of the driving forces behind the Reform, Dunstan, archbishop of Canterbury (959-88), and Oswald, bishop of Worcester (961-92) and archbishop of York (971-92), the latter himself trained in Fleury and one of the founders of Ramsey. An increased interest in the prognostics corresponding to that in the computus stands to reason in view of the incorporation of prognostics through associative attraction. Gneuss connected the prognostics with works pertaining to the Benedictine Reform outside the realm of the computus, which is unprecedented but which may indeed be the case.[135] Likewise,

---

[131] Gneuss (1997: 15).

[132] Clayton and Magennis (1994: 86). I owe this reference to Gneuss (1997: 15).

[133] Clayton and Magennis (1994: 86). Cf. Hollis (2001: 193).

[134] Cf. Stevens (1992: 137-41).

[135] A more detailed inspection of the links between eleventh-century prognostics and the Benedictine Reform can be found on pp. 88-92.

Clayton and Magennis noted that some texts in Tiberius A. iii, such as the Benedictine Rule, were staple fare in volumes produced during the Benedictine Reform; prognostics may belong in this category as well.

Titus D. xxvi, xxvii

The contents of Titus D. xxvi, xxvii are much more varied than is suggested by its cognomen, Ælfwine's *Prayerbook*. When Ælfwine was dean of New Minster, Winchester, he owned this volume, which was probably tailored to meet his needs. Although the manuscript now consists of two volumes, it was originally one: xxvii preceding xxvi. xxvii opens with a computus also containing prognostics, Ælfric's *De temporibus anni*, and the alphabet prognostic (folios 2-56), then turns into a prayerbook with miscellaneous notes, offices, devotions and prayers (folios 57-93). xxvi preserves the varied nature of the last part of xxvii, and consists of miscellaneous notes, devotions, prayers, a medicinal recipe, prognostics, a collectar, a litany and a charm.

In addition to the two main hands of the manuscript (i.e. xxvii and xxvi), nine other hands are attested.[136] The computistical part of Titus D. xxvii has already been introduced.[137] It contains a bloodletting lunary and calendar entries on the Egyptian Days and Dog Days (folios 2-8) in the first main hand, A, belonging to the scribe Ælfsige. A separate quire, folios 22-29, has four more Latin prognostics, with other texts intervening, in the other main hand, B. This quire starts with texts on the twenty-four Egyptian Days and the Dog Days, related to the two sets in Harley 3271.[138] The next prognostic is a year prognosis, followed (with other texts intervening) by a collective lunary different from those in Tiberius A. iii and Sloane 475. Finally, folios 55v-56v contain a guest text: the Old English alphabet prognostic written in hand C, which is not found elsewhere in Titus D. xxvi, xxvii. As Günzel deduced, the bifolium of folios 54-55 was added by hand A to enable him to complete Ælfric's *De temporibus anni*, followed by three short texts.[139] At a later date, hand C used the blank verso of folio 55 to write the alphabet prognostic, and it is he who introduced a singleton leaf, folio 56, to enable himself to complete the text. Hand D added two non-prognostic texts on folio 56v.

[136] Günzel (1993: 7).
[137] See pp. 29-35, 47.
[138] See pp. 38-39.
[139] Günzel (1993: 6).

Titus D. xxvi has a prognostic section on folios 3v-16r, all in the hand of scribe G. This scribe also contributed to Titus D. xxvi two encyclopedic notes immediately preceding the Latin prognostics. Seven scribes worked on xxvi, two of whom wrote the larger part of this volume.[140] Scribe G wrote all thirteen prognostics consecutively, on the first two quires (folios 2-17), but the prognostics do not open the first quire as they are preceded by the two short encyclopedic notes. Keynes pointed out that these two quires were inserted into the volume at a slightly later date to provide more writing space.[141] If this is the case, the prognostic section was added after the main part of the manuscript had been completed. Therefore, it is uncertain to what extent Ælfwine was able to influence the choice of texts in this part of the manuscript. As can be expected from a prognostic section, in contrast to prognostics in the computus, non-temporal prognostics are encountered. One is an encyclopedic note that makes mention of the colour of the moon as a predictive device, the other a dreambook. Dreambooks seem to be a standard ingredient of prognostic sections: Tiberius A. iii and Hatton 115 have dreambooks as well. Also present in this section are two fixed sequences of prognostics: first, the three Egyptian Days and three miraculous birthdays; second, a unit of four lunaries and a birth prognostic.[142] Two other noteworthy prognostics are a text on the twenty-four Egyptian Days uniquely attested in an Anglo-Saxon manuscript,[143] and a text on the Dog Days related to the one in Harley 3271, folios 123v-124r.

Titus D. xxvi, xxvii is a remarkable manuscript for several reasons. First, it contains the second-largest collection of Latin prognostics in any extant Anglo-Saxon manuscript. Second, Titus D. xxvi, xxvii is unique in that it has a prognostic section in addition to prognostics in the computus. Third, the manuscript preserves two texts not attested elsewhere: the alphabet prognostic and the prognostic by the colour of the moon. With the exception of the alphabet prognostic—a guest text—and possibly the collective lunary, the presence of (temporal) prognostics in xxvii can be explained by associative attraction triggered by the computistical

[140] There is an eighth hand, E, who wrote in the twelfth century, whereas the manuscript dates from the first half of the eleventh century (Günzel 1993: 6-7).

[141] Keynes (1996: 113).

[142] On these sequences, see pp. 60-62.

[143] This text does not list the dates in the formulaic manner customary for standalone Egyptian Days texts, but in calendric notation. I have not found this type in any other Anglo-Saxon manuscript, but there are continental analogues (see pp. 364-65).

texts.[144] The prognostic section in xxvi, on the other hand, may be the result of an interest in prognostic texts on the part of the scribe. Alternatively, Ælfwine may have requested their inclusion, if he actively participated in the production of Titus D. xxvi, xxvii, and if he had anything at all to do with the later insertion of the first two quires of xxvi. How could Ælfwine have accomplished this? For one thing, it has been argued repeatedly that Ælfwine partly wrote the manuscript, yet Günzel asserted that he is not to be identified as one of the main hands of the manuscript.[145] She dismissed the possibility that Ælfwine's is hand A, the scribe who wrote down his name as Ælsinus in a note in encoded writing on folio 13v of xxvii. This did not stop some scholars from speculating that hand B is Ælfwine's.[146] As it happens, speculation has not turned into fact, and there is no compelling reason to assign hand B to Ælfwine. There can be no doubt, however, that the manuscript was written for Ælfwine.[147] It is, therefore, conceivable that Ælfwine played a part in deciding on the type of texts to be included in xxvi and xxvii, but to what extent he selected the texts himself cannot be established. The fact that so many prognostics are included in Titus D. xxvi, xxvii would seem to indicate that he did not disapprove of the genre.

Sequences

Close observation of the manuscript evidence reveals certain fixed sequences of prognostics. These sequences form close-knit units: it is unusual to find other texts breaking them up. I have identified three such sequences of which the individual prognostics show strong thematic or structural coherence:[148]

[144] The presence of a collective lunary in xxvii is awkward (even though it is a temporal prognostic) because associative attraction usually pertains to short texts only.

[145] Günzel (1993: 3).

[146] Keynes (1996: 112-13). Pulsiano (1998a; 1998b: 99-103) remained skeptical, though he mentioned Ælfwine in connection with hand B.

[147] Günzel (1993: 2).

[148] In addition to the three sequences described here, there is one minor grouping the knowledge of which, like the β-sequence, did not travel widely. This grouping, an Old English dreambook and an agenda lunary, exists in two manuscripts: (1) Tiberius A. iii, fols 38r-40r (Christ Church, Canterbury), and (2) Hatton 115, fols 150v-53v (Christ Church, Canterbury?). I do not include this grouping with the main sequences because there is no structural or thematic connection whatsoever between the dreambook and the agenda lunary. Moreover, the dreambook-lunary sequence probably only

α a series of lunaries with a birth prognostic
β texts on the Egyptian Days and Dog Days
γ texts on the Egyptian Days and the miraculous birthdays

Sequence α consists of five texts in its most complete form: a bloodletting lunary (α1), a weekday birth prognostic (α2), birth, illness and dream lunaries (α3-5). The lunaries have a structural relationship, while the birth prognostic is thematically related to the birth lunary. These prognostics are all temporal and they depend upon lunar time.[149] There are seven representatives of the α-sequence in the corpus of Anglo-Saxon prognostics, two of which are complete:

(1) Titus D. xxvi, fols 6r-9v (α1-α5, in Latin)
(2) St. John's College 17, fol. 4r (α1-α5, in Latin)
(3) Lambeth Palace 427, fol. 3r (α1, α5, in Latin)
(4) Tiberius A. iii, fol. 65rv (α1-α4, in Latin)[150]
(5) CCCC 391, pp. 715-18, 720-21 (α2-α4, α5, in Old English)[151]
(6) Caligula A. xv, fols 131v-32r (α5, α3, in Old English)
(7) Hatton 115, fols 148r-49r (α5, α3, α2, in Old English)

The first five α-sequences adhere to the predominant order α1-α5, whereas the sequences in (6, 7) are not only incomplete, but they also lack this order. The scribe of (7) copied texts individually rather than wholesale, probably as they came to hand or caught his eye, which might explain why he did not write out whole sequences in the way that the scribes of (1-5) had done. Evidence of this scenario is presented by the incomplete state of α3 in (7),[152] a text which is followed immediately by a complete version of α2. The scribe of the α-sequence in (6) probably used an exemplar identical to very much like that of the Old English lunaries in the manuscript that hosts (4), i.e. Tiberius A. iii.

The α-sequence is attested in prognostic sections (1, 4, 5, 7) and in the computus (2, 3, 6). Incidentally, the existence of this sequence warrants

exists by virtue of the exemplar that the two manuscripts may have shared (the texts are very similar but neither can have been the exemplar of the other).

149 See pp. 30-31.

150 The illness lunary in Tiberius A. iii breaks off deliberately at the seventh day of the moon.

151 The α-sequence in CCCC 391 is interrupted by a γ-sequence which is placed between α4 and α5. The γ-sequence is directly followed by a Latin dream lunary in a, for Anglo-Saxon sources, unusual redaction (see p. 448).

152 The birth lunary in Hatton 115 breaks off deliberately at the fourteenth day of the moon.

the existence of bloodletting lunaries outside a computistical context, because such lunaries almost always precede the calendar or are found elsewhere in computistical sections.[153] Since the sequence came into being only towards the end of the Anglo-Saxon period in both the computus and prognostic sections,[154] it is unclear in which manuscript context the α-sequence may have originated. Nevertheless, since bloodletting lunaries appear out of place outside the computus in Anglo-Saxon manuscripts, and since the computus context antedates the development of prognostic sections, I assume that the computus is the place where the α-sequence evolved.[155]

The β-sequence is a unit of two, sometimes three, prognostics: a text on the twenty-four Egyptian Days (β1), one on the Dog Days (β2), and, optionally, one on the three Egyptian Days (β3). All three texts share a thematic feature in that they designate a number of days in the year on which it is dangerous to let blood or to take medicine. The first two genres are also the only ones found in a calendar context.[156] I have found three examples of the β-sequence:

(1) Harley 3271, fols 120v-21r (β1-β3, in Latin)
(2) Harley 3271, fol. 122rv (β1-β3, in Latin)
(3) Titus D. xxvii, fols 22r-23r (β1-β2, in Latin)

There are indications that β3 may not be an integral part of the sequence, as is shown by (1), where β1-2 are accidentally separated from β3 by a non-prognostic text,[157] and (3), which does not include the text on the three Egyptian Days at all. However, the exemplar of (1, 2) must have had the complete three-part β-sequence since β3 is present in both copies. No vernacular versions of the β-sequence have been identified. This sequence is attested in the computus (3) and in a prognostic section (1, 2).

Sequence γ is the most concise, with only two short prognostics: a text on the three Egyptian Days (γ1) and one on the three miraculous birthdays (γ2). The relationship between these texts is one of structure: both reveal three special days in the year. I have found five examples of the γ-sequence:

[153] See pp. 439-41.
[154] See pp. 77-92.
[155] The dichotomy of the two redactions of bloodletting lunaries in α-sequences might also suggest a parallel development (see pp. 439-41).
[156] See p. 26.
[157] See pp. 38-39.

(1) CCCC 422, p. 49 (γ1-γ2, in Latin)
(2) Titus D. xxvi, fols 3v-4v (γ1-γ2, in Latin)
(3) St. John's College 17, fol. 3va (γ1-γ2, in Latin)
(4) CCCC 391, p. 718 (γ2, γ1, in Old English)[158]
(5) Vitellius E. xviii, fol. 15r (γ2, γ1, in Old English)

The texts on the three Egyptian Days and the three miraculous birthdays must of necessity be complete to form a sequence at all, so there cannot be any fragmentary distributions. Remarkably, the sequence is reversed in Old English; I have not been able to discover the rationale behind this. As the prognostics in the γ-sequence are quite brief, the guest context in which they occur in (1) is not odd.[159] The γ-sequence is attested in the computus (3, 5) and in prognostic sections (2, 4).

The sequences described above testify to an attempt on the part of scribes or compilers to order prognostics thematically (α, β) or structurally (α, γ). The number of sequences by token—fifteen—, and the number of texts involved—forty-three out of a corpus of 174—, lead me to conclude that the effort of categorising prognostics played a considerable part in the later history and transmission of the Anglo-Saxon texts. If the period and place in which the sequences appeared are tabulated, the result is as follows:[160]

	first attested	place of origin
α	s. xi¹	Christ Church, Canterbury; Winchester; Worcester; *Ramsey
β	s. xi¹	New Minster, Winchester
γ	s. xi¹	Sherborne; New Minster, Winchester; Worcester; *Ramsey

table 3: sequence, date and origin

Aside from some variation in the place of origin of the sequences, both the earliest date and the overall origin strongly suggest that sequencing took place in the wake of the Benedictine Reform, a movement which proved pivotal in the spread of prognostic literature in Anglo-Saxon England. The growing interest in science and scholarship in this era provided a basis for a systematic approach to prognostics. The appearance of the α- and γ-sequences in manuscripts from all centres of the Reform would seem to indicate that the newfound knowledge was shared between the monasteries.[161]

158 This is the γ-sequence that interrupts the α-sequence of CCCC 391.
159 See p. 48.
160 On the designation '*Ramsey', see pp. 72-73.
161 I discuss the importance of the Reform movement more fully on pp. 88-92.

Conclusion

In this chapter I have analysed thirty-seven Anglo-Saxon manuscripts containing prognostics. The emphasis has been on Old English texts. In establishing the context in which prognostics are found, the Latin texts have been helpful. The fivefold contextual division outlined in this chapter proves satisfactory, since I have not yet encountered any English prognostic which defies classification in this structure.

My study of the manuscripts has brought to light a number of illuminating features of the transmission of Anglo-Saxon prognostics. First, prognostic material in calendars constitutes a considerable part of the entire prognostic corpus. Nevertheless, this prognostic material has remained virtually unstudied while it provides a wealth of information on the transmission of Egyptian Days and Dog Days. Second, there are several contexts in which one encounters prognostics, some of which create restrictions as to the type of prognostics they may contain. The most apparent limitation is that calendars can only incorporate prognostic material of genres in which a fixed date is assigned. The computus is less restrictive, though the process of associative attraction ensures that it draws in temporal prognostics only, notably texts on the Egyptian Days and Dog Days, and lunaries. The computus is the main source for Apuleian Spheres in English manuscripts. Non-temporal prognostics, such as dreambooks, are not found in this context. Third, in addition to restrictions on the type of prognostics included, the manuscript context determines to a certain extent the language in which prognostics are transmitted. Thus, prognostic material in calendars is almost exclusively in Latin. On one occasion only has a glossed entry for the Dog Days been recorded: in the calendar of CCCC 422. Computi contain Latin prognostics as well as Old English and glossed ones. The biggest share of the Old English prognostic corpus is encountered in prognostic sections. Fourth, medical manuscripts from Anglo-Saxon England would appear to differ from their continental counterparts: the number of prognostics found in English medical manuscripts is negligible compared to that in continental manuscripts. Apuleian Spheres, for instance, are frequently attested in continental medical volumes, but hardly ever so in English ones. The limited transmission of Anglo-Saxon medical manuscripts and their lack of prognostics has led to a situation in which the main sources for the prognostics are prognostic sections and computi. Continental medical manuscripts, on the other hand, are an important source of prognostics in their own right. Fifth, scribes who copied prognostics outside a computistical or medical context favoured separate sections for these texts. Whereas prognostics tend to be distributed almost randomly throughout the computus, these texts are gathered together in prognostic sections when outside of the computus, sometimes even in separate quires. The haphazard distribution of prognostics in computi and medical sections reflects the process of associative attraction rather than a genuine concern with the prognostics as a genre. On the other hand, the existence of prognostic sections in which large numbers of prognostics are collected and separated from the wider context reveal an attempt to gather and preserve the prognostics as a group. Finally, fixed sequences of prognostics would seem to indicate that the late Anglo-Saxon scribes were aware of structural and thematic correspondences between prognostic genres: they were able to recognise prognostics on the basis of their characteristics and group them together.

CHAPTER THREE

LANGUAGE, DATE AND PLACE OF ORIGIN OF ENGLISH MANUSCRIPTS CONTAINING PROGNOSTICS

The study of the language of the prognostics and the date and place of origin of the (parts of) manuscripts containing these texts is dependent upon a good understanding of the nature of the corpus of Anglo-Saxon prognostics. This inventory is anything but exhaustive for two reasons. First, manuscript survival is influenced by waves of material losses in the course of history, e.g. during the Viking raids and occupation, the Norman Conquest and the dissolution of the monasteries under Henry VIII.[1] These losses seem to have afflicted manuscript collections from specific foundations to a varying degree.[2] Second, the corpus of Old English and glossed prognostics is definitive, but the corpus of Latin prognostics in English manuscripts is larger than it is at present, as is evident from occasional new finds.[3] A discussion of the language, date and place of origin of the Anglo-Saxon prognostics must, therefore, allow for a certain margin of error. Yet although the inventory may be incomplete, the corpus as it stands leads to several new findings. First, the language in which prognostics are written is not haphazard but depends to a varying extent upon that of the immediate context. Second, the bulk of prognostics were copied in a few religious foundations only, notably those of Canterbury, Winchester and Worcester. Third, the period in which prognostics were disseminated is correlated to their context, e.g. prognostic material in calendars had enjoyed a long history by the time the first prognostic sections were being produced in the eleventh century.

The analysis presented in this chapter is dependent upon the exact size of the text corpus: thirty-seven (composite) manuscripts, segments and fragments, containing 174 prognostics in all. I refer the reader to appendix two for a brief survey of the pertinent data. In view of the limitations of a non-exhaustive text corpus, it is to be noted that all numbers in this chapter are soft, viz. they serve as indications rather than as definitive evidence.

[1] Gameson (1999: 14-19), Gneuss (1986: 645-48; 2001: 3).

[2] See Lapidge (2006: 31-126).

[3] See pp. 545-48.

Language

One of the recurring issues in the previous chapter has been the language in which prognostics were written. By language I do not mean dialect, but whether an English prognostic is in Latin, in Latin with Old English glosses, or in Old English. In this section I list and interpret the results of chapter two in terms of language. The quickest way to disclose the distribution of the languages in which the prognostics have been transmitted is to count the number of texts:

OE	L/OE	L	n
49	11	114	174

table 4: language

From the numbers in this table, it is evident that the majority of the prognostic texts are in Latin. The Old English and glossed prognostics constitute a closed corpus: it is highly unlikely that more of such texts will be discovered.[4] The contribution of Latin prognostics, however, may still grow. As the number of Latin texts increases, the proportion of Old English and glossed prognostics will diminish.

Since table 4 conveys no information other than the language distribution of the prognostics, it might prove more fruitful to differentiate according to the context as well. The lack of homogeneity frequently observed between the genres of individual texts in a manuscript makes it impossible for me to use the entire contents of these manuscripts as the basis for contextual research, as I illustrated in chapter two. So instead of employing the overall contents of a manuscript, in table 5 I make use of the direct context of the prognostics as elucidated in the fivefold division in chapter two, again using absolute numbers:

	calendar	computus	medicine	guest	prognostic section	n
OE	0	12	3	4	30	49
L/OE	1	3	0	0	7	11
L	36	39	8	5	26	114
n	37	54	11	9	63	174

table 5: language and context

[4] Ker (1957, 1976) and Healey and Venezky (1980) have exhaustively examined the corpus of Old English texts. Aside from manuscript fragments used as binding material for books, it is unlikely that many more Old English texts will come to light (but see Gretsch 2004). The chances of such fragments being prognostics are quite slim.

This table merits close inspection because it visualises a correlation between context and language. In order to structure my findings, I first analyse the various contexts in turn, after which I compare the various contexts and the influence the context exerted upon the choice of language for the prognostics.

Language and Context

There are no attestations of Old English prognostic material in calendars. This is not surprising since the calendar is in essence a Latinised context in which the vernacular, though not rare, is infrequent at least. An exception are the glossed Dog Day entries in the calendar of CCCC 422.[5] The calendar in question is preceded by a glossed bloodletting lunary, a prognostic genre of which I have found no other vernacular instances. The presence of relatively simple computistical material in Old English following the calendar gives the impression that the computus in which the calendar and the bloodletting lunary are embedded was intended to assist a student of time reckoning who was not yet fully at home in Latin computus texts.

Latin is also the predominant language of prognostics in the computus: thirty-nine texts are written in this language, against three glossed, and twelve Old English prognostics. There are five computi and calendars in which glossed and Old English prognostics are encountered.[6] The computi in these manuscripts have in common that they not only feature glossed and Old English prognostics, but that they have computistical texts in Latin and in Old English, as well as miscellaneous notes and charms in Old English. Henel compared the Old English computistical texts in four of the manuscripts above and Titus D. xxvii, and discovered that these texts are related to one another to a varying degree.[7] This knowledge coincides with the links I have found between some of the Old English prognostics in these manuscripts.[8] Computi which are written exclusively in Latin incorporate Latin prognostics only.[9] Titus D.

[5] The entries for the Egyptian Days also present in this calendar are not glossed.

[6] CCCC 422, Caligula A. xv + Egerton 3314, Vitellius C. viii, Vitellius E. xviii and Harley 3271.

[7] Henel (1934a: 40-70). Henel excluded Vitellius C. viii.

[8] See pp. 36-39.

[9] CTC O. 7. 41, Arundel 60, Tiberius C. i + Harley 3667, Tiberius C. vi, Vitellius A. xii, Lambeth Palace 427, Bodley 579 and St. John's College 17.

xxvii includes a number of computistical texts in Old English, but has prognostics in Latin only. These observations lead me to conclude that glossed and Old English prognostics are not unusual in computi, provided these sections contain computistical texts in the vernacular as well.

The medical context is one in which prognostics are not commonly found in Anglo-Saxon manuscripts.[10] Nevertheless, there are five medical sections and manuscripts containing prognostics. In these manuscripts, it is striking to see that the language of the prognostics agrees with that of the context. The absence of glossed prognostics in a medical context is explained by the absence of glossed medical sections.

The guest context is perhaps the most haphazard environment for prognostics, for there seems to be no contextual rationale underlying the choice of a prognostic as a guest text. Guest prognostics tend to follow the language of the context, but the alphabet prognostic in Titus D. xxvii is an exception to the rule.

Prognostic sections, finally, are contexts which contain the highest density of prognostics: all texts from prognostic sections (sixty-three) are found in five manuscripts in all, whereas fifteen manuscripts are needed for prognostics in the computus to number fifty-four. Moreover, prognostic sections are the main source of both Old English and glossed prognostics. It is also a context in which glossed and vernacular prognostics are attested more frequently than Latin ones.

The findings in this section show that the degree to which various languages are present can be differentiated according to the context in which the prognostic texts are encountered. Calendars are overwhelmingly Latinate, while prognostic sections tend to favour vernacular prognostics more than Latin ones. In between are the medical, guest and computistical contexts, which feature both Latin and Old English prognostics. In these contexts, the language of the prognostics often coincides with the language of the surrounding texts. In the next section I interpret these results to discover to what extent the language of the prognostics is determined by the language of the context, and whether it is possible to perceive differences in the treatment of the language of prognostics in the various contexts.

[10] See pp. 39-45.

Language Dependence

In the previous section I focussed on language and the individual contexts in which the prognostics are found. I now attempt to create some order on the basis of the results acquired. My main aim is to illustrate how the language of the context influences the language of the prognostics, which is what I understand by contextual language dependence. First, contextual language dependence is determined. Then this criterion will be used to interpret the frequency with which prognostics are attested in various contexts.

It has become apparent that the extent to which the language of the prognostics depends upon the language of the context may vary. In order to establish a weighted list of language dependence, it is important to discover the preferred language of the contexts themselves. All contexts for Anglo-Saxon prognostics can be in Latin, i.e. there are Latin calendars, computi, medical sections, texts surrounding guest material, and prognostic sections. In addition, some contexts can be in Old English, e.g. computi, medical and prognostic sections.

First, Latin is by far the language preferred in calendars. The absence of Old English prognostic material indicates strong language dependence, but a unique attestation of glossed prognostic material is observed. Second, Old English computistical texts are sometimes encountered, yet the number of computi in Latin is much more extensive. The attestation of a relatively large number of glossed and Old English texts always coincides with the presence of computistical texts in Old English, which points to strong language dependence. Third, prognostics in medical sections and manuscripts are without exception in the language of the context, so language dependence is very strong. This observation is confirmed by the absence of glossed prognostics in a medical context. Fourth, the language of guest material generally agrees with that of the immediate context, but the alphabet prognostic in Titus D. xxvii is an exception. Language dependence in a guest context is, therefore, on the same level as that of calendars. Fifth, prognostic sections tend to be either in Latin, in Old English, or glossed. There is virtually no mixing between prognostics of more than one language, a phenomenon which is frequently encountered also with other text genres, in homiletic collections, for instance. If texts in more than one language coexist in prognostic sections, they do not mingle. The first prognostic section in Tiberius A. iii, for instance, features a series of glossed prognostics followed by a series of Old English ones. Moreover, it seems that the language of the wider manuscript context is not important for the language of prognostic sections. Tiberius A. iii displays a sequence of glossed prognostics following the glossed *Regularis concordia*, yet the sequence of Latin prognostics in the second prognostic section is surrounded by texts which are glossed or written in Old English. The glossed prognostics in the first section are followed by vernacular prognostics. This would suggest that prognostic sections in themselves determine the language; the language does not depend upon the wider manuscript context. It is evident from the manuscripts that prognostic sections themselves set the standard for language. In Tiberius A. iii, the first section allows both glossed and Old English prognostics, but these are not mixed. The prognostic section in Hatton 115 contains Old English prognostics only, and was, in addition, conceived as a stand-alone booklet.[11] The latter also applies to the prognostic section in Titus D. xxvi, which is a separate unit inserted into the manuscript at a slightly later date.[12] The order of languages in prognostic sections suggests relatively strong internal language dependence.

The above considerations show that the language of the prognostics is dependent upon the language of the context. It proves hard to differentiate between the strength of language dependence in the five contexts, even if the number of exceptions is taken into account.[13] In all but the medical context, exceptions have been attested: (1) the glossed Dog Day entries in the calendar of CCCC 422; (2) the two glossed lunaries and the Apuleian Sphere in the computi of CCCC 422, Caligula A. xv + Egerton 3314 and Vitellius E. xviii, respectively; (3) the Old English alphabet prognostic as a guest text in a Latin environment in Titus D. xxvii; and finally, (4) the Latin lunary in the otherwise vernacular prognostic section of CCCC 391. Judging from the glossed prognostics in the computus, this context may select less strongly for language than the others do. The medical context has no exceptions for language preference, but as the number of Anglo-Saxon manuscripts incorporating prognostics is small anyway, this may not be significant. As it stands, the strength scale of contextual language dependence would be (from strong to less strong): (1) medical sections; (2) calendars, guest context and prognostic sections; (3) computi.

---

[11] See pp. 50-51.

[12] See pp. 57-59.

[13] Glossed prognostics are almost always exceptions as they occur mainly in contexts which are not glossed.

Place of Origin and Date

Two issues I have not yet addressed are the date and place of origin of the Anglo-Saxon manuscripts containing prognostics. Here, I am not concerned with the origins of the prognostic genres themselves.[14] My aim is to give an overview of the localities responsible for the dissemination of prognostics in Anglo-Saxon England and of the time when this took place. It will appear that there are only a few centres where the transmission of prognostics was undertaken on a significant scale. Moreover, the spread of prognostics throughout England can be pinpointed to certain limited periods, depending upon the context in which the texts are found. I use the data gathered in appendix one, at the same time cautioning the reader that the date and place of origin of the manuscripts, though based on manuscript catalogues, are not necessarily correct. More often than not, both date and place of origin have been, and still are, bones of contention; I have tried to weigh the pros and cons as well as I could. In contrast to the previous sections, where language was interpreted on the basis of individual prognostics, this section concerns itself with (parts of) manuscripts, and, therefore, deals with the number of manuscript sections containing prognostics, not the total number of prognostics contained in these sections.

Place of Origin

An inspection of the information available for the manuscripts containing prognostics elucidates that the question of origin cannot be answered without running into complications. The most salient problems are the undetermined place of origin of a number of manuscripts, notably that of medical ones; the place of origin of some manuscripts, which seems to waver between one place or another depending upon the scholar who determined it; the transfer of some manuscripts from their place of origin to another place where prognostics were added as guest texts, or where prognostic material was entered into the calendar.

[14] On the origins of the prognostic genres, see the introductions to the genres in the text edition.

An overview of the place of origin of Anglo-Saxon prognostics is given in table 6:[15]

Canterbury	Winchester	Worcester	*Ramsey	other	n
11	12	3	2	12	40

table 6: origin

Five preliminary remarks will clarify the contents of table 6. First, the data for this table pertain to the place in which prognostics were copied, which is not necessarily the place of origin of the entire manuscript. Second, the number of manuscripts listed in this table is forty, whereas the corpus comprises thirty-seven manuscripts. If a manuscript already contained prognostics and was then transferred to another place where more prognostics were added to the manuscript, I have counted the places of origin of both the manuscript and the later additions.[16] Manuscripts in which prognostics were added at a later date but which already featured prognostics have not been counted more than once if the manuscript remained in the foundation where it was originally written. The alphabet prognostic in Titus D. xxvii, for instance, was added at a later date in New Minster, Winchester, which is also the place the manuscript originated in. Third, I have noted those places individually from which two or more manuscripts containing prognostics have been attested. Fourth, the heading '*Ramsey' comprises two computi: Tiberius C. i + Harley 3667, and St. John's College 17. The first was copied in Peterborough, the second in Thorney. The reason why I have classed these manuscripts under '*Ramsey' is that parts of them can be traced to Byrhtferth's computus. In this case, I have favoured the origin of the exemplar rather than that of the manuscripts.[17] Nevertheless, one should be aware that grouping these manuscripts together in view of their relatedness is a matter of convenience rather than a confirmation of the prog-

[15] For comparison, see the following table, derived from Ker's findings (1957: lix-lx):

Canterbury	Winchester	Worcester	*Ramsey	other	n
17	16	19	5	55	112

These are the manuscripts containing Old English only!

[16] This pertains to CCCC 422 and CTC R. 15. 32. Digby 63, from Francia, is not taken into account, because although the Egyptian Days in the calendar were copied in Northumbria, the first set of prognostics was produced on the continent.

[17] This is done because some of the prognostics are so closely related that they must have been copied from a common exemplar. There are no other manuscripts containing prognostics for which this can be established so definitively.

nostics in these volumes having originally belonged to Byrhtferth's computus.[18] It is to be observed that the medical sections of St. John's College 17 (fols 1-2, 175-77) are definitely not considered to be part of Byrhtferth's original autograph, which is why these have been entered under 'other'.[19] Fifth, manuscripts from foundations appearing only once or of unknown origin have been categorised under the heading 'other'.[20] The place of origin of some manuscripts has not yet been established beyond doubt, but these are nevertheless listed under the most likely place of origin.[21]

Table 6 elucidates that twenty-eight manuscripts with prognostics hail from four places only whereas manuscript production took place throughout England:[22] Canterbury, Winchester, Worcester and *Ramsey. Of these, the first three produced twenty-six manuscripts containing prognostics. These places were the centres important in initiating the Benedictine Reform and responsible for the production of many manuscripts of a didactic, sentential or homiletic nature. The fact that twenty-six manuscripts containing prognostics originated in these places would seem to corroborate the idea that the Reform movement was instrumental in disseminating prognostics.[23] Of the Winchester foundations, New Minster was responsible for most of the prognostics; of the Canterbury foundations, Christ Church. The latter foundation, especially, was "an important source of supply of exemplars",[24] also of prognostics, Tiberius A. iii being a case in point. Worcester is mentioned separately even though only three manuscripts containing prognostics are of Worcester origin. The reason for this is that Worcester is not only responsible for the largest prognostic section in Old English, in CCCC 391, but also for

[18] Some texts, including a number of prognostics, in these manuscripts may not have been part of Byrhtferth's computus at all (see also p. 85).

[19] See p. 44.

[20] Of unknown origin are the medical manuscripts Harley 585, Harley 6258B and Sloane 475. Manuscripts from foundations appearing once in the prognostic corpus are CCCC 422 (prognostic material in the calendar is from Sherborne), CTC O. 7. 41 (Colchester), Vitellius A. xii (Salisbury), Harley 863 (Exeter), Digby 63 (Northumbria), Douce 296 (Crowland).

[21] I.e. Vespasian D. xiv (Christ Church, Canterbury? (or Rochester?)), Vitellius A. xviii (Wells?), Vitellius C. viii (Winchester?), Harley 3271 (New Minster, Winchester?), Lambeth Palace 427 (Winchester?), Hatton 115 (Christ Church, Canterbury?), Salisbury 150 (Shaftesbury?).

[22] See Ker (1957: xliii-lx).

[23] See pp. 88-92.

[24] Gameson (1999: 17).

the preservation of a prognostic section in Old English, i.e. booklet 5 of Hatton 115 (from Christ Church, Canterbury?). As I have shown in table 5, prognostic sections are the most important source of Old English prognostics, and we partly owe their survival to the efforts of the Worcester community in copying and preserving these sections.

If we look at the places where prognostics were copied, the context of the prognostics plays a role as well, as the case of Worcester has shown. The results of cross referencing origin with context are given here:

	calendar	computus	medicine	guest	prognostic section	n
Canterbury	8	2	0	1	3	14
Winchester	6	9	1	4	2	22
Worcester	2	0	0	0	1	3
*Ramsey	1	2	0	0	0	3
other	8	2	4	1	0	15
n	25	15	5	6	6	57

table 7: origin and context

In table 7, each instance of a context is counted separately. Some manuscripts contain more than one context. St. John's College 17, for instance, features prognostics in the medical section, the computus and the calendar. Tiberius C. i + Harley 3667, on the other hand, features prognostics in the computus only. These manuscripts account for the three examples of *Ramsey origin.[25]

The inclusion of prognostic material in calendars seems to have been popular mainly in Canterbury and Winchester. This practice may have to do with the fact that these are centres from which many computi have survived. The other calendars with prognostic material come from many different places. The combined group of calendars and computi points out that Canterbury, Winchester and *Ramsey were most beneficial for the propagation of prognostics in these contexts. Again, this may be indicative of the influence of the Benedictine Reform on the dissemination of computus material (and indirectly, prognostics). The exact origin of medical manuscripts and sections is hard to pinpoint. Of two manuscripts only, Royal 12. D. xvii and St. John's College 17, the place of origin has been established: Old Minster, Winchester, and Thorney Abbey, respectively. Three other manuscripts, Harley 585, Harley 6258B and Sloane 475 are of undetermined origin; the content

[25] Please note that the medical section of St. John's College 17 is not relegated to *Ramsey for reasons noted above.

of a medical manuscript does not offer many clues about the place of origin, in contrast to, for instance, computi and calendars. Prognostics as guest material seem to have been more in demand in Winchester than anywhere else in England. The importance of prognostic sections for the preservation of Old English prognostics cannot be denied. The sections preserved in Worcester have already been discussed. One of these, booklet 5 of Hatton 115, probably is from Christ Church, Canterbury. The same foundation was responsible for two other prognostic sections, both in Tiberius A. iii. What makes these sections interesting is that they contain Latin, glossed and Old English prognostics. The glossed prognostics are not found elsewhere in a prognostic section, and the Old English prognostics contain several uniquely attested texts. New Minster, Winchester, is home to one, possibly two, prognostic sections, in Titus D. xxvi and in Harley 3271.

That some foundations may have propagated vernacular prognostics more than others can be viewed from table 8:

	OE	L/OE	L	n
Canterbury	27	8	22	57
Winchester	9	3	45	57
Worcester	11	0	4	15
*Ramsey	0	0	20	20
other	2	0	23	25
n	49	11	114	174

table 8: origin and language

It is immediately visible that prognostics in Latin have been copied in all centres. Canterbury, Winchester and *Ramsey were earlier shown to be major sources for the transmission of prognostics. Worcester, too, was of importance in this respect. From table 8 it can be observed that these four places can be differentiated according to their treatment of the prognostics. *Ramsey focussed on Latin prognostics only, whereas Old English prognostics were mainly copied in Canterbury, Winchester and Worcester. Glossed prognostics are found solely in Canterbury and Winchester manuscripts. Canterbury and Worcester are the only places where vernacular prognostics constitute the majority of prognostics produced there. The Old English texts from Worcester have all been found in the prognostic section of one manuscript: CCCC 391. The Old English prognostics from Canterbury are also encountered in prognostic sections, in Tiberius A. iii and possibly booklet 5 of Hatton 115. In contrast to those from Worcester, Old English prognostics from Canterbury are contained in the computus as well, in Caligula A. xv + Egerton 3314. The glossed prognostics from Canterbury are likewise incorporated in prognostic sections (Tiberius A. iii) and in the computus (Caligula A. xv + Egerton 3314). Winchester computi, such as CCCC 422, Vitellius C. viii and Vitellius E. xviii also feature glossed and Old English prognostics, but prognostic sections from this location contain Latin prognostics exclusively.

The question is how it is possible for four places which have been responsible for most of the prognostic corpus to have acted so differently when it comes to the language of the prognostics. Prognostics were first brought into England in Latin, which remained the basic language for prognostics in Anglo-Saxon times. Vernacularisation never entirely replaced the Latin prognostic corpus, but table 8 illustrates that many prognostics were translated into the vernacular in Canterbury and Worcester, and, to a lesser extent, in Winchester. If the four places under discussion are graded according to the number of glossed and Old English prognostics, *Ramsey ranks lowest, followed by Winchester, Worcester and Canterbury.

In the case of Worcester, the Old English prognostics are contained in CCCC 391, of which it is sometimes said that it may have fulfilled a pastoral function in the hands of Wulfstan II.[26] This would explain why the prognostics are in Old English, i.e. they may have been intended for a lay audience which had little or no command of Latin. I do not deem this hypothesis likely, however, because prognostics were probably not used in a pastoral capacity at all.[27] Rather, vernacularisation was in vogue in the eleventh century, especially in the centres of the Reform movement.[28] Christ Church was responsible for all glossed and Old English prognostics from Canterbury, both those in prognostic sections and in computi. Prognostic sections, such as the ones in Tiberius A. iii from Canterbury, reflect a desire to gather a group of prognostics together, and may merely indicate that prognostics, whether glossed, in Old English or in Latin, were considered worthwhile to collect. The prognostic booklet 5 of Hatton 115 probably also originated in Christ Church, and was transferred to Worcester, thus lending support to the conclusion that in these two places especially, there was considerable interest in prognos-

[26] See pp. 51-53.
[27] See pp. 130-37.
[28] See pp. 88-92.

tics in the vernacular. Glossed and Old English prognostics in the computus are always accompanied by computistical texts in Old English. Therefore, such computi may have been intended for a monastic audience which was not yet skilled enough to fully grasp the complicated nature of time reckoning when presented in Latin. This applies to computi from Canterbury, but also to those from Winchester. The prospective audience for the prognostics, then, may have differed from place to place.

In this section I have concentrated on the place of origin of the manuscripts containing prognostics. While for some manuscripts the place of origin cannot be established beyond doubt, the results are, nevertheless, unambiguous. The large number of prognostics produced in Canterbury, Winchester and Worcester is significant in view of the role these places played in the Benedictine Reform. Manuscripts containing prognostics in computi and/or calendars from these religious establishments would seem to confirm this notion. Canterbury, Winchester and Worcester have been identified as the main places of origin for the glossed and Old English prognostics, and together with *Ramsey, for a large number of prognostics in Latin. Furthermore, Worcester played an important role in preserving prognostic sections in Old English, and Canterbury and Winchester did the same for glossed and Old English prognostics in prognostic sections and computi.

Date

Like the place of origin, the date attributed to a manuscript tends to differ from one scholar to the next. By using the latest manuscript catalogues available, those of Gameson and Gneuss,[29] I hope to be able to give a reasonably reliable insight into the production of prognostics throughout the Anglo-Saxon period and up to the twelfth century.[30]

From Ker's *Catalogue of Manuscripts Containing Anglo-Saxon*, it emerges that most Anglo-Saxon manuscripts that survive were produced in the eleventh century.[31] The transmission of prognostics would seem to mir-

[29] Gameson (1999), Gneuss (2001).

[30] Please note that I have not investigated the twelfth-century manuscripts exhaustively since the focus is on the Anglo-Saxon period (see p. 4).

[31] Ker (1957: xv-xix). I realise that Ker lists manuscripts containing Old English only.

ror this. In table 9, I list the date of the (portions of) manuscripts containing prognostics:[32]

ix	x	xi	xii	n
1	4	27	12	44

table 9: date

Two remarks will clarify the contents of this table. First, as in table 6, the total number of entries is higher than the total number of manuscripts because later additions, such as guest texts and the addition of prognostic material to the calendar, have been taken into account. CTC R. 15. 32, for instance, contains a calendar from 1035-36 with Dog Days, to which Egyptian Days have been added in s. xi^{ex}. Guest texts added around the time of composition of the manuscript—e.g. in Titus D. xxvii and Harley 3271—have also been counted separately. Second, texts written around the turn of a century have been entered for the later date. The calendar in Add. 37517, for example, has been dated to s. x/xi, in which case I have assigned it to the eleventh century.

Table 9 shows that prognostics were copied significantly more frequently in the eleventh century than in the centuries preceding.[33] Moreover, the decrease in transmission from the eleventh century to the twelfth is not as marked as the increase from the tenth to the eleventh (particularly when it is kept in mind that the manuscript evidence from the twelfth century is by no means exhausted[34]). Reasons for this are the expansion of manuscript collections in post-Conquest libraries soon after the Conquest,[35] a continued, though lessened, interest in prognostics in Latin, and the continued copying of prognostics in the vernacular in twelfth-century England.

In table 10, I differentiate the date according to context:

[32] For comparison, see the following table, derived from Ker's findings (1957: xv-xix):

viii	ix	x	xi	xii	n
1	5	23	133	25	189

This pertains to manuscripts containing Old English only.

[33] This corresponds to a significant increase in manuscript production in the eleventh century (see table in note preceding).

[34] Latin prognostics were more frequently copied in the twelfth century than is apparent from the prognostic corpus, e.g. in CPC 103, Egerton 821, Sloane 2839, Ludwig XII. 5 (see pp. 545-48). A large number of manuscripts from the twelfth century and after preserve calendars with prognostic material (see Wormald 1939-46).

[35] Gameson (1999: 5-20).

	calendar	computus	medicine	guest	prognostic section	n
ix	1	0	0	0	0	1
x	2	1	1	1	0	5
xi	17	10	2	2	5	36
xii	5	4	2	3	1	15
n	25	15	5	6	6	57

table 10: date and context

The total number of entries in this table is fifty-seven. As with table 7, this number is considerably higher than the total number of manuscripts because each context has been counted separately, as has the addition of guest texts or of prognostic material to the calendar. Thus, the calendar of CTC R. 15. 32 contains Dog Days original to the calendar of 1035-36, and Egyptian Days added by s. xi^{ex}.

It would appear that Anglo-Saxon prognostics got off to a late start compared to their continental counterparts. In the catalogues of medieval medical manuscripts by Beccaria and Wickersheimer, several instances can be found of continental stand-alone prognostics from the ninth century.[36] The sole Anglo-Saxon prognostic from the ninth century, however, was entered into the calendar of Digby 63 and does not constitute a stand-alone text. The number of manuscripts from ninth-century Anglo-Saxon England is small compared to those that have survived from the eleventh century, but whether this satisfactorily explains the extremely low rate of attestation of early prognostics is debatable. A more compelling reason might be that prognostics were not yet so well-known in Anglo-Saxon England in this period, simply because they were not yet imported frequently from the continent. The tenth century shows that prognostics were better known than in the ninth century, because a guest prognostic had been added to Royal 2. B. v by the end of the tenth century. The use of guest prognostics is a sure sign that there must have been sufficient prognostics around for one of them to be noticed and copied into another manuscript. Also from this century is the first Old English prognostic, embedded in a medical tract in Royal 12. D. xvii. Two calendars and one computus from the tenth century incorporate prognostics as well.

Ninth- and tenth-century prognostics are attested in limited contexts. Prognostic material in the form of Egyptian Day entries is first found in

[36] Beccaria (1956), Wickersheimer (1966).

the Roman calendar *Fasti Philocaliani*, dated to AD 354.[37] Since that time, calendars have featured entries on Egyptian Days and usually also on Dog Days.[38] That some of the earliest examples of Anglo-Saxon prognostics are found in calendars is not wholly unexpected in this light. The other context which ensures good transmission is the medical section. Prognostics are not often found in Anglo-Saxon medical manuscripts, but the one tenth-century example, in Royal 12. D. xvii, is embedded in a larger tract on bloodletting. Indeed, when we consider prognostics in English redactions in a medical context,[39] we see that out of five such texts, four are accommodated in tracts on bloodletting or on the humours. It stands to reason that the transmission of early Anglo-Saxon prognostics depended heavily on the context. The calendar and the context of a larger medical tract in which a prognostic is embedded, therefore, increased the chances of transmission for some of the earliest Anglo-Saxon prognostics.

The eleventh century witnessed a dramatic increase not only in manuscript production, but also in the dissemination of prognostics.[40] The computus and calendar, especially, abound with prognostics. This ties in with the growing interest in computi in the late tenth and early eleventh centuries and the accretion of non-computistical time-related material in the computus.[41] In the eleventh century prognostic sections were compiled for the first time. If such sections do indeed reflect an attempt at making a systematic collection of prognostics, these texts must have been available in sufficient numbers to make collecting them worthwhile. It should be noted that prognostic sections are almost exclusively an eleventh-century affair. In the middle of the twelfth century one more prognostic section was produced, in Old English.

The twelfth century saw a decline in prognostics in the calendar and computus, and a slight increase in guest prognostics. Furthermore, prognostic sections seem to have become extinct by the end of the twelfth century, after having experienced their prime in the eleventh century. Since I have refrained from investigating twelfth-century manuscripts systematically, the moderate yield for that century may not be indicative of a decline in interest in the prognostics.

[37] See pp. 330-35, 347-69.

[38] See pp. 26-29.

[39] I here exclude Sloane 475, fols 125-231, as the prognostics are atypical for the Anglo-Saxon medical context.

[40] See table 11 and below.

[41] See pp. 29-39.

Table 11 sheds light on the link between date and language:

	OE	L/OE	L	n
ix	0	0	1	1
x	1	0	5	6
xi	36	11	75	122
xii	12	0	33	45
n	49	11	114	174

table 11: date and language

As this table illustrates, the earliest surviving Anglo-Saxon prognostics (from the ninth and tenth centuries) are mostly in Latin, the only exception being the Old English medical tract with Dog Days in Royal 12. D. xvii, as remarked upon above. Except for this medical text and the guest prognostic in Royal 2. B. v, the other prognostics are encountered in calendars and a computus. Both the calendar and the pre-eleventh-century computi are Latinate contexts, so it is not surprising to find that early Anglo-Saxon prognostics are in Latin.

A sharp increase in the production of prognostics in Latin and Old English in the eleventh century is followed by a less pronounced decline in the twelfth. At least 122 prognostics date from the eleventh century, and at first sight it would seem that these came out of the blue in view of the mere six prognostics from the century preceding. Moreover, the tenth-century texts represent just a few of the prognostic genres known in Anglo-Saxon England, whereas the eleventh-century texts comprise the majority of prognostic genres and redactions. Since not one prognostic genre originated with the Anglo-Saxons (the prognostics are essentially Latin and Greek in origin), it is not the case that the Anglo-Saxon scribes of the eleventh century invented a wealth of prognostic genres. The popularity of prognostics in this era requires an explanation, therefore.

First, an influx of texts from the continent must have taken place because many prognostic genres, hitherto unknown to Anglo-Saxon scribes, are first attested in the eleventh century and quickly naturalised. Some prognostics occur in redactions unfamiliar to ones later known in Anglo-Saxon England, which strengthens the notion that they were imported from the continent, as illustrated by those found in Sloane 475.[42] Strong links existed between continental and English foundations in the

[42] See pp. 42-43. Ninth-century examples are the two stand-alone prognostics in Digby 63. This Frankish manuscript was transferred to and expanded in England.

second half of the tenth century,[43] which resulted in the importation of several continental manuscripts, some of which undoubtedly contained prognostics.[44]

Second, the computus, which harboured a growing corpus of prognostics, flourished in the eleventh century and was responsible for a wider dissemination of prognostics than before. This is clearly visible if we compare the contents of tenth-century computi to those of the next century. The prime example of a tenth-century computus is in Bodley 579. This computus contains Dog Day entries in the calendar, and two stand-alone prognostics. Caligula A. xv + Egerton 3314, from the eleventh century, on the other hand, features no less than twelve prognostics in the computus. This would seem to indicate that the accretive process was operating at full strength in the eleventh century.[45]

Third, in the eleventh century, prognostics were collected in separate prognostic sections for the first time. These collections varied from eight texts in Harley 3271, to twenty-two texts in the two prognostic sections of Tiberius A. iii. Even though there are only five prognostic sections from the eleventh century, these account for fifty-five individual texts, which is nearly half the total number of prognostics from the eleventh century.

Fourth, there is a possibility that a certain number of earlier exemplars may not have survived. The Anglo-Saxon prognostics were copied and translated from exemplars, and for some eleventh-century texts there are clear indications of their having been copied from lost exemplars. Evidence of copies from lost exemplars is manifold and visible in, among others, the Old English gloss of the dreambook in Tiberius A. iii, the prognostics in CCCC 391, and the β-sequence in Harley 3271.[46] I do not know whether these prognostics were copied from tenth- or eleventh-century exemplars, but a number of eleventh-century prognostics may indeed be copies of earlier texts.

[43] Baker and Lapidge (1995: xix-xxii), McGowan (2001a: 39-42).

[44] For instance, Wickersheimer (1966: 13-14 [II], 50 [XXXIII], 140-42 [XCII]) listed a number of Fleury manuscripts containing prognostics.

[45] See pp. 29-39.

[46] In the dreambook, some glosses do not correspond with the Latin. In addition, there are several 'wyn'/'p' mistakes. The prognostics in CCCC 391 show spacing between the syllables of words to such an extent that the final syllable of one word and the first syllable of the next sometimes seem to form a word. This practice would suggest dictation. The repeated β-sequence (see pp. 38-39, 61) in Harley 3271, finally, indicates that an exemplar was used since the second sequence cannot have been copied from the first. The same exemplar was probably used for the texts in Titus D. xxvii.

In the eleventh century, prognostics were glossed and translated into Old English on a large scale. Glossed prognostics, in particular, are only attested for this century. Glossed and Old English prognostics were made possible through the vernacularisation of computi in the eleventh century, which accounts for sixteen prognostics. Twenty-nine prognostics, either glossed or in the vernacular, are found in prognostic sections. One more Old English text occurs in Titus D. xxvii, which is the first guest prognostic in the vernacular. Harley 585, finally, contains the sole Old English prognostic from the eleventh century in a medical context. This century witnessed a rise in the popularity of prognostics, irrespective of language. Moreover, prognostics developed from a Latinate genre in the ninth and tenth centuries, to a Latinate and vernacularised genre in the eleventh century. The fact that computi came to be written partly in Old English in the eleventh century facilitated the transition from Latin to Old English prognostics. The emergence of prognostic sections, finally, guaranteed the large-scale production of prognostics in Latin, Old English, and with glosses. I have not found any significant differences between pre- and early post-Conquest manuscripts and their treatment of the language in which the prognostics were written.

Twelfth-century prognostics are fewer in number than eleventh-century ones, but this decline is not as pronounced as is the increase from the tenth to the eleventh century. One would have expected the twelfth-century prognostic corpus to be even more extensive than that of the eleventh century, because manuscripts from the first half of the twelfth century are more than twice as numerous as post-Conquest eleventh-century manuscripts.[47] Gameson has noted considerable growth in English libraries at the end of the eleventh century, owing to both import and production of manuscripts.[48] If the number of prognostics more than halved in the twelfth century and the production of manuscripts more than doubled compared to the later eleventh century, this disparity cannot be ascribed to accidental influences such as manuscripts losses.[49] Instead, there must have been a change in policy, such as extensive copying projects which took up so much time and effort that relatively less important genres such as prognostics did not receive the attention they held in the eleventh century.

[47] Gameson (1999: 5).

[48] Gameson (1999: 5-10, 14-19).

[49] Please note that a full investigation of twelfth-century English manuscripts may change the picture somewhat.

Gameson studied the frequency with which texts were copied in the period *c.* 1066-1130, and concluded that, in decreasing order of importance, English foundations focussed on: (1) patristic writings; (2) post-patristic theology; (3) biblical and (para-)liturgical books; (4) history; (5) hagiography; (6) texts in Old English; and (7) Latin classics.[50] Works outside these categories were produced in significantly smaller numbers, and comprise "Latin Christian poetry, grammatical and pedagogical works, medical texts, computistical treatises, decretals, and Rules".[51] The only contexts fit for prognostics in this group of writings are marginalised. Compared to eleventh-century scribes, those of the late eleventh and early twelfth centuries seem to have turned their focus elsewhere, and to have worked in a more programmatic manner. As a consequence, attention to the prognostics, a genre not covered by any of the major categories, flagged noticeably.

The first thing to be noticed is a lack of glossed prognostics from the twelfth century. Of the twelve prognostics in Old English, nine derive from the single prognostic section in booklet 5 of Hatton 115, a section which probably relied on an eleventh-century exemplar also used for Tiberius A. iii since some prognostics exist in closely related fashion in both volumes. The remaining texts in Old English are a prognostic component in a treatise on the humours and the Dog Days in the medical manuscript Harley 6258B, and two guest prognostics from Vespasian D. xiv. The medical context continued to exist in the twelfth century, though this context was never a popular vehicle for prognostics in Anglo-Saxon England.[52] Again, the late dates of Harley 6258B (s. xii$^{4/4}$) and Vespasian D. xiv (s. xii$^{2/4}$) may seem remarkable because both manuscripts contain texts in Old English. However, Elaine Treharne has convincingly argued a case for the continued dissemination of the Old English literary tradition well into the twelfth century.[53] In view of this verna-

[50] Gameson (1999: 20-27).

[51] Gameson (1999: 27).

[52] See pp. 44-45.

[53] Treharne (1998, 2001, 2003), Swan and Treharne (2000), particularly Treharne (2000) and Irvine (2000). Treharne and Swan (2000: 1-2) listed the following English writings attested in twelfth-century manuscripts: "the majority of texts are homiletic and hagiographical pieces written by Ælfric and anonymous authors. There are also two copies of the Gospels, a copy of the *Rule of St. Benedict*, Laws, apothegms and dialogue literature, prognostications, translations from Alfred's 'most necessary' books, and Psalters". It is striking that twelfth-century manuscripts containing prognostics are usually discussed in some detail, though without any noteworthy study of the prognostics contained in these volumes (an exception is Treharne 1998: 237-39).

cular tradition, therefore, it need not come as a surprise that Old English prognostics have benefited as well, albeit on a smaller scale than in the eleventh century.

There are three twelfth-century guest prognostics in Latin: two in CCCC 422 and one in Tiberius C. vi. Immediately following the prognostic in the latter manuscript is another guest prognostic in Anglo-Norman, probably the first of its kind in England. The majority of the Latin prognostics from the twelfth century, though, is found in calendars and computi. Two of these computi, Tiberius C. i + Harley 3667 and St. John's College 17, are assumed to be copies of Byrhtferth's computistical notebook, which he used in developing his computus and which he was working on between 988-96.[54] Before concluding that the prognostics in the computistical manuscripts mentioned above should, therefore, be placed in the late tenth century, it is to be noted that only three of the prognostics in St. John's College 17 (two of which also appear in Tiberius C. i + Harley 3667), formed part of Byrhtferth's computus with some certainty, to wit the entries on the Egyptian Days in the calendar, and two Apuleian Spheres.[55] The other prognostics in the manuscripts may not have formed part of Byrhtferth's computus, and may even date to a later period. The Latin text on the twelve Egyptian Days, in Tiberius C. i and St. John's College 17, for instance, is not attested in pre-twelfth-century English manuscripts. Moreover, there are several Old English representatives of the texts on the three and twenty-four Egyptian Days, but not one for the twelve Egyptian Days. If Byrhtferth had included a text on the twelve Egyptian Days, it would probably have made its way into eleventh-century manuscripts. This also applies to the Latin *Sortes Sanctorum* in St. John's College 17, of which no pre-twelfth-century copies have been attested either in Latin or in Old English. Between them, Tiberius C. i + Harley 3667 and the computus of St. John's College 17 harbour twenty prognostics in Latin. The remaining Latin prognostics are in a medical section, computi and calendars.

One final matter that requires study is the connection between date and place of origin, displayed in table 12:

[54] Baker and Lapidge (1995: xxvi).
[55] Baker and Lapidge (1995: xxv, 373-427).

	Canterbury	Winchester	Worcester	*Ramsey	other	n
ix	0	0	0	0	1	1
x	3	2	0	0	1	6
xi	42	52	15	0	13	122
xii	12	3	0	20	10	45
n	57	57	15	20	25	174

table 12: date and origin

The earliest Anglo-Saxon prognostic is a series of entries on the twenty-four Egyptian Days in the calendar of Digby 63. The opening quires of this manuscript were brought to England in the ninth century, and the scribe continued to work on the book in England. Thus, folio 36rv contains prognostics which were copied on the continent, while the calendar on folios 40-45 was compiled in England. Six prognostics from the tenth century are attested, five of which originated in Canterbury and Winchester. These were thus important places with regard to the early prognostics from Anglo-Saxon England.

Twenty-three prognostics dating from the eleventh and twelfth centuries derive from a number of places which are not major centres for the dissemination of prognostics. Prognostics from places here unspecified often concern entries in the calendar on the Egyptian Days or Dog Days. In addition, a number of prognostics in medical sections cannot be assigned a place of origin, which applies to those in Harley 585, Harley 6258B and Sloane 475. Canterbury, Winchester, Worcester and *Ramsey produced the majority of the eleventh- and twelfth-century prognostics: 144 texts in all. I have already analysed the texts from *Ramsey, so I shall not discuss these here.

Of the Canterbury prognostics, only five seem to have been copied at St. Augustine's, and these are all entries in the calendar on the Egyptian Days or Dog Days, in CTC R. 15. 32, CUL Kk. 5. 32 and Add. 37517. Gameson remarked that St. Augustine's is characterised by "a fairly barren stretch in the couple of generations before the Conquest", followed by "leisurely growth" and imports after the Conquest and in the twelfth century.[56] This certainly applies to the prognostics from this Canterbury foundation. The overwhelming majority of prognostics from Canterbury, however, hail from Christ Church.[57] This foundation had an

[56] Gameson (1999: 15).

[57] On the manuscripts owned by St. Augustine's and Christ Church, Canterbury, see James (1903: xix-lxxxvii).

extensive library which sustained heavy losses in the fire of 1067.[58] Nevertheless, twenty-five prognostics originated in Christ Church and antedate 1067. That this number is so high is mainly owing to the two prognostic sections in Tiberius A. iii, which contain twenty-two prognostics in all. The other three texts are in calendars. After the fire and the arrival of Lanfranc, archbishop of Canterbury (*c.* 1070-89), manuscript production increased and remained steady until well into the twelfth century.[59] Prognostics from Christ Church in this period, however, are not so numerous, amounting to twenty-four texts attested in calendars, computi, prognostic sections, and as guest texts. Caligula A. xv + Egerton 3314 and possibly booklet 5 of Hatton 115 deserve mention as major contributors of prognostics from post-Conquest Christ Church. This Canterbury foundation remained an important centre for the production of vernacular texts well into the twelfth century.[60]

Of the Winchester prognostics from the eleventh and twelfth centuries two derive from Old Minster, forty-nine from New Minster, and one from St. Mary's. A further three prognostics in computi from Winchester have not been assigned to a specific foundation. It is remarkable that so many prognostics have survived because Gameson speaks of "a comparative dearth of extant manuscripts" from Winchester in this period.[61] Prognostics are found in calendars and as guest texts. Additionally, computi and prognostic sections from Old and New Minster contribute many prognostics, indicating that such contexts received considerable attention in these foundations, see for instance Titus D. xxvi, xxvii, Vitellius E. xviii and possibly Harley 3271.

Eleventh-century prognostics from Worcester are concentrated in the prognostic section of CCCC 391; Dog Day and Egyptian Day entries in the calendars of CCCC 9 and Hatton 113 complete the picture. The eleven prognostics in Old English and the one in Latin in CCCC 391 are remarkable, because Worcester had no history of prognostics prior to these. This prognostic section appears out of the blue, whereas the prognostic genre was well-established in Canterbury and Winchester before these places started to produce prognostic sections and prognostics in the vernacular. As Gameson pointed out, Christ

[58] Gameson (1999: 16).
[59] *Ibid.*
[60] Treharne (2000: 11-12; 2003: 60).
[61] Gameson (1999: 18).

Church was an important source of exemplars.[62] There are links between booklet 5 of Hatton 115 (from Christ Church, Canterbury?) and the prognostics in CCCC 391, e.g. the otherwise unattested sunshine prognostic in the vernacular, and the α-sequence in Old English present in both manuscripts.[63] The Old English weekday brontology in CCCC 391 is also found in Tiberius A. iii and in Hatton 115, both probably from Christ Church, Canterbury. At the same time, the γ-sequence in CCCC 391 is attested in Old English in Vitellius E. xviii, from New Minster, Winchester. The origin of an exemplar for the Old English prognostics in CCCC 391 may, therefore, be posited either in Christ Church, Canterbury, or in New Minster, Winchester.[64]

The above study of the date of the prognostic corpus has elucidated that the genre experienced a slow start in ninth-and tenth-century England, enjoyed a peak in the eleventh century and suffered a moderate decline in the twelfth. It has been observed that prognostic sections are first attested in the eleventh century, which is also the only period in which prognostics came to be glossed. The role of Canterbury and Winchester as centres which propagated prognostics emerges in the late tenth century, accompanied by Worcester in the eleventh, and *Ramsey in the early twelfth century.

Late Anglo-Saxon Prognostics and the Benedictine Reform

A point I have not yet addressed is that of the rationale underlying the vernacularisation of a Latinate genre such as the prognostics. At several points in this chapter I have referred to Old English prognostics, their emergence, their place of origin and date. Three observations have been made: (1) prognostics flourish in the eleventh century; (2) they were vernacularised in the eleventh century; and (3) most of these texts originated in Canterbury, Winchester and Worcester. These observations seem to point at influences from the Benedictine Reform, an endeavour which

[62] Gameson (1999: 17).

[63] See pp. 51-52.

[64] The sole Latin prognostic in CCCC 391, a dream lunary is unlike any other such lunary from Anglo-Saxon England in that it has psalm verses at the end of each day of the moon. This set-up is more common in continental dream lunaries (see p. 448), which makes a continental exemplar for this particular prognostic likely.

Frantzen called "a movement without an official beginning".[65] The Benedictine Reform commenced around the mid-tenth century, during the reign of King Edmund (939-46), and gained new impetus under King Edgar (959-75). The latter assigned the archbishopric of Canterbury and the bishoprics of Winchester and Worcester to Dunstan (959-88), Æthelwold (963-84) and Oswald (961-92), respectively. These three prelates propagated a reform which led to the reinstatement of Benedictine monastic life, the foundation of new monasteries and an enlightenment in scholarship. Æthelwold's Winchester School employed both Latin and English in teaching, with the result that the vernacular gained a respectable foothold in education and learning.[66] This is best exemplified by the writings of Ælfric, which range from homilies and pastoral letters to linguistics, pedagogy and natural science, all in the vernacular.

It is in the period of the Reform that prognostics developed wide currency in Anglo-Saxon England. I must point out that monks working during and after the Benedictine Reform did not focus primarily on prognostics, but that prognostics gained interest indirectly, through learning and increased manuscript production. In the Reform period, prognostics were translated into Old English, and they flourished in calendars, computi and prognostic sections, as table 13 illustrates:

	calendar	computus	medicine	guest	prognostic section	n
OE	0	12	1	1	22	36
L/OE	1	3	0	0	7	11
L	26	16	0	2	25	69
n	27	31	1	3	54	116

table 13: language and context, s. x^2-xi^2

Out of the total corpus of 174 prognostics, 116 were copied in the era of the Benedictine Reform and its aftermath, i.e. from the second half of the tenth century to the second half of the eleventh century.[67] It cannot

[65] Frantzen (1983a: 122). I have consulted the following studies of the Benedictine Reform: Knowles (1949: 31-82), John (1963), Gneuss (1964: 94-99; 1986; 1992; 1996b: 8-13), Stenton (1971: 433-69), Stafford (1978), Wilcox (1994: 3-9), Gretsch (1999), Lenker (2000), Hill (2001). I realise that the way in which I represent the Benedictine Reform as a uniform movement with a common policy is somewhat simplistic and outdated, yet the scope of my argument does not allow a more exhaustive discussion.

[66] See Gretsch (2001), Stanton (2002).

[67] Stenton (1971: 456-57) noted that the importance of the Benedictine Reform is "misunderstood if it is dismissed as one of the many movements which have merely influenced a generation and then passed into history". Furthermore, the Reform "opened

be ascribed to coincidence that such a high proportion of prognostics was copied in this period. Instead, the Benedictine Reform must have inspired learning in many fields, including that of prognostication. Additional support for this idea is the vehemence with which a Reform writer such as Ælfric opposed some forms of prognostication, while slightly earlier homiletic collections such as the Blickling and Vercelli homilies do not mention prognostication even once.[68]

The three contexts which feature prognostics most extensively are calendars and computi (fifty-eight texts), and prognostic sections (fifty-four texts). Calendars and computi found a welcome audience in adherents to the Reform. Evidence for this conclusion is twofold: (1) that of the manuscripts themselves; (2) that of a concern with time reckoning exemplified by Ælfric and Byrhtferth. First, most Anglo-Saxon computi date from the eleventh century, which must be a direct result of the Benedictine Reform. I have already indicated that these eleventh-century computi show a higher concentration of prognostics than those from the tenth century and earlier.[69] Second, time reckoning proved of considerable interest to the Reformers. Oswald, one of the reformers, founded Ramsey. Oswald was trained in Fleury, and Ramsey maintained close ties with this place. At Oswald's request, Abbo of Fleury, an acclaimed computist, was invited to stay and teach at Ramsey. It is likely that Abbo brought computus manuscripts with him.[70] One of Abbo's pupils, Byrhtferth, wrote a computistical *Enchiridion*. For this purpose, he collected computistical writings, which included a number of prognostics, as exemplified in Tiberius C. i + Harley 3667 and St. John's College 17.[71] Another example of a concern with time reckoning is Ælfric's *De temporibus anni*. While Byrhtferth's computus displayed a certain affinity with prognostication, Ælfric's *De temporibus anni* strongly opposed the consultation of prognostics.[72] Nevertheless, we know from Ælfric's writings that he was familiar with several prognostic genres.[73] Perhaps more important than the fact that Reformers were timekeepers is the vernacula-

---

a new phase of English culture which survived the political catastrophe of the Norman Conquest".

[68] See pp. 114-26.

[69] See pp. 33-35.

[70] A good example of a continental computus containing prognostics is the ninth-century manuscript Harley 3017.

[71] See pp. 33-35, 85.

[72] See pp. 117-21.

[73] See pp. 98-101.

risation of computi. Both Byrhtferth's *Enchiridion* and Ælfric's *De temporibus anni* are in Old English. In addition, a number of computi were composed (partly) in the vernacular in the eleventh century, for instance, in CCCC 422, Caligula A. xv + Egerton 3314, Vitellius C. viii, Vitellius E. xviii and Harley 3271.[74] These five manuscripts also contain prognostics in Old English.

Prognostic sections first appear in the eleventh century.[75] They reflect an attempt at a systematic collection of prognostics that were probably culled from a variety of other contexts. Four eleventh-century manuscripts contain prognostic sections: CCCC 391, Tiberius A. iii, Titus D. xxvi and Harley 3271. Of these, Titus D. xxvi is the only one which does not contain any prognostics in Old English. The compilation of prognostic sections in the eleventh century cannot be ascribed to coincidence because we do not find such sections before, and only sporadically after, the eleventh century, e.g. booklet 5 of Hatton 115. This means that the emergence of these sections may be linked to the interest in learning promoted during the Benedictine Reform.

Before drawing conclusions, let us look at the monasteries which were responsible for the dissemination of prognostics during and immediately following the Benedictine Reform:

Canterbury	Winchester	Worcester	other	n
44	52	15	5	116

table 14: origin, s. x²-xi²

Table 14 illustrates that the foundations where prognostics were copied in large numbers are identical to those which played a crucial role in the Benedictine Reform. I have shown that the dissemination of prognostics in these centres compared to that in the rest of Anglo-Saxon England is not entirely haphazard.[76] Hollis has advanced the idea that the production of prognostics emanated from a single foundation, to which Liuzza assigned the name of Winchester.[77] Hollis's claim is based on the supposedly pastoral function of prognostics,[78] whereas Liuzza connects the rising popularity of prognostics with the development of the Winchester computus. I have already discussed the way in which prognostics were

[74] See pp. 36-39, 67-68.
[75] See p. 82.
[76] See pp. 71-77.
[77] Hollis (2001: 193), Liuzza (2001: 206, 210).
[78] See pp. 126-37.

transmitted via the computus.[79] Winchester computi with prognostics seem to take pride of place, but one should not rule out the Canterbury and Leofric-Tiberius computi (Canterbury and Winchester) and that of Byrhtferth (*Ramsey), all of which feature prognostics. Moreover, as I indicated, the contribution of prognostic sections should not be neglected. When it comes to prognostic sections in the vernacular, the foundations of Christ Church, Canterbury, and Worcester Cathedral played a seminal role in the production of prognostics. Even as late as the middle of the twelfth century, a prognostic section in Old English had been copied in Canterbury. Winchester is known for prognostic sections in Latin. The testimony of computi and prognostic sections, therefore, makes it improbable that any one of the foundations of Christ Church, Canterbury, New Minster, Winchester, Worcester Cathedral or *Ramsey, was alone responsible for the production and dissemination of prognostics. Furthermore, the ties with continental foundations— Dunstan's Canterbury with Ghent, Oswald's Worcester and Ramsey with Fleury—would seem to indicate that the prognostics may have entered English Reform centres from the continent via a number of different routes. These considerations indicate that all four centres seem to have played an equally important part in the propagation of prognostics.

I have focussed on the influence of the Benedictine Reform on the dissemination of Anglo-Saxon prognostics. Three facts substantiate my claim that prognostics gained acceptance and currency during and after the Benedictine Reform: (1) the period of production coincides with the Reform; (2) vernacularisation of the prognostics coincides with Reform practice of teaching and learning in the vernacular and in Latin; and (3) the overwhelming majority of prognostics originated in the religious foundations crucial to the impetus of the Reform.

Conclusion

In this chapter I have concentrated on some key issues in the transmission of Anglo-Saxon prognostics: the language, place of origin and date. Prognostics in the vernacular constitute only a small part of the entire corpus. The language of the prognostics tends to coincide with that of the context, and since all five contexts can be in Latin, this is the language for the majority of the prognostics. Computi, medical sections and

[79] See pp. 29-35.

the guest context also exist wholly or in part in Old English. This implies that prognostics in these contexts can be found in the vernacular. Prognostics in separate sections have been shown to be relatively free from outside influences when it comes to language. The fact that these prognostic sections have texts grouped together by language, e.g. in Tiberius A. iii, indicates that they adhere to internal language preferences. The prognostic corpus originated in a considerable number of places in Anglo-Saxon England, but in only a few of these were prognostics produced on a large scale. Christ Church, Canterbury, New Minster, Winchester, Worcester and *Ramsey appear to be the main centres for the dissemination of the prognostics. Calendars with prognostic material were produced in many English foundations, but particularly in Canterbury and Winchester. The computus seems to have enjoyed popularity in Canterbury, Winchester and *Ramsey. Medical manuscripts are hard to connect with a specific foundation, so that the prognostics contained therein cannot be assigned any definitive place of origin. The guest context was especially used for prognostics in Winchester. Prognostic sections, finally, were produced in Canterbury, Winchester and Worcester. The vernacularisation of prognostics seems to have been largely restricted to these same places. In investigating the date of the prognostics, I indicated that the genre reached a peak in the eleventh century. Prognostics were still a marginal genre in the ninth and tenth centuries. The popularity of the genre in the eleventh century can be explained by the influx of continental manuscripts; the increased production of manuscripts during and following the Benedictine Reform; a growing interest in the computus and the coming of age of the accretive process in computi; the emergence of prognostic sections; the possible loss of older exemplars. Even though manuscript production and import was twice as extensive in the first half of the twelfth century compared to the second half of the eleventh century, prognostics were apparently losing ground in the twelfth century. This may mainly be due to the programmatic manner in which twelfth-century scribes replenished libraries and may depend to a certain extent upon the language of the texts copied: utilitarian writings were dropped in favour of theology, history and Latin classics. Finally, I have advanced evidence for the popularity of the prognostics during the period of the Benedictine Reform and its aftermath.

CHAPTER FOUR

SUPERSTITION AND PROGNOSTICATION

It is evident by now that the prognostics can be grouped together in various ways, e.g. by context, language, genre, date and place of origin. The term 'prognostic', used to describe a genre, unifies many text types of a diverse nature, found in a variety of circumstances. Prognostics, therefore, do not seem to form a homogeneous group of texts. If the structure of prognostics is inspected, for instance, it appears that some are ordered by time sequences, others by the alphabet, numbered sequences or colours. Even within these broad categories, further distinctions can be made. Temporal prognostics may employ hours, days, months (absolute time), days of the moon (relative time), or systems of arbitrarily appointed days. Non-temporal prognostics may use the alphabet, as in the alphabet prognostic or dreambooks, numbered sequences, as in the *Sortes Sanctorum*, or colours, as in the prognostic on the colour of the moon. In spite of this diversity, prognostics can be accommodated within the larger framework of superstition.[1] In this chapter, it is my aim to clarify the status of prognostication as a superstitious practice. To accomplish this, I first investigate the authority that is voiced by the texts themselves, after which I examine an existing system to subdivide the field of superstition. The results are employed to determine the position of prognostication in Anglo-Saxon England, as gleaned from written sources, and the intended audience of the Anglo-Saxon prognostics.

Appeals to Authority

In the course of history, several prognostics changed from anonymous texts to ones written by historical or biblical figures, while some prognostics came to incorporate verbal echoes from learned or homiletic writings. These two features are a matter of authority: verbal echoes testify to the erudition of the writer and increases the status of the text; and texts

[1] It is to be noted that I use the term 'superstition' in an unprejudiced sense to denote a group of practices which fall outside a dominant religious system, with which they coexist. I elaborate upon the word 'superstition' on pp. 102-07.

supposedly written by authorities such as Hippocrates or Galen were thought to be more reliable than anonymous works. Moreover, a prognostic attributed to Augustine, for instance, was more likely to escape censure than if the same text were written anonymously.

Prognostics which disclose the name of the author are found repeatedly.[2] Swan wrote that medieval writers sometimes mentioned the authors of their source text, because "they are interested not in the authorial identity of the individuals named, but rather in the status of those individuals as authoritative sources which set up a chain of affiliation and validation for the text which names them".[3] There is no reason not to extend this chain of reasoning to scribes who added attributions to extant anonymous texts, as in the case of Apuleian Spheres. The earliest example of this genre, in a demotic papyrus, states that the Sphere is devised by Democritus. Medieval versions of this genre also mention Apuleius, Pythagoras and Petosiris as the author. The terms 'Apuleian Sphere' and 'Pythagorean Device' bear witness to these attributions, as does the so-called letter of the Egyptian astrologer Petosiris to Nechepso. The text on the development of the foetus was ascribed to Hippocrates, Galen and Augustine, among others, but was actually composed by Augustine's contemporary Helvius Vindicianus. Old Frisian redactions of this text name Augustine, which makes the text virtually impregnable to criticism. The Old English text, incidentally, carries no attribution. Medieval dreambooks were supposedly devised by Daniel. A wealth of alphabetical and thematic dreambooks has been transmitted in Greek and Arabic, notably those of Artemidoros, Astrampsychos, Daniel, Germanos, Nikephoros and Achmet bin Sirin. In Western medieval literature, Daniel's is the only alphabetical dreambook. The glossed dreambook in Tiberius A. iii, for instance, is entitled "**De somnior*um* diuersiitate** [*sic*] **sec*un*d*u*m ordinem abcharii** [*sic*] **danielis proph*ete***".[4] The alphabet prognostic was said to have been devised by Joseph. This, however, is a late medieval attribution. The earliest representative of this genre, in Old English but undoubtedly a translation, is unattributed and does not explain how the prognostic is to be used. The fact that late medieval alphabet prognostics are ascribed to Joseph and used oneirocritically has led modern scholars to describe this genre as the pseudo-Joseph dreambook. The year prognosis has been called the

[2] Attributions of prognostic genres are listed in full in the text edition.

[3] Swan (2001: 77-78).

[4] Text 7/4, ll. 2, 4.

Revelatio Esdrae de qualitatibus anni, after the prophet Ezra. It is to be noted that none of the Anglo-Saxon year prognoses carries a title or preface to this effect, but the earliest text witness from the continent does.

Two prognostic genres were not attributed to a specific author, but were identified with groups of people: the Egyptian Days and the *Sortes Sanctorum*. First, the three, twelve and twenty-four Egyptian Days have been known under this name throughout their existence. Medieval commentators claimed that the twenty-four Egyptian Days represent the nine or ten plagues suffered in Egypt, were relics of unlucky days from the Egyptian calendar or were unlucky days through an etymological link between Egypt and darkness.[5] Second, Klingshirn has argued that the name of the *Sortes Sanctorum*, a means of divination by dice, is probably a reference to the saints, from Col 1:12: "gratias agentes Patri qui dignos nos fecit in partem sortis sanctorum in lumine" (giving thanks to the Father who has made us worthy to share in the inheritance of the saints in the light).[6]

Some prognostics have been attributed to authorities by editors of medieval texts. The earliest Anglo-Saxon prognostic dates from the ninth century, but it would seem to have predecessors in the prognostics attributed to Bede; erroneously so, however. These pseudo-Bedan prognostics are:

> -*De tonitruis libellus ad Herefridum* (a collection of brontologies by compass directions, by month, by weekday)
> -*Pronostica temporum* (an astrological tract comprising a year prognosis and a prognosis of the year to come based on judicial astrology)[7]
> -*De natiuitate infantium libellus* (texts on foetal development, followed by the three miraculous birthdays and a weekday birth prognostic)
> -*De minutione sanguinis siue de phlebotomia* (a medical tract on bloodletting with Dog Days, three and twenty-four Egyptian Days, a bloodletting lunary and a moonbook)
> -*De tribus diebus periculosis* (a text on the three Egyptian Days)
> -*De Ægyptiacis diebus* (a text on the twenty-four Egyptian Days)
> -the hexameter verses on the twenty-four Egyptian Days in the calendar
> -*De diuinatione mortis et uitae* (an Apuleian Sphere of the Petosiris type)[8]

---

[5] "**S**i tenebre ęgyptiis [*sic*] greco sermone uocantur; / **I**nde dies mortis tenebrosos iure uocamus" (text 8.3/22, ll. 2-3).

[6] Klingshirn (2002: 82).

[7] This is not the same as a year prognosis! To my knowledge, judicial astrology was not practised in Anglo-Saxon England, see pp. 112-13.

[8] Collected in Migne (1861-1904: I.609-14, 759-86, 951-52, 955-56, 959-62, 963-66).

Of course, the attributions are entirely spurious, and although some of these prognostics—mainly bloodletting texts—came to be connected with Bede towards the end of the Middle Ages, most attributions are the work of Renaissance scholars.[9] Care should therefore be taken to distinguish between texts in which the alleged author is mentioned, and those that have been attributed to authorities by editors and collectors of medieval texts: the former shed light on contemporary reception, the latter do not.

Another method by which the authority of a text can be increased is by verbal echoes. An added bonus of verbal echoes, perhaps intended, is that they show the extent of learning of the writer or editor of the text.[10] I have collected three instances of this practice, from the sunshine prognostic, the Old English redaction of the twenty-four Egyptian Days and Ælfric's homily *Octabas et circumcisio Domini*.

First, one of the entries of the sunshine prognostic reads as follows: "if the sun shines on the fourth day [of Christmas], then the camels will carry off much gold from the ants which must guard the gold hoard".[11] This entry is clearly a reference to the story of the camels and the ants in the *Wonders of the East*,[12] which has been preserved in Anglo-Saxon manuscripts twice in Old English and once in Latin.[13] None of the analogues of the sunshine prognostic in other European vernaculars and in Latin includes this reference, so it is likely to be an addition made by the English translator.

Second, the Old English text on the Egyptian Days contains the following note: "nis þis nan wiglung. ac wise menn hit afunden þurh þone halgan wisdom swa heom god ælmihtig gedihte" (this is no divination, but wise men discovered it through the holy wisdom as almighty God revealed to them).[14] This quotation echoes a phrase from Ælfric's homily *Octabas et circumcisio Domini*: "nis þis nan wiglung ac is gecyndelic þing

[9] Jones (1939: 45-47, 73, 87-90).

[10] For instance, the appearance of a uniped in *Eirik's Saga* is said by Magnusson and Pálsson (1965: 101, n. 3) to be "symptomatic of the author's fondness for medieval learning".

[11] Translation of text 14/2, ll. 6-7.

[12] Förster (1906: 369, n. 1; 1912a: 65, n. 1). The relevant passage is in A. Orchard (1995: 177, 190-91 [§9]). The *Liber monstrorum* also refers to giant ants guarding a hoard of gold (A. Orchard 1995: 296-97 [II.15]).

[13] In Tiberius B. v and Vitellius A. xv (Gneuss 2001: 69 [373], 72 [399]); edited and translated by A. Orchard (1995: 175-203).

[14] Text 8.3/1, ll. 27-29.

þurh gesceapenysse" (this is no divination, but it is a natural thing through creation).[15] The phrase "þis nis nan wiglung" also figures in Ælfric's *De auguriis*.[16] The translator of the text on the twenty-four Egyptian Days must have been familiar with Ælfric's work, because the collocation "nis þis nan wiglung" is not found anywhere else and must have originated with Ælfric.[17]

The third instance of a verbal echo is transmitted from a prognostic to a homily rather than the other way round and merits close inspection for this reason. In the homily *Octabas et circumcisio Domini*, Ælfric remarked that many people "nellað heora þing wanian on monandæge".[18] Thorpe translated this as "will not undertake anything on Monday".[19] Meaney, however, saw in this phrase a verbal echo from the text on the three Egyptian Days, and translated it as "will not let blood from their livestock [on Monday]".[20] An Old English redaction of the three Egyptian Days contains the following statement: "Þry dagas syndon on geare... on þam natoþæshwon for nanre neode ne mannes ne neates blod sy to wanienne" (there are three days in a year... on which man's or cattle's blood should not, for any reason at all, be let).[21] These Egyptian Days are three Mondays, as explicated by the Old English and Latin redactions of this genre. Both the homily and the text on the three Egyptian Days would seem to contain references to the bleeding ((blod) wanian) of cattle (þing, neat) on Mondays. Meaney's supposition, therefore, has merit, but her translation is awkward because it would suggest that Ælfric focussed on the bleeding on Mondays of cattle only. The text on the three Egyptian Days, however, mentions bloodletting for both people and cattle. The phrase "heora þing wanian", translated by Thorpe as "undertake anything", features a third person plural pronoun in the genitive.[22] Meaney's reading "let blood from their livestock" preserves this pro-

[15] Clemoes (1997: 230/195-96). I return to this homily on pp. 117-20.

[16] Skeat (1881-1900: I.370/87).

[17] A proximity search in Healey and Venezky (2000) revealed that the phrase is exclusive to the two homilies from Ælfric and the twenty-four Egyptian Days.

[18] Clemoes (1997: 230/167-68).

[19] Thorpe (1844-46: I.101).

[20] Meaney (1984b: 124). Meaney was presumably unaware of the fact that Bosworth and Toller (1898: 1167, s.v. *wanian* I 3a) and Förster (1944: 60-61) already pointed out the connection between Ælfric's homily and the three Egyptian Days. Cf. Godden (1992: 149, n. 10), Liuzza (2001: 198, n. 83, 202).

[21] Text 8.1/4, ll. 1-3.

[22] Thorpe (1844-46: I.622) admitted that his translation was "purely conjectural".

noun. Förster has argued that "þing" is used indefinitely in conjunction with "wanian" to denote "blood", and that the phrase reads "diminish their blood", i.e. "bleed themselves".[23] Here, the verb "wanian" does not mean "to undertake", as Thorpe speculated, but "to weaken, reduce by medical treatment".[24] I prefer Förster's translation over Thorpe's or Meaney's because it is grammatical, and it moves the emphasis from the bleeding of cattle to that of people. Ælfric may have frowned upon the belief that some animals deteriorate through blessing,[25] but it is unlikely that the bleeding of cattle rather than people may have preoccupied him in the homily.

The passage from the homily continues as follows: "[many people] will not bleed themselves on Monday, because of the beginning of the week; but Monday is not the first day in the week, but the second".[26] It is to be noted that there are only three Egyptian Mondays in the year, whereas Ælfric would seem to suggest that every Monday is observed. Moreover, the texts on the three Egyptian Days do not state that these days are Mondays because of the primacy of this day. Meaney supposed a possible contamination of the three Egyptian Days with another kind of superstition, but there is no reason to support this view.[27] The superstition envisaged by Meaney would have to take the form of an agenda weekday prognostic (analogous to an agenda or bloodletting lunary), but such an agenda prognostic has not been attested in Anglo-Saxon manuscripts.[28] It is more likely that Ælfric spoke hyperbolically in order to

[23] Förster (1944: 61, n. 1).

[24] Bosworth and Toller (1898: 1167, s.v. *wanian* I 3a). To illustrate this denotation, Bosworth and Toller adduce the passage from Ælfric's homily, the text on the three Egyptian Days, and the tract on bloodletting and Dog Days (text 6/3, ll. 12-14): "Læcas lærdon þa þe wisoste wæron þ*æt* nan man on þam monþe ne drenc ne drunce ne ahwær his lichoman wanige butan hís nydþearf wære" (the wisest physicians taught that in this period no one is to drink [medicinal] potions nor to bleed his body except out of necessity). This quotation illustrates that "wanian" need not collocate with "blod"—as is the case in the homily—in order to mean "to let blood", although the collocation is more common. Another collocation is "blod lætan", cf. the collective lunary in Tiberius A. iii, where "sanguinem minere" is glossed by "blod lætan oððe wanian".

[25] Clemoes (1997: 230/171-74).

[26] "nellað heora þing wanian on monandæge, for angynne þære wucan, ac se monandæg nis na fyrmest daga on þære wucan, ac is se oðer" (Clemoes 1997: 230/167-69).

[27] Meaney (1984b: 125).

[28] However, a weekday bloodletting prognostic exists in Sloane 475, fols 125-231 (see pp. 245-46). Oddly, this prognostic reports favourable times for bleeding rather than unfavourable times, which cannot have been what Ælfric intended.

make the point that was the subject of the homily: the observation of wrongful times.[29] In addition to the circumcision of Christ, Ælfric's main concern in the homily was to denounce the custom of observing 1 January as the first day of the year.[30] The observation of the three Egyptian Mondays gave him the opportunity to deal with yet another "gedwylde" (error) along the same lines, that of Monday being the first day of the week. Ælfric, with considerable homiletic licence, amplified this error to denounce its practice. The ulterior motive, for which Ælfric used the three Egyptian Days as a scapegoat, was not only to display the gravity of the offence, but to point out a mistake in logic as well.[31]

In the above discussion I have introduced two methods by which a text gains in authority. Many prognostic genres are attributed to authorities in the form of historical or biblical figures or nations. These ascriptions were current in the Middle Ages, and will have contributed to the credibility and status of the text. The fact that the attributions are spurious does not negate the idea that the texts may have enjoyed a certain status in the Middle Ages precisely on account of these attributions. For one thing, the ascriptions reflect a desire on the part of the composer or scribe for these prognostics to be drawn into the canon of respectable texts. Verbal echoes function in the same way: they inherently augment the authority of the text because they reveal the amount of learning on the part of the composer.

---

[29] N.B. not the wrongful observation of times.

[30] Godden (2000: 45-47). For more information on the beginning of the year, see Harrison (1973), Harmening (1979: 120-45). Meaney (1984b: 124) remarked that Ælfric probably heard of the custom of observing 1 January "among the rural English", whereas Godden (1992, 2000: 46) ascribed this kind of knowledge to a learned environment. Meaney's claim is unsupported, especially in view of the evidence in favour of Godden's supposition. First, Ælfric himself mentioned that English time reckoning (gerim) starts on 1 January (Clemoes 1997: 228). Second, several sermons and Martin of Braga's *De correctione rusticorum* may have influenced Ælfric's ideas (Godden 2000: 46). Third, there are prognostics (a bookish genre) which use 1 January to predict the future. For instance, the year prognosis predicts the future based on the weekday on which 1 January falls. The many attestations of this prognostic testify to the popularity of this genre. Therefore, one does not need to presume a rural or heathen source for the observation of 1 January. Moreover, Meaney referred to Bede, who mentioned in *De temporum ratione* XV (Jones 1943: 211-12): "Incipiebant autem annum ab octauo kalendarium ianuarium die" ("They [the English people of the past] began the year on the 8th kalends of January [25 December]", Wallis 1999: 53). Interestingly, one of the year prognoses, 17/3, predicts the future based on the weekday of "middeswintres messedeg" (25 December) rather than on that of 1 January.

[31] Godden (2000: 52).

An Anatomy of Superstition

Superstition Defined

Judging from the writings of Wulfstan, Ælfric and others,[32] the late Anglo-Saxon church seemed to be aware of what constituted superstition. Someone living in the twenty-first century, however, is likely to understand the word 'superstition' only in a vague sense. Indeed, in a paper entitled "Superstitious Medicine", Payne wrote: "I hope you will not demand of me a definition of the word 'superstition,' for to frame one would be a difficult task. I take the word in the usual sense".[33] It is likely that a medieval person will have had a much more acute sense of superstition than we do. In this section, I attempt to provide a serviceable description of superstition. Moreover, it is my aim to provide a typology of superstition, of necessity anachronistic, in order to discover the vocabulary Anglo-Saxon writers may have used to signify prognostication.

Superstition is a phenomenon which is hard to grasp. The denotations of 'superstition' are manifold, and they all seem to be biassed. The *Oxford English Dictionary* gives the etymology of 'superstitio' as "standing over a thing in amazement or awe", and continues: "other interpretations of the literal meaning have been proposed, e.g. 'excess in devotion, over-scrupulousness or over-ceremoniousness in religion' and 'the survival of old religious habits in the midst of a new order of things'".[34] The following denotations are provided: (1) "unreasoning awe or fear of something unknown, mysterious, or imaginary, esp. in connexion with religion; religious belief or practice founded upon fear or ignorance"; (2) "an irrational religious belief or practice; a tenet, scruple, habit, etc. founded on fear or ignorance"; (3) "an irrational religious system; a false, pagan, or idolatrous religion"; (4) "a religious ceremony or observance of a pagan or idolatrous character"; (5) "religious observance"; and (6) "idolatrous or extravagant devotion".[35] It is to be observed that denota-

[32] See pp. 114-26.

[33] Payne (1904: 99).

[34] Simpson and Weiner (1992: s.v. *superstition*). On the etymology of superstition, cf. Hoffmann-Krayer, Bächtold-Stäubli *et al.* (1927-42, I.64-87, s.v. *Aberglaube*), Harmening (1979: 26-32).

[35] Simpson and Weiner (1992: s.v. *superstition*). After having written this chapter, I read Jahoda's *The Psychology of Superstition*, and discovered that he used the same dictionary approach to superstition as I have done here (1969: 2-3). The correspondence is entirely coincidental.

tions (1-3) pronounce a value judgement to the effect that superstition is regarded as irrational. I ignore the implications of "pagan or idolatrous", but the attribution of "fear or ignorance", in particular, does not do justice to the elaborate systems of superstition in existence in the Middle Ages.[36] Furthermore, the religious element in these denotations, in so far as religion itself is not understood as a system of observance, testifies to a belief in a higher power on the part of the compiler of the dictionary.[37] Harmening devoted some space to the meaning of 'superstition', but did not offer an acceptable sense other than the German translation 'Aberglaube'.[38] Since medieval superstition seems so hard to define even in studies that are devoted to the topic, I narrow it down to medieval prognosticatory superstition, which I describe as a system which, if properly applied, yields knowledge of the future. This working definition asserts that prognostication is a component of superstition. Prognostication is able to provide knowledge of the future from life till death, about which Christianity, for instance, is silent. Christianity, on the other hand, provides knowledge of the afterlife, with which prognostication does not deal. Moreover, the working definition makes clear that prognostication is systematic, not random, and that it relies on ritual and order.

In the twelfth-century *Decretum Gratiani*, many superstitious practices are denounced, including several kinds of prognostication.[39] It is striking to note, however, that this text makes no effort to distinguish between different types of superstition. The *Decretum Gratiani* is a source which could not have been known to an Anglo-Saxon audience, but Augustine's *Enchiridion*, for example, surviving in no less than seven pre-twelfth-century English manuscripts and one continental manuscript of English origin,[40] claims the following:

[36] For an overview of superstitions known in Germanic cultures, see Philippson (1929: 223-30), Hoffmann-Krayer, Bächtold-Stäubli *et al.* (1927-42).

[37] Religion implies a belief in a higher power, cf. Simpson and Weiner (1992: s.v. *religion*). The *Oxford English Dictionary* professes the primacy of Christianity among religions: a pagan, for instance, is "one of a nation or community which does not hold the true religion, or does not worship the true God" (Simpson and Weiner 1992: s.v. *pagan*).

[38] Harmening (1979: 14-25, 33-42, 259-316).

[39] Richter and Friedberg (1879-81: I.1044-46 [causa 26, questio 7, chapters 13-18]). The observation of times and divination in general is prohibited. Year prognoses, Apuleian Spheres, alphabetical dreambooks, *Sortes Sanctorum* are mentioned separately.

[40] Gneuss (2001: 40 [132], 46 [188], 87 [512], 103 [653], 111 [742], 112 [751], 119 [794.5], 141 [919.3]). Similarly, the pseudo-Gelasian decree *De libris recipiendis et non recipiendis*, in which the *Sortes Sanctorum* were declared apocryphal, is attested in six manu-

> For who would believe it to be such a great sin to observe days and months and times—as those do who on certain days, in certain months, or in certain years will or will not begin something, because they consider the time favourable or unfavourable in accordance with vain human doctrine—if we could not weigh the magnitude of this evil from the fear of the Apostle, who says: "I am afraid of you, lest perhaps I have laboured in vain among you" [Gal 4:11].[41]

In the *Expositio ad Galatas*, Augustine expressed himself in the same way.[42] It is clear from the quotation that Augustine opposed the observation of wrongful times. In view of the reputation Augustine's writings enjoyed in Anglo-Saxon England, the injunction not to observe times cannot have remained unnoticed. As we have seen, Ælfric concerned himself with this topic in the homily *Octabas et circumcisio Domini*, but in speaking of the Egyptian Mondays he did not denounce the practice on moral but on logical grounds.[43] The irony of resistance against the observation of wrongful times is that prognostics were a popular genre throughout the Middle Ages, despite the fact that nearly all of them deal with the observation of times. Between the vagueness of the *Decretum Gratiani*, and the specific injunctions by Augustine lie many categories of superstition.

Dieter Harmening's book *Superstitio* addressed the issue of superstition in the Middle Ages.[44] In doing so, Harmening devised a highly practical categorisation of superstitious practices, consisting of a threefold typology:[45]

---

scripts of English origin (Gneuss 2001: 55 [263], 94 [573], 109 [713], 112 [749.5], 119 [800], 121 [808.2]). On other writers which denounce superstitions, and which were familiar to Anglo-Saxon writers, see Meaney (1984b), Godden (2000: 46-47, 52).

[41] "Aut quis existimaret, quam magnum peccatum sit dies obseruare et menses et annos et tempora, sicut obseruant qui certis diebus siue mensibus siue annis uolunt uel nolunt aliquid inchoare, eo quod secundum uanas doctrinas hominum fausta uel infausta existiment tempora, nisi huius mali magnitudinem ex timore apostoli pensaremus, qui talibus ait: 'Timeo uos, ne forte sine causa laborauerim in uobis?'" (*Enchiridion* XXI.79; Evans 1969: 93).

[42] Divjak (1971: 103 [35.1-3]). Ambrose, Augustine's teacher, already denounced the observation of times (Zelzer 1982: 223-24). Cf. Harmening (1979: 76).

[43] See pp. 99-101.

[44] Harmening (1979).

[45] Harmening (1979: 46-48). There are more ways of dividing superstition into categories (e.g. Thomas of Aquinas, *Summa theologiae* II.2.92-96, cf. Harmening 1979: 310-16), but the present one can be implemented successfully with regard to the Anglo-Saxon data.

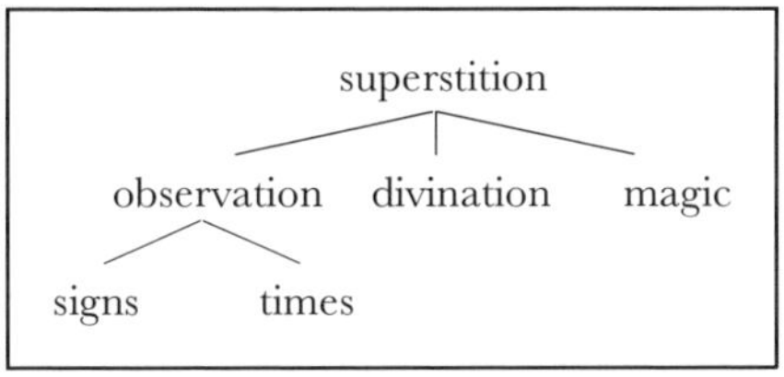

figure 1: typology of superstition

I describe each group and indicate where the various prognostic genres belong.[46]

First, the observation of signs and times simply entails observing properly and interpreting the results.[47] This branch of superstition requires an observer who interprets the findings, but this observer need not participate in any activity to disclose that which is to be observed. A sign that can be observed is, for instance, the behaviour of animals. Omens such as the call of birds or the neighing of horses do not require an elaborate system of knowledge, and can be interpreted fairly easily once the questioner knows what to look for. The same applies to the observation of comets. Signs for which more insight is needed are dreams. The knowledge required for interpreting dreams correctly is contained in the prognostic genre of dreambooks, texts which can run to impressive length. Another prognostic genre that belongs to the observation of signs is the text on the colour of the moon.

The group of observation of times contains all temporal prognostics, which make up the larger part of the English prognostic corpus. Time is a diverse subject, and may involve days of the moon (lunaries), weekdays (year prognosis), dates (Egyptian Days), and periods (Dog Days). Again, this group of superstitions entails observing and interpreting. Some prognostic genres rely on the observation of both signs and times. Examples are the Apuleian Sphere, which uses a system of days of the moon and weekdays (times) combined with the letters in one's name (signs), and the sunshine and wind prognostics, which predict the future based on sunshine or wind (signs) on the twelve days of Christmas (times).

Second, divination is a type of superstition that is more elaborate to practise and requires more knowledge.[48] Divination necessitates a participant who is more than an observer, and who must carry out an action

[46] The branch of superstition of each prognostic is indicated in the text edition.
[47] Harmening (1979: 76-177).
[48] Harmening (1979: 178-216).

before the information to be observed is disclosed. This action needs to be performed in a proper fashion and as prescribed. Examples of divination are judicial astrology,[49] prophecy,[50] lot-casting, geomancy, aeromancy, necromancy and haruspex. For each type of divination, rules exist which must be followed in order for the consultation to be successful. Two Anglo-Saxon prognostics which exemplify divination are the alphabet prognostic and the *Sortes Sanctorum*. The purpose of the alphabet prognostic is lost to us as the text is not prefaced by an explanation of its use, but it may have served as a rhapsodomantic device. The *Sortes Sanctorum* are a form of astragalomancy. In order for this prognostic to work, it is necessary for the participant to throw three dice, sort the numbers of the throw from high to low, and consult the text. These *sortes* show that we are dealing not with observation, but with divination. The distinction lies in the fact that the former requires a questioner who merely observes, and the latter a questioner who participates to disclose what is to be observed.

Third, the superstitions belonging to magic are exceedingly hermetical and ritualistic.[51] Examples of magic practices are the use of amulets,[52] incantations, potions and witchcraft. If divination is more intricate than observation because the participant needs to disclose the information to be observed, magic is the culmination of superstition in that it requires an even more hermetic procedure which must be followed to the letter for it to be a success. Moreover, magic is not merely a means to foresee the future. More often than not it is a way to influence the future, i.e. to accomplish a desired result in the time to come. There are no prognostics which belong to this group of superstitions, which is why I shall not discuss magic any further.

Superstition was, and still is, a rather amorphous subject which lacks clearly marked boundaries in early writings on this topic. The *Decretum Gratiani*, for instance, does not distinguish between different types of superstition. Augustine's *Enchiridion*, on the other hand, shows that the observation of times was a major issue in some circles. Based on Har-

[49] It is to be noted that the words 'divination', 'astrology', 'prognostication' and 'superstition' must not be confused with each other, as they all have different meanings.

[50] Prophecy is a form of superstition which is particularly interesting because it features extensively in the Bible and is an integral part of the religious experience.

[51] Harmening (1979: 217-58).

[52] Amulets, used without magic, have been classed under observation by Harmening (1979: 47). The purpose of an amulet is, however, to influence the future of the wearer, so I do not consider it as belonging to observation.

mening's book *Superstitio*, I have outlined a threefold typology of superstitious practices: observation, divination and magic. Observation requires an observer, divination requires a participant to disclose what is to be observed, and magic requires a participant who must follow a strict protocol to influence the future.[53] These three types of superstition reflect increasing stages of participation and knowledge. Prognostication seems to occupy a place somewhere between observation and divination,[54] of which the observation of times is represented most frequently due to the primacy of temporal prognostics.

An Old English Vocabulary of Observation and Divination

In the section on authority, we saw that Ælfric used the word "wiglung" to distinguish lunar influence which is natural (gecyndelic þing) from that which lies outside Creation (wiglung). "Wiglung" is not the only word employed in writings on superstition. In this section, I introduce an Old English vocabulary of observation and divination, compiled with the help of the *Thesaurus of Old English*, Bosworth and Toller's *Anglo-Saxon Dictionary*, and the *Old English Corpus Online* from the *Dictionary of Old English Project*.[55]

---

[53] Thorndike (1923-58: I.512) wrote that "prediction of the future and attempting to influence events go naturally together", and also "that arts of divination cannot be separated either in theory or practice from magic arts". I strongly disagree with this notion, because there is a fundamental difference in purpose between observation/divination and magic: even though all may end up influencing the future, this is not the primary aim of observation and divination.

[54] In terms of purpose, the boundary between observation and divination is not as clear-cut as that between magic on the one hand, and observation and divination on the other. Both observation and divination aim to foretell the future, while magic is used to influence the future. In view of the hermetic nature of superstition, Harmening (1979: 46-48, 178-79) contrasted observation with divination and magic. In general, the latter two require more knowledge than observation does, but I do not agree with Harmening (1979: 179) that, for this reason, observation belongs to 'Volkskultur' (popular culture) and divination and magic to 'Hochkultur' (high culture). Kieckhefer (1989: 85-90) distinguished magic from divination. He used the terms 'observational' and 'experimental divination' for observatory and divinatory superstition. Although Kieckhefer's terminology differs somewhat from mine, the distinction is the same.

[55] Roberts, Kay and Grundy (2000), Bosworth and Toller (1882-1972), Healey and Venezky (2000).The reader might also wish to consult Bonser study of "Survivals of Paganism" (1963: 117-57). An outstanding early appreciation of the vocabulary of superstition is Serjeantson (1936).

Five preliminary remarks will help delimit the subject at hand. First, this survey is not exhaustive. Second, the superstitions of magic are not included because I am interested in prognostication, which is limited to the fields of observation and divination.[56] Third, items relating to prophecy have been omitted. Prophecy is a type of divination which is condoned by the church since many aspects of the religious experience are tied up with prophecy. Examples include the prophets of the Old Testament, biblical typological allegory, the fifteen signs before Judgement Day, and the many prophecies uttered by saints. Arguably, one could distinguish between those kinds of prophecy which are (1) inspired by God or Satan and their minions; (2) "gecyndelic"; and (3) examples of "wiglung"—lacking divine or infernal inspiration and not "gecyndelic" either. In practice, however, most, if not all, words relating to prophecy must be interpreted as inspired. The part of the vocabulary that covers prophecy will, therefore, not be included.[57] Fourth, although I make a distinction between observation and divination, it should be kept in mind that this may not be how the Anglo-Saxons would have perceived it. Thus, compounds signifying the observation of birds all make use of elements meaning 'diviner' rather than 'observer'. This means that some words for divination might also be used for observation. Fifth, it will appear that most words are culled from glosses and glossaries. The findings from glossaries in particular are highly ambiguous if one does not place them in their original context.[58] Since I merely intend to introduce the vocabulary of superstition (and do not analyse the semantic field), I admit to using the glosses and glossaries without relating them to their context. The following is an example of a problem encountered in glossary material.

[56] Divination includes the mantic arts, notably necromancy, which belong to divination but which are sometimes linked with magic in Anglo-Saxon England. See, for example, Bosworth and Toller (1882-98: 833, s.v. *scin-lac*).

[57] This is a (non-exhaustive) checklist of lemmas for prophecy: ærcwide, andbecnian, andgiettacen, awitegian, boda, bodian, bydel, deofolwitega, forebeacen, forebicnung, forecweðan, forecwide, forecyþan, foregewis, foregleaw, foremanian, foresceawian, foresceawodlice, foresceawung, foresecgan, foreseon, foretacn, foretacnian, forewarenian, forewarnian, forewis, forewitan, forewitegian, forewitegung, forewitig, forewitol, forewittiendlic, forhradian, fortin/fertin, fyrngidd, geryne, gesegen, gespræc, giedd, gieddung, godspræce, niþwundor, sagu, tacn, tacnian, tacnung, weatacen, witedomlic, witega, witegdom, witege, witegestre, witegian, witegiende, witegung, witegungboc, witigendlic (cf. Roberts, Kay and Grundy 2000: I.384-85, 660-61, 670).

[58] With regard to glosses and glossaries, the articles collected in Lendinara (1999) on this topic have proved very helpful.

The Old English *hapax legomenon* "wigbedwiglere" (one who divines from altars)[59] glosses Latin "ariolus" in one of the Plantin-Moretus glossaries.[60] In another of the Plantin-Moretus glossaries, "ariolus" is a secondary gloss to "augur", which is glossed in Old English by "wicca".[61] There are more *interpretamenta* for "ariolus" in glossaries and glosses: "diuinos" and "sacerdotes idolorum" (for "ariolos"), "diuinus" and "ereptícius" (for "ariolus"), "qui in ara coniecturam faciunt" (for "arioli"), and Old English "dreas" and "wigleres" (for "arioli"), "wicca" (for "ariolus"), and "witgan" (for "ariolos").[62] I do not need to pursue this matter further for anyone to realise that there is no end to this exercise and that the chain connecting unrelated words by means of glosses is potentially endless. "Augur", for instance, is glossed as, among others, Latin "auspex",[63] Old English "fugelweohlere", "hælsere", "wiglere" and "wielare".[64] We started out with "wigbedwiglere" (one who divines from altars), which would seem, through "ariolus", to be correlated somehow to observers, e.g. "fugelweohlere" (diviner from birds, i.e. observer of bird omens), diviners, e.g. "wiglere" (diviner), "witega" (prophet), and magicians, e.g. "drea" (sorcerer), "wicca" (witch). A "wigbedwiglere", however, is not necessarily a magician, and certainly not an observer of bird omens. It is important, therefore, to realise the limitations of glossary material as used in this survey. A large part of the Old English vocabulary of superstition consists of *interpretamenta* from glosses and glossaries. Words such as "wigbedwiglere" and "fugelweohlere" are uniquely attested. While it is possible to determine what they mean, I do not establish whether they are accurate glosses.

---

[59] Bosworth and Toller (1882-98: 1220, s.v. *wigbed-wiglere*). Bosworth and Toller use the word "sacrifices" instead of "altars", the latter being the correct translation of Old English "wigbed". "Wigbedwiglere" literally means "diviner" (wiglere) "from altars" (wigbed, i.e. weofod). This collocation relies on a mistaken reading of "ara-" (altar) in the word "(h)ariolus". This mistake has also been made in the secondary gloss "qui in ara coniecturam faciunt" (Hessels 1890: 21/a823).

[60] Wright and Wülcker (1884: I.108/10).

[61] Wright and Wülcker (1884: I.183/31).

[62] Oliphant (1966: 142/d742, 22/a42); Hessels (1890: 20/a800), Oliphant (1966: 156/e320); Hessels (1890: 21/a823); Wright and Wülcker (1884: I.79/15), Rhodes (1889: 75/12); Wright and Wülcker (1884: I.189/22); Oliphant (1966: 142/d742).

[63] Wright and Wülcker (1884: I.108/12).

[64] Wright and Wülcker (1884: I.108/12), Hessels (1890: 23/a953), Wright and Wülcker (1884: I.312/38, 540/22).

The following is an overview of the Old English vocabulary of observation and divination :[65]

Observation of signs:
-birds:[66] fugelhwata[go], fugelweohlere[go] (diviner by birds), wigol(fugel)[go] (divinatory bird)[67]
-dreams: swefenracu[o] (interpretation of dreams), swefen reccan[o] (to interpret dreams), swefenrecerre[go] (interpreter of dreams)[68]
-omens: hæl[o] (omen), hwatu[o] (omen)[69]

Observation of signs and times:
cepan (to observe, to regulate by)[70]

Divination:
-general: friht[o] (divination), frihtere[o] (diviner), frihtrian[go] (to divine), frihtrung[go] (divination), hælsend[go], hælsere[go] (diviner), hælsian[go] (to divine), hælsung[go], hwata[o],[71] hwatung[o], wamfreht[go], wigle[go] (divination), wiglere (diviner), wiglian (to divine), wiglung (divination)[72]

---

[65] In this list I follow the conventions of the *Thesaurus of Old English* (Roberts, Kay and Grundy 2000: I.xxi-xxxi) by using the following flags: superscript [g] = a word mainly found in glosses and/or glossaries, superscript [o] = a word infrequently used (including *hapax legomena*), or a word rarely used in the applicable denotation. One should be aware that a word can have more than one denotation, in which case I have chosen the denotation having to do with superstition. "Hælsian" and derivatives can mean both "to exorcise" and "to divine", the former is the more usual denotation, the latter is rare (Bosworth and Toller 1882-98: 500, 505, s.v. *hælsian*, *halsian*; Toller 1908-21: 497, 503-04, s.v. *hælsian, halsian*). Abbreviations used for reference works: BT = Bosworth and Toller (1882-98), C = Campbell (1972), C*ea* = Cameron *et al.* (1980-), T = Toller (1908-21), Th = Thorpe (1840: II).

[66] BT (343, s.v. *fugel-hælsere*) adduce the spurious compound *fugelhælsere*.

[67] BT (343, s.v. *fugel-hwata*, *fugel-weohlere*; 1222, s.v. *wigol*).

[68] BT (946, s.v. *swefen-racu*; 945-46, s.v. *swefen* II; 946, s.v. *swefen-reccere*).

[69] BT (499, s.v. *hæl*), T (496, s.v. *hæl*; 579, s.v. *hwatu*).

[70] T (122, s.v. *cepan* Ia, II), Henel (1942: 98), C*ea* (fiche C 1.2, s.v. *cepan* B.1.c).

[71] BT (572, s.v. *hwat*, *hwata*) give the denotation of "hwata" as "diviner" instead of "divination". "Hwata" can mean both, but as a simplex it has not been attested as "diviner" (in compounds this denotation exists, e.g. "fugelhwata").

[72] Th (glossary, s.v. *fyrht*), BT (353, s.v. *fyrht*), T (267, s.v. *friht*); BT (338, s.v. *frihtere*); C (28, s.v. *frihtrian*); BT (337, 338, s.v. *frictrung*, *frihtrung*), T (267, s.v. *frihtrung*); BT (500, s.v. *hælsend*), T (497, s.v. *hælsend*); BT (500, s.v. *hælsere*), T (497, 503, s.v. *hælsere*, *halsere*); BT (500, 505, s.v. *hælsian*, *halsian*), T (497, 503-04, s.v. *hælsian*, *halsian* II); BT (500, 506, s.v. *hælsung*, *halsung*), T (497, 504, s.v. *hælsung*, *halsung* II); Th (glossary, s.v. *hwata*), BT (572, s.v. *hwat*, *hwata*), T (579, s.v. *hwatu*); Th (glossary, s.v. *hwatung*), BT (572-73, s.v. *hwatung*; 1164, s.v. *wamm-freht*; 1221, s.v. *wigle*), T (746, s.v. *wigle*); Th (glossary, s.v. *wiglere*), BT (1221, s.v. *wiglere*), T (746, s.v. *wiglere*); BT (1221, s.v. *wiglian*; 467, 1221-22, s.v. *ge-wig-*

-astrology:[73] byrdwiglere^go, byrdwitega^go, dægmælsceawere^go (astrologer); mearcung^go, reonung^go (astrology), steorgleaw^go (skilled in astrology), steorsceawere^go (astrologer), steorwigle^go (astrology), steorwiglere^go (astrologer), steorwiglung^go (astrology), tidsceawere^go, tidymbwlatend^go, tunglere^go (astrologer), tungolcræft^o (astrology), tungolcræft(ig)a^go (astrologer), tungolgescead^go, tungolspræc^go (astrology), tungolwitega^go (astrologer)[74]
-sortilege: behleotan^o, gehleotan^o (to appoint by lot), gehlytta^o (chosen by lot), gehlytto^o (a lot), hleotan^o (to cast lots), hliet^o, hlot^o (a lot), hlot sendan^o, hlot weorpan^o (to cast lots), hlyta^o, hlytere^o (diviner by lots), hlytm^o (casting of lots), hlytman^o (to allot), ta^o (a lot), tan^o (a twig used in casting lots), tanhlyta^go, tanhlytere^go (diviner by lots), tohleotan^o (to divide into parts for which lots are to be cast)[75]

The above list contains some sixty words, compounds and collocations for observation and divination. If the words for prophecy and the mantic arts were included, this number would be about doubled. This seems a

lung, wiglung), T (746, s.v. *wiglung*).

[73] Some Anglo-Saxons distinguished between astrology and astronomy, also called "lex astrorum" (tungolæ) in Aldhelmian glosses: "'astraloia', þæt ys þonne tungolcræft, and 'astronomia', þæt ys tungla gang" (astrology, that is star-craft, and astronomy, that is [knowledge of] the course of the stars) (Kotzor 1981: II.258/17-19). Lemmas which are used for astronomy only are not included. This pertains to "tungolæ" and "tungolcræftwise" (BT 1020, s.v. *tungol-æ, tungolcræft-wise*), which Roberts, Kay and Grundy classed under astrology (2000: I.660, s.v. 16.01.04.06.01). Some words are used for both astronomy and astrology, e.g. "tungolcræft", while others are also used to denote astrologers or the three magi, e.g. "tungolcræf(ig)a", "tungolwitega" (BT 1020, s.v. *tungolcræft, tungol-cræfta, tungol-cræftiga, tungol-witega*). More information on natural versus judicial astrology is provided below.

[74] BT (378, s.v. *ge-byrd-wiglære*), *Cea* (fiche B 1.9, s.v. *byrd-wiglere*); BT (378, s.v. *ge-byrd-witega*), *Cea* (fiche B 1.9, s.v. *byrd-witega*); BT (193, s.v. *dæg-mel-sceawere*), Wright and Wülcker (1884: I.108, n. 1, 188, n. 2), T (144, s.v. *dægmæl-sceawere*), *Cea* (fiche D 1.1, s.v. *dægmæl-sceawere*); BT (674, s.v. *mearcung*), T (634, s.v. *mearcung* III), C (47, s.v. *mearcung*); T (686, s.v. *reonung*), C (52, s.v. *reonung*); BT (917, s.v. *steor-gleaw*; 918, s.v. *steor-sceawere* I), T (711, s.v. *steor-sceawere*); BT (918, s.v. *steor-wigle*); T (711, s.v. *steor-wiglere*); BT (918, s.v. *steor-wiglung*; 983, s.v. *tid-sceawere, tid-ymbwlatend*), T (721, s.v. *tid-ymbwlatend*); BT (1020, s.v. *tunglere, tungol-cræft, tungol-cræfta, tungol-cræftiga, tungol-gescead*); T (726, s.v. *tungol-spræc*); BT (1020, s.v. *tungol-witega*).

[75] C (8, s.v. *behleotan*), *Cea* (fiche B 1.3, s.v. *behleotan*); BT (401, s.v. *ge-hleotan*), T (344, s.v. *ge-hleotan*; 344, s.v. *ge-hlytta* II; 344, s.v. *ge-hlytto* I); BT (542, s.v. *hleotan*), T (551, s.v. *hleotan*); Th (glossary, s.v. *hlyttas*), BT (543, 546, s.v. *hlet, hlyt*), T (553, s.v. *hlit*); BT (401, 544-45, s.v. *ge-hlot, hlot*), T (553, s.v. *hlot*); BT (544-45, s.v. *hlot*), T (553, s.v. *hlot*); BT (544-45, s.v. *hlot*; 546, s.v. *hlyta*), T (555, s.v. *hlyta*); BT (546, s.v. *hlytere*), T (553, s.v. *hlitere*); BT (546, s.v. *hlytm*); T (555, s.v. *hlytman*); BT (966, s.v. *ta*; 971, s.v. *tan* II, *tan-hlyta, tan-hlytere*; 999-1000, s.v. *to-hleotan*).

considerable vocabulary, but if we look at the incidence by type of these lemmas compared to the entire vocabulary of Old English, they are almost negligible. Most of the lemmas (in observatory or divinatory denotations) are rare, *hapax legomena* or culled from glosses and glossaries:

	gloss + rare	rare	unrestricted
n	31	25	4
incidence	51.7%	41.7%	6.7%

table 15: vocabulary for observation and divination

This table shows that over fifty percent of the Old English vocabulary of observation and divination stems from glosses and glossaries, while over ninety-three percent is rare.

The observation of signs, and divination by astrology are almost entirely confined to glosses. The former can be considered a marginal issue,[76] whereas the latter seems to have been rather popular to judge by the eighteen lemmas that have come down to us. This conclusion, however, is deceptive because most lemmas are *hapax legomena* or rare, and are furthermore found mainly in glosses to Aldhelm's prose *De laude uirginitatis*.[77] We could conclude, then, that Aldhelm took an interest in astrology, which is somewhat surprising because no astrological texts have been transmitted in Anglo-Saxon manuscripts.[78] The signs of the zodiac were known,[79] but these were not linked with prediction and, therefore, do not constitute divination by astrology. In this respect, it is important to distinguish between "astrologia naturalis" (astrology in the sense of astronomy for computational purposes) and "astrologia superstitiosa" (judicial astrology).[80] When Aldhelm (*c.* 639-709) wrote his *De laude uirginitatis*, he would have been familiar with the concepts of both natural and

[76] The vocabulary of observation of birds and dreams consist of *hapax legomena*.

[77] Lemmas which are typically attested in Aldhelmian glosses are, for instance, "steorglæw", "steorwigle", "steorwiglung", "tungolgescead" and "tungolspræc".

[78] Astrology is a highly codified form of divination, which means that textual evidence of its existence must be attested.

[79] In the calendars of Arundel 60 and St. John's College 17, for instance.

[80] Harmening (1979: 181-82). Systems of propitious and unpropitious times, such as the Dog Days, lunaries and the sunshine prognostic, are classed under observation rather than under divination, because their ulterior astrological basis derived from natural astrology, not judicial astrology. Prognostication in the form of Egyptian Days and Dog Days was a calendric matter in Anglo-Saxon England, witness the frequent entries of such days in calendars (see pp. 26-29). Cf. Liuzza (2001: 192-93, n. 64).

judicial astrology through learning.[81] It is unlikely, however, that he, or any other Anglo-Saxon for that matter, had first-hand experience with judicial astrology. While astrology with an aim to predict the future was known in classical times and in Byzantine, Syriac and Arabic cultures, it surfaced first in Western Europe through Arabic science via Córdoba and Catalonia in France, in the late tenth, and eleventh centuries.[82] Subsequently, texts on judicial astrology made their way to England via ties with continental monasteries (Fleury and Chartres, for instance), presumably already in the eleventh century.[83] The first manuscript evidence of judicial astrology in England advanced by Burnett are the twelfth-century Anglo-Norman manuscripts Wellcome, MS 21 and Sloane 2030.[84] This agrees with the earliest English examples of judicial astrology I have encountered in the form of zodiacal prognostics, in the twelfth-century manuscript Egerton 821.

A lemma in a gloss or glossary must not be considered evidence of the contemporary existence of the conventions implied by the lemma. Old English words for astrology, for instance, do not prove the existence of judicial astrology in Anglo-Saxon England. Moreover, the vocabulary of superstition must be related to evidence of superstitious practices. In the case of astrology, eighteen *interpretamenta* have been attested, but there is no evidence, documentary or otherwise, that judicial astrology was ever practised in Anglo-Saxon England.[85]

[81] From Aldhelm's letter to Leuthere (Lapidge and Herren 1979: 152-53, 199, n. 4), written *c.* 670-72 while the former studied at the Canterbury school of Theodore and Hadrian (Lapidge and Herren 1979: 137-38), it appears that Aldhelm was familiar with natural astrology from his study of the computus, cf. Hollis (2001: 188). The kind of astrology Aldhelm referred to here was auxiliary to the computus rather than a form of judicial astrology. Michael Herren informed me that Aldhelm derived his knowledge of judicial astrology from Cicero's *De diuinatione*.

[82] Burnett (1997: 2-5). Byzantine, Syriac and Arabic astronomical learning showed a marked interest in judicial astrology. For an outstanding overview of the introduction of Arabic knowledge into Western Europe and subsequently into England, see Burnett (1997) and the following: Haskins (1915), Singer (1917: 108-09; 1928: 71-85), Thorndike (1923-58: I.697-718), Bonser (1963: 156-57), Talbot (1967: 24-37), Wedel (1968: 49-89), Rubin (1974: 189-92), Jones (1984: 69), North (1986a; 1986b: 96-107, 114-22), Kieckhefer (1989: 86, 116-50), Hugonnard-Roche (1996), Getz (1998: 36-44).

[83] Burnett (1997: 5-10).

[84] Burnett (1997: 10, 88, n. 26).

[85] Similarly, the Old English vocabulary for sortilege exceeds direct evidence of the practice of sortilege in Anglo-Saxon England. It has never been proven conclusively that sortilege was anything more than a topos in Anglo-Saxon literature. An instance of a typical, imaginative approach to sortilege can be found in Elliott (1989: 82-90). Even if

The reverse need not apply: a considerable corpus of prognostics has survived, but a specific vocabulary for this group of superstitions is almost non-existent. Nevertheless, the Anglo-Saxons had a clear conception of the boundaries of the genre of prognostics as a whole, so including all genres which we are able to distinguish today. Indications for this are the premeditated inclusion of different types of prognostics depending upon the manuscript context, and the creation of prognostic sections. Calendars feature temporal prognostics using absolute time, while computi include temporal prognostics which employ structures of absolute and relative time, and tabular material, such as Apuleian Spheres. Medical sections, on the other hand, have medical prognostics with a focus on bloodletting. Prognostic sections, finally, incorporate both temporal and non-temporal prognostics, and show a wider range of temporal prognostics than in computi. Therefore, Anglo-Saxon compilers were able to tally genre and context. The collection of texts in prognostic sections is the strongest kind of evidence we have. The fact that compilers gathered a wide variety of prognostic genres in sections which are sometimes even on separate quires, strongly suggests that these collectors knew that such texts belonged to one larger genre.

In this section I have compiled an Old English vocabulary of observation and divination. With the help of the words for astrology I have shown that the vocabulary should be handled with care if it is to serve as evidence for superstitious practices in Anglo-Saxon England. In order to investigate the lexicon, it will prove necessary to view the lemmas in their proper context. This is what I do in the next section with regard to the vocabulary of prognostication.

References to Prognostication in Anglo-Saxon Sources

There can be little doubt that the late Anglo-Saxon church, represented by Ælfric and Wulfstan, was concerned with the repression of superstition. Ælfric was so preoccupied with the topic of divination, it seems, that he even used the word "wiglere" in his *Grammar* to illustrate a gramma-

one is willing to acknowledge actual uses of sortilege in Anglo-Saxon England, one must be careful to distinguish between references to prognostic, biblical (e.g. Acts 1:26) and runic sortilege. Unfortunately, most defenders of Anglo-Saxon runic sortilege do not discriminate between these categories, nor do they find it reprehensible to get their evidence from widely different periods, cultures and countries.

tical construction: "ân ðissera is *COMMVNIS GENERIS*: *hic et haec augur* þes and ðêos wiglere".[86] Like Ælfric, Wulfstan had a predilection for alliterative lists of enemies of the faith (based on Deut 18:10-11,[87] and 1 Cor 6:9-10), and included these in a number of homilies and laws, always featuring "wigleras" (diviners).[88] The tenacity with which Ælfric and Wulfstan, the laws and the penitentials, opposed all forms of superstition must be interpreted as a policy or programme on the part of the Anglo-Saxon church.[89] The topicality of the subject of superstition in late Anglo-Saxon England need not be questioned, therefore. I presume the reader to be familiar with Anglo-Saxon writings pertinent to this issue, so I shall not repeat these here.[90] Instead, I focus on texts in which prognostication is mentioned explicitly. To this purpose, the writings of the Anglo-Saxons are a poor source of information. There are Old English words which denote divination, but there is no collective designation for prognostication.

The first mention in the vernacular of prognostication is found in the writings of Ælfric. About three centuries before Ælfric, Bede had narrated in his *Ecclesiastical History* that St. John of Beverley was called upon to heal a nun who fell ill after having been bled:

> Then [John] asked when the girl had been bled and, on hearing that it was on the fourth day of the moon, he exclaimed, "You have acted foolishly and ignorantly to bleed her on the fourth day of the moon; I remember how Archbishop Theodore of blessed memory used to say that it was very

---

[86] Zupitza (1880: 48/17-49/2). Ælfric could have chosen from a number of Old English nouns of more than one gender (cf. Kitson 1990).

[87] Cited below.

[88] See, for instance, Ælfric's homilies *Sermo ad populum, in octavis pentecosten dicendus* (Pope 1967-68: I.435/371-436/383), and *Feria secunda, Letania maiore* (Godden 1979: 189/285-90); Wulfstan's homilies *De temporibus Anticristi*, *Be hæðendome* (Napier 1883: 194/17-20, 203/21-204/4, 309/21-26), and *De fide catholica* (Bethurum 1957: 163/128-34); and the laws Edward and Guthrum [§9], VI Æthelred [§7], and II Cnut [§4] (Liebermann 1903-16: I.134, 248, 310). Likewise, lists of superstitious practices enjoyed great popularity, cf. Ælfric's homilies *Natiuitas Sanctae Mariae Virginis* (Assmann 1889b: 28/93-100), *Dominica x post Pentecosten*, *Saul and the Witch of Endor* [=addition to *De auguriis*] (Pope 1967-68: II.550/72-83, 796/124-25), [addition to] *Dominica secunda post Pasca* (Clemoes 1997: 542/245-48); Wulfstan's homily *Sermo de baptismate* (Bethurum 1957: 184/165-68); and the latter's *Canons of Edgar* [§16] (Fowler 1972: 4, 5).

[89] Frantzen (1983a: 142-48) observed that the normative efforts of Ælfric and Wulfstan were central to the Benedictine Reform on all levels of the ecclesiastical hierarchy.

[90] The most recent overview of Anglo-Saxon opinions on superstition is Liuzza (2001: 190-98).

> dangerous to bleed a patient when the moon is waxing and the Ocean tide flowing. And what can I do for the girl if she is at the point of death?"[91]

Of course, John, having holy qualities that other people lacked, healed the girl. The passage of St. John of Beverley healing a nun has become a *locus classicus* for our knowledge of medical practice in the relatively undocumented earlier stages of Anglo-Saxon history. It is customary to draw attention to this passage for one of two reasons: (1) the text comments upon the medical practice of bloodletting in Bede's time and upon the study of medicine at Theodore's Canterbury school; or (2) the text seems to offer evidence that prognostication was practised in Bede's time, apparently against the express directions of an authority such as Theodore.[92] While it is warranted to point out that bloodletting was indeed practised in Bede's time on the basis of the above quotation, it is not valid to read a commentary on prognostication into the passage.[93] This passage may at first glance call to mind a bloodletting lunary because mention is made of days of the moon and bleeding. Many bloodletting lunaries agree that the fourth day of the moon is good for bleeding "in matutina" (in the early morning).[94] St. John of Beverley, however, is not made to refer to a bloodletting lunary, but to an opinion

[91] "Interrogans autem ille, quando flebotomata esset puella, et ut cognouit, quia in luna quarta, dixit: 'Multum insipienter et indocte fecistis in luna quarta flebotomando. Memini enim beatae memoriae Theodorum archiepiscopum dicere, quia periculosa sit satis illius temporis flebotomia, quando et lumen lunae et reuma oceani in cremento est. Et quid ego possum puellae, si moritura est, facere?'" (*Historia Ecclesiastica* V.3; Colgrave and Mynors 1991: 460). Translation Colgrave and Mynors (1991: 461).

[92] Payne (1904: 13-15), Singer (1928: 147-48), Jones (1939: 88-89), Grattan and Singer (1952: 48-49), Bonser (1963: 297), Talbot (1967: 11), Rubin (1974: 64-65, 100, 140), Cameron (1993: 27), Stevenson (1995: 50-52), Getz (1998: 13), Liuzza (2001: 202).

[93] Grattan and Singer (1952: 49), Bonser (1963: 297) and Stevenson (1995: 51) mentioned the passage in connection with Egyptian Days, but there is absolutely no basis for assuming that it has anything to do with Egyptian Days. It is striking that some of the more sensible writers on Anglo-Saxon medicine and/or prognostics fail to interpret the passage correctly. Liuzza (2001: 202) seems to be under the impression that "such belief served to permit, with, as it were, Bede's *imprimatur*, a broader range of less rational medical calendars". Likewise, Cameron (1993: 27) saw evidence of the existence of bloodletting lunaries in the seventh century in the passage from Bede. With regard to the spurious attribution of the bloodletting prognostics to Bede, Jones (1939: 89) had already pointed out that "blood-letting according to Egyptian Days is definitely superstition uncharacteristic of Bede".

[94] For instance, in CCCC 422, Arundel 60, Tiberius A. iii, Titus D. xxvi, Titus D. xxvii, Harley 3271, and St. John's College 17.

on nature held by Archbishop Theodore, his erstwhile teacher.[95] This notion expounds the growing and dwindling influence of the waxing and waning of the moon upon the sublunar, a theory current in medieval science. The waxing moon is said to have detrimental effects on bloodletting. In this light, it is dangerous to let blood on the fourth day of the moon. This idea, however, stems from natural science, not from an arbitrary listing of dangerous days of the moon in a bloodletting lunary; in the words of Payne: "the reasons assigned by the bishop for avoiding certain days were physical facts, not superstitions".[96] Therefore, the above passage from Bede's *Ecclesiastical History* cannot be used as a commentary upon prognostication.

The influence of the moon on the earth and its inhabitants is not one of prognostication, but must be relegated to the field of natural science. This becomes evident from its inclusion in such writings as Bede's *De temporum ratione*, Ælfric's *De temporibus anni*, and Byrhtferth's *Enchiridion*.[97] Indeed, lunar influence upon the sublunar has been expounded from classical times onwards.[98] Wallis remarked that "medieval thinkers... were careful to distinguish this natural or 'environmental' [lunar] influence from astrological determinism".[99] Ælfric is quite specific on the distinction between natural science and prognostication:

> Every bodily creature which the earth produces in creation, however, is according to nature, fuller and stronger in full moon than when the moon is waning. Therefore, trees also, if they are felled during full moon, are harder and more lasting for building, and especially if they are made sapless. This is no divination, but it is a natural thing through creation.[100]

In this passage from the homily *Octabas et circumcisio Domini*, Ælfric distinguishes between "wiglung" (divination) and that which is "gecyndelic

[95] Jones (1939: 88-89), Wallace-Hadrill (1988: 176).

[96] Payne (1904: 15).

[97] Jones (1943: 231-32 [XXVIII]), Henel (1942: 64 [VIII.13-14]); Baker and Lapidge (1995: 144 [III.2.124-28]), respectively.

[98] Jones (1943: 362), Wallis (1999: 306-07)

[99] Wallis (1999: 306).

[100] "Is hwæþere æfter gecynde on gesceapenysse ælc lichamlic gesceaft þe eorðe acenð fulre 7 mægenfæstre on fullum monan þonne on gewanedum. Swa eac treowa gif hi beoð on fullum monan geheawene hi beoð heardran 7 langfærran to getimbrunge 7 swiþost gif hi beoð unsæpige geworhte. Nis þis nan wiglung ac is gecyndelic þing þurh gesceapenysse" (Clemoes 1997: 230/191-96).

þing" (a natural thing). A bloodletting lunary relates to "wiglung" as lunar influence does to "gecyndelic þing".

Ælfric used the word "wiglung" for "divination". I have already shown that the same word was used to assert that the text on the Egyptian Days did not represent divination.[101] So far, though, no specific mention has been made of prognostication. The homily *Octabas et circumcisio Domini*, however, does contain several references to prognostication:

> Now foolish men practise many divinations on this day [1 January], with great error, after heathen custom, against their Christianity, as if they could prolong their life or their health, with which they provoke the Almighty Creator. Many are also possessed with such great error that they regulate their journeying by the moon and their acts according to days, and will not bleed themselves on Monday, because of the beginning of the week; though Monday is not the first day in the week, but the second. Sunday is the first in creation, in order and in dignity.[102]

Again, the word "wiglung" (and its derivative "wiglian") is used, but now Ælfric links it with 1 January. This is an overt reference to the observation of times. In addition, Ælfric speaks of people who "cepað be ðam monan heora fær, 7 heora dæda be dagum" (regulate their journeying by the moon and their acts according to days). This is an unambiguous reference to lunaries, in particular to the agenda lunary (Förster's 'Tagwähllunare'![103]) which tells the questioner what actions are to be undertaken on each day of the moon. Two fragmentary agenda lunaries from Anglo-Saxon England have come down to us, and agenda components are included in collective lunaries.[104] Finally, Ælfric displayed his knowledge of the three Egyptian Days in the phrase "nellað heora þing wa-

[101] See pp. 98-99.

[102] "Nu wigliað stunte men menigfealde wigelunga on þisum dæge, mid micclum gedwylde æfter hæðenum gewunan ongean hyra cristendom, swilce hi magon heora lif gelengan, oððe heora gesundfulnysse mid þam ðe hi gremiað þone ælmihtigan scyppend. Sind eac manega mid swa micclum gedwylde befangene, þæt hi cepað be ðam monan heora fær, 7 heora dæda be dagum, 7 nellað heora þing wanian on monandæge, for angynne þære wucan, ac se monandæg nis na fyrmest daga on þære wucan, ac is se oðer, se sunnandæg is fyrmest on gesceapenysse 7 on endebyrdnysse, 7 on wurþmynte" (Clemoes 1997: 229/162-70).

[103] Förster (1912c: 37).

[104] A fragmentary redaction of the agenda lunary exists in Tiberius A. iii and Hatton 115. The agenda component in collective lunaries can be found in Tiberius A. iii, Titus D. xxvii and Sloane 475.

nian on monandæge".[105] I have already quoted a passage from the same homily in which Ælfric explained the influence of the moon. Immediately preceding this passage, Ælfric denounced divination with these words:

> The Christianity of a man who lives with devilish divination is void. He appears as a Christian, but is a wretched heathen, just as the same apostle [Paul] says about such a man: "I believe that I laboured in vain when I turned you to God. Now you observe days and months with vain divinations".[106]

More interesting than the phrase "mid deoflicum wiglungum" is Ælfric's free rendering of Gal 4:10-11, which runs in the original: "Dies obseruatis et menses et tempora et annos. Timeo uos ne forte sine causa laborauerim in uobis". I have already shown that Augustine used the same quotation from Paul's letter to the Galatians to denounce the observation of times.[107] Ælfric goes one step further when he translates Gal 4:10 as "nu ge cepað daga 7 monða *mid ydelum wiglungum*".[108] There cannot be any doubt how "cepað" should be interpreted here, because Ælfric added the phrase "mid ydelum wiglungum". Moreover, Ælfric regularly employed the verb "cepan" in connection with observatory superstitions, particularly those relating to the observation of times.[109] With four references, the *Octabas et circumcisio Domini* is the richest Anglo-Saxon source of evidence for prognostication.

Ælfric's concern with prognostication does not end here. In *De temporibus anni*, modelled upon Bede's computistical writings, Ælfric added an injunction against divination by the moon, not present in Bede's computus: "No Christian must divine anything from the moon; if he does so, his faith is void".[110] This is the second instance where Ælfric is not content simply to translate his source, but where he adds a reference to superstition. In a note to the above passage, Henel commented as follows:

[105] See pp. 99-101.

[106] "Nis þæs mannes cristendom naht þe mid deoflicum wiglungum his lif adrihð; he is gehiwod to cristenum menn, 7 is earm hæþengilda, swa swa se ylca apostol be swylcum cwæð: Ic wene þæt ic swunce on ydel þa ða ic eow to gode gebigde. Nu ge cepað daga 7 monða mid ydelum wiglungum" (Clemoes 1997: 230/186-91).

[107] See pp. 103-04.

[108] Emphasis is mine.

[109] Cf. Henel (1942: 98).

[110] "Ne sceal nan cristenman nan ðing be ðam monan wiglian; gif he hit deð, his geleafa ne bið naht" (*De temporibus anni* VIII.7; Henel 1942: 60).

> he [Ælfric] mentions only one type of such prognostication, forecasting the weather by the *position* of the moon in the sky. In his own time, this particular type does not seem to have been known; at least no texts explaining it have come to light in English MSS. of the tenth or eleventh centuries. But in the homily on the Octave of the Lord... Ælfric also mentions that people avoid doing business on Monday..., and that they will not undertake journeys on certain days of the moon. The latter type, superstitious beliefs and forecasts connected with the *phase* of the moon, was very common in Anglo-Saxon England. This is attested by a surprisingly large number of entries, both in Latin and Old English, in MSS. about coeval with Ælfric, or a little later.[111]

Henel then continues with a list of the many prognostic genres known in England in Ælfric's days. It is unfortunate that Henel sought to distinguish between "position" and "phase" of the moon when there is absolutely no need to. There is no mention of the position of the moon in the phrase "Ne sceal nan cristenman nan ðing be ðam monan wiglian". Rather, the reference is to the phase (i.e. day) of the moon, viz. to lunaries, exactly as in the homily Henel adduced: "many are also possessed with such great error, that they regulate their journeying by the moon".[112]

The homily *De auguriis* is, as the title leads us to suspect, a rich source of references to superstition. The first mention of prognostication is:

> Likewise, he who believes in divination either from birds, or snores, or horses or dogs, he is no Christian but a wicked apostate. Neither must any one observe days on which day one travels, or on which one returns, because God created all seven days which succeed in the week until the end of this world.[113]

Ælfric is once more concerned with "cepan be dagum", a topic which he also introduced in the homily *Octabas et circumcisio Domini*. He opposed not only the observation of times, but also the observation of signs, which is evident from the phrase "wiglungum oððe be fugelum oððe be fnorum

[111] Henel (1942: 97-98). Emphasis is Henel's.

[112] "Sind eac manega mid swa micclum gedwylde befangene, þæt hi cepað be ðam monan heora fær" (Clemoes 1997: 229). See above for a discussion of this passage.

[113] "Eall swa gelice se ðe gelyfð wiglungum oððe be fugelum oððe be fnorum oððe be horsum oððe be hundum, ne bið hé ná cristen, ac bið forcuð wiðersaca. Ne sceal nan man cepan be dagum on hwilcum dæge he fare, oððe on hwylcum he gecyrre, forðan þe god gesceop ealle ða seofan dagas, þe yrnað on þære wucan oð þysre worulde geendunge" (Skeat 1881-1900: I.370/88-94).

oððe be horsum oððe be hundum". Ælfric's inspiration for mentioning both types of superstition comes from a sermon of Caesarius of Arles, a source which he used extensively in composing *De auguriis*.[114] It is, therefore, questionable to what extent Ælfric was merely copying his source, or commenting upon actual practice. The reference to the observation of birds is not unfamiliar, because there are three *hapax* glosses in Old English which cover the same subject.[115]

There is another type of observation of signs which belongs to the field of prognostication, i.e. dream interpretation. It will not come as a surprise that Ælfric's name appears once more in connection with this type of prognostication. In the hagiographic text *Natale Sancti Swyðuni Episcopi*, Ælfric relates the story of a bedridden old thane from the Isle of Wight. With the oneiric intercession of Saint Swithun, the man was healed, whereupon "he went very quickly to Winchester, and told the venerable bishop Æthelwold how he was healed through the holy Swithun".[116] Before we are to conclude that all dreams have oneirocritical value, Ælfric continues: "now it is to be known that we must not at all observe too much from dreams, because they are not all from God".[117]

In addition to the previous reference to dream interpretation, I have found four more examples. First, the uniquely attested "swefenrecerre" glosses "coniectorem" in one of the Cleopatra glossaries.[118] Second, another *hapax*, "swefenracu", is found in a note to Thorpe's edition of the *Confessionale pseudo-Egberti*: "on canone hit cwyð, se ðe halsunga 7 galdorcreaftas 7 swefenraca behealdað, þa beoð on hæðenra manna gerime" (in the Canon it says that he who practises divination, magic, and dream interpretation is reckoned among heathen men).[119] The Old English

---

[114] Meaney (1985: 477), Godden (2000: 52), Liuzza (2001: 196), Miles, Jayatilaka and Godden (2002: s.v. *Aelfric, Lives 17 (On Auguries)*).

[115] See p. 110.

[116] "he ferde.... to winceastre forraðe, and cydde aðelwolde þam arwurþan bisceope, hu he wearð gehæled þurh þone halgan swiþun" (Skeat 1881-1900: I.466/399-401).

[117] "Nu is to witenne þæt we ne sceolan cepan ealles to swyðe be swefnum, forðan þe hi ealle ne beoð of gode" (Skeat 1881-1900: I.466/403-04).

[118] Wright and Wülcker (1884: I.366/12).

[119] In the index of *Ancient Laws and Institutes of England*, Thorpe (1840: II) mentioned "swefenracu", and cross-referenced it to the *Canons of Edgar* 16, n. 2, erroneously so. The quotation is located in the *Confessionale pseudo-Egberti* 19 (Thorpe 1840: II.154, n. 4). The edition of the latter cited by Healey and Venezky (2000, bibliography search for Conf 5 (Mone) or Cameron B11.5) was not available to me. Spindler's edition of the *Confessionale pseudo-Egberti* (1934: 184/273-74 [19e]) does not refer to Thorpe's reading.

Confessionale pseudo-Egberti, more accurately entitled *Scrift boc*, is adapted from, among others, the *Poenitentiale Theodori*.[120] The Canons referred to (those of the Council of Ancyra?, *c*. 314) seem to have served as a model for all references to dream interpretation in continental and Anglo-Saxon penitentials.[121] Third, "swefen reccan" (in the sense "to interpret dreams") occurs once, in the Old English *Orosius*. Here, Joseph tells that he learned sorcery in Egypt, and that "he mihte swa wel swefn reccan, 7 eac þæt he of ðæm cræfte Pharaone þæm cyninge swa leof wurde" (he was able to interpret dreams very well, and also that he became dear to Pharaoh because of this art).[122] Fourth, dreams feature extensively in the Bible, especially in connection with Joseph and Daniel, who were famed dream interpreters.[123] Below, I list three excerpts:[124]

> (1) Gen 40:8: They [Pharaoh's baker and butler] answered: "we have dreamed a dream, and there is nobody to interpret it to us". And Joseph said to them: "does not interpretation belong to God? Tell me what you have dreamed".[125]
>
> And they said to Joseph: "we dreamt a dream but do not know any one who can tell us what it meant". Then Joseph said: "tell me what you saw".[126]
>
> (2) Lev 19:26: You shall not eat with blood. You shall not divine nor observe dreams.[127]
>
> You shall not eat blood, nor practise divination or interpret dreams.[128]

---

[120] McNeill and Gamer (1938: 243-44), Raith (1964: iv), Frantzen (1983a: 133-37).

[121] Cf. McNeill and Gamer (1938: 198, n. 102). See also Keskiaho (2004). See the *Poenitentiale Martenianum* XLVIII, (addition VII following) *Vindobonense b.*, *XXXV capitulorum* XVI.2, *pseudo-Theodori* XII.24 (Wasserschleben 1851: 291, 496-97, 516, 598), *Theodori* I.xv.4, *Cummeani* (*excarpsus*) VII.16, *Cummeani* (*Remense*) IX (Wasserschleben 1851: 201, 482, 504; Schmitz 1883: 537-38, 633-34, 652).

[122] Bately (1980: 23/29-30 [I.v]).

[123] Their fame extends to the attribution of alphabetical dreambooks to Daniel, and the alphabet prognostic to Joseph (see p. 96). More prognostics attributed to Daniel in non-Western sources are in DiTommaso (2005: 279-98).

[124] The translation of the Vulgate is taken from the Douai-Rheims version.

[125] "qui responderunt somnium uidimus et non est qui interpretetur nobis dixitque ad eos Ioseph numquid non Dei est interpretatio referte mihi quid uideritis".

[126] "& cwædon to Iosepe: Wit gesawon swefn, ac wit nyton hwa hit unc atelle hwæt hit behealde; ða cwæþ Iosep: Secgaþ me hwæt gyt gesawon" (Crawford 1922: 180).

[127] "non comedetis cum sanguine non augurabimini nec obseruabitis somnia". The King James Version reads "times" instead of "dreams".

[128] "Ne ete ge blod, ne ne gyman hwata ne swefna" (Crawford 1922: 296).

(3) Deut 18:10-11: Neither let there be found among you any one that shall expiate his son or daughter, making them to pass through the fire: or that consults soothsayers, or observes dreams and omens, neither let there be any wizard, nor charmer, nor any one that consults pythonic spirits, or fortune tellers, or that seeks the truth from the dead.[129]

Take heed that you do not practise magic, nor observe dreams or practise divination or vain incantations, and neither must you request the counsel of a witch or seek guidance from the dead.[130]

Notwithstanding the free translations into the vernacular,[131] the Old Testament is an important historical source of information on dreams in Anglo-Saxon England. The reference to dream interpretation in Ælfric's *Natale Sancti Swyðuni Episcopi*, the three Old English words for dream interpretation and the quotations from the Bible illustrate that the concept of dream interpretation was known to the English. Of all types of prognostication, this is the superstition most frequently mentioned.

References to prognostication appear to be almost exclusively the domain of Ælfric and the Bible. There is another group of writings concerned with this topic: the Anglo-Saxon penitentials.[132] These are largely based on older penitentials and continental sources,[133] such as the sermons of Martin of Braga and Caesarius of Arles. Caesarius's works proved a popular source in England, witness Ælfric's use of one of Caesarius's sermons for his *De auguriis*, and the (fragmentary) attestation of Caesarius's writings in sixteen Anglo-Saxon manuscripts.[134] Like the writings of Ælfric and Wulfstan, penitentials abound in condemnations

[129] "nec inueniatur in te qui lustret filium suum aut filiam ducens per ignem aut qui ariolos sciscitetur et obseruet somnia atque auguria ne sit maleficus ne incantator ne pythones consulat ne diuinos et quaerat a mortuis ueritatem".

[130] "WARNA ðe ðæt ðu ne gyme drycræfta ne swefna ne hwatena, ne idelra galdra, ne ne axa nane wiccean rædes, ne sece ðu riht æt deadum" (Crawford 1922: 354).

[131] The Old English translation of (1) does not reveal that dream interpretation belongs to God, while that of (3) omits the prohibition to let children go through a fire and preserves six out of eight superstitious practices mentioned in the Vulgate.

[132] I inspected several editions and studies of the penitentials, of which the following were helpful: Wasserschleben (1851), Schmitz (1883), McNeill and Gamer (1938), Raith (1964), Kottje (1980), Frantzen (1983a, 1983b), Körntgen (1993), Meens (1994).

[133] On the history and sources of the penitentials known (though not necessarily developed) in Anglo-Saxon England, cf. Wasserschleben (1851: 13-52), McNeill and Gamer (1938: 23-50), Frantzen (1983a, 1983b), Meens (1994: 30-36, 55-69, 289-91).

[134] Gneuss (2001: 48 [215], 73 [409], 92 [555], 93 [559], 94 [574], 95 [583], 99 [628], 108 [690], 109 [699, 710], 119-20 [800, 801], 121 [808, 808.2], 123 [814], 140 [914]).

of superstition. These injunctions may have originated on the continent or in Ireland, and found their way into English penitential literature.[135] Censure of prognostication is aimed at three types: dream interpretation,[136] *Sortes Sanctorum* and the observation of times.

The *Poenitentiale Theodori*, chapter XII [27], forbids a number of superstitions without attempting to provide any kind of structure: divination by birds is named alongside idolatry, magic, astrology and fancy dress parties on 1 January.[137] One particular type of divination denounced in this chapter is lot-casting: "if anybody consults *sortes* which contrary to reason are called *sanctorum*, or consults any kind of lots, or casts lots with whatever evil intent, or divines from them, he must do penance for three years, one on water and bread".[138] In fact, most medieval penitentials oppose the *Sortes Sanctorum*.[139] Finally, the Old English penitential forbids the observation of times:

> It is certainly not permitted for a Christian to practise vain divinations, as heathen men do (i.e. that they believe in the sun, the moon and the course of the stars, and seek divination of the times at which to begin their business).[140]

[135] Frantzen (1983a: 74).

[136] Condemnations of the observation of dreams and the *Sortes Sanctorum* are found in continental, but not in the Irish and Welsh penitentials, to my knowledge.

[137] Thorpe (1840: II.32-34) presented this as the *Poenitentiale Theodori*, whereas Wasserschleben (1851: 595-98) called it the *Poenitentiale pseudo-Theodori*.

[138] "si quis sortes habuerit, quas Sanctorum contra rationem uocant, uel aliquas sortes habuerit, uel qualicunque malo ingenio sortitus fuerit, uel diuinauerit, iii. annos pœnitat, i. in pane et aqua" (Thorpe 1840: II.33 [XXVII.12]), cf. Wasserschleben (1851: 597 [XII [27].12]).

[139] See Schmitz (1883: 327-28), McNeill and Gamer (1938: 41, 229, n. 66, 276 [28], 288 [VII (104)], 305-06 [37]), Raith (1933: 54 [IV.15]), Klingshirn (2002: 106-08), the *Capitula et fragmenta Theodori* (Thorpe 1840: II.84 [De incantatoribus, maleficis, et sortilegis]), the *Poenitentiale pseudo-Bedae* XXX.3, *pseudo-Romanum* VI.4, *Hubertense* XXIX, *Mersenburgense a.* XXVI, *Bobiense* XXVI, *Vindobonense a.* XXIX, *Sangellense* VI.17, (addition VII following) *Vindobonense b.*, *XXXV capitulorum* XVI.1, *pseudo-Gregorii III* XXVI, *Corrector Burchardi* LII, LVIII (Wasserschleben 1851: 272, 368, 381, 394, 409, 419, 428, 496-97, 516, 544-45, 643-44), *Poenitentiale Valicellanum I* CXI, *Valicellanum II* LVIII, *Casinense* LXIX, *Arundel* XCI, *Romanum* XXXVII, *Cummeani* (*capitula iudicorum*) XVI.1 (Schmitz 1883: 327, 379, 414, 462, 479, 665), *Egberti* VIII.1, *Cummeani* (*excarpsus*) VII.4, *Parisiense* XX, *Mediolanense* I (Wasserschleben 1851: 239, 481, 414, 707; Schmitz 1883: 581, 632, 684, 811).

[140] "Homini Christiano certe non est permissum uana auguria facere, uti gentiles faciunt, (id est, quod credant in solem et lunam, et in cursum stellarum, et auguria temporum exquirant, ad negotia sua incipienda)" (Wasserschleben 1851: 327 [II.23]). "Nis na

This penitential is an adaptation of the penitential of Halitgar, bishop of Cambrai (817-31), with additions from other penitentials.[141] The excerpt is remarkable in that it mentions the observation of times explicitly. The reading of Halitgar in Schmitz's and Raith's editions prohibits the observation of times, but in a different way: "Christians are not permitted to observe the traditions of heathens, ... either the moon or the course of the stars, or the vain delusion of the signs for building a house".[142] Likewise, the *Corrector Burchardi*, from Burchard of Worms (d. 1025), prohibits observation of the new moon to build a house.[143] I have not seen the observation of times referred to in any other penitentials but the *Corrector* and the Arundel penitential.[144] Whoever compiled the Old English penitential must have linked the injunction to an agenda lunary. Agenda lunaries list appropriate actions for each day of the moon. One of these actions is building a house, another to undertake business.[145] If the compiler had been unaware of the link between the injunction and agenda lunaries, he would not have changed the example from building a house into undertaking business. Halitgar's source for this particular injunction are the canons of the first Council of Braga (563),[146] one of which forbids astrology, as a counter-argument to the Priscillian heresy.[147] This decree, however, does not mention the observation of times, so Halitgar must have added this himself, after which it underwent a revision at the hands of the compiler of the Old English penitential.

---

soðlice nanum cristenum men alyfed þæt he idela hwatunga bega swa hæðene men doð, þæt is þæt hi gelyfen on sunnan 7 on monan 7 on steorrena ryne 7 secan tida hwatunge hira þing to beginnenne" (Raith 1933: 30 [II.23a]).

[141] Wasserschleben (1851: 40-52), Schmitz (1883: 565-73), McNeill and Gamer (1938: 295-97), Raith (1964: iii-iv, xxiv-xl), Frantzen (1983a: 133-34, 137-39).

[142] "non liceat christianis traditiones gentilium obseruare, ... aut luna aut stellarum cursum, aut inanem signorum fallaciam pro domu facienda" (Raith 1964: 30-31), cf. Schmitz (1883: 727 [IV.26]).

[143] Wasserschleben (1851: 643 [LIII]), McNeill and Gamer (1938: 330 [61]). The same chapter also preserves the reference to the sun, the moon, and the stars. On the variation between the contents of the *Corrector* in various manuscripts, cf. McNeill and Gamer (1938: 41-43, 321-23).

[144] Schmitz (1883: 463 [XCV]).

[145] The collective lunary in Tiberius A. iii (9.1/1), for instance, reads: "in domum nouam. intrare" (l. 105), and "omnibus rebus agendis utilis est" (e.g. l. 3).

[146] Schmitz (1883: 727 [IV.24])

[147] "Si quis duodecim signa de sideribus, quae mathematici obseruare solent, per singula animi uel corporis membra disposita credunt et nominibus patriarcharum adscripta dicunt, sicut Priscillianus dixit, anathema sit" (Barlow 1950: 108).

I have come to the end of a perhaps not comprehensive, but representative survey of Anglo-Saxon documentary sources pertaining to prognostication. Superstition was a major concern in the Anglo-Saxon church, yet prognostication received little attention. Ælfric and Wulfstan inveighed extensively against superstition, but only the former mentioned prognostication explicitly.[148] The sources which I have adduced are threefold: Ælfric's homilies, the Bible and penitentials.[149] All three have in common that their perspective on prognostication did not originate in England. In his homilies, Ælfric is known to have used older, continental sources on which he based, among others, his views on superstition.[150] Ælfric, however, was personally familiar with some prognostic genres at least.[151] Three types of prognostication were singled out in this section: dream interpretation, the observation of times and the *Sortes Sanctorum*. Evidence of the existence of the first two goes back to the Bible and patristic writings, but the third is an odd one out in Anglo-Saxon England. The *Sortes Sanctorum* had been known on the continent long before the English encountered them: the first text witness in an English manuscript is in St. John's College 17, from *c.* 1110; the earliest continental evidence dates from the fifth century.[152] This seems to suggest that references to this kind of prognostication in the English penitentials were copied from older sources without any regard for the currency of such superstitions in England at the time.

Attitudes towards Prognostication

Folklore or 'Mönchsaberglaube'?

If we are to believe Aldhelm, Ælfric, Wulfstan and the penitentials, superstition was rife in Anglo-Saxon England. The enthusiasm and fre-

[148] Ælfric seems to have busied himself with correct doctrine, in which prognostication cannot have been regarded favourably. Wulfstan devoted his efforts to making policy and placing doctrine within an administrative perspective. As such, opposing superstition in general sufficed.

[149] The popularity of these writings is illustrated by the number of Anglo-Saxon manuscripts in which they are attested. Cf. Gneuss (2001: 150, s.v. Ælfric, 157, s.v. Bible, 176, s.v. Penitential literature).

[150] Godden (2000: xxxviii-lxii).

[151] Ælfric knew the agenda lunaries and the three Egyptian Days. See pp. 98-101.

[152] See pp. 476-79.

quency with which superstition was denounced, especially in the Reform writings of Ælfric and Wulfstan, provides a picture of a clergy battling against hosts of astrologers, observers, diviners and magicians. Tempting though this image may be, it should be kept in mind that most Anglo-Saxon views on superstition did not originate in late Anglo-Saxon England. Furthermore, the frequency with which Ælfric and Wulfstan repeated themselves over the same issue (and in the same words!) makes it seem that they used stock phrases. The same applies to the penitentials, which are sometimes mere variations on a theme. The penitentials forbid *Sortes Sanctorum* whereas such prognostics are first attested in English manuscripts in the twelfth century. Likewise, Aldhelm's *De laude uirginitatis* mentions judicial astrology, a type of divination not practised in Anglo-Saxon England. These considerations serve to illustrate that one should not rely on documentary evidence alone.

Many types of superstition are literary phenomena, which is particularly true of prognostication, judicial astrology and magical rituals, such as incantations and formulae. Of these categories, prognostics are attested most frequently, but they are referred to least often in contemporary commentaries. Nevertheless, with regard to the presence of Apuleian Spheres and other prognostics in the computus of Vitellius E. xviii, Pulsiano wrote: "the intersection of secular knowledge and divine operation... at once provides a view of beliefs and practices and, given the relative frequency with which such prognosticative texts, charms, and remedies occur in other manuscripts, a sense, although at best still vague, of how commonplace and thus how embedded these beliefs and practices were within at least the monastic circle and possibly within the lay community as well".[153] Granted that the dissemination of prognostics reached a head in eleventh-century Anglo-Saxon England, and that Ælfric strongly forbade prognostication, who were the people most likely to have consulted prognostic texts?

People who believed in divination are called "stunte men" (foolish men) by Ælfric.[154] Moreover, these people are "possessed with such

[153] Pulsiano (1998b: 97).

[154] Clemoes (1997:229 / 162). A proximity search in Healey and Venezky (2000) elucidates that the phrase "stunte men" is an Ælfrician coinage. Ælfric's worries over "stunte men" went so far that they figured in his *Grammar*: "*corrigo* ic bête sume lêase bôc oððe ic stŷre sumum stuntum menn" (I emend a mistake in writing, or I correct foolish men) (Zupitza 1880: 173/9-11).

great error" that they ordered their life by prognostication.[155] Judging from the attestation of prognostics as written texts from antiquity onwards, such knowledge must be considered a literary manifestation. An indications of the bookish nature of prognostication is that text witnesses of one redaction of a prognostic genre can sometimes be linked with each other even though they may hail from different places. Moreover, these texts are sometimes so similar as to preclude oral transmission. Finally, all Old English prognostics are translations, and the texts resemble each other so closely at times that they must all have derived from the same translation yet are found in manuscripts hailing from different places. Thus, when Ælfric spoke of 'foolish men', he was in all likelihood not speaking of illiterate people. In fact, there are strong indications that these 'foolish men' must be sought in the religious establishment. First, the texts were copied in a monastic environment. Second, the manuscripts were kept in libraries accessible to monks in particular. Third, literacy was elementary in monastic, clerical and court environments, but not necessarily so outside these milieus. Fourth, the attributions to authorities and the verbal echoes in prognostic texts will have been lost on less educated laymen. Fifth, most prognostic genres are closely dependent upon a correct observation of time. The number of computi and calendars in Anglo-Saxon manuscripts testifies to an ecclesiastical preoccupation with timekeeping.[156] I could advance more reasons, but it is understood that the Anglo-Saxon prognostics are essentially a literary phenomenon.

The importance of natural science in the wake of the Benedictine Reform resulted in a corresponding interest in prognostics. Furthermore, it is in this period that prognostication is forbidden by Ælfric. This is a curious convergence of facts which leads to the conclusion that the transmission of prognostics was on the rise in Anglo-Saxon England during the Reform, as were the 'foolish men'. Prognostication was not the domain of 'Volkskunde' (folklore), which had its place among lay people. Rather, it was a manifestation of what Henel termed 'Mönchs-

[155] "mid swa micclum gedwylde befangene" (Clemoes 1997: 229/166). The notion of superstition as a persistent error is widespread. Ælfric's term "gedwylde" signifies an error of a religious nature, while Singer's many denouncements of Anglo-Saxon medicine and prognostication are accusations of an error of primitiveness.

[156] Granted that farmers must also observe proper times for sowing, harvesting and so on, these times are seasonal and readily observable, and less dependent upon times arbitrarily arrived at, such as Egyptian Days (or Easter for that matter).

aberglaube' (monkish superstition).[157] Henel contrasted this type of learned superstition with folklore and advanced the notion that prognostication must have received considerable clerical support despite resistance from people such as Ælfric.[158] This is indeed true if we consider the large corpus of prognostic texts that has come down to us from the eleventh century, and the fact that manuscripts connected with churchmen such as Wulfstan II, Leofric, Ælfwine and Byrhtferth contain collections of prognostics.[159] Ælfric, then, responded to a development in superstitious practices which had become topical in his own time, and which was an integral part of the learning prevalent in England during the Benedictine Reform.[160] The 'foolish men' may have been Ælfric's fellow brethren, and should certainly not be sought among the laymen of Anglo-Saxon England.[161] In this respect, it is a strange irony to see that some of the scribes who copied Ælfric's works must have been 'foolish men' themselves, because many prognostics are found in manuscripts also containing Ælfric's works, notably his *De temporibus anni*.[162]

[157] Henel (1934-35). The word 'Volkskunde' was employed by Förster (1908a: 43-44) to avoid the connotations the term 'superstition' would have evoked in speaking of the prognostics. Moreover, Förster has argued that prognostication started out as a literary, learned phenomenon, which penetrated lay culture in the later Middle Ages. It is to be noted, however, that Förster's ideas do coincide with Henel's notion of 'Mönchsaberglaube' with regard to prognostication in the early Middle Ages and in Anglo-Saxon England.

[158] Henel (1934-35: 329-31).

[159] See p. 53.

[160] See pp. 88-92.

[161] Godden (1992: 150). Cf. Förster (1908a: 43-44), Henel (1934-35: 329-31), Godden (2000: 46), Liuzza (2001: 210).

[162] In the case of Ælfric's *De temporibus anni*, this need not be marvelled at, because this treatise is found in the same computistical context as many of the prognostics, e.g. Caligula A. xv + Egerton 3314, Tiberius A. iii, Titus D. xxvii and Vitellius C. viii. Henel already remarked upon the co-occurrence of prognostics and Ælfric's *De temporibus anni* (1942: xii-xiii). In addition, Henel (1942: xxxviii) recognised close links between those manuscripts contain both *De temporibus anni* and prognostics (Henel's manuscripts A, D, and E). Six manuscripts of English origin contain works by Ælfric as well as prognostics (Gneuss 2001: 67-68 [363], 70 [380], 73 [404], 74 [411], 77 [435], 100 [637]). One continental manuscript which was in England by s. xi[in], likewise features Ælfric's works and prognostics (Gneuss 2001: 91 [541]).

The Pastoral Hypothesis

Recently it has been argued that prognostics were copied not because monks or the clergy had any use for them, but because these texts fulfilled a pastoral function.[163] Despite the bookish nature of prognostics, these texts would then have been accessible to a very different audience from monks and churchmen, viz. the lay community. On the basis of current research, I see no compelling reason to credit the pastoral hypothesis with regard to prognostication, but since analysis of the pastoral functions of late Anglo-Saxon manuscripts is becoming more topical now,[164] and since some of these manuscripts also contain prognostics, I discuss the hypothesis here.

In a chapter entitled "Encouraged Magic", Flint has argued that 'Christian' magical practices, especially those dealing with sickness and health, were propagated to displace 'pagan' ones.[165] It is to be noted that Flint's 'Christian' magic incorporates the whole range of observatory, divinatory and magical superstitions.[166] Flint envisaged a clergy actively at work to prevent a pagan community from practising intolerable superstitions by replacing such practices with superstitions sanctioned by the church:

> These magical healing practices are transformed, in this light, from unwelcome remnants of a religion wholly to be dispossessed into welcome and amenable holders of a ground that Christianity wanted badly to annex, and to annex securely. They were preserved then, even cherished, in the English material, as residents of areas within which compromise

[163] Flint (1991: 301-328), Hollis (2001: 192-93, 197), Liuzza (2001: 209-10); Gittos (2005: 75).

[164] See, for instance, Tinti (2005), specifically the analyses of CCCC 422, part B, and Laud Miscellaneous 482 by Gittos (2005) and Thompson (2005), respectively.

[165] Flint (1991: 254-328).

[166] Flint (1991: 314-24). On the terminology of superstition, see pp. 102-07. Flint's terminology proves exceedingly vague. She used 'astrology' to describe lunaries (Flint 1991: 131-35, 145), while the words 'witchcraft' and 'magic' seem to cover the whole gamut of superstitions. This practice leads to bewildering statements (I have added the threefold system of superstition in square brackets), e.g. "when speaking of the rescue of astrology [i.e. divination], I suggested that contemporary witchcraft [i.e. magic] was the context for the compilation of lunaria [i.e. observation of times]" (Flint 1991: 321). Flint subsequently links this statement with the attestation of Anglo-Saxon lunaries, but such prognostics descended from a line of lunar prognostication antedating the Christian era. Lunaries are, therefore, not compiled under the influence of 'contemporary witchcraft', whether on the continent or in Anglo-Saxon England.

> was still possible, and as a means by which (like the *Sortes Sanctorum*) waverers, especially wavering leaders, might still be won over, bringing their followers with them.[167]

Flint concluded that this is how, among others, prognostication, was employed, viz. in pastoral ministration.[168] I object to this train of thought for a number of reasons. First, to what extent this echo from Gregory the Great's advice to Augustine of Canterbury was still applicable in eleventh-century England (the heyday of the prognostics), and exactly how untouched by Christianity the population was at the time, is a matter of debate. It seems to me, however, that the intensified pastoral ministration of the clergy following the Benedictine Reform, targetted local, Christian communities, which is, in effect, preaching to the converted. These communities can hardly be expected to have reverted entirely to paganism in the period preceding the Reform, despite the Viking raids and settlements. Second, the wavering (heathen?) leaders mentioned by Flint would not be won over by pastoral work, but by missionary activity. Third, Flint sees a polarity which relies heavily upon a happy coincidence: of the many superstitions available, pagans practise those which are most abject to Christians, while the latter propagate (not practise!) precisely those superstitions which are not practised by pagans. I cannot think of a way to justify a polarity as clear-cut as this one, in which one group of people has an intuitively bad taste, so to speak, and the other has not. Fourth, one would expect a prognostic vocabulary in the vernacular to have come into existence, and this did not happen.[169] Fifth, clerical opposition to superstition covered the whole range of superstitious practices,[170] except that on which Christianity itself is based. To judge from the writings of Ælfric and Wulfstan, the laws and the penitentials, this opposition was a matter of policy, which makes it impossible for any promotion of 'Christian' superstition to be encouraged on the programmatic scale Flint suggests. Her example of the *Sortes Sanctorum* in the quotation above is particularly ill-chosen because lot-casting, notably the *Sortes Sanctorum*, were condemned explicitly in the penitentials.[171] In addition, text witnesses of the *Sortes Sanctorum* have not been attested in English manuscripts before the twelfth century, which makes it unlikely that

[167] Flint (1991: 324).
[168] Flint (1991: 324-25).
[169] See pp. 113-14.
[170] See pp. 114-26. Cf. Liuzza (2001: 210).
[171] See p. 479. Cf. Hollis (2001: 193).

this type of lot-casting was known at first hand in pre-Conquest England, let alone that it was being propagated by the clergy on any scale.

An example of the workings of the pastoral hypothesis as outlined by Flint was first voiced by Singer and has been repeated uncritically by Jordan,[172] who wrote the following with regard to the Apuleian Sphere in Bodley 579:

> The figure [of Death] is part of a chart called the *Sphera Apulei* or the Sphere of Life and Death, which was used in the following manner. When visiting a sick person, the priest would add the numerical equivalents of the letters in the patient's given name with the day of the moon on which the patient fell sick and divide the total by thirty. If the remainder from this answer appeared on the scroll held by Satan-Mors the priest would administer extreme unction; if the number was held by the adjacent crowned figure of Christ-Vita... no special preparations were necessary, for the patient would live.[173]

The above description of how an Apuleian Sphere works is entirely factual,[174] but I have not found any reference to priests and extreme unction in the texts of the Apuleian Spheres, nor in any of the other Anglo-Saxon prognostics.[175] The framework of pastoral ministration added to the Apuleian Sphere is in fact a fabrication by present-day scholars.

As a thought experiment, let us credit the pastoral hypothesis. Contrary to what I concluded in the previous section, this would turn Ælfric's 'foolish men' into lay people, and the prognostics bookish tools for the lay community through the mediation of parish priests. The things to do are (1) to find evidence that the prognostics were meant for a lay audience; (2) to investigate which manuscripts may have been used in a pastoral capacity; and (3) to discover the role of vernacularisation.

First, it can be argued that some prognostics were not intended for monks or clergymen. What would a monk profit from consulting birth prognostics or year prognoses, for instance? A monk might profit from this more than we think: the income and supplies of a monastery depended to a certain extent upon the surrounding, lay community, so naturally the success or failure of a harvest was an issue of interest to farmers and monks alike. Likewise, the character of new candidates for the clergy could be gleaned from birth prognostics. Furthermore, Liuzza

[172] Singer (1928: 146). Cf. Sigerist (1942: 292), Liuzza (2005: II.29).
[173] Jordan (1986: 290, 293).
[174] See pp. 181-95.
[175] See text 2/10 and the other Apuleian Spheres.

pointed out that "many churchmen, after all, were born and raised in the towns and villages and farms of their own region, and certainly shared with their lay neighbours a worldview which included a belief in celestial influence on earthly life, the existence of days of various qualities, and a desire to use knowledge of such things to one's advantage whenever possible".[176] This means that monks and the clergy were just as curious about the future as laymen. Bloodletting prognostics, to give another example, might be equally important to the lay community and to monks and churchmen, because both groups would need medical assistance at times. A monk would benefit from consulting prognostics just as much as a lay person would. I even think that monks gleaned more from prognostics than parish clergy and laymen, because the learned nature of many of the prognostics could not be appreciated to the full extent by an uneducated or less educated audience. This learned aspect of prognostics is borne out by the authorities mentioned in some prognostics and the ecclesiastical preoccupation with elaborate methods of timekeeping displayed in both prognostics and computi. Conversely, it has in fact been argued that the authority of prognostics is not negated by a pastoral function, but that "their [i.e. the prognostics'] possible adoption as part of the pastoral duties of the monastic priest working amongst the laity, or the parish priest himself, illustrates their utility and authority within a Christian context".[177] There is some truth in this perspective, but as it hinges precisely on the debatable pastoral functions of prognostication, I find it hard to credit.

Second, if a claim for a pastoral use of prognostics is not necessarily substantiated by the texts themselves, the text carriers must be taken into account. In a lucid analysis of the pastoral functions of the Red Book of Darley (CCCC 422, part B), Gittos has argued that "even vernacular medical remedies and prognostics are at last recognised as having a place in the highest churches in the land".[178] She wrote this to indicate that the vernacular is a respectable language of learning in its own right in late Anglo-Saxon England, yet it inadvertently weakens the case for the use of prognostics in a pastoral capacity. When the "medical remedies and prognostics" referred to are in Old English, does this mean that they are representative of monastic learning in the vernacular "in the highest churches in the land" (i.e. prognostics as a literary manifestation

[176] Liuzza (2001: 209).
[177] Treharne and Pulsiano (2001: 7).
[178] Gittos (2005: 75). Gittos referred to Liuzza (2001).

of learning), or are these same texts, some of which are in CCCC 422, used in a pastoral capacity? While the vernacular may be relevant for the liturgical texts, such as masses, rites and blessings, this is not evidently so for the prognostics in CCCC 422. This is precisely the problem in the analysis of the function and intended uses of manuscripts: instead of a holistic approach, certain categories of text material are singled out.[179] In the case of CCCC 422, the texts pertaining to the liturgy of the parish church are singled out, but what about prognostics, the calendar and the Easter tables on pages 27-49? Were these primarily intended to be shared with the parish community, or were they the tools with which the parish priest verified the passage of time to ascertain that he followed the liturgy properly. Psalters, office books prayer books, sacramentaries, confessionals and penitentials are of immense value to the study of pastoral ministry, but prognostics in such manuscripts often appear in small numbers (e.g. in calendars) or are isolated from the material that was primarily intended pastorally, viz. either in the computus or in prognostic sections (e.g. CCCC 391, Titus D. xxvi, xxvii, Vitellius E. xviii).

With the preceding in mind, let us see which manuscripts are viable pastoral volumes. Hollis discerned five manuscripts which she linked to pastoral ministry, to wit: CCCC 422, Titus D. xxvi, xxvii, Vespasian D. xiv, Vitellius E. xviii and Hatton 115.[180] She categorised Caligula A. xv, Tiberius A. iii and Harley 3271 as manuscripts used in the education of priests.[181] Liuzza, on the other hand, distinguished CCCC 391, CCCC 422 and Titus D. xxvi, xxvii as devotional manuscripts, and Tiberius A. iii as representative of manuscripts employed in pastoral ministry.[182] Of the devotional manuscripts, Liuzza wrote that their "primary use appears to have been securely within the monastic walls".[183] A comparison between Hollis's and Liuzza's lists illustrates that there is as yet no agreement on the function of the above manuscripts.

In speaking of the relevance of pastoral manuscripts with reference to prognostics, one should take into account the type of manuscript and the immediate context of the prognostics. Manuscripts such as CCCC 422, Titus D. xxvii and Vitellius E. xviii feature prognostics in the computus.

---

[179] Obviously, this makes research on the prognostics difficult as well, which is why I analysed the prognostics in their immediate context rather than in the light of the manuscripts in their entirety.

[180] Hollis (2001: 191-93).

[181] Hollis (2001: 193).

[182] Liuzza (2001: 209-10)

[183] Liuzza (2001: 210).

It can be justified that a priest would use prayers for pastoral purposes, but would this priest also explain the foundations of time reckoning to a lay audience, and at the same time communicate the prognostics present in the computus? Vespasian D. xiv and Hatton 115 contain homilies and prognostics in Old English, which would make these manuscripts likely candidates for pastoral work. In Vespasian D. xiv, the prognostics were added at the slightly later date perhaps for a very different, utilitarian, purpose, though: to fill blank spaces.[184] Moreover, the manuscript "does not show obvious signs of having been used in this way [i.e. in pastoral ministry]".[185] Hatton 115 can be disqualified for a different reason: the manuscript as it is now did not exist as such in the twelfth century.[186] The prognostic section (booklet 5) was copied in the middle of the twelfth century (in Christ Church, Canterbury?) and was bound with four homiletic booklets in Worcester, probably in the first half of the thirteenth century. The twelfth-century pastoral manuscript Hatton 115 advanced by Hollis, then, did not exist.[187]

Liuzza mentioned "collections of prognostics" such as those in Tiberius A. iii associated with pastoral ministry.[188] This volume has been described as a reference book containing texts of, among others, religious instruction.[189] The manuscript itself may not have functioned in a pastoral capacity at all but as an instructional manuscript for monks or clergymen. Scragg emphasised that Tiberius A. iii is a monastic production, while "the audience intended for such material [viz. prognostics] is much harder to assess".[190] Among the devotional manuscripts listed by Liuzza are two which are numbered among the pastoral manuscripts by Hollis: CCCC 422 and Titus D. xxvii.[191] The remaining volumes are Titus D. xxvi and CCCC 391.[192] If I were to select pastoral manuscripts which contain prognostics that may actually have had a pastoral func-

[184] See p. 46.

[185] Treharne (2001: 410).

[186] See pp. 50-51.

[187] Hollis (2001: 193).

[188] Liuzza (2001: 209). I acknowledge that Liuzza did not explicitly link this manuscript with pastoral ministry.

[189] Budny (1997: I.631-32). See also pp. 53-57.

[190] Scragg (2001: 275). In the same volume, Treharne and Pulsiano (2001: 7) also referred to Tiberius A. iii as a "monastic manuscript".

[191] The unlikelihood of prognostics in the computus being used for pastoral work has been pointed out.

[192] The former is a pastoral manuscript according to Hollis, while she does not mention the latter.

tion as well, CCCC 391 would have been my only choice on the following grounds. In contrast to those in Titus D. xxvi, the prognostics in CCCC 391 are in Old English, which makes it easier to communicate them to a lay audience. Moreover, the prognostics are conveniently gathered together in a prognostic section, and not scattered throughout the computus. Finally, it has been suggested that CCCC 391 was used in a pastoral capacity by Wulfstan II.[193] However, as definitive support for the pastoral function of CCCC 391 is lacking, and since I consider prognostic sections the effort of collectors rather than of pastoral workers,[194] I exclude even this one manuscript.

Third, another aspect of the pastoral hypothesis is that it hinges on language as a means to reach a lay audience. Such an audience would hardly have benefited from instruction in Latin. The Benedictine Reform made the vernacular, if not an alternative to Latin, a feasible step on the way to learning in Latin at least, as appears from the large output of scientific writings in Old English in this period. In the eleventh century, Latin prognostics are being glossed and translated into Old English. Translations of prognostics must have had a purpose and a prospective audience. It is tempting to ascribe this development to pastoral ministration and a lay audience, but before I do so, let us look at the evidence. During the Benedictine Reform, new monasteries were founded and Benedictine monks and oblates replaced a secularised clergy in old foundations where monastic life had declined. It was in the places mentioned last that prognostics gained their popularity, i.e. in a predominantly monastic setting. In other words, monks copied and translated the texts. Apart from booklet 5 of Hatton 115, there are hardly any indications that manuscripts containing prognostics ever left the scriptoria in which they were produced. Some manuscripts containing prognostics in Old English, such as Tiberius A. iii, may have been intended for the instruction of priests. Moreover, computi in the vernacular containing prognostics in Old English may have been used in teaching time reckoning. However, since instruction in the vernacular was possible in late Anglo-Saxon England, selected material in Old English, such as computi and grammatical works, could be used for the education of monks, just as well as for parish priests and other churchmen who had contact with the lay community.

---

[193] But see pp. 51-53.

[194] See pp. 150-53.

In conclusion, a case for the pastoral hypothesis with respect to prognostics cannot be made. There is no incontrovertible support for the theory advanced by Flint. The arguments she proposed are tenuous and depend upon a polarity between allowed and disallowed superstition which may not have existed. It is clear from all kinds of sources (laws, homilies, penitentials, even Ælfric's *Grammar* and *De temporibus anni*), that superstition was proscriptively rejected by the late Anglo-Saxon church. This same church would hardly propagate 'Christian' superstitions to displace 'pagan' ones, which is a feature of the early missionary church, rather. I have put the pastoral hypothesis to the test, and found that (1) prognostics may have been appreciated at least as much by monks as by secular clergy or the lay community; (2) there is no compelling manuscript evidence which corroborates Flint's theory; and (3) the fact that prognostics exist in the vernacular does not prove they were intended for a non-monastic audience. It would require extensive research into the uses of Anglo-Saxon manuscripts and the mind-set of Anglo-Saxon priests and laymen to render support for the pastoral hypothesis when it comes to prognostication. Therefore, I maintain for now that Ælfric addressed the clergy as 'foolish men', and that the prognostics are a bookish type of superstition which appealed more to the monastic than to the lay mind.

Conclusion

In this chapter I have discussed the status of prognostication as a component of superstition. I have studied the use of authorship and verbal echoes in the Anglo-Saxon prognostics. These served to heighten the authority and credibility of the prognostics, while at the same time they are an indication that the intended audience of the texts must be sought among the educated. Next I discussed the concept of superstition in the Middle Ages. The threefold typology of superstition developed by Harmening has been introduced: observation, divination and magic. Prognostication seems to belong mainly to the category of observation, with branches into divinatory superstition. Strangely enough, the Old English vocabulary of observation and divination does not reflect the fact that prognostication is the only superstitious genre which is attested abundantly in Anglo-Saxon manuscripts. The larger part of the vocabulary is rare and/or found in glosses and glossaries. The terminology for judicial astrology, for instance, occurs almost exclusively in Aldhelm's *De laude uirginitatis*, but this form of astrology was not practised in Anglo-Saxon England. It has become apparent that, although superstition is a major concern in late Anglo-Saxon orthodoxy, prognostication was a type of superstition that did not receive much focussed attention. In fact, prognostics were particularly in demand during and following the Benedictine Reform. The final issue studied in this chapter is that of the intended audience of the Anglo-Saxon prognostics. Ælfric called prognosticators 'foolish men', and there are strong indications that these men were to be found among his own colleagues. This would seem to negate the pastoral hypothesis, i.e. the notion that prognostics were used in pastoral ministration. I have found no reasons to support the pastoral hypothesis.

CHAPTER FIVE

INTENDED USE OF PROGNOSTIC TEXTS

The prognostic genre has been relegated to such diverse disciplines as magic, medicine, arithmetic, or combinations thereof in the form of medico-magic and magico-medicine, or iatromathematics.[1] Recent studies of prognostics have allowed for a certain margin of functional ambiguity, but the medical basis of many of the Anglo-Saxon prognostics is still emphasised.[2] Since it is not my intention to provide a definitive answer as to the intended use of the prognostics, I discuss some of the uses prognostics may have had in Anglo-Saxon England. In this respect, it is important (a) to distinguish between actual use (signs of use of the physical text) and theoretical use (indications of possible use revealed by the contextual setting and type of prognostic), and (b) to distinguish between text-internal and contextual implications, and the opinions of scholarship. Below, I focus on three main areas: signs of use, function and context, and shape and context.

Signs of Use

It would be interesting to find signs of actual use on a page on which a prognostic is written. An example of this is in Vercelli, Bibliotheca Capitolare, MS CLXXVII (Arab. 42). Folio 143r of this tenth-century manuscript contains an Apuleian Sphere which actually seems to have been consulted.[3] In the right hand margin, a medieval person noted down the following two sequences: "iii xxi xxiiii xv xxiii v xv xxi v viiii" and "xxx xxx xxx xxx xxvi".[4] The first sequence presumably represents a proper

[1] The terms 'medico-magic' and 'magico-medicine' were used extensively in Singer's writings on Anglo-Saxon medicine. The term 'iatromathematics' was employed among others by Gundel and Gundel (1959) and Wallis (1995), and has found its way into accepted use in speaking of prognostics, see Liuzza 2005: II.29.

[2] See, for instance, Wallis (1995), Hollis (2001), Liuzza (2001).

[3] Sigerist (1942: 297-300). A reproduction of fol. 143r can be found in Sigerist (1942: 298, fig. 2).

[4] The second sequence actually reads "xxx xxx xxx xxx xx vi", with a line break between "xx" and "vi".

name, the second a reduction of the numerical outcome of the proper name by decrements of thirty.[5] On the basis of the first sequence, Sigerist reconstructed several possible names of the person who copied the numbers into the margin, the most likely one being Aldemuelus.[6] The second sequence shows that this Aldemuelus obeyed the instructions in the text of the Apuleian Sphere, "and gather this into one and divide by thirty and look up that which remains".[7] Aside from the discrepancy between the outcome of sequence one (141) and two (146),[8] which may be resolved by taking the day of the moon into account, these marginal notes establish beyond doubt that someone actually consulted the Apuleian Sphere in the Vercelli manuscript and lived to tell the tale, as "xxvi" is listed in the top half of the diagram.

Unfortunately, the example just given is not from an Anglo-Saxon manuscript. The only signs of actual use present in English manuscripts, apart from the copying of prognostic texts, are indirect and constitute emendations or alterations of, and additions to the texts. I list the more noteworthy examples. First, the Apuleian Sphere in Caligula A. xv received the following thirteenth-century(?) addition: "littera duplari. non uult nec bis num*er*ari" (double letters should be counted twice).[9] Moreover, yet another late hand added several scribbles to the diagram and altered the explanatory text.[10] A number was noted down in the margin, which may possibly testify to a consultation of the Apuleian Sphere, but which is more likely to be a correction of the text. Second, the bloodletting lunary in St. John's College 17 has undergone extensive revisions in a hand identical to, or resembling that of the main scribe. These revisions are not in the manner of emendations, but amount to a switch from a familiar English redaction of the text, to a redaction of which I have found no other representatives whatsoever. The original readings have been expunged and supplanted by new readings on the same line, e.g. "**L**una **xxviii.**[**N**on *est* bona.] `Ab .vi. usq*ue* sera*m* b*ona*´" (On the twenty-eighth ⟨day of the⟩ moon [It is not good ⟨to let blood⟩] `From sext to evening it is good´), where the reading in square brackets is

[5] On the working principle of Apuleian Spheres, see pp. 181-95.

[6] Sigerist (1942: 299). 'a'=iii, 'l'=xxi, 'd'=xxiiii, 'e'=xv, 'm'=xxiii, 'v'=v, 'e'=xv, 'l'= xxi, 'v'=v, 's'=viiii.

[7] "& sic in unum colligis & partire in triginta & quicquid remanserit respicies" (Sigerist 1942: 299).

[8] On which see Sigerist (1942: 299-300).

[9] See notes to text 2/3.

[10] *Ibid.*

the expunged original, and the transposed reading the new text.[11] Third, the Latin alphabetical dreambook in Titus D. xxvi has several interlinear emendations to the text. These emendations do not pertain to the contents of the dreambook, but to the language. Thus, "**I**n piscina*m* ce`*ci*´disse gaudiu*m* s*ignificat*" (To fall into a fishpond signifies happiness), and "**Q**ui `*se*´ currere non posse uidit: inpedictione*m* s*ignificat*" (If you see `yourself´ unable to run, it signifies hindrance).[12] Fourth, the first β-sequence in Harley 3271, folios 120v-21r, was so poorly executed that it was repeated in its entirety on folio 122rv.[13] Fifth, several 'nota' signs have been added in the margins of Bald's *Leechbook* in the early thirteenth century, also next to the tract on bloodletting that also deals with Dog Days and contains a moonbook.[14] Sixth, the text on the three Egyptian Days in Vitellius C. viii shows punctuation of a later date.

The examples above provide evidence that, after having been copied, these prognostics were perused at least once, though not necessarily in the Anglo-Saxon period. The reasons for modifying the texts vary: some were emended in view of content or language, some were overhauled completely, others were changed to remedy poor composition or were marginally annotated. There can be no doubt that the alterations were designed to improve the texts, probably with the aim to facilitate consultation of the prognostics, for why else would anyone revise, enhance or emend a text but to increase its legibility or facilitate its use?[15] Nevertheless, such changes are rather indirect signs of use, because there are no further indications that the prognostics under discussion have actually been used as predictive devices. As to the rest of the prognostic corpus, the fact that these texts have been copied in such great numbers testifies to their popularity, but direct evidence of actual use is lacking. However, it would have been a pointless exercise for these texts to have been transmitted without the express intent of consultation.

[11] Text 9.2.3/10, l. 28.

[12] Text 7/5, ll. 87, 137.

[13] See pp. 38-39, 61.

[14] Wright and Quirk (1955: 24-26), Ker (1957: 332 [264]), Hollis and Wright (1992: 213). Wright and Quirk, and Ker dated the 'notae' to s. xii/xiii.

[15] Ker (1957: xlviii) noted that "the old [i.e. Anglo-Saxon] manuscripts were valued and commonly consulted until at earliest the end of the twelfth century". The extensive investigations of Elaine Treharne have elucidated that the use of Old English was no marginal issue in post-Conquest England (Treharne 1998, 2001, 2003; Swan and Treharne 2000).

If we are to credit Ælfric's comments on prognostication, some prognostics, such as agenda lunaries and Egyptian Days, were quite well-known.[16] Moreover, genres relating to bloodletting will have been highly practical in a society where bleeding was standard medical procedure, so it is reasonable to assume that such prognostics will have been consulted occasionally at least. Whichever way these findings are interpreted, it must be kept in mind that indirect evidence of the use of Anglo-Saxon prognostics is the strongest kind of evidence we have.

Function and Context

I have shown that there are no unambiguous signs that the Anglo-Saxon prognostics have ever been turned to actual use. In view of the number of prognostics transmitted, this is somewhat puzzling. In the following sections, I try to discover how the context may throw light upon the intended use of prognostics. I do not think all prognostics should be treated alike, but that their use may depend upon the context in which they are attested.

It is perhaps instructive to sketch the chronological development of prognostics in various manuscript contexts. There are some prognostic genres which go back a long way into the pre-Christian era, e.g. alphabetical dreambooks, but aside from an Apuleian Sphere in a demotic papyrus of the fourth century and the appearance of Egyptian Days in a continental calendar of AD 354, not much is known of the early history of prognostics. In the eighth century they surface incidentally in continental manuscripts,[17] in the ninth century in larger numbers in continental medical and computistical manuscripts, and in English calendars. In the tenth century, prognostics find their way into English computi, and they are occasionally used as guest texts. The eleventh century is the age when prognostic sections are first attested, in England exclusively. Below, I investigate the shift from one context to another, after which I give an example of how the shift operated on the textual level.

---

[16] See pp. 98-101, 117-21.

[17] Some of the earliest text witnesses are in Vossianus Lat. Q. 69 (s. viii^{ex}: text on the development of the foetus and year prognosis) and Vossianus Lat. F. 96A (s. viii^{ex} or ix: twenty-four Egyptian Days), see pp. 223-28, 347-69, 491-94.

The Medical Context

The *Oxford English Dictionary* defines 'medicine' as "that department of knowledge and practice which is concerned with the cure, alleviation, and prevention of disease... and with the restoration and preservation of health".[18] This denotation is at most about a century old, but there is no reason to assume that the term 'medicine' meant something else in Anglo-Saxon times.[19] Many genres of prognostics, as diagnostic tools for health and illness, can be encountered in a medical context. This is borne out by the etymological relationship between the medical term 'prognosis' (πρόγνωσις), and the generic name of the observatory and divinatory superstitions under discussion, 'prognostic' (προγνωστικόν).[20] There is one important way, however, in which prognostics differ from (other) medical texts: the former cannot offer a cure for illness. At most, prognostics warn of impending health hazards—eating gooseflesh on the Egyptian Days, for instance—, or of situations which may necessitate medical assistance or precautions. Therefore, prognostics are not part of curative medicine, but of diagnostic or preventative medicine. I distinguish three mutually non-exclusive categories of medical prognostics: (1) prognostics of overtly medical intent; (2) prognostics which refer explicitly to medical practice; and (3) not necessarily medical prognostics in a medical context.

Browsing through the prognostic genres known in Anglo-Saxon England, it appears that the majority of these texts deals with illness and health. There are genres which primarily serve a medical purpose: those which are concerned with bloodletting (bloodletting lunaries, moonbooks, Dog Days, Egyptian Days),[21] those which deal with dietary concerns (regimens), birth prognostics, Apuleian Spheres and illness lunaries. These are indeed the types of prognostics mentioned most frequently in studies on Anglo-Saxon medicine.[22] In view of the many medical

[18] Simpson and Weiner (1992: s.v. *medicine* n[1]).

[19] Indeed, even an outstanding study such as Cameron's *Anglo-Saxon Medicine* (1993) does not offer a definition of medicine which does not agree with that of the *Oxford English Dictionary*.

[20] Simpson and Weiner (1992: s.v. *prognosis*, *prognostic* n[1]).

[21] The role of bloodletting as a medical procedure is outlined in Cameron (1993: 159-68).

[22] The following is a selective checklist of prognostics discussed in studies of medieval medicine: Payne (1904: 16-20): various prognostic genres with a focus on bloodletting prognostics (particularly the pseudo-Bede *De minutione sanguinis, siue de phlebotomia*, see pp.

prognostic genres, it is not surprising to encounter prognostics in a medical context. This is the case with continental prognostics, but the Anglo-Saxon prognostics only marginally feature in medical sections.[23] Despite the medical status of many prognostics, therefore, English texts seem to have moved from there to new pastures.

Before providing an overview of the opinions of scholarship on the medical status of prognostics, let us turn to the prognostics and their contexts. The bloodletting prognostics must have been put to medical use, as is sometimes reflected in the texts themselves. First, marginal 'nota' signs in Royal 12. D. xvii were entered against the bloodletting instructions of the text on the Dog Days, thereby implying that this part of the text deserved particular notice.[24] Second, in the same manuscript, the Dog Days are introduced as follows: "The wisest doctors taught that in this period [i.e. the Dog Days] no one should drink any [medicinal] potion or bleed his body at any time, except when it is necessary".[25] Likewise, the text on the twenty-four Egyptian Days in Caligula A. xv contains a reference to medical practice:

> The doctors of old wrote in Latin books that there are always two days in each month on which it is very hurtful to drink any [medicinal] potion or to let blood, because there is a time on each of these days that if one opens a vein on this time, it will cause death or protracted pain. A doctor knew this and bled his horse on such a time, and it lay dead immediately.[26]

The last quotation is all the more remarkable because it refers to medical experiment, while I have not been able to trace any reference to this subject in Latin analogues of the Dog Days and twenty-four Egyptian

97-98, 278-79), and Egyptian Days; Singer (1917: 110, 116, 120-21; 1928: 144-46): Egyptian Days, Apuleian Spheres, Dog Days in the medical sections of St. John's College 17; Smith (1919-33: I.70): a study on veterinary literature which makes mention of the veterinary aspects of the Egyptian Days (see quotation below); Grattan and Singer (1952: 38-49): Egyptian Days, Apuleian Spheres; Bonser (1963: 157, 265, 270, 296-99): Apuleian Spheres, birth prognostics, Egyptian Days, moonbooks, Bonser's chapter "Prognostic Methods" (1963: 288-89) is hardly worth mentioning; Talbot (1967: 20, 125-28): birth prognostics, prognostics in later medieval medical times; Rubin (1974: 64, 67-68, 142): Egyptian Days, birth prognostics; Jones (1984: 65-69): several genres cursorily introduced; Deegan (1987: 22-23): birth prognostics; Cameron (1993: 27, 161-65, 183-84): bloodletting lunaries, Dog Days, Egyptian Days, and some birth prognostics; Stevenson (1995: 50-52, 55): Egyptian Days and Apuleian Spheres.

[23] See pp. 44-45.

[24] See pp. 40-41.

[25] Translation of text 6/3, ll. 12-14.

[26] Translation of text 8.3/1, ll. 1-5.

Days.[27] Doctors, on the other hand, are also mentioned in the Latin texts on the Dog Days, e.g. "it is dangerous to accept a potion or let blood according to [the opinion of] doctors of old".[28]

Not all prognostic genres are medically inclined.[29] It is debatable whether brontologies, dreambooks, lunaries (except for bloodletting and illness lunaries), and texts on the unlucky days, for instance, serve a medical purpose. Moreover, there are only eleven prognostics in the corpus which are attested in a medical context, viz. about 6.3% of all texts under discussion.[30] Nevertheless, the meagre contribution of prognostics in medical sections is somewhat remedied by the number of medical prognostics in a non-medical context. The text on the twenty-four Egyptian Days quoted above is an example of a medical prognostic in a non-medical context. However, the fact that such texts of medical intent are attested outside a medical context (they move from a natural to a more artificial environment) may be relevant to the changing purpose these prognostics fulfilled.

Many studies have been conducted on the field of medicine in Anglo-Saxon England, and it is rare for these studies not to mention prognostics at all.[31] Cockayne was the first to present the larger part of the vernacular corpus of English medicine.[32] He edited a substantial body of medical literature and the majority of the Old English prognostics. Cockayne placed prognostics in the category of starcraft, preceded by volumes on wortcunning and leechdoms. The incorporation of three diverse fields in one study is indicative of the way in which Cockayne perceived these topics. The emphasis in his work is on the popular science side of Anglo-Saxon literature, a quaint, folkloric, vernacularised branch of learning

[27] See, for instance, the Latin text on the twenty-four Egyptian Days in Caligula A. xv, fols 129v-30r (the pages preceding the Old English redaction!).

[28] Translation of text 6/12, ll. 8-9. References to doctors are quite common in medical writings, as Bald's *Leechbook* testifies to (see Rubin 1974: 99; Nokes 2004: 59-61). Nokes found it hard to justify the fact that the doctors appealed to in text 6/3 are anonymous, but then the Latin texts on the Dog Days do not identify the doctors either.

[29] With regard to many of the prognostics published by Cockayne (1864-66), Payne (1904: 17) commented succinctly: "but as they are not medical, I do not say more about them". The exclusion of prognostics from Payne's list of medical contents of Cockayne's *Leechdoms* is significant as well (1904: 36-37).

[30] See table 5.

[31] Getz's *Medicine in the English Middle Ages* (1998) is one of the few studies on medicine in which prognostics are not mentioned at all.

[32] Cockayne (1864-66).

at that, witness the title of his trilogy.[33] The folkloric views of Cockayne were succeeded by the 'medico-magical' or 'magico-medical' predilections of Grattan and Singer, which in turn made way for the ultra-rational approach of Cameron. All three views present differing opinions on Anglo-Saxon medicine, subject to academic fashion, and the English medical prognostics share this fate. The view held by Singer is that prognostics belong to a degenerate, medico-magical branch of medicine, which is epitomised by the phrase "a mass of senseless prognostications".[34] Cameron successfully tried to reinstate medicine as a rational branch of medieval science, going so far as to rationalise some of the more irrational recipes and charms.[35]

Wallis, Hollis and Liuzza investigated the Anglo-Saxon prognostics with ample consideration.[36] They took care to take the manuscript context into account, but they did not always recognise the implications of a changing context on the intended use of the prognostics. Wallis made the important observation of the transition of temporal prognostics and other time-related or time-structured texts from a medical context to the computus.[37] She called these iatromathematical texts, stressing both their medical and arithmetical side. Hollis distinguished several types of prognostics, including medical ones, and regarded the inclusion of prognostics in the computus a "'superstitious' analogue to computus study".[38] She perceived the difference between some of the contexts in which prognostics are transmitted, but calls all 'medical' prognostics medical irrespective of the context.[39] Liuzza, finally, offered a more balanced view, where texts in the computus serve a time-related function, and texts in a medical manuscript serve a medical purpose.[40]

[33] To what extent Cockayne promoted prognostics as a vernacular genre is apparent in his edition of the glossed collective lunary in Tiberius A. iii, "glossing a Latin text" in his words (1864-66: III.184). Cockayne's edition of the largest glossed dreambook, Tiberius A. iii, fols 27v-32v, is preceded by the casual note "the Saxon glosses some Latin" (1864-66: III.199). See also Cockayne (1864-66: III.ix-x).

[34] Singer (1961: I.xxvi); cf. Singer (1928: 144-46, 166; 1961: I.xxiv-xxvi).

[35] Cameron (1983, 1993). For an overview of opinions on Anglo-Saxon medicine held by Cameron and earlier scholars, see chapters 1, 12, and 13 of Cameron's *Anglo-Saxon Medicine* (1993: 1-4, 117-58).

[36] Wallis (1995), Hollis (2001), Liuzza (2001).

[37] Wallis (1995:107-09).

[38] Hollis (2001: 192).

[39] Hollis (2001: 197).

[40] Liuzza (2001: 196-209).

It is remarkable that prognostics are usually assigned an overbearing medical status, which obstructs ideas on other possible uses of these texts. If we look at the facts, the eleven prognostics in a medical context do not speak in favour of an overall medical status of Anglo-Saxon prognostics. Medical prognostic genres, in particular, were taken out of this context in Anglo-Saxon England, and incorporated in calendars, computi and prognostic sections.[41] Certain prognostic genres may have had an explicitly medical purpose, but in some cases this function was overridden by other considerations, such as the structure of the texts (in calendars and computi), the brevity of the texts (in a guest context), and the contents of the texts (through a general concern with the future in prognostic sections), as I demonstrate in the next sections.

The Arithmetical Side: Calendars and Computi

The medical status of many of the Anglo-Saxon prognostics has been discussed above, but there is another side to prognostics: an arithmetical component. This arithmetical aspect is expressed in the structure of prognostics and through the incorporation of prognostics in the calendar and the computus. All prognostics use a highly structured framework which serves as a formula for the interpretations. This observation applies to both non-temporal prognostics, such as alphabetical dreambooks and directional brontologies, and to temporal prognostics. The latter group in particular uses arithmetical systems by which the text is constructed, such as the thirty days of the moon, or two Egyptian Days per month. The importance of the arithmetical component is corroborated by the wholesale inclusion of temporal prognostics in the calendar and computus.

Calendars are rather abstract contexts in which bare numbers and events are recorded. The contribution of Dog Days and Egyptian Days, ferial days, seasonal markers and saints, is reduced to a rigid system which leaves no room for elucidation. The user of a calendar must be familiar with the theoretical background of the categories of information. The dangerous nature of Dog Days, for instance, is not explained in the calendar, but the period in which the Dog-star is visible is included in the calendar. Likewise, the Egyptian Day verses which often head calendars require some inside knowledge, otherwise a mnemonic line such as

[41] See pp. 29-33.

"Terc*us* *in* maio lup*us* e*st* & septim*us* anguis" may seem meaningless.[42] Consulting a calendar, therefore, is a matter which required (and still requires) initiation into the knowledge contained therein. Prognostics such as Dog Days and Egyptian Days, which assign fixed dates in the year, are particularly well-adapted to feature in calendars, because the dates can be taken from a text and can be entered directly into the calendar.

Once at home in the art of calendar reading, there is a practical side to calendars in that users have access to a wide range of data, among which prognostic material. To what extent this prognostic material was actually put to practice is a question hard to answer. The indications available argue as much against as in favour of practical application. Whereas early medieval calendars were in need of information to avoid a vacuum or blank space, later Anglo-Saxon calendars did not suffer from a lack of information, so prognostic material must have been included for a purpose.[43] Moreover, a number of Anglo-Saxon calendars had prognostic material added in the post-Conquest period, which means that such information was supplied intentionally. These two facts can be used to conclude that (1) a tradition came into existence which stipulated that calendars without prognostic material were somehow incomplete; (2) the purposeful introduction or addition of prognostic material into the English calendar probably meant it was to be used. A condition of (2) is that the user of the calendar knew what Dog Days and Egyptian Days are and what to avoid on these days. Although these two prognostic genres are the most popular ones in Anglo-Saxon manuscripts, it cannot be established how many of the users of a calendar recognised prognostic calendar entries and knew what to expect on these dates.

Computi exhibit a host of temporal prognostics through an accretive process, and through the transmission of prognostics from one computus to the next.[44] It is, therefore, evident how computi came to include prognostics. It is not clear, however, what purpose these inclusions served. According to Wallis, associative attraction drew medical texts of a diverse nature into the computus: "humoral physiology and pathology, prognostics, therapeutics, regimen, and herbal pharmacy".[45] Prognostics are here mentioned as a branch of medicine, but it should be realised

---

[42] Text 8.3/5, ll. 17-18.

[43] See pp. 26-29.

[44] See pp. 29-35.

[45] Wallis (1995: 111).

that medical texts need not be structured by time, whereas I have shown that the prognostics are almost without exception temporal in a computistical context.[46] The virtual absence of non-temporal prognostics can only be explained by the observation that time-ordered prognostics are favoured. This preference would seem to imply that the medical status of prognostics is ignored, because the emphasis had shifted from the content to the structure of the text. If structure were of no importance, one would expect to find in the computus non-temporal prognostics just as frequently as temporal prognostics. Remarkably, none of the catalogues and manuals of Anglo-Saxon writings perceived a connection between function and structure.[47] In this respect, it is instructive to consult Edwards's *Middle English Prose*, in which prognostics are discussed in the chapter "Utilitarian and Scientific Prose", not in the chapter "Medical Prose".[48]

The intended use of prognostics in the computus is open to debate. Non-prognostic medical texts contained in computi show that the computus may have been consulted for various reasons, including time reckoning and medical issues. Nevertheless, the exclusion of non-temporal prognostics and the emphasis on the structure of prognostics would seem to indicate that these texts specifically were incorporated on the basis of their time-ordered, arithmetical construction. This makes it hard to say anything concrete with regard to the practical use of prognostics in the computus. It is clear, though, that in moving from a medical context to the calendar and the computus, prognostics were no longer favoured because of their medical content, but because of their arithmetical structure.

The Utilitarian Approach: Prognostics as Guest Material

A marginal group of nine prognostics found its way into Anglo-Saxon manuscripts as guest material.[49] It is impossible to assert that these guest prognostics may have fulfilled a medical purpose, for the simple reason

[46] See pp. 29-33.

[47] See pp. 8-14.

[48] Braswell (1984) and (Voigts 1984), respectively. Please note that in the latest *Companion to Middle English Prose* (Edwards 2004), the distinction is less apparent as the two topics are merged into "Scientific, Medical and Utilitarian Prose" (Keiser 2004).

[49] See table 5.

that the context in which they appear is unpredictable and invariably non-medical.

A pragmatic reason to add guest material to an existing manuscript is to make good use of blank spaces. Such blank spaces may exist at the end of a longer text, which was the case in the Regius Psalter, Royal 2. B. v, where guest texts were entered immediately following the canticles, in at least four different hands. The first series of additions concerns a group of encyclopedic texts and a month brontology. Another possibility is the addition of texts on blank spaces of quire endings, as happened in Vespasian D. xiv. This homiletic collection in Old English boasts two prognostics inserted by the main hand at two different quire endings. These examples will suffice to indicate the process of adding guest texts.[50] Additions such as these served a utilitarian purpose, viz. to eliminate blank space. In addition, there may have been contextual considerations which led a scribe to add a particular text, but in the case of the prognostics, I have not been able to discover a link between text and context in terms of content. There are several practical constraints which determine not the genre of the text, but the type of text to be added. The most important of these are the brevity of the text, the language of the context, and the availability of texts which meet the former two requirements.[51] There are prognostic genres which fit this description quite well, so it need not come as a surprise that prognostics were among the types of texts entered as guest material. The primary function of these prognostics as guest material may have been more relevant than either their content or their structure.

Concerns with the Future: Prognostic Sections

The last context to be examined is that of the prognostic section. Over a third of the entire prognostic corpus is encountered in such sections.[52] This proportion is significant enough to presume some sort of deliberate intent on the part of the compilers of prognostic sections. Since the contents of manuscripts which feature prognostic sections vary, the larger manuscript context need not reveal the function of the prognostics con-

[50] See pp. 45-49 for more examples.
[51] See pp. 45-49, 67-70.
[52] See table 5.

tained therein.[53] A miscellany (Tiberius A. iii) will have served a different use from that of a psalter (CCCC 391) or a prayerbook (Titus D. xxvi, xxvii). Instead, let us examine the prognostic section and its contents in isolation.

Prognostic sections feature many different prognostic genres. Not only do they include temporal prognostics, as computi do, but non-temporal texts such as alphabetical dreambooks are also attested. In fact, many of the Anglo-Saxon non-temporal prognostics owe their survival exclusively to prognostic sections. In prognostic sections, medical prognostics, such as illness lunaries, occur side by side with all manner of non-medical genres, such as the sunshine and wind prognostics. Two types of medical prognostics are only infrequently represented in prognostic sections, viz. the bloodletting prognostics, and Apuleian Spheres.[54] If one were to make a distinction—which I do not(!)—between those prognostics which might be of more use in practice and those which are less useful, bloodletting texts would belong to the former category, and their relative absence in prognostic sections might be indicative of the level of intended use of these sections.

The flexibility with which prognostic sections incorporate both temporal and non-temporal prognostics illustrates that this context did not put any strong demands on the type of prognostic included. If the structure or type of prognostic does not influence its presence or absence in a prognostic section, what does? I have already argued that the only real constraint in prognostic sections is the language of the texts.[55] Beyond that, the selective procedure may have relied mainly on the discretion of the compiler since he chose which prognostics to include. For prognostic sections, these texts often turn out to be non-temporal or semi-temporal, such as sunshine prognostics, thereby complementing a taste for purely temporal prognostics in computi. Moreover, there is a relative lack of bloodletting prognostics in prognostic sections, whereas these texts abound in computi and calendars. These observations give the impression that prognostic sections complement the range of prognostic genres in the computus. It would seem, therefore, that prognostic sections are compositions arranged with meticulous care and insight.

---

[53] Nevertheless, manuscripts that feature prognostic sections seem to display a greater variety in genres, just as prognostic sections allow a greater variety of genres.

[54] The only notable exception to this are the prognostics in Harley 3271.

[55] See pp. 68, 69-70.

The density of prognostics is by necessity heaviest in prognostic sections, but the number of prognostics in these sections is also quite high. In other words, prognostic sections run to quite some length. Booklet 5 of Hatton 115 numbers eight folios, six of which contain prognostics. The prognostic section in CCCC 391 comprises nine pages. This may not amount to much in comparison to the length of a psalter, for instance, but it should be kept in mind that prognostics never enjoyed the attention that psalters did.

Prognostic sections allow considerable freedom in arrangement and genre selection. Nevertheless, some genres are attested significantly more often than others. Dream lunaries and year prognoses, infrequently found in other contexts, and brontologies and alphabetical dreambooks, not often found in other contexts and not at all in computi, are four genres prominent in prognostic sections. Although we do not today appreciate dream lunaries as much as an Anglo-Saxon audience would,[56] dreams have always held people's fascination. Knowing that we still use direct descendants of the dreambooks popular in classical times, the focus of prognostic sections on dreambooks is not unusual. These dreambooks may have known practical applications, because, unlike the arithmetical side to many of the temporal prognostics, there is nothing in dreambooks that could hold the attention of a reader but its value as a predictive device. Year prognoses and brontologies are bound by a focus on the weather as a predictive device. All four genres are united in their concern with directly observable phenomena, which is not the case with many of the prognostics prevalent in computi. Six prognostics are found exclusively in prognostic sections, viz. the semi-temporal wind and sunshine prognostics, the non-temporal prognostic on the colour of the moon, the temporal month prognosis, and the prognostics on the development of the foetus and the prediction of the gender of the unborn child. The latter two may have felt better at home in a medical section, but the fact that they are found in a prognostic section rather than in a medical context may be indicative of the multifarious role of prognostic sections. In addition, the existence of four non-medical and rare prognostics would seem to appoint a preservative role to prognostic sections.

Although prognostic sections allow for a great deal of freedom with regard to the range of prognostic genres they can contain, the preva-

[56] Without wishing to anthropologise, I do think the primacy of the solar calendar, and an increased reliance on artificial methods of timekeeping, does play a role in the waning interest in lunar time in Western-European society.

lence of certain genres does point in the direction of a programmatic, or at least systematic, approach to collecting prognostic texts. Earlier, I indicated that the transmission of prognostics in computi is, to a certain extent, a spontaneous process.[57] This is not so in prognostic sections, where some genres are favoured over others. Examples are the alphabetical dreambooks and year prognoses adduced above: three out of six extant Anglo-Saxon prognostic sections feature these two genres. Moreover, some genres feature repeatedly in a single prognostic section. The first prognostic section in Tiberius A. iii, for instance, boasts no less than three dreambooks and two year prognoses. Some prognostic sections do not show such a multiplicity of identical prognostic genres, but rather a diversity of certain types of prognostics. CCCC 391 includes four brontologies, but each represents a different genre. The preference for some genres, and the aim of completeness with regard to others, e.g. brontologies, testify to a taste for collecting prognostics, not only with an aim to gather a large range of prognostic genres in separate sections, but also to collect some prognostic genres in particular. This would indicate a systematic approach on the part of the compiler.

I have sketched an image of prognostic sections as compositions arranged with care and deliberation and with a collector's insight. It seems as if these sections complement the range of prognostic genres encountered in computi, because they repeat only a small part of the computistical prognostics, and they consist of a large non-temporal component. Moreover, the emphasis on readily observable signs such as dreams and thunder, and times, such as New Year's Day (for the year prognosis) and the twelve days of Christmas (wind and sunshine prognostics), point to the practicality and immediate usability of prognostics in separate sections.

TEXTUAL SHAPE AND CONTEXT

In the preceding sections, I have tried to shed light upon the way the context may have influenced the intended use of prognostics. As yet, I have drawn no conclusions because another matter requires discussion first: that of the relationship between the shape of a prognostic and its context. There are only a few genres in which context and shape are linked, but when this occurs, it also affects the reception of the text.

[57] See pp. 33-35.

Apuleian Spheres are absent in a medical context in English manuscripts, where the appearance of this genre is restricted to the computus. On the continent, however, Apuleian Spheres are attested in medical manuscripts. This is one example of how a prognostic is transferred from one context to another. For Apuleian Spheres, the phases in the transition from a medical context to the computus are lost to us, because the prognostic itself largely remains the same.[58] Moreover, there is no intermediate context through which it passed on its way to the computus. Therefore, Apuleian Spheres are not good examples to illustrate the relationship between textual shape and context.

Fortunately, one prognostic genre does change its appearance depending upon the context: the Dog Days. Texts on the Dog Days are found embedded in medical tracts, extracted as a set of dates in the calendar, as stand-alone texts in computi, and as stand-alone texts in prognostic sections. The development of the genre is displayed in this diagram:

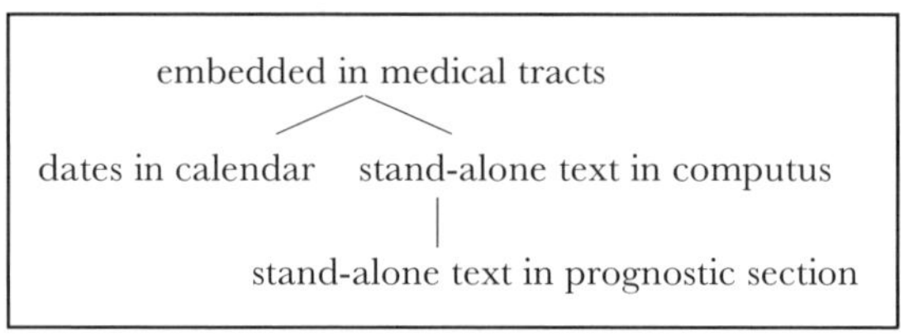

figure 2: Dog Days in context

In classical times, the Dog Days were known as a period in which disease was rife.[59] Therefore, texts dealing with Dog Days dictate hygienic measures to prevent illness in the period when the Dog-star is visible. These texts were intended as medical advice, and were often embedded in medical tracts pertaining to bloodletting, dietary rules and occasionally the humours. Therefore, Dog Days must be placed, in origin, in a medical context. English examples of Dog Days in medical tracts are in Harley 6258B, Royal 12. D. xvii and St. John's College 17. In the Royal manuscript, the prognostic is integrated into Bald's *Leechbook*, though it forms an individual recipe in a collection of consecutively numbered recipes. The other two texts were copied in the twelfth century: medical

[58] An exception is text 2/11 (in St. John's College 17), which consists of a diagram unaccompanied by the explanatory text and conversion tables (see pp. 30-31).

[59] See pp. 273-75.

tracts on the humours and dietary concerns do not seem to have been in great demand in Anglo-Saxon England.[60]

The Dog Days comprise a fixed period in the solar year. As such, they are excellent material to be reduced to a bare set of dates which can be transferred to a calendar. This is what happened to the twenty-four Egyptian Days in AD 354, and also to the Dog Days at some point in time. The transition shows how the medical knowledge of the Dog Days is turned into a calendric affair. There are no fewer than eighteen English calendars with Dog Days. In this format, the entire medical intent of the text is dropped to the extent that a bare set of dates is all that remains. Where the medical texts on the Dog Days may contain information on dietary and hygienic precautions during the Dog Days and the way in which blood should be let in case of an emergency, Dog Days in calendars dispose of the arguments and consist of three entries at most: one at the beginning of the Dog Days, one at the end of the Dog Days, and sometimes one introducing the appearance of the Dog-star. In contrast to the overtly medical redactions of the Dog Days, references to these days in the calendar are meaningless if the user of a calendar does not know what the entries refer to, or what one should do or avoid doing on these days.[61] If the Dog Days in the calendar are not just ornamental, seasonal markers, a certain level of in-depth calendric knowledge on the part of the user must be assumed. This, in turn, necessitates the typical user of a calendar to have been familiar with the medical background of the Dog Days.[62]

Finally, the information focussing on the Dog Days, embedded in medical tracts, was stripped of its immediate context, i.e. the tracts on bloodletting, the four humours or the dietary rules. This text, which focussed on the Dog Days exclusively, started to function on its own, sometimes accompanied by a moonbook, another prognostic genre.[63] Such distinct, stand-alone redactions of the Dog Days were drawn into the computus, as in Vitellius E. xviii and Titus D. xxvii, and thence into prognostic sections, in Titus D. xxvi and three times in Harley 3271. Texts on the Dog Days transmitted in the computus moved from this context into that of prognostic sections without any significant changes in shape. Prognostic sections are a final stage in the development of prog-

[60] See pp. 32-33.
[61] See pp. 147-49.
[62] See pp. 143-49.
[63] See pp. 276-80.

nostic contexts in that they are the last novel context for prognostics to appear in. The period in which prognostic sections were developed coincides with the heyday of prognostics in the computus, yet their intent differs in that computi attract temporal prognostics on the basis of their time-ordered or arithmetical structure, whereas prognostic sections are a phase of specialisation in which texts were collected on the basis of their common aim: foreknowledge of the immediate future.

The example outlined above shows that the textual shape of information on the Dog Days changed depending on the context: from an integral part of a medical tract to a bare set of dates in the calendar, or to a stand-alone text in the computus and in prognostic sections. The same prognostic genre may be attested in various contexts in the same period, as the Dog Days attest.[64] This coexistence implies that the move of a prognostic from one context to another does not prevent the older context from containing such a prognostic. It does indicate, however, that the intended use of such a prognostic varied, depending upon the context in which it was encountered.

The development from context to context can be witnessed in other prognostic genres as well. Although evidence from English manuscripts is lacking, the twenty-four Egyptian Days follow a similar route: from calendars to a medical context (or vice versa, in continental manuscripts), computi, and from there into prognostic sections (in Anglo-Saxon manuscripts).[65] Again, the textual shape changed depending upon the context. Most prognostic genres did not change their outward appearance, but still moved from context to context. At the same time, some non-temporal prognostic genres, such as alphabetical dreambooks, have no place in the computus or in a medical context and are restricted to a specific context. Remarkably, the only other prognostic genre besides the Dog Days which moved from a medical context to the computus and prognostic sections in English manuscripts is the text on the three Egyptian Days. The implication is that Anglo-Saxon scribes did not regard the majority of prognostic genres as proper medical material at all. I have already referred to the two medical birth prognostics uniquely attested in a prognostic section.[66] In this light, the traditional and widespread view of prognostics as medical, medico-magical or

[64] Dog Days are found in medical manuscripts, calendars, computi, and prognostic sections composed of the same period.

[65] See pp. 358-69.

[66] See pp. 150-53.

iatromathematical is untenable, that is, if these terms relate to the use of prognostics.[67] Rather, prognostics may adapt themselves in intent, if not in shape, to the context in which they are incorporated.

I conclude from the above that the majority of prognostic genres had a medical status, but that the intended use of the texts depended upon the context. The following stages can be distinguished: (1) a medical application; (2) an implicit application in the calendar;[68] (3) a structure-driven, time-related incorporation in the computus; (4) a utilitarian, space-consuming role as guest material; (5) a role in the collective effort at gathering texts dealing with foreknowledge of the future in prognostic sections. These various applications, however, may at most influence the chances of a prognostic being put to use. A guest prognostic in a homiletic collection, for instance, may have been included to fill a blank space, not as a predictive device. Nevertheless, it is unacceptable to rule out the possibility that if a prognostic was copied, this may have been done with the express intention of its being used, irrespective of the context. To copy a text in order to ignore its purpose entirely would be an act which goes against common sense. Even if prognostic sections were the work of collectors, these compilers must have appreciated the potential of the texts they copied or the curiosity which these texts elicited.

The influence of the context is twofold. First, it bears on the preference for certain types of prognostics in a certain context, which is evident from the presence of temporal prognostics in the computus, for instance. Second, the chances of a prognostic being put to use after its codification is also influenced by the context. A prognostic placed in a context which lends itself to frequent perusal has a higher chance of being consulted or read than a prognostic in some forgotten tome. In other words, if the setting is favourable, prognostics may have been consulted. Moreover, the context might push the reader of a text into a mode of appreciation which is not stable for that particular prognostic genre or type of text, but which depends upon the context as a whole.

[67] There is no harm in considering a bloodletting lunary as a text with a medical status, which is not the same as envisaging a medical use for every bloodletting lunary, regardless of the context.

[68] Implicit in the sense that the precautions necessary on the Dog Days, for instance, are not explained in the calendar, which presupposes familiarity with the genre on the part of the reader.

Conclusion

In this final chapter I have tried to elucidate the intended use of the Anglo-Saxon prognostics. I have done so on the basis of three criteria: (1) actual signs of consultation; and a possible relationship between (2) function and context, and (3) shape and context. First, there are no definitive signs of use of the Anglo-Saxon prognostics beyond changes to the text, such as emendations, corrections and additions. However, there are indications that prognostics were (intended to be) consulted. Three such pointers are Ælfric's commentary on the contemporaneous belief in some prognostics, the practical design that must be inferred when a text has been copied, and the changes made to existing texts after having been copied. Second, the context may influence the way a text is employed to such an extent that the emphasis of this text shifts. In the case of prognostics, the move from a medical context to computi and prognostic sections, for instance, may shed light on the intentions of the compiler. A medical prognostic may be included in a computus on the basis of its arithmetical structure, and in a prognostic section because it deals with the immediate future. In determining the intended use of such texts, therefore, the context should be taken into consideration as well. Third, in some cases, the context influences the physical shape of a text. This is clearly visible in texts on the Dog Days, which start to discard all kinds of medical knowledge on their way from a medical context to calendars, computi and prognostic sections. This change in shape is not a matter of preference on the part of the compiler, but purely utilitarian: a calendar can accommodate a set of dates for the Dog Days, but not a long piece on the medical precautions on these days.

CONCLUSION

When struck by a thunderbolt it is unnecessary to consult the Book of Dates as to the precise meaning of the omen.[*]

Prognostication in Anglo-Saxon England represents a brief but important phase in the history of the future. Prognostication is a practice which, in its codified form, dates back more than four thousand years. Despite their respectable age and everlasting relevance, the English prognostics from before the thirteenth century have remained in relative obscurity. The prognostics under discussion have been actively studied for a period of roughly a century, from the second half of the nineteenth century to the first half of the twentieth, after which interest in these texts flagged.

Prognostics have always been considered in the light of their status as either folkloric or learned texts. Förster viewed prognostication in Anglo-Saxon England as an exponent of 'Volkskunde' (folklore), whereas Henel regarded it 'Mönchsaberglaube' (monkish superstition). The opinions of modern scholarship are apparent through the place of prognostics in indices and bibliographies. Ker relegated prognostics to the realm of folklore, as did Greenfield and Robinson, and, arguably more importantly, the makers of the *Old English Corpus* and the *Dictionary of Old English*. The Anglo-Saxon prognostics, therefore, run the risk of misrepresentation until the next dictionary of Old English appears. Throughout this study, I have pointed at many indications that the prognostics are a form of science in Anglo-Saxon England: prognostics are codified; they contain learned allusions and appeals to authority; they were brought from the continent in manuscripts of learning; they were translated into Old English in manuscripts containing science such as the computus; they were gathered into prognostic sections in Reform manuscripts which may never have left the medieval scriptoria. In short, while Förster may be correct in assuming that prognostication moved into the field of folklore in the later Middle Ages and in the Renaissance, it was a form of learning of interest particularly to monks in the Anglo-Saxon period.

[*] Ernest Bramah, *The Wallet of Kai Lung*.

In order to investigate the status of prognostication, it is necessary to know what prognostics are. Therefore, it is rather ironic that none of the scholars who busied themselves with prognostics provided a definition. The meaning of prognostication apparently is self-evident, which makes it understandable that scholars continue to misinterpret prognostication as a form of folklore. With the help of the characteristics of prognostics known in Anglo-Saxon England, I have defined prognostics as a codified means of predicting events in the life-time of an individual or identifiable group of individuals, using observation of signs and times, or mantic divination.

Prognostics establish a causal or synchronic link between an event in the future and a specific sign or point in time. To accomplish this, they make use of a threefold structure which consists of the identification of what is to be observed, the subject of the query and the outcome. The subjects to be queried are varied but have in common that they pertain to and take place within the life-time of an individual. Popular subjects are health (especially bloodletting and the outcome of an illness), birth and death, the relevance of dreams, agriculture and the weather.

It is possible to categorise prognostic genres on the basis of their structure. Structural features have been used to organise genres into larger groups, but many of these systems are haphazard by being too inclusive, too vague, or by showing overlap in genre descriptions. Moreover, in the categories proposed by Ker, Cameron, Hollis and Wright, and, most recently, Liuzza, a core of prognostics is distinguished, and a number of texts placed are outside this core. This categorisation gives the misleading impression that some genres are more 'prognostic' than others. Of the many systems that categorise prognostics, Förster's is still most useful, because it merely lists the genres without trying to create an order of precedence or centrality. I have adopted this system and added the factor of (non-)temporality to each genre, which proves useful in explaining the manuscript context in which specific genres appeared.

Inspection of the manuscript context reveals that Anglo-Saxon prognostics were not written down at random, but appear in a limited number of contexts, to wit in calendars, computi, medical sections, as guest texts, and in separate sections. Calendars have come to incorporate entries on Egyptian Days and Dog Days, i.e. temporal genres which are structured by a system of concrete dates. As has been pointed out by Wallis, early medieval ecclesiastical calendars included extra information in addition to saints' days to fill up conspicuous gaps. Calendars from Anglo-Saxon and early post-Conquest England, however, tended to include prognostics out of tradition rather than of necessity.

The medieval computus, a system of time reckoning for ecclesiastical purposes, gradually drew in text genres which were not essential to time reckoning itself, but which testified to an interest in time keeping. This is certainly true for the Anglo-Saxon computus, because in this context no fewer than fifty-four prognostics are attested. Several types of computi were known in late Anglo-Saxon England, but it is striking that prognostics were not copied from one copy of a specific computus to the next. Instead, prognostics were transmitted vertically, i.e. between different types of computi. It is likely that non-computistical material was included in the computus if it came to hand during the production of a particular manuscript. Nevertheless, a certain degree of selection is apparent in the preference for temporal over non-temporal prognostics.

The presence of prognostics in medical sections is to be expected since many prognostic genres concern health issues. However, Anglo-Saxon medical sections rarely feature prognostics. The level of integration of a prognostic in a medical context depends upon the way in which it is incorporated. Prognostics embedded in tracts on bloodletting, for example, are usually more fully integrated into the context than a prognostic which was copied into a medical section without regard for its position or purpose. In comparison with medical sections from continental manuscripts, the English medical context is a poor source of prognostics. Some genres which occur in a limited context only in English manuscripts, e.g. Apuleian Spheres in the computus, are often attested in medical sections in continental manuscripts. Moreover, some genres, such as regimens, are rare in Anglo-Saxon manuscripts but common in continental medical manuscripts.

It sometimes happened that a scribe had some blank space left after a certain part of a manuscript had been finished. Such areas proved good environments for guest material, i.e. texts added at a later date to make optimal use of blank spaces. Guest texts need have no bearing upon the immediate context into which they are placed. Thus, guest prognostics may appear among homilies, in a psalter or a computus. There are no obvious contextual motivations which can sufficiently explain what type or genre of guest text was chosen, other than practical considerations such as the brevity of the text in view of the space available.

The final context is the prognostic section, a hitherto unnoticed gathering specifically designed to contain prognostics. These sections are an English phenomenon and may be linked to the Benedictine

Reform because the manuscripts containing prognostic sections were all produced in centres which played key roles in the Reform. No continental representatives have been found, and prognostic sections were unknown in England before the eleventh century. The rationale behind the existence of prognostic sections is obscure, but there are strong indications that they were consciously intended as collections of material dealing with the future. The range of prognostics that could be incorporated into prognostic sections is considerable, varying from temporal genres also present in computi, to (non-)temporal prognostics rarely encountered elsewhere. Prognostic sections often survive as independent units within a manuscript. Manuscripts such as CCCC 391 and Titus D. xxvi feature prognostic sections in separate quires, while the composite manuscript Hatton 115 features an entire booklet devoted to prognostics, a booklet which is totally unrelated to the others in the manuscript. Tiberius A. iii is an important manuscript because it has no fewer than two prognostic sections, the first of which contains a large number of prognostics in Old English, and in Latin with running glosses in the vernacular. Prognostic sections are the most important source of prognostic texts in the vernacular.

The transmission of prognostics in fixed sequences shows that sometimes these texts were copied in batches of which the content proved quite stable. These sequences were compiled on the basis of structural or thematic links, which is an indication that the makers of these sequences recognised the common features of a number of prognostic genres.

The transmission of prognostics in English manuscripts took place in Latin with or without glosses in Old English, and in the vernacular. The language of choice is not random or a matter of taste, but depends heavily upon the language of the manuscript context. The calendar is a Latinate context which does not allow for prognostic material in the vernacular. The only exception is the calendar in CCCC 422, which contains some glossed items, including entries for the Dog Days. The computus is fairly tolerant for prognostics in Latin, with glosses, or in Old English, i.e. if the computus in question is composed in the vernacular at least in part. Computi in Latin only do not allow the inclusion of prognostics in the vernacular. A number of eleventh-century computi contain computistical texts in Old English, and it is in these computi that prognostics with glosses or in Old English are encountered. Still, prognostics in the vernacular are a minority in computi as compared to ones in Latin. The medical context is very strict with regard to language:

prognostics in a medical context always follow the language of the context. Prognostics as guest texts generally adhere to the language of the context, although the Old English alphabet prognostic in Titus D. xxvii illustrates that this is not invariably the case. The language preferred in prognostic sections, finally, is independent of that of the immediate manuscript context. However, the language choice inside a prognostic section is closely adhered to. Prognostic sections are very important in that they are the only context in which prognostics in the vernacular and with glosses are more common than prognostics in Latin. Moreover, the majority of prognostics in the vernacular and with glosses hail from prognostic sections.

Most manuscripts containing prognostics hail from Canterbury, Winchester, Worcester and *Ramsey. Calendars and computi were mainly produced in Canterbury, Winchester and *Ramsey, medical sections and guest texts in Winchester, and prognostic sections in Canterbury, Winchester and Worcester. Prognostics in Latin were copied in all four places, glossed ones in Canterbury and Winchester, and vernacular texts in all places but *Ramsey. Prognostics were first incorporated into English manuscripts in the late ninth, and tenth centuries. In the eleventh century, they were copied on a large scale. The twelfth century saw a moderate decline in the transmission of prognostics. The facts with regard to language, place of origin and date point to a correlation between the incorporation of prognostics in computi and prognostic sections in the eleventh century, the vernacularisation of prognostics in the same period, and the Benedictine Reform.

It has generally been assumed that prognostication went against orthodox Christianity in Anglo-Saxon England, but there are strong indications that this is not the case. Several prognostics include references to authorities, which was intended to sanction the texts from a medical or religious perspective. In addition to authorities, verbal echoes were employed to link prognostics to a tradition of learning present in the *Wonders of the East*, for instance, but also to Ælfric's homilies.

With the help of Harmening's threefold system of superstition, it has been possible to define prognostics as observatory and divinatory superstitions: prognostics make use of the observation of times and signs or mantic arts such as the use of letters or dice. Therefore, they should be placed in the categories of observation and divination and do not belong to the superstitions of magic. A study of the Old English semantic field of superstition significantly shows that there are no Old English words which adequately describe prognostication, except for the verb "cepan". Moreover, most words for observation and divination are rare or exist solely as glosses. My analysis of the vocabulary of superstition has revealed that prognostication received only little attention in the Anglo-Saxon period, even though Wulfstan and Ælfric inveighed extensively against superstition. Homilies, the Bible and penitentials sometimes refer to prognostication, but none of these sources specifically reveals that prognostication was being practised in Anglo-Saxon England. It is impossible, therefore, to maintain that prognostication was in opposition to Christian practices in Anglo-Saxon times. In fact, it is likely that prognostic texts were popular mainly in a monastic setting during the Benedictine Reform. The audience for prognostics in Anglo-Saxon England is sometimes sought outside monastic libraries with the idea that prognostics played a role in the pastoral activities of the Anglo-Saxon clergy. However, there is no evidence that would support this pastoral hypothesis. Prognostics were just as useful inside as outside a monastery. Moreover, there is no agreement over which manuscripts also containing prognostics may have been used in a pastoral capacity, and even if such manuscripts can be identified, it is debatable to what extent the entire contents of these volumes have been used in pastoral care.

Aside from incidental additions and corrections, there are no physical signs that the prognostics have ever been used. The intended use of Anglo-Saxon prognostics has been explored to examine to what extent these texts were actually manifestations of medico-magic or iatromathematics. The intended use of prognostics should probably be linked to the context in which the texts are found. Thus, the medical context attracted prognostics which are overtly medical in intent. Nevertheless, most prognostics with a medical status, such as bloodletting texts, are encountered in contexts other than medical sections. This might indicate that the medical status of such prognostics was of secondary importance in view of other features, e.g. the structure of the texts (in calendars and computi), or a general concern with the future (in prognostic sections). Calendars and computi proved attractive contexts for prognostics. The incorporation into a time reckoning context may have come about by a concern with the often tabular structure of prognostics, or the temporal aspects which are prominent in most prognostics. The guest context does not reveal anything about the intended use of prognostics other than that prognostics were useful as guest material on account of their brevity. Prognostic sections reveal a concern with texts that deal with the future. Here, prognostics were not necessarily valued for their tabular or temporal aspects, because prognostic sections include a wealth of genres which are not structured by time and are not as rigidly tabular as lunaries. These sections are probably the work of text collectors.

The shape of a prognostic may be an indication that the function of the text in question was not invariably the same. Information on the Dog Days, for instance, was first embedded in a medical context in longer tracts on the humours and bloodletting. After this, the Dog Days were stripped of all information but their start and finish, in order for the genre to be included in calendars. At the same time, the Dog Days were taken out of the context of medical tracts and incorporated into computi and thence into prognostic sections. This example reveals that a prognostic could be lifted from its original context to other contexts, and that the demands of these other contexts actually changed the shape of the text depending upon what was considered relevant.

My study of the Anglo-Saxon and early post-Conquest prognostics adds new perspectives to what had already been discovered many decades ago by Cockayne, Förster and Henel. From the first substantial edition of prognostics by Cockayne in the mid-nineteenth century, knowledge of the prognostics took a flight in the writings of Förster. Förster's idea of the Anglo-Saxon prognostics as a form of folklore was countered by Henel's view of the genre as a form of monkish superstition. Regrettably, Henel's observations went unheeded. My book has substantiated that the Anglo-Saxon prognostics are indeed a form of 'Mönchsaberglaube' which gained an audience as a result of the Benedictine Reform. Moreover, the newly developed division of the manuscript context has proved its worth in analysing the placement of the prognostics, the language in which they were written, and the date and place of origin of the manuscripts in which they were transmitted.

Throughout this study I have regarded prognostics as a corpus of texts, but did the Anglo-Saxons do so as well? This is a difficult question to answer, but I would be inclined to answer in the affirmative. The purposeful introduction of prognostics into the computus is a sign that Anglo-Saxon scribes were able to recognise prognostics on the basis of their structure. The fact that temporal prognostics only were included shows the existence of a selective procedure. Furthermore, prognostic sections are indicative of an attempt to assemble a group of texts which share a set of distinctive features. Again, a selective procedure must have existed.

The co-occurrence of both temporal and non-temporal texts shows that prognostics were not gathered on the basis of their structure only, but that the compilers of prognostic sections knew that an alphabetical dreambook and a year prognosis, for instance, belonged to the same group of texts. Finally, the attestation of fixed sequences of prognostics in which texts were put together on the basis of structural or thematic similarities is yet another indication that the Anglo-Saxon compilers were aware of the common ground between these texts.

TEXT EDITION

The following pages contain an introduction to and text edition of the corpus of English prognostics which form the basis for my study. For the edition, I initially turned to existing publications of the prognostics, which I then compared to microfilms, microfiches, photographs and facsimiles. In December 2002 and April 2006, I was able to inspect all manuscripts in person from London, Cambridge and Oxford libraries, except for Bodley 579, which was not in a condition to be inspected.

Introductions to the Texts

The prognostics known in England before the second half of the twelfth century can be grouped into thirty-two genres.[1] These genres are here presented in alphabetical order. For each genre, the attestations are listed by language, library and manuscript (not in order of chronology or place of origin). Detailed information on the individual texts in the manuscripts can be found in appendix one. For each genre, I provide a full survey of the structure, aim and history in the descriptions.

The descriptions focus on the Anglo-Saxon and early post-Conquest period. An account of superstitious practices in the classical, pre-Christian period can be found in Jastrow, Gundel, Bottéro and Reiner.[2] The transition of prognostication from pre-Christian times to the early medieval period is obscure and still requires considerable research. The early and high Middle Ages are studied by Thorndike.[3] The introduction of Arabic judicial astrology in Western Europe is examined by Budge, Haskins, Thorndike, North, Hugonnard-Roche and Burnett.[4] Prognostication in the later medieval period is discussed by Wedel, Weißer, Braswell, Voigts and Kurtz, Taavitsainen and Means.[5] After the Middle

[1] See pp. 14-15 for a complete list.

[2] Jastrow (1905-12), Gundel (1907, 1927), Gundel and Gundel (1959, 1966), Boll, Bezold and Gundel (1966), Bottéro (1974), Reiner (1995).

[3] Thorndike (1923-58).

[4] Budge (1899, 1913), Haskins (1915), Thorndike (1923-58: I.697-718), North (1986b), Hugonnard-Roche (1996), Burnett (1997).

[5] Wedel (1920), Weißer (1982), Braswell (1984), Voigts (1984, 1986, 1994, 1995), Taavitsainen (1987, 1988, 1994), Means (1992, 1993, 1994), Voigts and Kurtz (2000).

Ages, prognostics were transferred to the domain of almanacs and folklore. This development is beyond the scope of this book.[6]

In researching the genres presented here, I have made use of a wealth of studies, editions and encyclopedic sources. The most relevant of these are listed for each prognostic genre under the heading 'literature'. In addition to the works mentioned, I recommend *Paulys Real-Encyclopädie der classischen Altertumswissenschaft*, the inaptly named *Handwörterbuch des deutschen Aberglaubens*, and Harmening's *Superstitio*.[7]

I have not tried to place prognostics into stemmatic relationships, but I do occasionally refer to redactions and versions. The term 'redaction' describes prognostic texts of one genre which share a number of features from which it may be concluded that they are related. Texts which diverge in phrasing, structure, vocabulary or content can be said to form separate redactions. Within a redaction, I speak of 'versions', texts which display small variation in, for instance, phrasing, but which have enough in common to form one redaction. I use no hard and fast rules to establish redactions and versions, but then I do not offer authoritative stemmas either. Therefore, my efforts in the field of textual relationships are to be regarded as indicative rather than definitive.

Edition of the Texts

My aim has been to provide a thorough description of the prognostic genres and a reliable working edition, i.e. an edition which is faithful to the texts as they appear in the manuscripts, but which is not burdened by exhaustive explanatory notes.[8] The working edition is neither diplomatic nor critical. I do not uncritically offer manuscript readings, yet this does not mean that I provide grammatically correct texts for this reason. Emendations, deletions and additions have been based on readings from

[6] Förster included many editions and references to the post-medieval folkloric almanac tradition in his articles on the prognostics (1903, 1908a-c, 1910, 1911, 1912a-c, 1916, 1921, 1925-26, 1929, 1936, 1944).

[7] Wissowa *et al.* (1894-1978), Hoffmann-Krayer, Bächtold-Stäubli *et al.* (1927-42), Harmening (1979).

[8] In view of the large number of texts and the amount of research that went into the introductions to the prognostic genres and the study, it has proved unfeasible to provide exhaustive commentaries upon the content, and the language, morphology and phonology of the texts themselves, for which I refer the reader to Förster's editions (1903, 1908a-c, 1910, 1911, 1912a-c, 1916, 1921, 1925-26, 1929, 1936, 1944).

other witnesses rather than on dictionaries and grammars, and have all been accounted for.

I have presented each text individually even if a specific redaction is attested more than once, because this does justice to the fact that each prognostic has been valued individually in the study. This working edition is the first ever to offer a representative sample of English prognostic texts in one volume, containing all prognostics in Old English, all Latin prognostics with Old English glosses and a fair share of Latin prognostics, from a wide range of manuscripts dating from the ninth to the twelfth centuries. Researchers are now in a position to consult these texts without first having to compile a small library of (outdated) books and articles.

Editorial Procedure

The original texts have been represented as closely as possible to allow for the demands that different researchers might have concerning the texts, and to provide the reader with a good understanding of the state of the texts when they were copied into the manuscripts. My main consideration has been to keep the text edition as free from editorial intrusion as possible. Editorial intrusion in the main text is limited to the transposition of displaced writing when this is indicated in the manuscript, and the addition of letters or words which were lost through accidental damage, all of which are accounted for in the apparatus.

If there are variant readings available from similar redactions or related texts, I have used these to shed light on obscure passages, mistakes or omissions in the texts in the apparatus. The Apuleian Sphere in Tiberius C. i, for instance, opens with: "**R**atio sperę pitagori philosophi que*m* apulet*us* scripsit. ut de quacu*m*q*ue* scire uolueris *u*e*l* *con*sulere".[9] From similar texts in Vitellius E. xviii and St. John's College 17, it is evident that the text should have read "Ratio sperę pitagori philosophi quem apuleius descripsit. ut de quacumque re scire uolueris uel consulere". Similarly, the weekday brontology in CCCC 391 has the meaningless collocation "becland begena" for "becnað landbegengena",[10] the latter being the intended form supported by readings from other brontologies

[9] Text 2/4, ll. 1-2.
[10] Text 5.1.3/1, l. 5.

of the same type. In each case the main text features the manuscript reading, the notes the emendations suggested.

It has not been my aim to correct the grammar of the texts, but I signal cases where scribes or compilers ran into problems. For instance, the three scribes who copied the texts on the Dog Days in Titus D. xxvii and Harley 3271 had difficulty in making sense of the final sentence:

> Titus D. xvvii, fols 22v-23r: "**A**utenticorum in his medicorum cohibentur diuersorum potionum dictione. seu flebotomatum usus adhibenda"[11]

> Harley 3271, fols 120v-21r: "Autenticor*um* in hís medicor*um* cohibent*ur* diuersor*um* potionu*m* dictione. Seu flebotomatu*m* usus adhibendi"[12]

> Harley 3271, fol. 122v: "Autenticor*um* in his medicor*um* cohibent*ur* diuersoru*m* potionu*m* dictione. seu flebotómatu*m* usus adibenda."[13]

All three texts were probably derived from a common exemplar. They were copied in the period 1023 x 1032, most likely in New Minster, Winchester. The scribe of the second text is the least critical towards his material yet supplies the correct reading "adhibendi". The scribe of the Titus text erroneously wrote "adhibenda", while the scribe of the third text initially wrote "adibendi" but bethought himself and changed '-i' in '-a'.[14] Similarly, the Apuleian Spheres in Harley 3667 and St. John's College 17 are copies of one exemplar, but where the former reads "q*uo*d si i*n* media luna co*m*putes", the latter reads "q*uo*d si in media luna co*m*pot*us* es", wrongly so.[15] Another example is the bloodletting prognostic uniquely attested in Sloane 475. The scribe who copied the text had little understanding of most of the material he copied,[16] and in the bloodletting text this is clearly visible. The text lists certain hours per weekday on which bloodletting is beneficial. The structure of the entries is "die... hora... bonum est". The entry for Wednesday, however, reads "**Die mercur .iii. h*or*a .iiii. & vii. x** bona e*st*", which gives the impression that the third, fourth, seventh and tenth hour are good.[17] It is

[11] Text 6/14, ll. 10-11.

[12] Text 6/19, ll. 8-9.

[13] Text 6/20, ll. 9-10.

[14] In a more logical order, the sentence reads "usus potionum seu flebotomatum cohibentur adhibendi dictione medicorum diuersorum autenticorum in his". Similar statements are found in 6/12, ll. 8-9, 6/21, ll. 10-11, 6/26, ll. 10-11.

[15] Texts 2/8, ll. 13-14, and 2/13, l. 14, respectively.

[16] See pp. 42-43.

[17] Text 4/1, l. 5.

likely that the scribe misinterpreted two of the minims preceding "hora" as hours (adding a third for some reason), whereas they properly form the inflection of the weekday: "die mercurii". Therefore, the text should have read "Die mercurii hora .iiii. & vii. x bona est". Confusion over the gender of nouns, as displayed in the bloodletting prognostic ("bona" versus "bonum") is also apparent in hexameter verses on the twenty-four Egyptian Days, sometimes even within a single line: "Aprilis decima est undena a fine minatur", versus "Aprilis decima est undeno a fine minatur", versus "Aprilis decimo est undeno a fine minatur", versus "Aprilis decima est undene a fine minatur".[18] Finally, medieval scribes do not adhere to the old rules for declining the names of the months in Latin, but generally employ the ablative after 'mense', and the genitive after kalends, nones and ides, but even so, variation is frequent.[19]

From the examples given above it is clear that scribes were sometimes faced with problems in understanding the texts and concomitant grammatical issues. In these and all other instances, emended readings and readings suggested by other text witnesses are supplied in the critical apparatus.

Presentation of the Texts

The edition of the text is presented in the main body of the page. Line numbers are supplied in the left margin, numbered by threes. The text is mostly kept free from editorial signs, except for transpositions (in apostrophes) and the insertion or indication of text lost through accidental damage (indicated in round brackets when the text can be reconstructed, or with raised stops when reconstruction is impossible). Manuscript foliation is presented in the critical apparatus. Manuscript punctuation, capitalisation and spelling have been retained.[20]

The texts are exceedingly simple in content and often consist of items in consecutive order which are unambiguous in content and structure. There are no complex sentences whose understanding would benefit from implementing modern punctuation or capitalisation. I have subdivided the texts according to their text-internal structure. This division replaces the need for imposing modern punctuation and capitalisation

[18] '-a, -a' 8.3/7,17,22; '-a, -o' 8.3/16,19,21,24-26,28; '-o, -o' 8.3/5,10,23; '-a, -e' 8.3/30.

[19] See, for instance, 3.1.2/4; 8.2/1,2; 8.3/12-14; 12/1; 15/3; 17/4-8.

[20] Cf. Godden (1977), Mitchell (1980). The *punctus elevatus* is represented by a colon.

because it brings out the internal order of the prognostic texts, the interpretation of which leaves room for little or no ambiguity. Word division has been modernised because it is often unclear from the manuscript whether compounds are written as one word or not. Moreover, some scribes practise a peculiar word division in which single words are broken up and the final syllable of one word is connected to the first syllable of the next.[21]

Most prognostics are structured in a systematic framework, such as the twelve months, the days of the moon, the weekdays or the alphabet. I have used this division to structure my edition, irrespective of whether the text itself is divided accordingly on the manuscript page or whether the text is continuous. In this respect, I have followed Förster, who edited a large number of prognostics.[22] In comparing existing editions, I noticed that the structure of the prognostics, an important aspect of the genre, was clearer in Förster's editions than in Cockayne's.[23] Cockayne, for instance, reproduced the entries for a dreambook containing 302 entries consecutively, which makes finding a specific entry an arduous task.[24] Förster applied a numbered structure to the same dreambook and thus presented a text that can be studied with far more ease than Cockayne's.[25] Whenever the manuscript presents the text as anything other than continuous (e.g. in tabular form as some lunaries do), this is indicated in the apparatus.

Abbreviations and ligatures have been expanded. Expansions are indicated in italics. Idiosyncratic abbreviations were sometimes employed for words which were used repeatedly in a single text. This practice is most widespread in dreambooks, where "getacnað" is soon abbreviated to "gē" or "ḡ", and "significat" to "s̄".[26] I have expanded the abbreviation "ł" to "*ue*l" in Latin texts and to "*oððe*" in Old English texts.[27] The signs "7" and "&" have not been expanded, except when they occur as part of a word, as in "surg&" for "surg*et*". Rubricated letters are indicated in bold type.

---

[21] For instance, the scribe of Sloane 475, fols 125-231.

[22] Förster (1903, 1908a-c, 1910, 1911, 1912a-c, 1916, 1921, 1925-26, 1929, 1936, 1944).

[23] Cockayne (1861, 1864-66).

[24] Cockayne (1864-66: III.198-214).

[25] Förster (1910: 47-70).

[26] See text 7/4.

[27] See Förster (1908b: 303, n. 2). In text 7/2, for instance, "ł" is used alongside "oððe" (ll. 14, 22).

Critical Apparatus

Despite the common practice to divide the critical apparatus into textual notes, lexical variants from other manuscripts, phonological and spelling variants from other manuscripts, and explanatory notes,[28] I have chosen not to make a physically layered system for two reasons. First, I have not made collated editions of the prognostics, so representing variants from other manuscripts does not apply. Second, most of the texts are quite brief, which makes a layered apparatus cumbersome. The apparatus contains information on damage and omissions when this cannot be represented in the main text; alterations and corrections by the scribe or later hands; and comments on obscure readings, mostly on the basis of related text witnesses.

Editorial Signs

⟨ ⟩	indicates editorial additions: dates to texts on the Dog Days and Egyptian Days, numbered entries to alphabetical dream-books, foliation in the notes, the presence of diagrams.
[ ]	indicates erasure or deletion through expunction: "[s]tan".
( )	indicates loss through accidental damage: "ni(ht)um".
< or >	indicates alteration: "ær] æ- < [h]". The alteration is italicized if it is not in the main hand.
` ´	indicates addition or alteration to the text. The addition or alteration is italicized if not in the main hand: "**B**`*i*´rru*m*". Apostrophes also indicate transposition from another part of the text when this transposition is indicated in the manuscript (which will be clarified in the apparatus).
]	follows a lemma: "winð] *read* wind" (i.e. the manuscript reads "winð", but one should read "wind").
~	substitutes for a lemma in the apparatus: "hoc] *read* in ~" .
. . .	indicates approximate number of letters lost where erased or damaged text cannot be read, e.g. "uolueris ···· nit".

[28] Cf. Gneuss (1994: 21-23).

1 Alphabet Prognostic

Literature

Brand (1849-55: III.336-38); Martin (1867: 348-50); Steinmeyer (1874); Schönbach (1875, 1890); Sievers (1875, 1877); Birch (1878: 507-09; 1892: 278-80); Tobler (1883: 86); Camus (1891: 205-06); Gaster (1891: II.57-58); Bradley (1897); Skeat (1897); Dieterich (1901); Bolte (1901-06: IV.276-341); Pradel (1907: 32-33, 70-71, 142); Schneegans (1908: 586); Salvioni, Subak and Schneegans (1909: 336); Förster (1910: 39-40; 1936); Heinevetter (1912); Wilhelm (1914-18: I.113); Thorndike (1923-58: II.294-95); Dobbie (1942: lxxxiii-lxxxv); Schmitt (1966: 195-96); Martin (1977: 18); Fischer (1982a: 7); Hunt (1987: 180, n. 127); Kieckhefer (1989: 88); Hollis and Wright (1992: 266); Kruger (1992: 8); Günzel (1993: 61-63); Epe (1995: 55); Liuzza (2001: 189-90, 220, n. 132); Haag (2003: 46)

Alias

pseudo-Joseph dreambook, dream alphabet, *sortes biblicae*

Attribution

medieval: Joseph

Branch of Superstition

divination: literamancy, stoicheiomancy (with letters), rhapsodomancy, bibliomancy (with books or the Bible), oneiromancy (with dreams)

Text

OE: 1. London, British Library, Cotton Titus D. xxvii, fols 55v-56v

Description

In the past, (1) has been called an enigma, which is an appropriate designation to this day. Little is known of the origin and purpose of this particular alphabet prognostic. The aim of (1) can only be stated in a tentative manner. The text is structured in the order of the Roman alphabet, the use of which implies that the text derives from a Latin exemplar, rather than a Greek or Germanic source.[1] Each letter is followed by a response. For instance, the response of the letter 'i' is: "commence whatever you want and it will be accomplished for you".[2] The response of the letter 'z' is an alliterative *Gloria*, printed as a separate text by Dobbie, and entitled

[1] Hollis and Wright (1992: 266) queried whether the runic alphabet was "employed as an organizing principle in prognostic texts". I have not come across any instances of such practice. It is not likely that a prognostic structured by the runic alphabet will ever be found, because this kind of superstition is essentially non-Germanic.

[2] Translation of text 1/1, l. 9.

"The Gloria II".[3] The *Gloria*, however, is an integral part of the alphabet prognostic in as far as it constitutes the response of the letter 'z'. This, and the fact that (1) is the oldest alphabet prognostic hitherto attested, is all that can be said with certainty.

(1) has received little attention. Most of our knowledge of the genre has derived from continental alphabet prognostics. Several redactions in Greek, Latin and the vernacular (Middle High German, English, Welsh, Old French, Sicilian) have been attested, dating from the twelfth to the eighteenth centuries.[4] Förster posited the following time-line for the dissemination of the alphabet prognostic: Greek genesis (seventh century at the latest), Greek redaction in Southern France (seventh to eighth centuries), Latin redactions (eighth to ninth centuries), vernacular redactions (ninth century and after).[5] Remarkably, the attested texts mirror this time-line exactly in that the vernacular redactions are oldest (starting with the Old English one), after which follow Latin redactions, and finally a sixteenth-century Greek alphabet prognostic. Text (1) is a translation of a Latin alphabet prognostic no longer extant, and is not an immediate descendant of a Greek original.[6]

A number of alphabet prognostics have introductions which instruct the reader to open a psalter at random, retrieve the first letter on the page and consult the prognostic to find the outcome of a dream.[7] Some of these texts are attributed to Joseph, which has led Förster and others to call the alphabet prognostic a pseudo-Joseph dreambook,[8] just as the ascription of the alphabetical dreambooks to Daniel has led scholars to regard these as pseudo-Daniel dreambooks.[9] Introductions that explain the use of the text are not found in the earliest witnesses: (1) and a twelfth-

[3] Dobbie (1942: 94). Dobbie (1942: lxxxiii-iv) acknowledged the fact that the poem is not independent of the entire text.

[4] Martin (1867: 368), Steinmeyer (1874), Schönbach (1875, 1890), Sievers (1875), Tobler (1883: 86), Camus (1891: 205-06), Gaster (1891: II.57-58), Pradel (1907: 32-33, 70-71, 142), Schneegans (1908: 586), Salvioni, Subak and Schneegans (1909: 336), Förster (1910: 39-40, n. 1-8; 1936: 234-37), Wilhelm (1914-18: I.113), Thorndike (1923-58: II.294-95), Thorndike and Kibre (1963: 740), Martin (1981: 15, 34, 36, 56, 58), Tschann and Parkes (1996: fol. 48r, art 16). For manuscript sources, see Förster (1936: 237-40 nn. 1-7).

[5] Förster (1936: 229).

[6] Förster (1936: 240 n. 6).

[7] See (Schönbach 1875: 81; 1890: 2), Sievers (1875: 297).

[8] Förster (1910: 39-40; 1936: 233), Thorndike (1923-58: II. 294-95).

[9] Alphabetical dreambooks (see pp. 290–96) are not to be confused with alphabet prognostics.

century Middle High German text lack such an introduction.[10] Therefore, these oneirocritic introductions may be later additions.[11] The earliest evidence of the use of the alphabet prognostic as a dream device is in the thirteenth-century Dorset manuscript Cleopatra B. ix.[12] Another thirteenth-century alphabet prognostic with a dream purpose explained in an introduction is in Digby 86.[13] Remarkably, this text is in Anglo-Norman. The absence of other early alphabet prognostics makes it difficult to substantiate an original oneirocritic use for this prognostic genre. Where Schönbach has reservations, Förster opined that (1) is "without doubt to be considered a dream alphabet".[14]

In 1936, Förster edited two Welsh alphabet prognostics which he claimed were intended for 'Psalterwahrsagung' (psalter soothsaying).[15] This notion is a marked change from his earlier appellation pseudo-Joseph dreambook. Förster now focussed on the intended use of the texts.[16] The late date of the explanatory introductions to the genre also obscures the rhapsodomantic side: the earliest witnessess of the alphabet prognostic do not explain how the text is to be used, whereas introductions from later redactions do. The latest view on (1), by Liuzza, agrees with Förster that alphabet prognostics were intended as *sortes biblicae*.[17]

Steinmeyer suggested that the alphabet prognostic was intended for casting lots: the letters were supposedly carved onto sticks which functioned as *sortes*.[18] He did not speculate as to the occasions on which these lots were used. There is no medieval historic, archeological or textual evidence whatsoever to support Steinmeyer's hypothesis, nor is there any indication in the text itself that it should be applied in this manner, although the Greeks are known to have forecast the future through astragalomantic letter oracles.[19]

Sortilege, dream prediction and psalter sortilege are not the only explanations that have been given to the alphabet prognostic. Sievers was

[10] Steinmeyer (1874).

[11] Schönbach (1875: 82), Günzel (1993: 61-63).

[12] Hunt (1987: 180, n. 127).

[13] Tschann and Parkes (1996: xviii-xix [16], fol. 48r).

[14] "unzweifelhaft als Traumalphabet anzusprechen" (Förster 1936: 239 n. 6).

[15] Förster (1936: 228, 232-33). The attribution to psalters relies entirely upon the instructions provided in later alphabet prognostics.

[16] Förster (1910: 39-40).

[17] Liuzza (2001: 189-90, 220, n. 132).

[18] Steinmeyer (1874). Cf. Bradley (1897: 683), Förster (1936: 231-33).

[19] Dieterich (1901), Bolte (1901-06: IV.276-341), Heinevetter (1912), Förster (1936: 230-31).

the first to publish (1), followed by Birch, Skeat and Günzel.[20] Whereas Sievers did not elaborate upon either the purpose or the origin of (1), Birch offered an explanation of its use which should be rejected on account of its highly conjectural nature: "[the letters] may be descriptive of a set of illustrations which had been prepared for an alphabet of illuminated initial letters".[21] The fact that (1) is a later addition to the manuscript, which had no more room left for a set of illuminated initials anyway, considerably weakens Birch's conjecture. Moreover, there are practical obstacles: how would one, for instance, effectively depict the response of 't' in an initial: "do not fear those who live in sin and intend evil"?[22] Günzel remained skeptical with regard to the oneirocritic attribution to (1) for two reasons: first, the aforementioned complication of a possibly late oneirocritic attribution which postdates (1); second, the syntax and subject matter of (1) differs compared to oneirocritic, continental redactions.[23] Text (1) has complete sentences with finite verbs, whereas the continental texts contain short statements. Furthermore, the subject matter of (1) is overtly Christian whereas the continental texts tend to reflect on life in general.[24] The continental alphabet prognostics, in contrast to (1), are in Günzel's eyes comparable to alphabetical dreambooks both in syntax and subject matter.[25] Despite these reservations, Günzel does not offer an alternative purpose for (1).

In 1897, Skeat published (1), under the title "An Anglo-Saxon Enigma". This title reveals his reception of the text: he proposed that the text is a riddle and that the letters of the alphabet are to be expanded to an applicable solution based on the sentence that follows the letter, e.g. "A⟨vis⟩. He gangeð 7 biþ his siðfæt gesund" (Bird: he goes and his journey will be safe), "B⟨onum⟩. God þu fintst gyf ðu hit onginst 7 þe bið wel" (Good: you will find good [things] if you proceed, and you will be well).[26] Still in the same year, Bradley rejected Skeat's interpretation, offering in-

---

[20] Sievers (1877: 189-90), Birch (1878: 508-09; 1892: 279-80), Skeat (1897), Günzel (1993: 121-22).

[21] Birch (1878: 507).

[22] Translation of text 1/1, l. 19.

[23] Günzel (1993: 61-63).

[24] *Ibid.*

[25] Hollis and Wright (1992: 266) noted that "the possibility of a connection with the alphabetically organized Dreambooks does not seem to have been explored". There are, however, no connections discernable between these two genres beyond those observed by Günzel and the fact that both are arranged in alphabetical order.

[26] Skeat (1897: 543).

stead a novel explanation: the original Latin alphabet prognostic integrated the letter of the alphabet into the first word of the sentence. Bradley reconstructed a Latin redaction, e.g. "Ambulabit, et salvum erit iter ejus" (He will go and his journey will be safe) for Old English "A⟨mbulabit⟩. He gangeð 7 biþ his siðfæt gesund".[27] A Middle High German alphabet prognostic exists which corroborates Bradley's idea, e.g. "D demut" (humility), "F vrede" (peace),[28] but Förster banished an alphabet constructed along the same lines from the corpus of alphabet prognostics.[29] A parallel to the alphabetical constructions advanced by Skeat and Bradley is found in the early tenth-century Durham, Cathedral Library, MS A. IV. 19. This manuscript received a number of additions, among which a text in alphabetical order focussing on biblical characters and Christian living, an issue also addressed in (1).[30] The Durham alphabet is structured in the same way as proposed by Bradley, e.g. "Adam is the first man created by God".[31] There are no direct links between (1) and the Durham alphabet, and there is no reason to assume that the Durham alphabet influenced (1), but future investigation of alphabetical texts such as these may shed some more light on their genesis and function.

Bradley thought (1) a *sors*, and he related alphabet prognostics to the *Sortes Sanctorum*.[32] However, the comparison is inapt because it revolves around forecasting by means of books, and the *Sortes Sanctorum* which were known in medieval Western Europe are not rhapsodomantic devices (although Greek ancestors of the genre were). Moreover, the Greek letter divinations use dice, but alphabet prognostics do not.

From the above, it appears that the purpose and usage of (1) remains enigmatic. It is likely that the genre is of Latin (and perhaps ultimately Greek) extraction, as all prognostics are, although affixing a date of ori-

[27] Bradley (1897: 683). Note the agreement between the Old English and a fifteenth-century Latin alphabet prognostic: "A significat prosperum iter et uiam felicem" (Sievers 1875). The other responses in this Latin redaction do not coincide with the Old English. Bradley already commented upon this.

[28] Martin (1867: 368).

[29] Förster (1936: 239 n. 5).

[30] Gneuss (2001: 49 [223]), Brown, Wormald, Ross, and Stanley (1969: 15-17). The alphabet can be found on fol. 88v. The text was added *c.* 970.

[31] "Adam primus homo factus est a domino..." (Brown, Wormald, Ross, and Stanley 1969: fol. 88v).

[32] Bradley (1897: 683). For a similar view, see Förster (1936: 231-32). The *Sortes Sanctorum* are described on pp. 476-79.

gin to this genre is impossible. (1) is as yet the oldest representative of the genre. The purpose of (1) is not clear: it has variously been interpreted as a means of divination by lot (either as lots to be cast or as *sortes biblicae*), a manual for illustrating initials, a riddle, and an aid in dream interpretation. The last suggestion has been put forward most often, which is why this text is included in the prognostic corpus. There is something to say in favour of an oneirocritic and rhapsodomantic application in that it is more probable for one or a few (intermediate) texts of this prognostic to omit an introduction to this effect, than it is for an introduction to be affixed to one text which is subsequently disseminated widely in many different languages.[33] Whether it is an intended ambiguity of the alphabet prognostic or not, I do think there is a riddling aspect to (1) which might appeal to readers who are not prognostically inclined.

Edition

1/1 London, British Library, Cotton Titus D. xxvii, fols 55v-56v/1

A. He gangeð 7 biþ his siðfæt gesund.
B. God þu fintst gyf ðu hit onginst 7 þe bið wel.
C. bliðnysse getacnaþ nis hit on þissum leohte.
D. Ne gewealdest þu þæs ðu wilt ne þu hit æfre fintst.
E. becume blisse ðe: 7 þu bist symble gesund.
F. tacnað deaþ fram deaþe on þyssum geare bide god godes.
G. þu scealt geðeon be þisse geþohtunge.
H. ð ðe ne biþ geseald þenc þu on oðer.

Each entry starts on a new line. Skeat (1897) and Bradley (1897) suggested that the letters of the alphabet stand for the first letters of Latin words, making this text a riddle or a puzzle rather than a prognostic. Skeat's and Bradley's solutions are given below (except for the letters 'f' *and* 'z'*, which lacked solutions).* **1** A *may signify Latin* auis *or* ambulauit*; both would agree with the Old English interpretation* | **2** B *may signify* bonum, *Old English* god | **3** C *may signify* caecitas *or* caelum. *Bradley translated the Old English into* C significat felicitatem non esse in hoc mundo. *The Latin text edited by Sievers (1875) has* C cecitatem cordis. *If Old English* bliðnysse *(*happiness*) is a mistake for* blindnysse *(*blindness*), a reconstruction along the lines of Bradley would read* significat cecitatem non esse in hoc mundo, *which would agree in spirit with the redaction printed by Sievers* | **4** D *may signify* desiderium, *Old English* wilt | **5** E *may signify* ecclesia *or* eueniet, *Old English* becume | **7** G *may signify* gratiam *or* gaudium, *Old English* geðeon | **8** H] ~ *may signify* honos, *which fits the Old English description; Bradley's suggestion* hoc *is less convincing* | ð] *read* ðæt.

[33] Förster (1936: 230) mentioned that no less than twenty-six alphabet prognostics contain introductions stating an oneirocritic and rhapsodomantic purpose.

I. ongin þ*æt* þu wille þ*æt* þe bið geendod.
K. beorh þe þ*æt* þu ne gange on frecnysse.
L. hera ðu god on ealla tíd þines lifes.
M. God þe gemiclað þ*æt* ðe forþ gespewð þ*æt* þu don wilt.
N. hylt þu ð to dónne ne bið seald þínu*m* dǽdu*m*.
O. ealle friðsumaþ god on eallu*m* his mihtum.
P. Gyf þu riht nimst nelt ðu wifes wesan.
Q. forþam micel gód is 7 nergendlic swyðe 7 þu fintst blisse.
R. forlǽt al ða syn.
S. þu bist hal gyf þu to gode gehwyrfst se sit hal 7 mihtig.
T. ne fyrhteð þa þe on synnum lyfiað 7 yfel þencað.
V. Blis seo ðe biþ geseald 7 weg on geweald.
X. Blisse 7 weg 7 éce líf.
Y. Býcna sibbe 7 gesynta.
Z. Wuldor sy ðe 7 wurðmynt   wereda driht*en*
fæder on foldan   fægere gemǽne
mid sylfan sunu   7 soðu*m* gaste.
amen::

9 I *may signify* initium *or* incipio, *Old English* ongin | **10** K *may signify* kaue, *Old English* beorh | **11** L *may signify* lauda, *Old English* hera | **12** M *may signify* magnificat, *Old English* gemiclað | gespewð] ~ ‖ ⟨*f. 56r*⟩ | **13** N] ~ *may signify* nuta, *Old English* hylt; *Bradley suggested Old English* nyle *for* hylt, *Latin* noli | ð] *read* ðæt | **14** O] ~ *may signify* omnia, *Old English* ealle | **15** P] ~ *may signify* probitatem *or* puritas, *which would fit the Old English description* | **16** Q] ~ *may signify* quaere *or* quoniam, *Old English* forþam | **17** R] ~ *may signify* relinque *or* renuncia, *Old English* forlǽt | **18** S] ~ *may signify* salus *or* saluus, *Old English* hal | **19** T] ~ *may signify* timete *or* terrebit, *Old English* fyrhteð | **20** V] ~ *may signify* uita, *which would fit the Old English description* | Blis seo] ~ *may be a mistake for* Blisse; *the manuscript reading* Blis seo *is grammatically correct, but the sequence of a noun followed by its demonstrative pronoun is awkward* | **21** X] ~ *may signify* Christus, *which would fit the Old English description* | **22** Y] ~ *may signify* ymnus *according to Skeat, which seems reasonable* | Býcna] *read* Býcnað | **23-26** Z] ~ *is the last letter of the Latin alphabet, and may, therefore, be equated with* 'Ω', *the last letter of the Greek alphabet (cf. Rev 1:8, where God is said to be the Alpha and the Omega, the beginning and the end). The letter* 'z' *is followed appropriately by an Old English* Gloria Patri, *known as* The Gloria II | **24** foldan] *Günzel read* soldan, *but the* 'f' *has an unambiguous horizontal stroke and alliteration clearly requires an* 'f' | gemǽne] ~ ‖ ⟨*f. 56v*⟩.

2 Apuleian Sphere

Literature

Migne (1861-1904: I.963-66); Riess (1891-93: 382-83); Budge (1899: 229-30; 1913: I.458-59, II.539); Jenkinson (1908: 31); Förster (1912c: 45-49); Lehmann (1914); Wickersheimer (1914: 164-74); Singer (1917: 120; 1928: 144-46, 167; 1961: I.xxv); Thorndike (1923-58: I.682-85, I.692-94); Preisendanz (1928-31: II.81); Vyver (1936: 674-76); Jones (1939: 90); Sigerist (1942); Grattan and Singer (1952: 38-42, 48); Wormald (1962: 125-26); Bonser (1963: 157, 289); Gundel and Gundel (1966: 27-36, 69-71); Heimann (1966: 39-46); Desham (1977: 166-71); Jones (1984: 65-69); Murdoch (1984: 310); Betz (1986: 165-66); Jordan (1986: 290, 293); Voigts (1986, 1994); Hunt (1987: 161, 171); Braekman (1988: 83-111); Stevenson (1995: 51-52); Burnett (1997: 8, fig. 3); Pulsiano (1998b: 93-97); Liuzza (2001: 189; 2005); Iconclass (2002 [49D36, 58B2, 58BB1, 98B(APULEIUS)3])

Alias

Sphere of Democritus, of Petosiris, of Pythagoras, of life and death

Attributions

medieval: Apuleius (Platonicus), Democritus, Nechepso, Petosiris, Pythagoras; post-medieval: Bede, Columba, Hippocrates, Plato[1]

Branches of Superstition

observation of times: weekdays, days of the moon

[1] Singer (1928: 145; repeated Grattan and Singer 1952: 42) wrote: "During the Dark and Middle Ages this diagram [i.e. Apuleian Sphere] is common in the English manuscripts, where it is variously assigned to Hippocrates, Democritus, Apuleius, Apollonius, Pythagoras, Columcille, Bede, Petosiris, Nechepso, and Plato". This wealth of attributions is not attested in Anglo-Saxon manuscripts, however. I have not come across ascriptions to Apollonius and Hippocrates. The former is probably a misinterpretation of the opening line of some Apuleian Spheres: "Ratio spere pythagori philosophi quam appollogius [read apuleius] descripsit" (see text 2/6). The ascription to Columcille (also in Förster 1912c: 48; Bonser 1963: 157) is erroneous, and is based upon Columcille's Circle (in Vitellius E. xviii, fol. 15v). The diagram of Columcille's Circle indeed resembles that of an Apuleian Sphere, but the Circle is actually a charm, not a prognostic device. The ascription of Apuleian Spheres to Columcille (Columba) is not medieval, but the work of Singer and affiliates. Plato is mentioned in Apuleian Spheres, but only as part of the name Apuleius Platonicus. Nechepso, finally, is the recipient, not the writer, of the so-called Letter of Petosiris to Nechepso, the designation for a certain redaction of Apuleian Spheres (see below). This Letter has been wrongfully ascribed to Bede (see below). The attribution of writings to Nechepso and Petosiris is discussed in Gundel and Gundel (1966: 28, n. 1).

divination: arithmomancy (with numbers), onomatomancy, (with the (values of the) letters in a name), literamancy, stoicheiomancy (with letters)

Texts

L/OE: 1. London, British Library, Cotton Vitellius E. xviii, fol. 16r
L: 2. Cambridge, Trinity College, O. 7. 41, fol. 1r
3. London, British Library, Cotton Caligula A. xv, fol. 125va
4. London, British Library, Cotton Tiberius C. i, fol. 7v
5. London, British Library, Cotton Tiberius C. vi, fol. 6v
6. London, British Library, Cotton Vitellius E. xviii, fol. 14v
7. London, British Library, Harley 3667, fol. 4va, 4vc
8. London, British Library, Harley 3667, fol. 5r
9. London, British Library, Sloane 475, fols 132v-133v
10. Oxford, Bodleian Library, Bodley 579, fols 49v-50r
11. Oxford, St. John's College, MS 17, fol. 8rb
12. Oxford, St. John's College, MS 17, fol. 41ra
13. Oxford, St. John's College, MS 17, fol. 41rb

Description

When Grattan and Singer printed a diagram and an alphabetical list of letters with numerical values for an Apuleian Sphere, part of the caption read: "it is not clear what is to be done with the numbers when obtained, but the point is not worth prolonged study".[2] The number of scholars who have subsequently studied Apuleian Spheres have proved Grattan and Singer wrong. The most recent analysis is Liuzza's.[3]

The purpose of the Apuleian Sphere is to help predict the outcome of an illness, while predictions concerning other issues are occasionally found, such as the outcome of a fight or the chances of recovering a fugitive slave or lost or stolen property.[4] This prognostic genre was transmitted from Greek via Latin,[5] and some scholars have posited an Egyptian origin.[6] Bonser claimed a Pythagorean Greek origin for Apuleian Spheres, while "Celtic influence is seen in the treatment of the earlier examples, Byzantine in the latter".[7] The supposed 'Celtic influence' is not supported by the texts themselves, but Bonser was probably thinking of

[2] Grattan and Singer (1952: 39, fig. 18).
[3] Liuzza (2005).
[4] Thorndike (1923-58: I.683), Braekman (1988: 95-96).
[5] Thorndike (1923-58: I.682-83).
[6] Singer (1928: 144).
[7] Bonser (1963: 157).

Columcille's Circle, a charm in Vitellius E. xviii, fol. 15v, which was sometimes mistaken for an Apuleian Sphere. An ultimate Greek descent is substantiated by the use of Greek writing and names in some of the Anglo-Saxon Apuleian Spheres (2, 3, 8, 11, 13).[8] The oldest Apuleian Sphere in Greek hitherto attested dates back to the fourth century,[9] in a demotic papyrus at the Leiden Museum of Antiquities.[10] The earliest Latin translations are sometimes thought to have been composed in the sixth century, and despite the fact that no pre-ninth-century Spheres have been found, some scholars adhere to this date.[11] Jones assigned an eighth-century *terminus post quem*.[12] Singer made mention of "a large number of early manuscripts from the eighth century onwards", whereas he had earlier indicated that the earliest text is found in Paris, Bibliothèque nationale, Lat. 11411, fol. 99r (s. ix^1).[13] Stevenson recently has argued that the Apuleian Sphere in Lat. 11411 constitutes evidence of the presence of this genre in Anglo-Saxon England at the time of Archbishop Theodore, describing the manuscript as "an eight-century Anglo-Saxon manuscript from Echternach".[14] In the same passage, she connected Apuleian Spheres with Egyptian Days, and with the medical knowledge of Theodore.[15] These connections, however, are illusory at best. From the ninth century onwards, this genre is attested increasingly more frequently in Western manuscripts.[16]

[8] The text redactions I have termed continental Petosiris, and English Petosiris I and II (see below) use Greek names in Greek script as a basis for their examples. The compartmentalised circular diagrams (see below) employ Greek qualifications in addition to Latin.

[9] Haelst (1976: 336, item 1079).

[10] Thorndike (1923-58: I.682, n.4) refers to the text in Leemans (1843-85: II.35), but there is a more recent edition: Preisendanz (1928-31: II.81). The diagram itself is reproduced in Budge (1899: 230).

[11] Sigerist (1942: 293), Murdoch (1984: 310). The former claimed that "the Sphere of Democritus was translated into Latin probably around the 6th century AD when such translations were made in large numbers", although not one sixth-century Sphere has been attested.

[12] Jones (1984: 65).

[13] Singer (1928: 144-145). Facsimile in Singer (1928: 145, fig. 54), Grattan and Singer (1952: 39, fig. 18). On the manuscript, see Jenkinson (1908: xxxi), Wickersheimer (1966: 123 [LXXVIII]).

[14] Stevenson (1995: 52).

[15] Stevenson (1995: 51-52, 55).

[16] For editions, studies and manuscripts, see Jenkinson (1908: xxxi, 31), Förster (1912c: 47-49), Wickersheimer (1914; 1966: 29 [XIX], 35 [XXV], 50 [XXXIII], 64 [LIV.3], 88 [LXIX], 123 [LXXVIII.1], 134 [LXXXVI], 140 [XCII.1], 141-42 [XCII.

Despite the huge popularity of this prognostic device in the Middle Ages, vernacularisation set in rather late, as the sole rudimentarily glossed Anglo-Saxon Apuleian Sphere (1) attests.[17] This may have to do with the (Latinate) computistical context in which this genre is usually found in Anglo-Saxon England, but even computi partly in the vernacular do not include vernacularised Apuleian Spheres while they do contain translations of other prognostics.[18] The computus which contains (1), for example, includes five other prognostics in Old English and four in Latin, one of which being yet another Apuleian Sphere (6).[19] I have not encountered any early medieval continental manuscripts containing Apuleian Spheres in the vernacular. In the later Middle Ages, translations of are less exceptional, as evidenced by several Middle English redactions as well as a Syriac Sphere.[20]

At the heart of the Apuleian Sphere lies a diagram without which the prognostic is useless. In addition to a diagram, Apuleian Spheres consist of a variable set of elements, which may include: (a) an explanatory text of the procedure to be followed, (b) a set of numerical values for the letters of the alphabet, (c) a list of numerical values for the days of the week, and, sporadically, (d) a list of numerical values for the days of the moon. The tabular material and explanatory texts show great variation which makes a discussion of Apuleian Spheres rather complicated, in contrast to the simplicity of purpose of this genre. The order and presence of the components of Apuleian Spheres varies.

The explanatory text informs the enquirer how to predict the outcome of an illness, for instance. The procedure to be followed is a form of divination by numbers: the numerical values for the letters in one's name are added up to the numerical value for the weekday and the day of the moon on which the illness started. If a table of numerical values for the days of the moon is present, this table should be consulted. Otherwise one may simply add the value of the day of the moon itself to the calculation. From the sum, thirty is subtracted as many times as possible until

5]), Thorndike (1923-58: I.692-94), Singer (1928: 144-45), Sigerist (1942), Grattan and Singer (1952: 39), Beccaria (1956: 213 [55.24], 382 [134.4]), Hunt (1987: 161, 171), Burnett (1997: 8, fig. 3).

[17] Some prognostic genres, e.g. lunaries, were translated in relatively large numbers.

[18] See pp. 30-31, 36-39, 67-70.

[19] See pp. 37-38.

[20] Middle English Spheres are printed and discussed in Voigts (1986, 1994), Braekman (1988: 88-111), the Syriac one in Budge (1913: I.458-59, II.539).

one arrives at a number between 1 and 30,[21] which can be compared to the list of numbers in the diagram. The reason behind the choice of the number thirty is not revealed. The importance of the lunar calendar in this prognostic (see below) may have been of influence. Redactions exist which use the number twenty-nine instead of thirty.[22]

The phrasing of the explanatory text takes two main shapes: a six-line verse and a prose description. These two formulations are not mutually exclusive. There are Apuleian Spheres which have both a verse and prose explanation (3, 9, 10), while in exceptional cases the explanatory text is lacking altogether (11). In its archetypical form, the six-line verse is as follows:

Collige per numeros quicquid cupis esse probandum.
Iunge simul nomen feriam lunamque diei.
Collectamque una summam partire trigenos.
Quodque superfuerit rotulus discernet uterque.
Quos retinet uitae necnon et mortis imago.

---

[21] Following the Latin phrases "diuide per triginta" or "partire trigenos" (see verse text below), most scholars represent the instructions as "divide by thirty [and look up the remainder in the sphere]". This is slightly misleading to the modern reader as 'remainder' is reminiscent of long division, which was not practised in the early medieval West. Indeed, the demotic Greek Sphere has "see how many times thirty there are" (Betz 1986: 165, n.90).

[22] There are prognostic genres similar to Apuleian Spheres which also use numerical values for names and a subtraction process. Budge edited and translated a twelfth-century Syriac manuscript which included a method to discover which hand contains an object, who has stolen something from the questioner, who will die first, and what the course of an illness will be (1913: II.524-25, II.526-27, II.531-41). See also Braekman's study of the *Secreta secretorum* (1981: 105-11). An unusual illness prognostic which shows some similarities with the calculations of Apuleian Spheres but which does not use a diagram is found in the eleventh-century manuscript Dijon 448: "Cum quis aegrotare coeperit, quo die egrotauerit require, uel nomen egroti computabis et numerum diem addes, ex numero tres partes facit; si unus aut duo remanserit, conualescit egrotus" (Wickersheimer 1966: 30-31 [XXII.2]). Another prognostic without a diagram but with a list of numerical values for the letters of the alphabet is in Cleopatra B. ix, fol. 10v (s. xiii^2), and Egerton 843, fol. 31v (s. xiii^2), text from the latter: "Si uis scire quis prius moriatur, uir an mulier, computa nomina illorum et prospice numerum litterarum suarum et diuide per nouem. Si par numerus superfuerit, mulier condet uirum; si impar. uir mulierum" (Hunt 1987: 171 [9]). Finally, Vindicianus' *Gynaecia* contains a numerical method to predict the gender of an unborn child: "Viri et mulieris nomina litteraliter iunge, si pares sunt littere, masculum pariet mulier. Item pueri nati et matris nomina simili modo iuncta sexum futuri partus indicant, ut praedictum est" (Cilliers 2005: 184). Many numerical divinations are included in the twelfth-century Syriac manuscript edited and translated by Budge, see, for instance (1913: I.cxiv-cxvii, II.622-26).

Si supra fuerit uiuet morietur et infra.[23]

This verse is frequently encountered (3, 5, 9, 10). Text (10) constitutes the earliest example ever found of the six-line verse, but there is no reason to posit an Anglo-Saxon origin.[24] Since the verse is a mnemonic device, the content does not show great variation, except for copying mistakes, e.g. "discernat" for "discernet" (5); garbling of the order of the verse lines (9); grammatical variation, e.g. "numerum" for "numeros" (10); and some textual variation, e.g. "lunam feriamque" for "feriam lunamque".[25]

The prose explanations vary extensively, and a number of separate textual redactions can be distinguished based on the opening lines, the number used in calculations, and the presence or absence of an example.[26] The first redaction I distinguish is the Apuleian, of which the opening line runs: "Spera apulei platonici de uita uel de morte uel de omnibus negotiis & quicquid inquirere uolueris" (1, 3, 10). This type requires subtraction of the number thirty and does not give an example of how the calculations should be carried out. The second redaction is the Pythagorean, which has the opening line "Ratio spere phytagori phylosophi quem apuleius descripsit ut de quacumque re scire uolueris uel consulere" (4, 6, 9, 12). The Pythagorean redaction also uses the number thirty and does not give an example. The third redaction, that of Petosiris, uses the numbers twenty-nine and thirty, and provides examples. Continental Petosiris Spheres are presented as letters from Petosiris to Pharaoh Nechepso: "Petosiris Nechepso regi salutem. De his, quae a me ad humanae uitae cautelam inuenta sunt".[27] Calculations are based on the number twenty-nine exclusively, and this variant uses as example the names of Hector and Achilles.[28] These names are usually in Greek characters, which makes a list of numerical values for the letters of the alphabet redundant. Petosiris's Letter to Nechepso has wrongfully been

[23] "Count by numbers whatever you wish to be examined. / Take together the [values for] name, weekday and moon of the day. / And divide the single, gathered sum by thirty. / Whatever remains both [i.e. halves] of the circle will differentiate. / The image of life and also that of death holds them. / If it is above, he will live; if below, he will die".

[24] Voigts (1986: 298).

[25] The latter is attested in the early fifteenth-century Harley 3719 (Voigts 1986: 301).

[26] See table 27 for a quick reference guide to the prose explanatory texts.

[27] Riess (1891-93: 382).

[28] Migne (1861-1904: I.963-66), Riess (1891-93: 382-83), Wickersheimer (1914: 166-67), Vyver (1936: 674-76).

attributed to Bede in the sixteenth century, as have a number of other prognostic genres.[29]

I distinguish two Petosiris redactions in English manuscripts. In English Petosiris I redactions, the opening paragraph was replaced by one resembling the Pythagorean, but the example of the Petosiris variety has been retained. This is most readily seen in the numbers used in calculation: thirty is referred to in the opening paragraph, twenty-nine in the example. The opening line of the Petosiris I redaction is an abbreviation of the Pythagorean: "De quacumque re scire uolueris uel consulere" (8, 13). The explanation, therefore, refers to subtractions of thirty, but the example adduced uses the number twenty-nine. The example calculates the outcome of a fight between an unknown person (Hector in continental Petosiris redactions) and Achilles, and uses the numerical values for the letters of the Greek alphabet.[30] Moreover, the name of Achilles is written in Greek in the examples. The second English redaction, Petosiris II, has an opening line identical to the Pythagorean (2). The Pythagorean opening quickly shifts to an explanatory text of the Petosiris variety, which is apparent because the number mentioned is twenty-nine exclusively (in contrast to Petosiris I!). The example in Petosiris II concerns calculations of a number of names of Greek deities, whose names are written in Greek. The diagram that accompanies Petosiris I is a rhomboid, that of Petosiris II a regular circular one.[31] Both English Petosiris redactions differ from the other redactions in some respects: calculations are based on the number twenty-nine (but note that the explanatory text of Petosiris I also mentions thirty); there is no list of numerical values for the letters of the alphabet; there is no list of numerical values for the days of the week.[32] Jones observed that the continental Letter of Petosiris to Nechepso was common in Fleury computi.[33] This observation is inte-

[29] Jones (1939: 90). A Sphere of the Petosiris redaction is printed in Migne's edition of Bede's works (1861-1904: I.963-66). On spurious attributions to Bede, see pp. 97-98.

[30] See notes to 2/8,13.

[31] On the diagrams, see below. Wickersheimer (1914: 167) noted that one of the continental Petosiris redactions made use of a rectangular diagram. The diagram of the English Petosiris II text 2/2 is odd in that it supplies a list of numerical values for the letters of the alphabet, which is superfluous because Petosiris redactions make use of Greek letters. Therefore, the regular circular diagram of 2/2 may well have replaced an older rhomboid or rectangular diagram.

[32] On the list of numerical values for the weekdays, see below.

[33] Jones (1939: 90).

resting because the English Petosiris I texts are attested in Byrhtferth's computus, which is indebted to the computus of Abbo of Fleury.[34]

Some scholars consider the Petosiris redaction to be a prognostic genre in its own right. Wickersheimer, for instance, thought that what he described as the Apuleian/Pythagorean Sphere "does not at all derive from the Sphere of Petosiris, but from another Greek figure like the one seen in Leiden papyrus V".[35] This may be the case for the older, continental Spheres of Petosiris, but the English Petosiris I Spheres are crossovers which incorporate elements from the Pythagorean redaction. In general, English witnesses of Petosiris redactions have much in common with other redactions, Petosiris II more so than Petosiris I. The following diagram clarifies the types and redactions of explanatory texts:

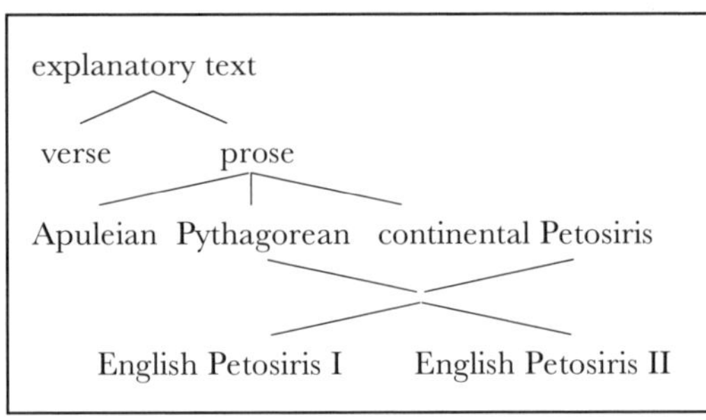

figure 3: explanatory texts of Apuleian Spheres

As the example of the Petosiris redactions illustrates, it is possible to recognise a number of discrete prognostic genres in Apuleian Spheres, rather than separate redactions of one main genre.[36] Doing so, however, has far-reaching consequences: there are at least four different types of diagrams in seven redactions, three types of lists of numerical values for the letters of the alphabet in eight redactions, two redactions of the list of numerical values for the weekdays, and two redactions of lists of numerical values for the days of the moon in two redactions.[37] Combinations of

[34] See pp. 29-39 for a study of the transmission of prognostics in the computus.

[35] "ne dérive point de la sphère de Petosiris mais d'une autre figure grecque que l'on rencontre dans le papyrus V de Leyde" (Wickersheimer 1914: 167). He referred to the Sphere in the Leiden papyrus introduced above. Singer (1917: 120) also considered the Sphere of Petosiris a genre in its own right.

[36] See below for more information on this issue.

[37] These findings pertain to Apuleian Spheres from English manuscripts solely. See pp. 559-63.

different types and redactions of these lists, explanatory texts, and diagrams are frequently encountered, which makes contemplating the number of distinct prognostic genres rather academic.[38] So instead of seeing a host of prognostic genres, for pragmatic reasons, I only recognise Apuleian Spheres, consisting of a number of flexible components.

If the Greek alphabet is used, as in the Petosiris redactions, for instance, there is no need for a separate list of numerical values for the letters of the alphabet. Indeed, the earliest attestation of an Apuleian Sphere, in the Leiden papyrus, does not include such a list as the text is in Greek. The transition of this genre from Greek to Latin necessitated a conversion table, because most of the letters of the Roman alphabet do not have a fixed numerical value. The list present in Latin Spheres links the twenty-three letters of the Roman alphabet to a set of arbitrary numbers. I distinguish three types of lists for the letters of the alphabet: those which are or should have been absent because the letters follow the Greek system (2, 8, 13), those which convey small values (1-7, 10, 12), attested in seven redactions, and those which convey large values (5, 10), attested in one redaction.[39] The purpose of the latter list is unknown, but it may have been intended for the initial letter of a name. Some texts have more than one list of small numerical values for the letters of the alphabet (4, 6, 12). The placement of the list varies: it may be found written in columns alongside the text and diagram (1, 5, 7, 10), in a table around the diagram (4), in an outer ring of the circular diagram (2, 6, 12), and inside the diagram (3).[40]

The days of the week all have a value which must be included if the calculation is to be relied upon. These values are arbitrary and the list should, therefore, always be present in the text. Petosiris redactions lack these lists, but (2), a Petosiris II type, features a list added in a later hand. This list deviates from those in English Apuleian Spheres, in which there are two redactions of the list of numerical values for the weekdays.[41]

In the Middle Ages it was believed that the day of the moon on which something happened was of great importance, witness the large number of medieval lunaries. In Apuleian Spheres, accordingly, the days of the

[38] Theoretically, there are at least 7*8*2*2=224 different configurations possible. Add to this attested irregularities such as two diagrams for one text, diagrams without text, lists of values for the letters of the alphabet where none are needed, and the number of prognostic genres becomes too large to contemplate.

[39] See table 30.

[40] See table 26.

[41] See table 28.

moon play an essential part. There are two types of lists of numerical values for the days of the moon: those which do not exist because the values equals that of the synodic days of the moon (1-6, 9, 12); and those which are present because the values of the days of the moon are arbitrary, ridiculously large numbers (7, 10). Continental Petosiris texts employ such lists,[42] but this is not the case for English Petosiris redactions. In fact, English witnesses of this list of lunar values are linked to the diagrams of *uita/mors* rather than the explanatory text. There are two redactions of the list of arbitrary lunar values.[43]

Diagrams lie at the heart of the genre of Apuleian Spheres since the outcome of the query is revealed in the diagram in the form of a set of numbers from one to thirty, placed in different sections of the diagram. All diagrams comprise an auspicious and inauspicious component, but the shape and style of the diagram exhibits great variation. There are four basic types: regular and compartmentalised circular diagrams, rhomboid diagrams, and figures of, literally, life and death:

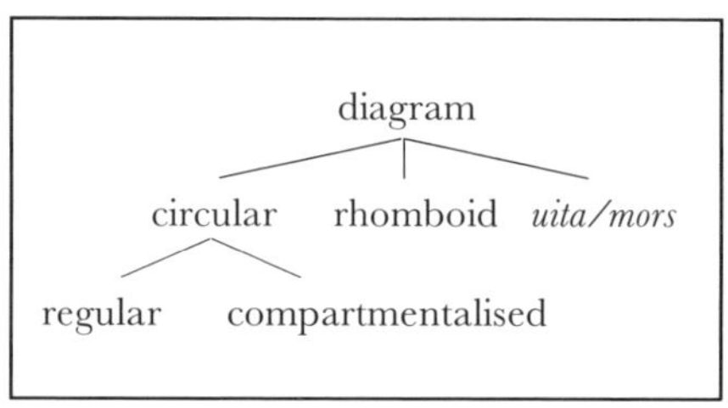

figure 4: diagrams of Apuleian Spheres

Some Apuleian Spheres have more than one diagram (4, 7, 10, 12). The regular circular diagram is the most basic type and consists of a circle subdivided into a top and bottom half (1, 2, 4 [twice], 6, 7, 12 [twice]).[44] If the number of the outcome is retrieved from the top half of the diagram, it means that the questioner will live; numbers in the bottom half signify death. The compartmentalised circular diagram is more intricate in that the top and bottom half are subdivided into compartments indicating the quality of life and death (3, 11). The labels for these compartments are in Greek, sometimes transliterated into Latin script and with

[42] Cf. Riess (1891-93: 383), Wickersheimer (1914: 166-67).

[43] See table 29.

[44] 2/9 has a dry-point circle that indicates the place where the diagram should have been drawn.

glosses in Latin, e.g. "ZωH MIKPA", "zoe micra *id est* uita minor" (3). Sometimes coded writing has been added to heighten the hermetic nature of this prognostic genre, e.g. "ΘANAΘOC MHΓAC", "m···rs c··t· [i.e. mors cita]" (11). Like compartmentalised circular diagrams, rhomboids are compartmentalised as well (8, 10).[45] Whereas rhomboids are sometimes found in Petosiris I redactions, which employ Greek writing, the compartments in these diagrams are labelled exclusively in the Roman alphabet, in contrast to compartmentalised circular diagrams. The rhomboids of (8) and (10) have little in common beyond their shape. The distribution of the numerical values they contain does not correspond. In addition, rather than the top half of (8) signifying life and the bottom half death, the left side means death and the right side life.[46] Finally, the figures of life and death, i.e. the *uita/mors* diagrams, may have been an Anglo-Saxon invention because it is found in three English manuscripts but not once in a continental volume (5, 7, 10). Instead of listing the sets of numbers in a geometrical figure, such as a circle, rhomboid or rectangle, they are listed in banners carried by a heavenly figure and a denizen of the netherworld. The heavenly figure carries a banner containing the set of numbers corresponding to life, and the fiend a banner with the numbers for death.

In addition to the four basic shapes of the diagrams, mention should be made of the set of numbers these diagrams contain. There are three main types of numerical sets, which coincide with the types of diagrams: four redactions for regular circular and *uita/mors* diagrams, one redaction for compartmentalised circular diagrams, and two redactions for rhomboids.[47] The only diagrams to show some overlap, then, are the regular circular and the *uita/mors* ones. The distribution of numbers in the *uita/mors* diagrams of (7), for instance, does not correspond to that of (5, 10), but to the first regular circular diagrams of (4, 7, 12).

So far, I have concentrated on the component parts of Apuleian Spheres. The number of combinations possible if one were to assemble an Apuleian Sphere has led scholars to distinguish several prognostic genres instead of redactions of Apuleian Spheres, as I have already hinted at before. Wickersheimer and Sigerist made a distinction between the Sphere of Democritus, Pythagoras or Apuleius, the Sphere of Peto-

---

[45] The diagram of 2/13 has been cut out (see p. 543), but the relatedness of this text to 2/8 indicates that the diagram of 2/13 will have been a rhomboid.

[46] A sinister/dexter reorientation?

[47] See table 31.

siris, and the *tetragonus subiectus*, a Sphere with a rectangular diagram.[48] Likewise, Thorndike saw distinct genres in the Sphere of Democritus, the Sphere of Petosiris, and the Sphere of Apuleius or Pythagoras.[49] He thought that the latter had replaced the older Sphere of Democritus. Such genre distinctions are based upon the supposedly diverse origins of Spheres of life and death, and the various shapes and divisions of the diagrams. Thus, the rectangular diagram of the oldest Sphere of Democritus was thought to have changed into a compartmentalised circular one (the Apuleian or Pythagorean Sphere), whereas the Sphere of Petosiris retained its original, regular circular shape. There are no indications for these developments to have taken place at all. Therefore, I prefer to regard all instances of the Sphere of Life and Death as variations upon one genre. How and why a number of different redactions came into being is a question which cannot be answered, but like everything that evolves, such developments sometimes took place gradually over time and abruptly at certain points in time.[50]

There are only two sets of Anglo-Saxon Apuleian Spheres which closely resemble each other, to wit (4, 12), and (8, 13). Both redactions are incorporated in copies of Byrhtferth's computus, probably from a common exemplar,[51] and the redactions of their components agree in every way. It seems likely, therefore, that both sets are related. With regard to other redactions, proving relatedness is not so easy. The most obvious examples are the three Apuleian Spheres which have *uita/mors* diagrams (5, 7, 10). It is impossible for these diagrams to have been conceived of independently. The earliest of the three (10) inspired the other two,[52] but the transmission caused some modifications to the overall composition of the texts, as the following table illustrates:

[48] Wickersheimer (1914: 164-74), Sigerist (1942: 292-93). The earliest Apuleian Sphere had a rectangular diagram. Such a *tetragonus subiectus* was more common in continental Apuleian Spheres (cf. Wickersheimer 1966: 35 [XXV], 141-42 [XCII.5]). I have found no English instances. A picture of a rectangular diagram is published in Wickersheimer (1966: pl. ix).

[49] Thorndike (1923-58: I.682-83).

[50] The comparison between texts 2/5,7,10 below will illustrate this.

[51] See pp. 35, 72, 85.

[52] Voigts (1986: 295-96) mentioned a tentative link between the diagrams of 2/5,10 (the link with 2/7 had not yet been discovered at the time). Most writers have focussed on the iconographical connections of the diagrams of these two Spheres (Wormald 1962: 125-26; Heimann 1966: 39-46; Desham 1977: 166-71). All conclude that the similarities indicate that 2/5 is a direct copy of 2/10.

	text	letter values	weekday values	lunar values	values for outcome
5	verse	small 5 + large	absent	absent	rc/um 4
7	absent	small 7	absent	redaction 1	rc/um 3 (2*)
10	verse + Apuleian	small 5 + large	redaction 1	redaction 2	rc/um 4 + r 2

table 16: redactions of components of Apuleian Spheres with *uita/mors* diagrams

Let us assume that the chronological order of the texts reflects the stages of transmission: (10) is from the 980s, followed by (5) from s. xi$^{3/4}$, and finally (7) from *c.* 1122. Text (10) represents the most complete phase: an Apuleian Sphere with an explanatory text in both verse and prose, a set of numerical values for the letters of the alphabet, and one for the capitals, a list of values for the weekdays, and one for the days of the moon, *uita/mors* diagrams and a rhomboid, each diagram containing its own set of values. In the process of transmission to (5), components were lost, including the prose explanation, the values for the weekdays and the days of the moon, and the rhomboid with its set of values. Three components, however, were retained: the *uita/mors* diagrams, the set of numerical values in the diagram, and the otherwise unattested list of values for the capitals. The latter, in particular, has been copied very closely.[53] It may be possible, therefore, that (5) as a whole is a direct copy of (10), albeit poorly executed. Text (7), however, cannot have derived directly from either (10) or (5), because it has totally different redactions of values for the letters of the alphabet, and for the days of the moon (already lost by (5) and unattested elsewhere). Moreover, (7) gained a regular circular diagram in addition to its *uita/mors* diagrams, and both diagrams have the same redaction of numerical values, a redaction which is not found in the *uita/mors* diagrams of (10). The only thing that (7) and (10) have in common are the *uita/mors* diagrams themselves.

Where, then, do the other components of (7) come from? The redaction of the numerical values in both diagrams of (7) is identical to that of the first regular circular diagrams of (4) and (12).[54] The diagrams of (7) even replicates some of the numerical ambiguities present in those of (4) and (12), which may have its cause in the fact that (4) and (7), while no longer so now, used to be in the same manuscript.[55] A direct link

[53] The set of values for the capitals 'I', 'M', 'V', 'X', and 'Z', in both 2/5,10, read '$\bar{\text{I}}$', '$\bar{\text{I}}$', '$\bar{\text{V}}$', '$\bar{\text{X}}$', and '$\bar{\text{I}}$', respectively, whereas the numerical values for the first set and the other letters in the second set do not have any dashes over them.

[54] See table 31.

[55] See pp. 518-19.

between the values for the diagrams of (7) and (4) is, therefore, not unthinkable. This link does not solve all problems in the transmission of (7): the redactions of the values for the letters of the alphabet and the days of the moon are not encountered elsewhere in English manuscripts, but they must have come from somewhere. Moreover, the compiler must have made a conscious choice to incorporate a list of values for the days of the moon and he must have had access to such a list, despite their rarity in English manuscripts. No other type of Anglo-Saxon Apuleian Sphere uses values for the days of the moon but the texts accompanying the *uita/mors* diagrams of (7) and (10). In continental manuscripts, on the other hand, values for the days of the moon do occur with Spheres of the Petosiris type, which makes a continental source probable. This is in fact very likely in view of the association of the Sphere of Petosiris with the Fleury computus, and on account of the use Byrhtferth made of Abbo's computistical work in compiling his own computus, in which (7) is found.[56] If we add up the findings, it appears that (7) is a composite of *uita/mors* diagrams derived from (10), a regular circular diagram inspired by (4), numbers for both diagrams of (7) taken from the first diagram of (4), and continental influences in the values for the letters of the alphabet and for the days of the moon.

A comparison of all Anglo-Saxon Apuleian Spheres would make it seem as if these prognostics are DIY kits which can be constructed from a choice of components, often offering more than one alternative for each part.[57] Needless to say, this cannot have been the case, because these texts were transmitted with a certain default configuration of components. It is unlikely that anything such as a manuscript or booklet ever existed in the early Middle Ages which listed all the readings and diagrams possible at the time. Nevertheless, a certain degree of variation was feasible, as the composition of (7) illustrates. Text (7), however, is based in part upon sources which were capable of exerting considerable influence (10, 4), and in part upon a source no longer traceable but which must have furnished the list of values for the days of the moon since such a list cannot have appeared out of the blue.

This short review has introduced the nature, purpose and origin of Apuleian Spheres. The earliest Sphere dates from the fourth century, but there are no attestations of the genre in a Western source before the ninth century. At this time, the Sphere gained in popularity and numer-

[56] See pp. 187-88.

[57] For the redactions of the component parts, see tables 26-32.

ous texts appeared. The genre did not lend itself to vernacularisation until the later Middle Ages, and even then on a small scale only. The basic make-up of Apuleian Spheres is a diagram accompanied by tabular material and an explanatory text. The basic requirements for an operational text are a diagram with a set of numbers, a set of numerical values for the letters of the alphabet, and for the days of the week. Apuleian Spheres may be accompanied by more tabular and explanatory material, depending upon the redaction and the type of diagram. In view of the complexity inherent in this genre, Apuleian Spheres deserve to be the subject of prolonged study.

Edition[58]

2/1 London, British Library, Cotton Vitellius E. xviii, fol. 16r/9-39

VITA VEL DE MORTE:–

Spera apulei platonici de uita uel de morte uel de om*n*ibus negotiis. & quicquid inquirere uolueris. sic computabis per om*ne*s litteras. utputa de nomine ęgri. Adde luna*m* quota fuerit die. qua decubuerit & quotiens potueris diuide per triginta. & quicquid superauerit reuerteris ad organiolum infra scriptum. & si superiori conuenerit parti numerus uitalis erit. sin autem inferiori conuenerit mortis pręsagium est. sic ętiam & de omnib*us* negotiis. **R**atio in sanitate hominis.

A iii
B iii
C xxii
D xxiiii
E xv
F iii
G vii ⟨DIAGRAM⟩

The bottom margin is damaged; text illegible in the bottom left-hand corner | **1 VITA**] *read* DE ~ | **2** uel$_1$] & *2/3* | **5** si] si[c] | **6** sin] *read* si | **14** ⟨DIAGRAM⟩ *this regular circular diagram is placed to the right of the list of numerical letter values. The diagram has three concentric rings around a central circle. No writing is placed in these rings. The central circle is divided into two parts by two parallel horizontal lines. The top part (N) has six rows (r) of numbers and text in five columns (c), and the bottom part (S) has five rows in three columns: Nc1r4/c5r4* **VI/TA**; *Nc2r1-6* i ii iii iiii vii ix; *Nc3r1-6* xi xiii xiiii xvi xvii xix; *Nc4r1-6* xx xxii xxiii xxvi xxvii x; *Sc2r5* **MORS**; *Sc1r1-4* v vi viii xii; *Sc2r1-4* xv xviii xxi xxiiii; *Sc3r1-4* xxv xxviii xxviiii xxx.

[58] Order of the texts: 1, 3, 10, 5, 7, 2, 9, 4, 12, 6, 8, 13, 11.

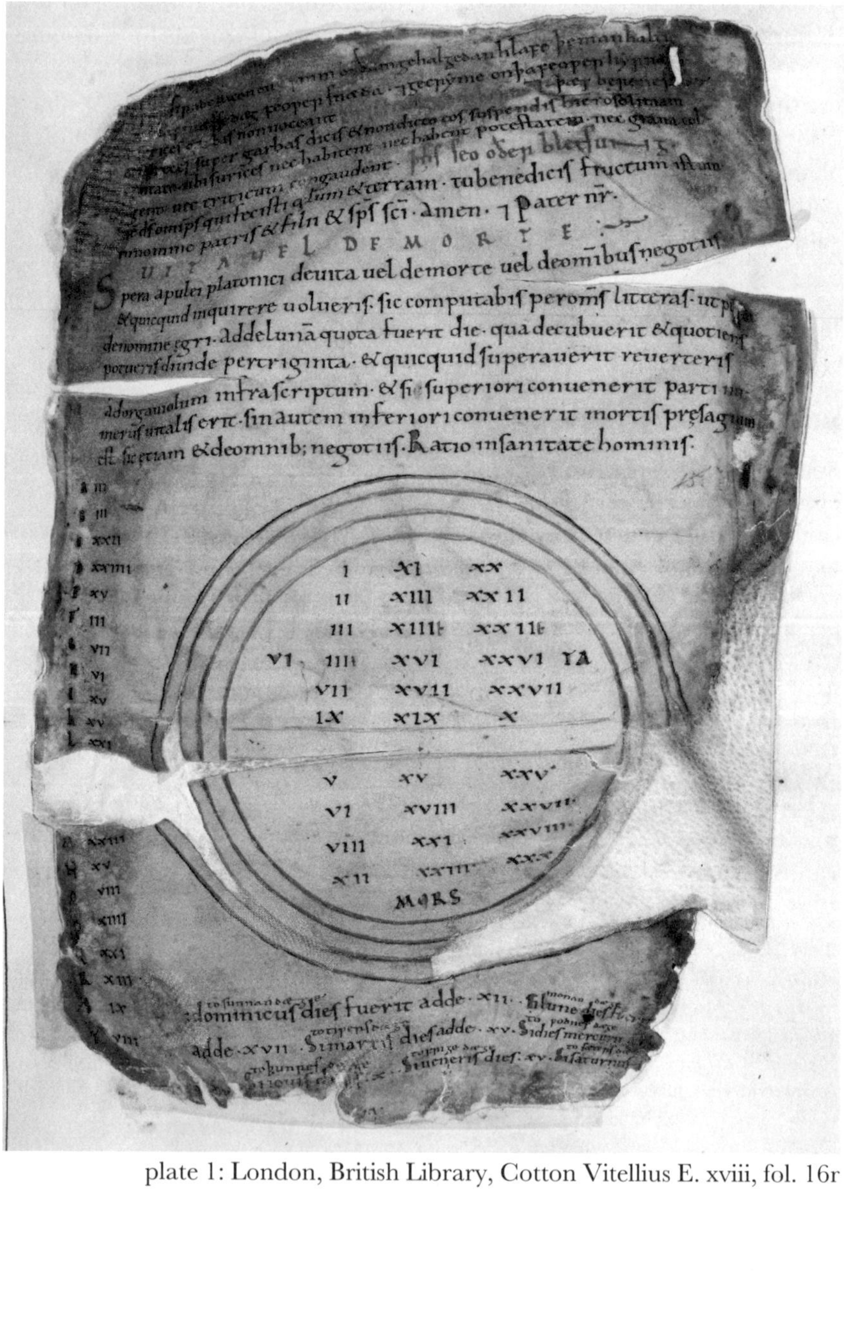

plate 1: London, British Library, Cotton Vitellius E. xviii, fol. 16r

H vi
I xv
K xv
L xxi
M xxiii
N xv
O viii
P xiiii
Q xxi
R xiii
to sunnandæge monandæge
S ix **Si** dominicus dies fuerit adde .xii. **si** lune dies fuerit
to tiwersdæge to wodnesdæge
T viii adde .xvii. **Si** martis dies adde .xv. **Si** dies mercurii adde
to þunresdæge to frigedæge to sætersdæge
(**V**) v xxv. **Si** iouis dies .x. **Si** ueneris dies .xv. **Si** saturnus d(ies
X vi adde .xxvi.
Y iii
Z iii)

25 monandæge] *read* to ~ | **26** .xii.] *read* .xiii. | **28** .xvii.] *read* .xviii. | **30** (**V**) v] *edges damaged, text partly illegible* | .x.] *read* .xi.

2/3 London, British Library, Cotton Caligula A. xv, fol. 125va

Collige p*er* numeros quicquid cupis esse p*ro*bandu*m*.
Iunge simul nom*en* feria*m* luna*mque* diei.
Collecta*mque* una summa*m* partire trigenos.
Quodq*ue* sup*er*fuerit rotulus discern*et* uterq*ue*.
Quos r*e*tin*et* uitę necnon & mortis imago.
Si sup*ra* fuerit uiu*et* mori*e*tur & infra.

Directly above the diagram, added in a thirteenth-century(?) hand: littera duplari: non uult nec bis numerari. *For a list of additions and changes to the diagram, see relevant notes. I have examined the text under UV lighting in the hope of getting a better reading of the additions, but to no avail. The verse is written in continuous lines* | **1** numeros] numerum *2/10*.

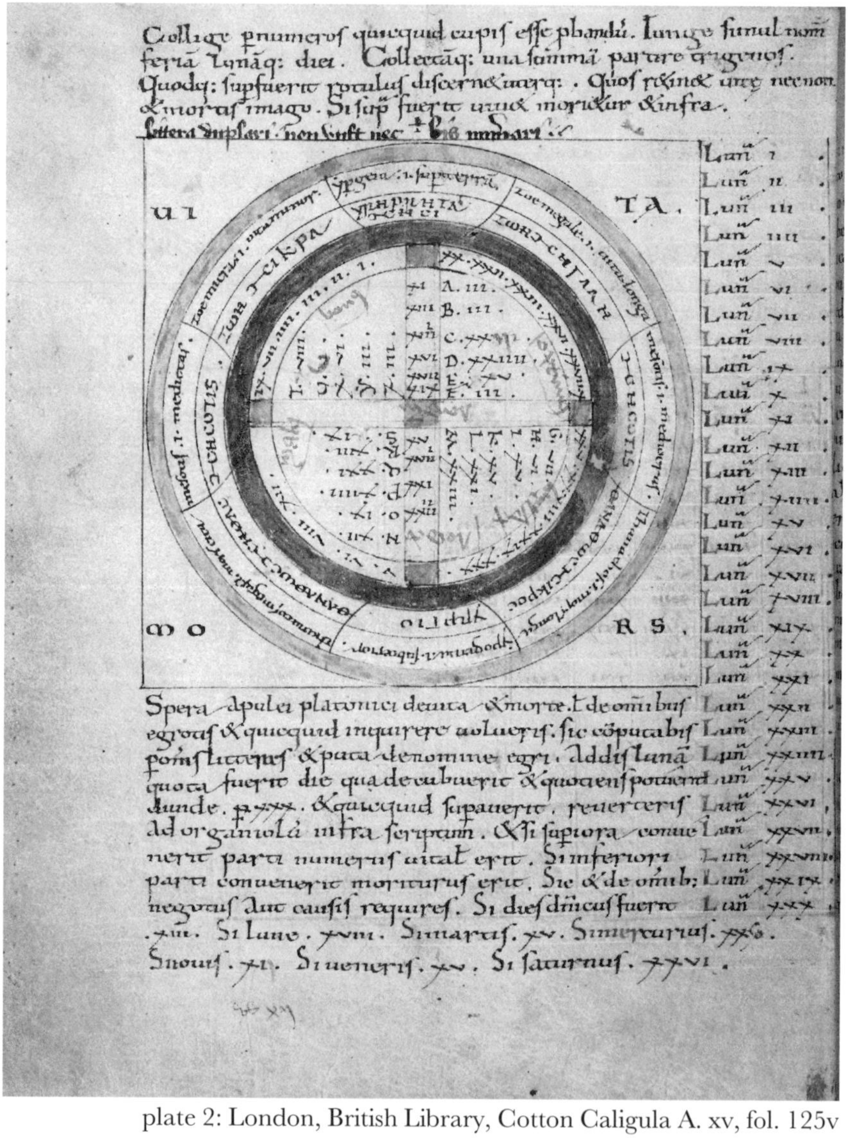

plate 2: London, British Library, Cotton Caligula A. xv, fol. 125v

⟨DIAGRAM⟩

Spera apulei platonici de uita & morte. *ue*l de om*n*ibus egrotis & quicquid inquirere uolueris. sic co*m*putabis p*er* om*ne*s litteras & puta de nomine egri. Addis luna*m* quota fuerit die qua decubuerit & quotiens potúerit diuide .p*er* xxx. & quicquid sup*er*auerit. reuerteris ad organiolu*m* infra scriptum. & si sup*er*iora conuénerit parti numerus uital*is* erit. Si inferiori parti conuenerit moriturus erit. Sic & de om*n*ib*us* negotus aut causis requires. Si dies d*omi*nicus fuerit .xiii. Si lune .xviii. Si martis .xv. Si mercurius .xxv. Si iouis .xi. Si ueneris .xv. Si saturnus .xxvi.

7 ⟨DIAGRAM⟩ *this compartmentalised circular diagram is placed between the* Collige *verse and the explanatory text. The diagram has five concentric rings around a central circle. The central circle (0) contains numbers and numerical letter values. The ring verging on the central circle (1) contains numbers. Rings 2 and 5 are empty, while ring 3 contains Greek writing and ring 4 writing in Greek and Latin, both in Latin script. Overall, the diagram is compartmentalised into eight parts, the top half for life and the bottom half for death. Outside the diagram, at the top left and right is written:* VI/TA.*; at the bottom left and right:* MO/RS. *The numerical letter values (in columns) are: NE0* A .iii. B .iii. C .xxii.* D .xxiiii. E .xv. F .iii.*; SE0* G .vii. H .vi. I .xv. K .xv. L .xxi. M .xxiii.*; SW0* N .xii.** O .ix. P .xiiii. Q .xxi. R .xiii. S .ix.****; NE0* T .viii.† V .v.†† X .vi. Y .iii. Z .iii. *The numbers of the diagram are subdivided into groups designated by the Greek writing, as follows: W3* MHCOTIS.*; W4* mesotis i*d est* medietas.*; NW3* ZωH MIKPA*; NW4* zoe micra i*d est* uita minor. *NW1* ix . vii . iiii . iii . ii . i .*; N3* YΠHPΠHTA††† MHCI*; N4* yp*er*geia i*d est* sup*er*terra*m*.*; N0* xi xiii xii \`i´i xvi xvii xix*; NE3* ZωH MHΓΑΛΗ*; NE4* Zoe megale i*d est* uita longa.*; NE1* xx . xxii . xxiii . xxvi . xxvii . x .*; E3* MHCOTIS.*; E4* mesotis i*d est* mediocras‡*; SE3* ΘANAΘωC MIKPOC*; SE4* Thanathos i*d est* mors longa*; SE1* xxv . xxviii . xxix . xxx .*; S3* YΠPΓIO‡‡*; S4* ypogeina‡‡‡ i*d est* subterior*; S0* xv xvi \`i´i xxi xx\`ii´ii*; SW3* ΘANAΘωC MHΘAC§*; SW4* thanatos megas i*d est* mors cita*; SW1* v . vi . viii . xii . *A later hand has added several scribbles in the central ring, in lighter ink: NW0* bon*us; NE0* optim*us; SE0* pessim*us; S0* peior*; SE0* mal*us; and in the centre* melior | * .xxii.] .xx[iii]. -[iii] > ii *by later hand* | **.xii.] *read* .xv. | *** .ix.] .[x]ix. | † .viii.] .[x]viii. | †† .v.] *a later hand has added a long stroke to the left-hand ascender of, thereby turning it into a sign for the number* 6 | ††† YΠHPΠHTA] *read* YΠHPΓHIA | ‡ mediocras] *read* mediocritas | ‡‡ YΠPΓIO] *read* YΠOΓHIO | ‡‡‡ ypogeina] *read* ypogeia | § MHΘAC] *read* MHΓAC | **10** potúerit] *read* potúeris | **11** sup*er*iora] *read* sup*er*iori | **13** negotus] *read* negotiis | **14** .xxv.] -v < [x] *by later hand* | .xi.] xi[i]. *Added in the bottom margin, directly below* .xi. *and in a later hand*: i*d* e*st* xii.

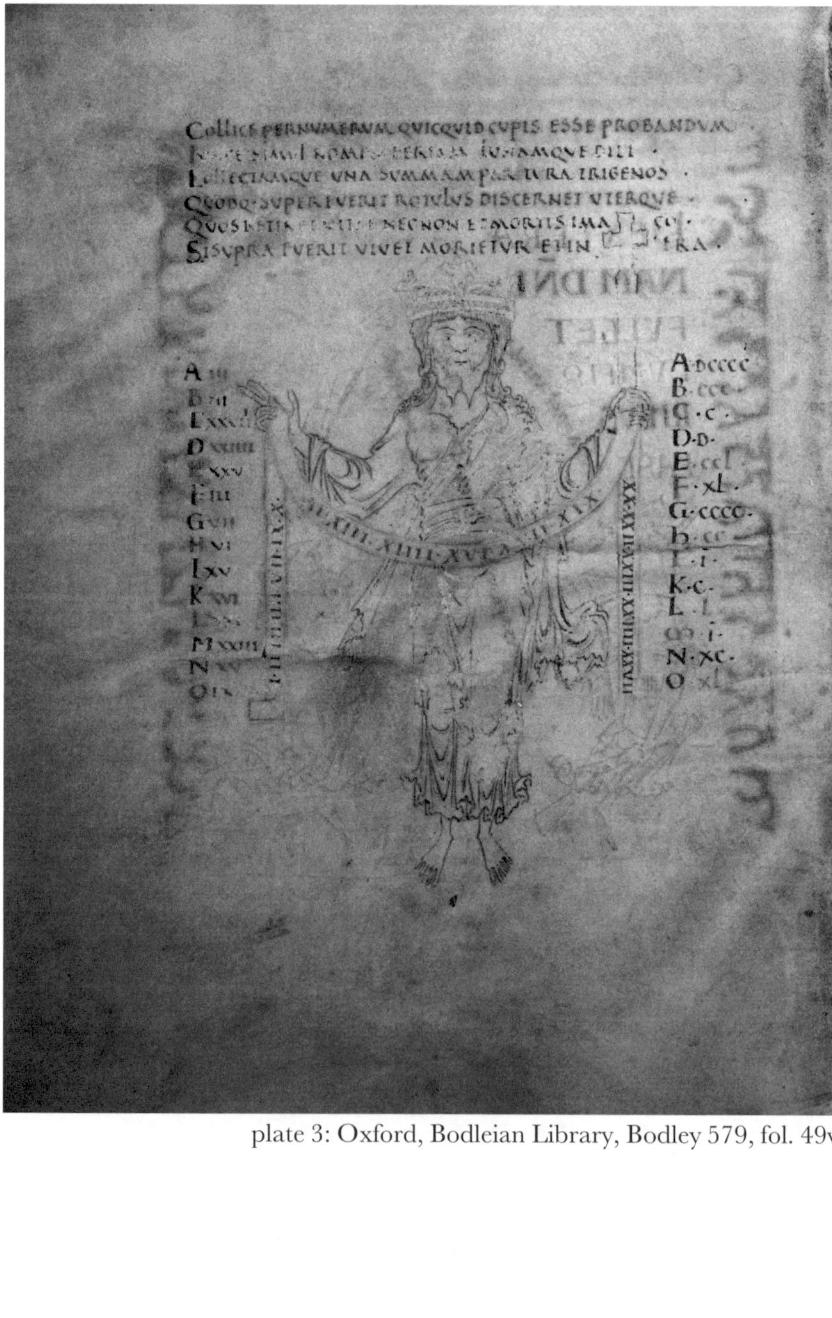

plate 3: Oxford, Bodleian Library, Bodley 579, fol. 49v

2/10 Oxford, Bodleian Library, Bodley 579, fols 49v-50r

COLLIGE PER NVMERVM QVICQVID CVPIS ESSE PROBANDVM.
IVNGE SIMVL NOMEN FERIAM LVNAMQVE DIEI.
COLLECTAMQVE VNA SVMMAM PARTIRA TRIGENOS.
QVODQ*VE* SVPERFVERIT ROTVLVS DISCERNET VTERQVE.
QVOS RETINET VITAE NECNON ET MORTIS IMAGO.
SI SVPRA FVERIT VIVET MORIETVR ET INFRA.

A	**iii**		**A**	**.dcccc.**
B	**iii**		**B**	**.ccc.**
C	**xxvii`i´**		**C**	**.c.**
D	**xxiiii**		**D**	**.d.**
E	**xxv**		**E**	**.ccl.**
F	**iii**		**F**	**.xl.**
G	**vii**	⟨DIAGRAM VITA⟩	**G**	**.cccc.**
H	**vi**		**H**	**.cc.**
I	**xv**		**I**	**.ī.**
K	**xvi**		**K**	**.c.**
L	**xxi**		**L**	**.l.**
M	**xxiii**		**M**	**.ī.**
N	**xv**		**N**	**.xc.**
O	**ix**		**O**	**.xl.**

SPERA APVLEI PLATONICI DE VITA DE MORTE. VEL DE OMNIB*VS* NEGOTIIS. ET quicquid inquirere uolueris. sic co*m*putabis p*er* omnes litteras. utputa de nomine ęgri. addis luna*m* q*uo*ta fuerit die q*ua* decubuerit. & quoties potueris diuide p*er* .xxx.^{ta} & q*ui*cq*ui*d sup*er*auerit reuerteris ad organiolu*m* infra scriptu*m*. & si sup*er*iori conuenerit parti numerus uitalis erit. Sí inferiori parte conuenerit moriturus erit. Sic & de omnib*us* negotiis aut causis requires. Si dies d*omi*nic*us* fuerit adde xiii.^{cim} Si lunę .xviii.^{cim} Si martis .xv.^{cim} Si mercurius .xxv. Si iouis .xi.^{cim} Si ueneris .xv.^{cim} Si sat*urn*us .xxvi.^{sex}

1 NVMERVM] numeros *2/3,5,9* | **4 PARTIRA**] **PAR**[·]**TIRA**, **-I-** < **V**; *read* Partire | **14** ⟨DIAGRAM VITA⟩ *this figure is placed between the first and second list of numerical letter values on fol. 49v. The figure holds a dangling banner in its hands, on which is written:* **i . ii . iii . iiii . vii . ix . x. / xi . xiii . xiiii . xvi . xvii . xix. / xx . xxii . xxiii . xxiiii . xxvii.** | **21 .xl.**] ~ ‖ ⟨*f. 50r*⟩ | **25** quoties] *read* quotiens | **27** parte] *read* parti.

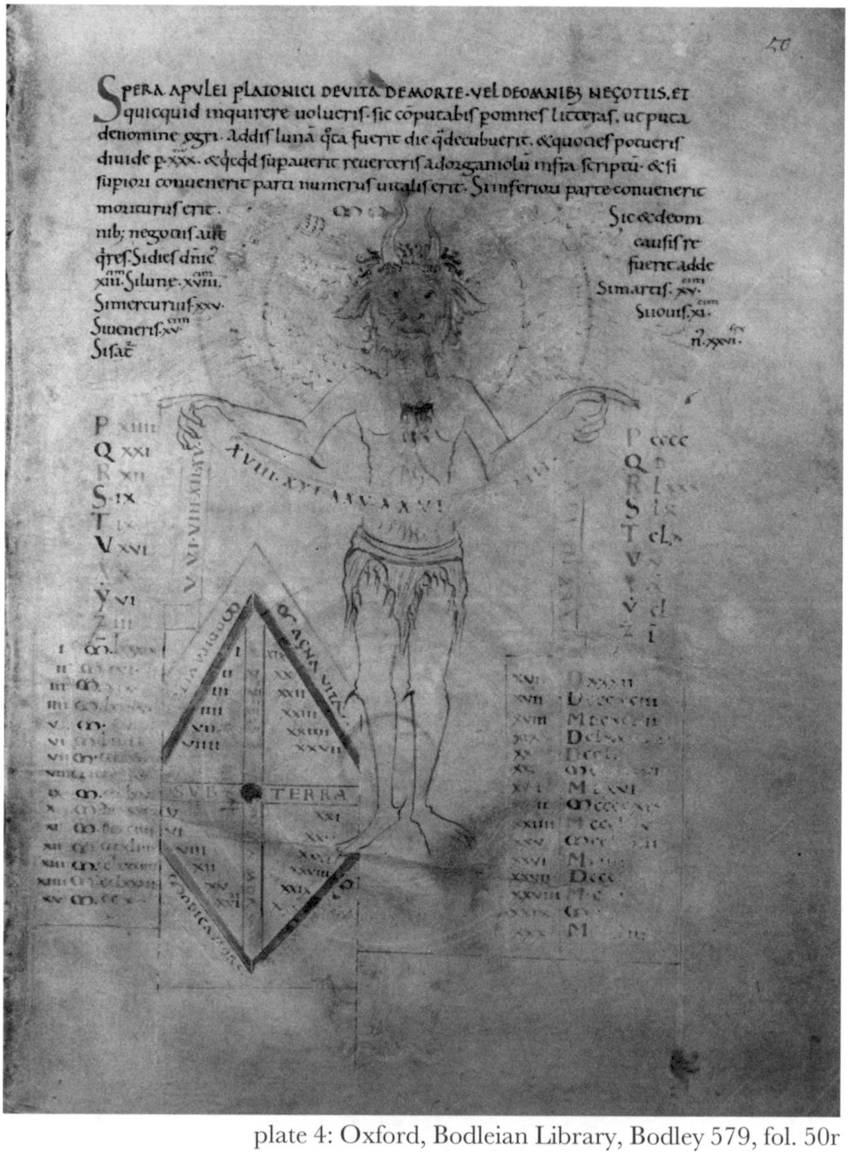

plate 4: Oxford, Bodleian Library, Bodley 579, fol. 50r

P	**xiiii**		**P**	**cccc**
Q	**xxi**		**Q**	**d**
R	**xii**		**R**	**lxxx**
S	**ix**		**S**	**lx**
T	**ix**		**T**	**clx**
V	**xvi**		**V**	**.v̄**
X	**x**		**X**	**.x̄**
Y	**vi**		**Y**	**cl**
Z	**iii**	⟨DIAGRAM MORS⟩	**Z**	**ī**

i	**M̄.lxxxix.**		**xvi.**	**Dxxxii**
ii	**M.cvi.**		**xvii**	**.Dcccxciii**
iii	**M.xix.**		**xviii**	**Mdcxciiii**
iiii	**M.lxxxv.**		**xix**	**Dclxxxviii**
v	**M.xv.**		**xx**	**Dccli**
vi	**M.liiii.**		**xxi**	**Mclxxxvi**
vii	**M.ccccxxxix**		**xxii**	**Mdxvi**
viii	**Mccccclvi**	⟨DIAGRAM⟩	**xxiii**	**Mccccxix**
ix	**M.ccclxv.**		**xxiiii**	**Mccclxv**
x	**M.dccxxix.**		**xxv**	**Mcclxiiii**
xi	**M.dcxciiii.**		**xxvi**	**Mciiii**
xii	**M.cccxliii.**		**xxvii**	**Dccclxxx**
xiii	**M.cclxxxiiii.**		**xxviii**	**M.cvi**
xiiii	**M.cclxxxii.**		**xxix**	**Mcv**
xv	**M.ccx.**		**xxx**	**Mcxliiii**

38 ⟨DIAGRAM MORS⟩ *this figure is placed between the first and second list of numerical letter values, and those for the days of the moon. To the right and left of the head is written:* MO/RS. *The figure holds a dangling banner in its hands, on which is written:* **v . vi . viii . xii . xv. / xviii . xxi . xxv . xvi . xxviii. / xxviiii . xxx.** | **46** ⟨DIAGRAM⟩ *this rhomboid diagram is placed between the first fifteen values for the days of the moon and the legs of the figure of death. The diagram is unusual in that some of the numbers for death are entered into the top half. The diagram consists of a central area divided into two parts (N0 and S0) by two horizontal lines, in between is written:* **SVB / TERRA**. *Around the central part are two rhomboid rings, the first (i.e. innermost) of which is empty and coloured. The central area (0) contains numbers and designations for the quality of life or death. Ring 2 contains designations for the quality of life or death, while the pertinent numbers are provided in the central area. Overall, the diagram is compartmentalised into 8 parts (designated by the points of the compass): NW2* **MODICA VITA.**; *NW0* **i ii iii iiii vii viiii**; *NE2* **MAGNA VITA.**; *NE0* **xix xx xxii xxiii xxiiii xxvii**; *SE2* **MAGNA MORS.**; *SE0* **xxi xxv xxvi xxviii xxix xxx**; *S0* **MEDIA MORS.**; *N0* **x xi xii`i´ xii`ii´ `x´vi xvi`i´**; *SW2* **MODICA MORS.**; *SW0* **v vi viii xii xv xvi`ii´**.

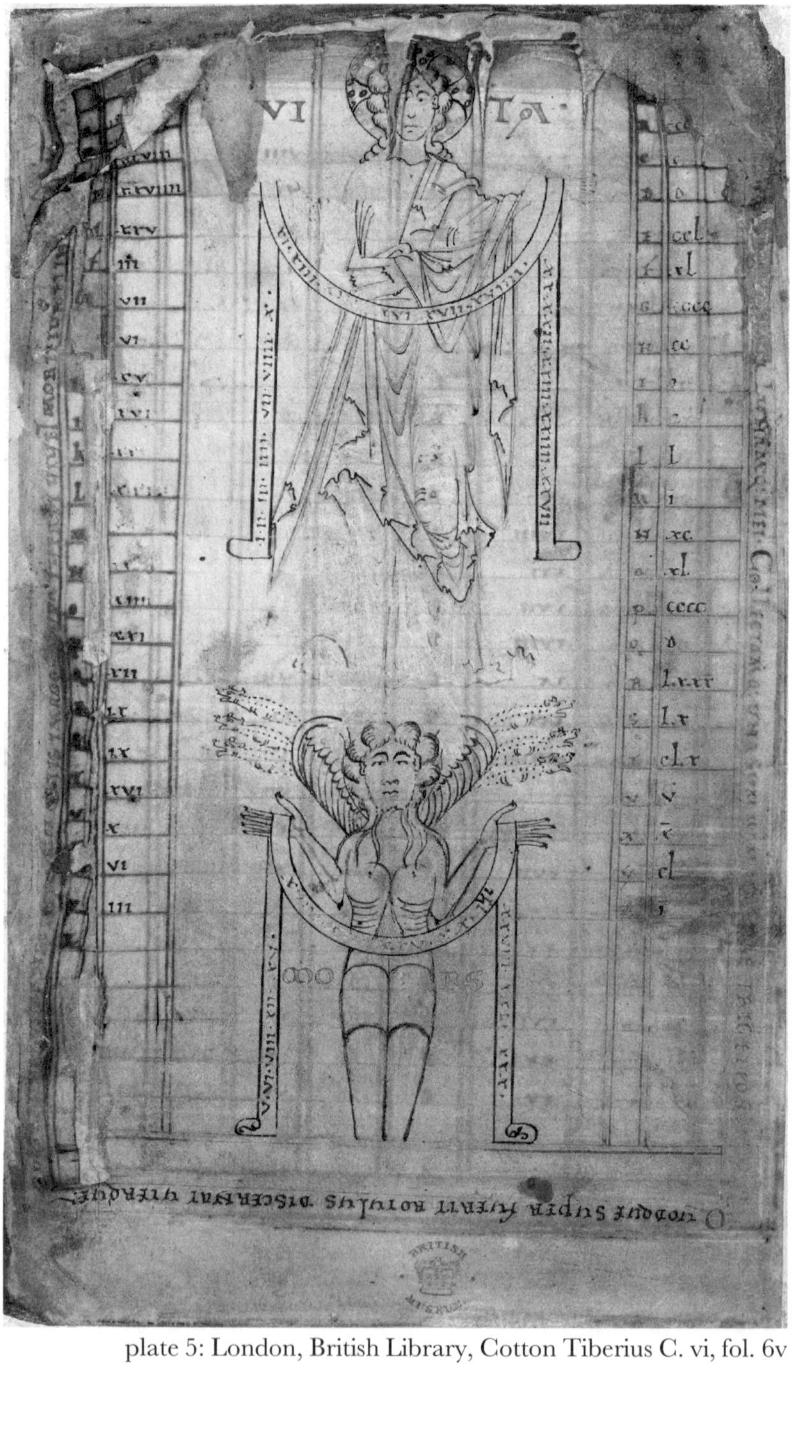

plate 5: London, British Library, Cotton Tiberius C. vi, fol. 6v

2/5 London, British Library, Cotton Tiberius C. vi, fol. 6v

COLLIGE PER NVMEROS QVICQVID CVPIS ESSE PROBAND(**VM.**)
(**IVNGE SIMVL NOMEN FERIAM**) **LVNAMQ*VE* DIEI**.
COLLECTAMQ*VE* VNA SVMMAM PARTIRE TRIGENOS:–
QVODQVE SVPERFVERIT ROTVLVS DISCERNAT VTERQVE:–
QVOS RETINET VITAE NECNON ET MORTIS IMAGO.
SI SVP*RA* FVERIT VIVET MORIETVR ET INFRA:–

A	**ii**(**i**)		**A**	(**dcccc**)
B	**ii**(**i**)		**B**	**ccc**
C	**xxviii**		**C**	**c**
D	**xxviiii**		**D**	**d**
E	**xxv**		**E**	**ccl**
F	**iii**		**F**	**xl**
G	**vii**	⟨DIAGRAM VITA⟩	**G**	**cccc**
H	**vi**		**H**	**cc**
I	**xv**		**I**	ī
K	**xvi**		**K**	**c**
L	**xxi**		**L**	**l**
M	**xxiii**		**M**	ī
N	**xv**		**N**	**xc**
O	**ix**		**O**	**xl**
P	**xiiii**		**P**	**cccc**
Q	**xxi**		**Q**	**d**
R	**xii**		**R**	**lxxx**
S	**ix**		**S**	**lx**
T	**ix**	⟨DIAGRAM MORS⟩	**T**	**clx**
V	**xvi**		**V**	**v̄**
X	**x**		**X**	**x̄**
Y	**vi**		**Y**	**cl**
Z	**iii**		**Z**	ī

The verse written along the page margins, starting at the top left. Lists of numerical letter values are in columns | **5** DISCERNAT] *read* discernet | **11 xxviiii**] *read* xxiiii | **14** ⟨DIAGRAM VITA⟩ *this figure is placed between the first and second list of numerical letter values from* 'a' *to* 'n'. *To the right and left of the head is written:* **VI/TA**. *The figure holds a dangling banner in its hands, on which is written:* **i . ii . iii . iiii . vii . viiii . x. / xi . xiii . xiiii . xvi . xvii . xviiii. / xx . xxii . xxiii . xxiiii . xxvii.** | **26** ⟨DIAGRAM MORS⟩ *this figure is placed between the first and second list of numerical letter values from* 'r' *to the bottom margin. To the right and left of the legs is written:* **MO/RS**. *The figure holds a dangling banner in its hands, on which is written:* v . vi . viii . **xii . xv. / xviii . xxi . xxv . xx**`vi´**.*** **/ xxviii. xxix .** xxx. | * **xx**`vi´**.**] **xx . ii.**, **ii.** > `vi´.

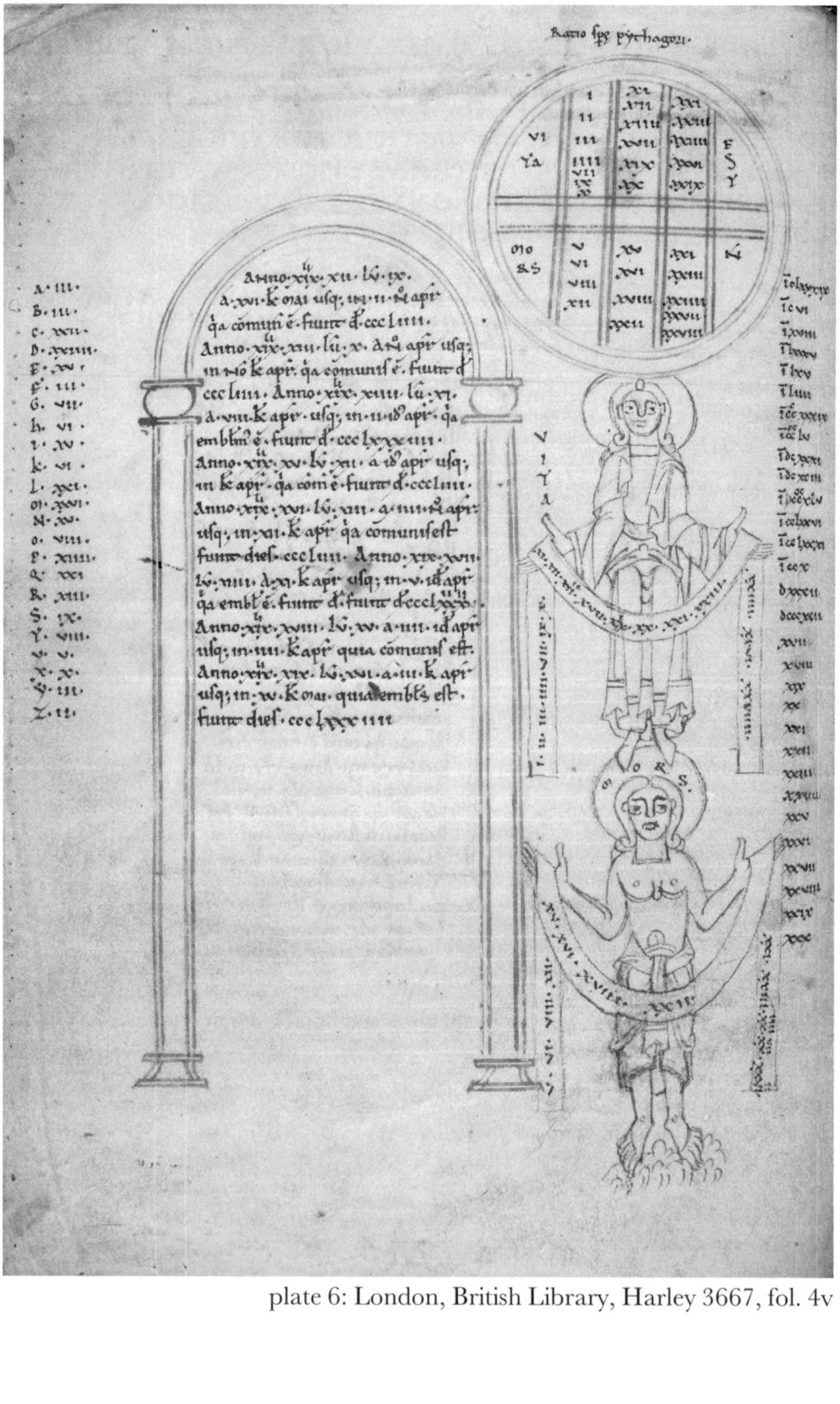

plate 6: London, British Library, Harley 3667, fol. 4v

2/7 London, British Library, Harley 3667, fol. 4va, 4vc

Ratio sper*ę* pythagori.
⟨DIAGRAM⟩

A	.iii.		īclxxxix
B	.iii.		īcvi
C	.xxii.		īxviii
D	.xxiiii.		īlxxxv
E	.xv.		īlxv
F	.iii.		īliiii
G	.vii.		īcc`c´xxxix
H	.vi.		īcc`cc´lv
I	.xv.		īdcxxxi
K	.vi.		īdcxciii
L	.xxi.		īcc`cc´lxv
M	.xxvi.		īcclxxvi
N	.xv.		īcclxxxi
O	.viii	⟨DIAGRAM VITA⟩	īccx
P	.xiiii.		dxxxii
Q	.xxi.		dcccxcii
R	.xiii.		xvii
S	.ix.		xviii
T	.viii.		xix
V	.v.		xx
X	.x.		xxi
Y	.iii.		xxii
Z	.ii.		xxiii

This incomplete Apuleian Sphere consists of diagrams (fol. 4vc), a list of numerical letter values (fol. 4va), and a list of values for the days of the moon. Fol. 4vb contains a computistical table | **2** ⟨DIAGRAM⟩ *this regular circular diagram is placed underneath the header mentioned in the text and to the left of the list of values for the days of the moon (extending to the day 5). The diagram has one concentric ring around a central circle. No writing is placed in the ring. The central circle is divided into a top and bottom part by two sets of double horizontal lines. Both parts are subdivided into five columns (c) by parallel vertical lines. The top part (N) has seven rows (r) of numbers and text, and the bottom part (S) has five rows: Nc1r3-4, c5r4-6* **VI/TA / E/S/T***; Nc2r1-7* i ii iii iiii vii ix x*; Nc3r1-6* xi xii* xiiii xvii xix xx*; Nc4r1-5* xxi xxiii xxiiii xxvi xxix*; Sc1r1-2, c5r1* MO/RS / Ń*; Sc2r1-4* v vi viii xii*; Sc3r1-4* xv xvi xviii xxii*; Sc4r1-5* xxi xxiii xxiiii xxvii xxviii | * xii] *read* xiii | **13** īcc`cc´lxv] ī[d]cc`cc´lxv | **16** ⟨DIAGRAM VITA⟩ *This figure is placed between the computistical table and the list of values for the days of the moon, and extends from days 6 to 22. To the left of the body is written vertically:* VITA. *The figure holds a dangling banner in its hands, on which is written:* i . ii . iii . iiii . vii . ix . x. / xi . xii* . xii`ii´ . xvii . x`i´x . xx . xxi . xxiii. / xxiiii . xxvi . xxviiii. | * xii] *read* xiii | **19** xvii] ~ *and further: instead of listing the values for the days of the moon, the list erroneously continues with the days themselves* | **25** .ii.] *read* .iii.

xxiiii
xxv
xxvi
xxvii
xxviii
xxix
⟨DIAGRAM MORS⟩ xxx

32 ⟨DIAGRAM MORS⟩ *this figure is placed to the left of the list of values for the days of the moon, and extends from day 23 to the bottom margin. In the aureola is written:* MORS. *The figure holds a dangling banner in its hands, on which is written:* v . vi . viii . xii. / xv . xvi . xviii . xxii. / xxi . xxiii . xx`iiii´ . xx`vii´ . xxvi`ii´.

2/2 Cambridge, Trinity College, O. 7. 41, fol. 1r

Racio sperę pytagorice qua*m* apulei*us* descripsit. de q*ua*cu*m*q*ue* re scire uolueris. utputa de egris qua die ebd*omade* euenerit. q*uo*ta luna fuerit scire debes. Adde nom*en* ipsi*us* de q*uo* inq*ui*ris. p*er* litt*er*as in hac pagina scriptas. 7 in num*er*o colligens partire p*er* .xxix. 7 q*ui*cq*ui*d remanserit. in sp*er*a respicies. si sursu*m* in media linea i*n*ueneris: eger cito co*n*ualesc*et*. Si aut*em* i*n* lat*er*alib*us*: longa egritudine p*er*ibit. similit*er* de o*mn*ib*us* reb*us*. Multis modis hoc scriptu*m* repp*er*i. s*ed* sic*ut* hic annotaui ueru*m* e*ss*e p*ro*baui. Exceptis dieb*us* egiptiacis. It*eru*m si uis cu*m* litt*er*is grecis nom*en* ho*min*is 7 num*eru*m feriaru*m* hic descriptu*m*. & luna*m* diei co*m*puta 7 partire p*er* .xxix. & q*uo*d remanserit: in sp*er*a respicies sic*ut* sup*ra*. NVMER*VS* F*ERIARVM*.

ccc .xviii. ccci ccc ix ccc liii. dcxii
HΛYOC. CYNΛHNH. APHC. HPMHC. ZHYC.

A fourteenth-century(?) hand has added (1) a Collige *verse in ring 3 of the diagram (see below), (2) several numerical values to correct or expand those provided for the letters of the alphabet in ring 2 of the diagram (see below), and (3) the numerical values of the weekdays after the diagram* | **9-10** NVMER*VS* F*ERIARVM*.] *the numerical values of the weekdays are not included in the original text. The later hand responsible for all additions also added the list of values after the diagram:* Dies sol*is* .xvi. D*ies* Lune .xvii. D*ies* m*ar*t*is* .xv. D*ies* m*er*curi*us* .xxv. D*ies* iouis .xi. Dies uen*er*is .xv. Dies sat*ur*n*us* xvii | **11** ccc liii.] *read* ccc lvi. | **12** HΛYOC] *Helios = (8+30+10+70+200) = 318, i.e. if upsilon (400) is counted as iota (10)* | CYNΛHNH] *read* CYΛHNH, *Selene = (200+5+30+8+50+ 8) = 301, i.e. is upsilon (400) is counted as epsilon (5)* | ARHC] *Ares = (1+100+8+200) = 309* | HPMHC] *Hermes = (8+100+40+8+200) = 356* | ZHYC] *Zeus = (7+5+400+200) = 612, i.e. if eta (8) is counted as epsilon (5).*

dc ccc xciii dx

ΑΦΡωΛΥΘΗ. ⟨DIAGRAM⟩ ΚΡωΝωC.

14 ΑΦΡωΛΥΘΗ] *read* ΑΦΡωΔΥΤΗ, *Aphrodite = (1+500+100+70+4+10+300+8) = 993, i.e. if omega (800) is counted as omicron (70), and upsilon (400) as iota (10)* | ⟨DIAGRAM⟩ *this regular circular diagram is placed underneath the examples of Greek deities. The diagram has three concentric rings around a central circle. The central circle is divided into two main parts by two parallel horizontal lines. Both parts are subdivided into three columns (c) by parallel vertical lines. The top and bottom part (N0 and S0) have six rows (r) of numbers each: N0c1r2-6* ii x iii vii ix*; N0c2r1-6* xi. xiii. xiiii. xvi. xvii. xix.*; N0c3r2-6* xx xxii xxiii xxvi xxviii*; S0c1r1-5* v vi viii iiii xii*; S0c2r1-3,r6* xv xviii xxi xxiiii*; S0c3r1-3,r5* xxv xxvii xxix i. *A cross is placed at the top in rings one and two (counting outwards from the central circle). The letters of the alphabet are placed in ring 1, the corresponding numerical values in ring 2 (from the top, clockwise):* A iii. B iii.[*] C xxv.[**] D xxiii.[***] E xv. F iii. G vii. H v.[†] I xv.[††] K xv. L xx.[†††] M xxvi.[‡] N xv. O ix. P xiiii. Q xxi. R xiii.[‡‡] S ix.[‡‡‡] T viii.[§] V v.[§§] X vi. Y iii. Z iii. *A later hand added an incomplete* Collige *verse in ring 3 (from the top, clockwise):* Collige p*er* num*erum* q*ui*cquid cupis e*ss*e pr*o*bandu*m*. Iu*n*ge sim*u*l feria*m*[§§§] lunam*que* diei. Collecta*mque* sim*ul*[¶] su*m*ma*m* par*t*íre t*r*igenos: Quodq*ue* sup*er*fuerit rotulus det*er*net[¶¶] ut*er*go.[¶¶¶] | [*] iii.] *underneath ~ in a later hand* .ii. | [**] xxv.] *read* xxii., *underneath ~ in a later hand* .xxvii. | [***] xxiii.] *underneath ~ in a later hand* xxviii. | [†] v.] *read* vi., *underneath ~ in a later hand* .vi. | [††] xv.] *underneath ~ in a later hand* .vii. | [†††] xx.] *read* xxi., *underneath ~ in a later hand* xxi. | [‡] xxvi.] *underneath ~ in a later hand* .xxii. | [‡‡] xiii.] *underneath ~ in a later hand* xii. | [‡‡‡] ix.] *underneath ~ in a later hand* xx. | [§] viii.] *underneath ~ in a later hand* ix. | [§§] v.] *underneath ~ in a later hand* vi. | [§§§] feria*m*] ~ [· · ·]; *read* nomen ~ | [¶] sim*u*l] read una | [¶¶] det*er*net] *read* discernet | [¶¶¶] ut*er*go.] *read* ut*er*que. Quos retinet uite necnon & mortis imago. Si supra fuerit uiuet morietur et infra. | ΚΡωΝωC] *Kronos = (20+100+70+50+70+200) = 510, i.e. if omega (800) is counted as omicron (70).*

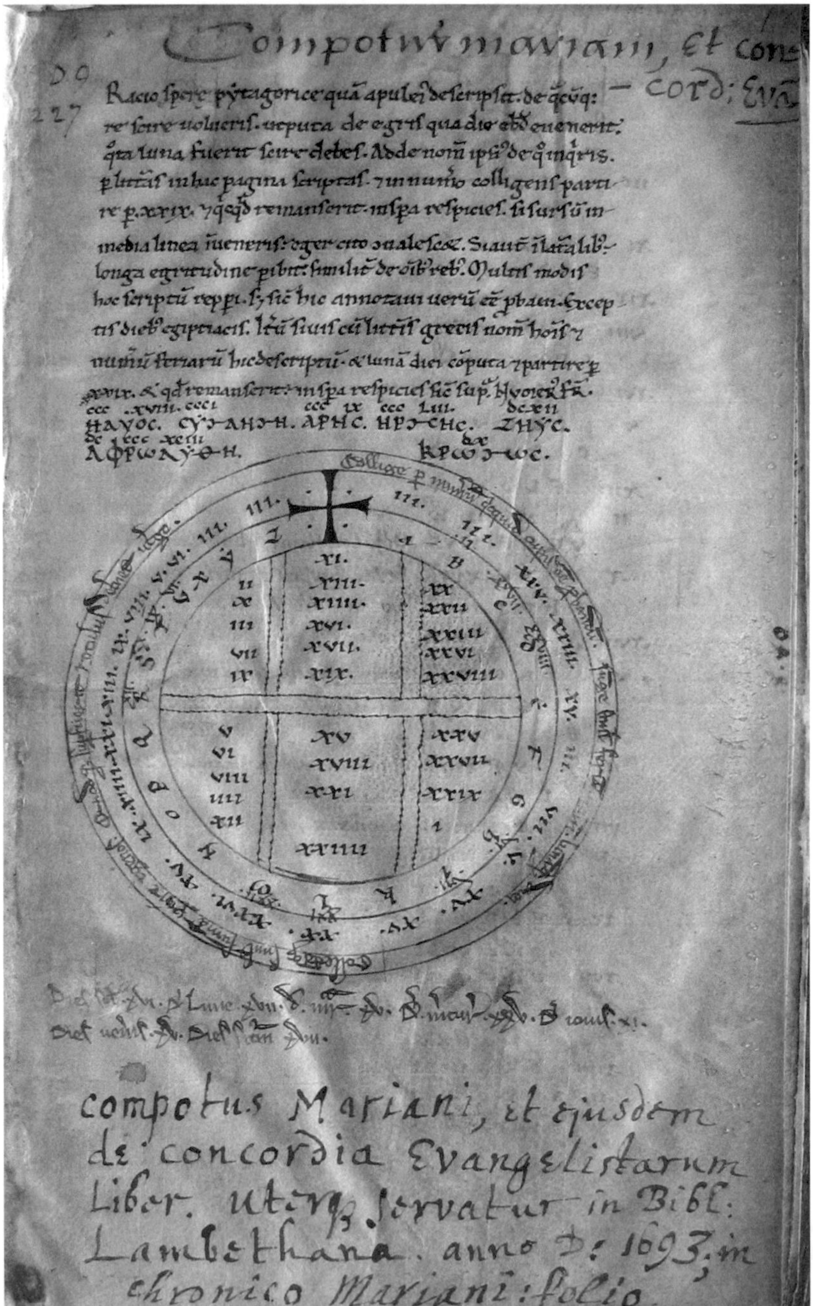

plate 7: Cambridge, Trinity College, O. 7. 41, fol. 1r

2/9 London, British Library, Sloane 475, fols 132v-133v/11

& partíris in trigintas **.xxx.** partes & quicquit remanserit in spera res pisties. & síc inuenies & sic rursum inueneris uiu*et*. & prosperum erit. síc autem infra fuerit morietur síc & de omib*us* negotus. aut causis requires. Sí dominicus. dies fuerit ponis **xiii.** Si lune **.x.viii.** Si martis **.xv.** Si mercurius **.xxv.** Si iouis **.xi.** Si ueneris **.xv.** Si saturnus **.xxvi.**

prima littera nomini uirit & posterior nominis puelle. uel pueri illius cuius asignatur posterior uere nomini uiri & auterior nominis pueri uel puelle aquo sub alator prima littera in prima pagina. & auterior in postrema linea & prima & nonna*m* media litera adiuguntur cum positis rotet. & sine errore. resspiciens quocumque. uolueris;

Quodque sup*er*fuerit. rotulus discern*et* \`uterque´
Collige p*er* numeros quicquit cupis esse \`p*ro*bandum´
Quodre tim*et* uite néc. inon & mortis \`in mago´
Iunge simul nomen feria*m* luna*m*que *id est* \`*id est* diei´
Supra fuerit uiu*et* morietur & infra
Collectamque una*m* su*m*man partire. tragenos.

Text lacks diagram and opening lines. The six-line verse is jumbled, the correct order is: Collige *[...]*, Iunge *[...]*, Collectamque *[...]*, Quodque *[...]*, Quos *[...]*, Si supra *[...]*. *A dry-point circle on fol. 132v indicates that a diagram should have been drawn* | **1** &] ‖ ~ ⟨*f. 133r*⟩ | trigintas **.xxx.**] *delete* trigintas *(dittography)* | res pisties] *read* respicies | **2** sic] *read* si | rursum] *read* sursum | inueneris] -ne- < [··] | síc$_2$] *read* si | **3** omib*us*] *read* omnibus | negotus] *read* negotiis | **6** nomini] *read* nominis | uirit] *read* uiri | **7** nomini] *read* nomine | auterior] *read* anterior | **7-8** aquo sub alator] *read* a quo subdatur | **8** pagina] -n- < ti | auterior] *read* anterior | **9** nonna*m*] nonnā; *read* nonna, *i.e.* nona | media] *read* in ~ | litera] *read* linea | adiuguntur] adiu‖guntur ⟨*f. 133v*⟩ | rotet] *read* rote | resspiciens] *read* respicies | **10** quocumque] *read* quidcumque | uolueris;] *read* inuenere ~ | **11** \`uterque´] *transposition from line below indicated* | **12** \`p*ro*bandum´] *transposition from line above indicated* | **13 Quodre tim*et***] *read* Quos retinet | néc. inon] *read* necnon | \`in mago´] *read* imago; *transposition from line above indicated* | **14** *id est* \`*id est* diei´] *transposition from two lines above indicated; read* diei | **15** Supra] *read* Si supra | **16** su*m*man] *read* summam | tragenos] *read* trigenos.

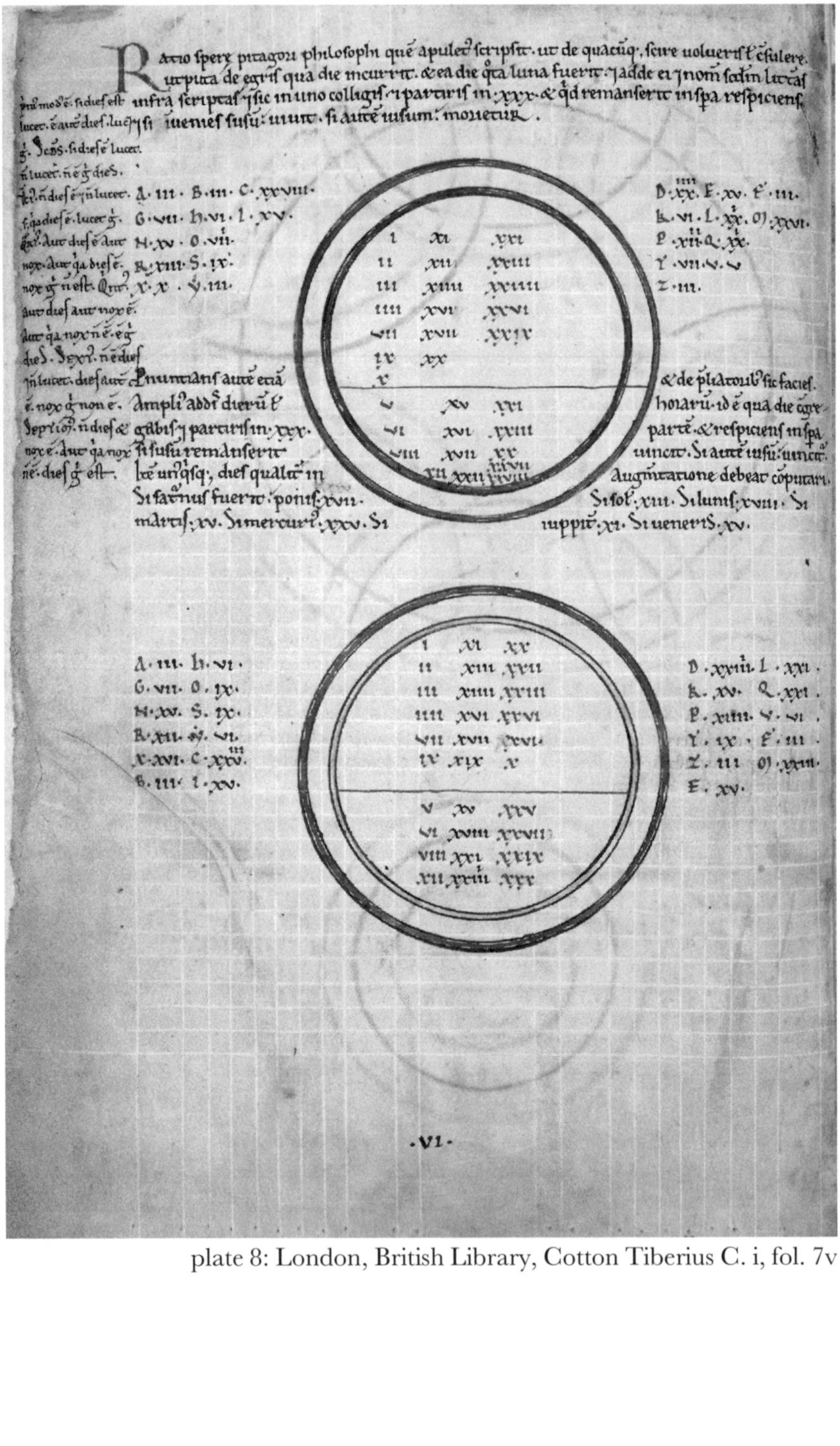

plate 8: London, British Library, Cotton Tiberius C. i, fol. 7v

2/4 London, British Library, Cotton Tiberius C. i, fol. 7v

Ratio sperę pitagori philosophi que*m* apulet*us* scripsit. ut de quacu*m*q*ue* scire uolueris *uel* *con*sulere. utputa de ęgris qua die incurrit. & ea die q*uo*ta luna fuerit. 7 adde ei 7 nom*en* *secundum* litt*er*as infra scriptas 7 sic in uno colligis. 7 partiris in .xxx. & q*ui*d remanserit in sp*er*a respiciens. 7 si i*n*uenies susu*m*: uiuit. si aute*m* iusum: morietur.

A.iii.	**B**.iii.	**C**.xxviii.		**D**.xx`iiii´.	**E**.xv.	**F**.iii.
G.vii.	**H**.vi.	**I**.xv.		**K**.vi.	**L**.xx`i´.	**M**.xxvi.
N.xv.	**O**.vii`i´.		⟨DIAGRAM⟩	**P**.xii`ii´.	**Q**.xx`i´.	
R.xiii.	**S**.ix.			**T**.vii.	**V**.v	
X.x.	**Y**.iii.			**Z**.iii.		

P*ro*nuntians aute*m* etia*m* & de p*re*liatorib*us* sic facies. Ampli*us* addis dieru*m* *ue*l horaru*m*. id e*st* qua die *con*gregabis 7 partiris in .xxx. parte*m*. & rescipiens in sp*era* si susu*m* remanserit uincit. Si aute*m* iusu*m*: uincit*ur*. Ite*m* un*us*q*ui*sq*ue* dies qualit*er* in augm*en*tatione debeat co*m*putari. Si sat*ur*nus fuerit: ponis .xvii. Si sol*is* .xiii. Si lunis .xviii. Si martis .xv. Si mercuri*us* .xxv. Si iuppit*er* .xi. Si ueneris .xv.

A.iii.	**H**.vi.		**D**.xxiii`i´.	**L**.xxi.
G.vii.	**O**.ix.		**K**.xv.	**Q**.xxi.
N.xv.	**S**.ix.	⟨DIAGRAM⟩	**P**.xiiii.	**V**.vi.
R.xii.	**Y**.vi.		**T**.ix.	**F**.iii.
X.xvi.	**C**.xxv`iii´.		**Z**.iii.	**M**.xxiii.
B.iii.	**I**.xv.		**E**.xv.	

1 apulet*us*] *read* apuleius | scripsit] *read* descripsit | quacu*m*q*ue*] *read* ~ re | **3** ei] *read* eis | **4** si$_1$] si[c] | **8** ⟨DIAGRAM⟩ *this regular circular diagram is placed between the first list of numerical letter values and between the second paragraph of explanatory text. The diagram has one ring around a central circle. No writing is placed in the ring. The central circle is divided into two parts by a single horizontal line. The top part (N) has seven rows (r) of numbers in three columns (c), and the bottom part (S) has four rows in three columns: Nc1r1-7* **i ii iii iiii vii ix x**; *Nc2r1-6* xi xii* xiiii xvi** xvii*** xx; *Nc3r1-5* **xxi xxiii xxiiii xxvi xxix**; *Sc1r1-4* **v vi viii xii**; *Sc2r1-4* xv xvi xvii† xxii; *Sc3r1-4* **xxi xxiii xx†† `xxvii´ xxviii** | *xii] xii[i]; *read* xiii | **xvi] xvi[i]; *delete* ~ | ***xvii] *add* xix | †xvii] *read* xviii | ††**xx**] *read* xxiiii | **9** .vii.] *read* .viii. | **13** uncit*ur*] *read* uincetur | **14** .xvii.] [xxv] *written over* ~ | **18** ⟨DIAGRAM⟩ *this regular circular diagram is placed underneath the second paragraph of explanatory text and between the second list of numerical letter values. The diagram has one ring around a central circle. No writing is placed in the ring. The central circle is divided into two parts by a single horizontal line. The top part (N) has six rows (r) of numbers in three columns (c), and the bottom part (S) has four rows in three columns: Nc1r1-6* **i ii iii iiii vii ix**; *Nc2r1-6* xi xiii xiiii xvi xvii xix; *Nc3r1-5* **xx xxii xxiii xxvi xvi.* x**; *Sc1r1-4* **v vi viii xii**; *Sc2r1-4* xv xviii xxi xxii`i´i; *Sc3r1-4* **xxv xxvii** **xxix xxx** | ***xvi**] [**x**]**xvi**; *read* xxvii | ****xxvii**] *read* xxviii.

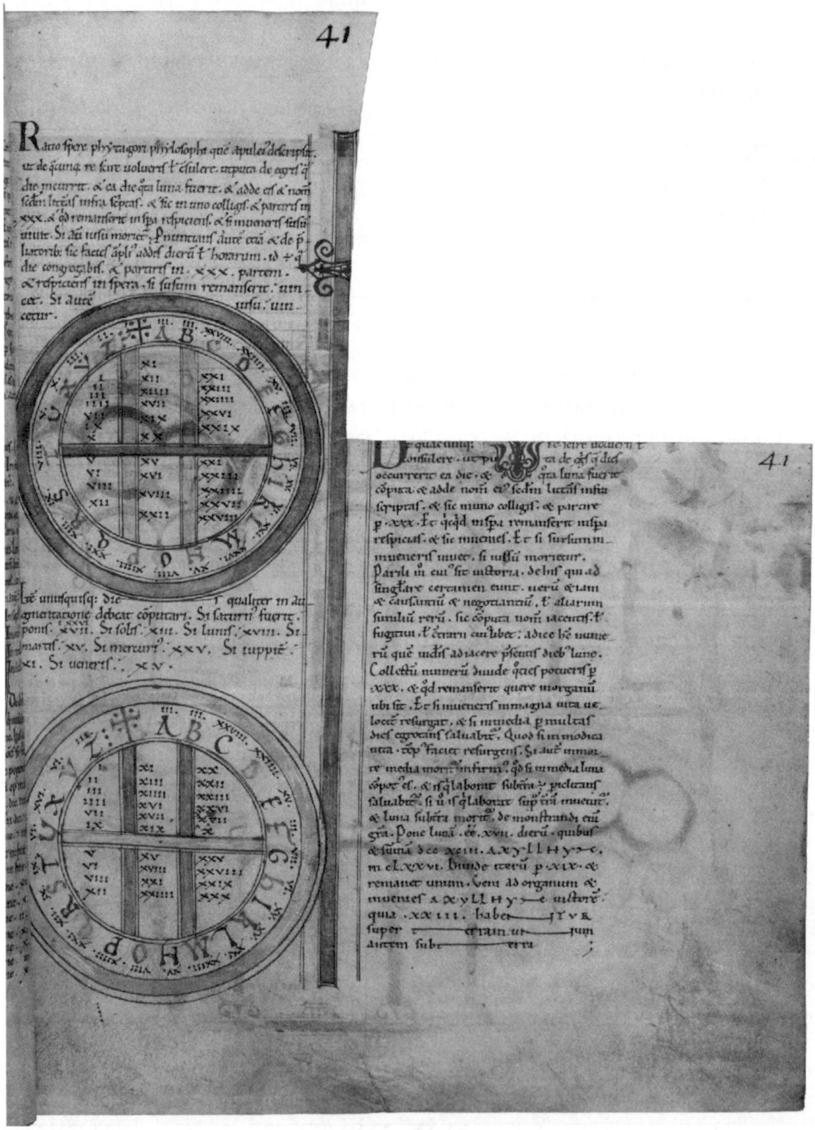

plate 9: Oxford, St. John's College, MS 17, fol. 41r

2/12 Oxford, St. John's College, MS 17, fol. 41ra/1-16

Ratio sperȩ phytagori phylosophi que*m* apulei*us* descripsit. ut de q*ua*cunq*ue* re scire uolueris *ue*l co*n*sulere. utputa de ȩgris q*ua* die incurrit. & ea die q*uo*ta luna fuerit. & adde eis & nom*en* *secundum* litteras infra sc*ri*ptas. & sic in uno colligis. & partiris in .xxx. & q*ui*d remanserit in sp*er*a respiciens. & si inueneris susu*m* uiuit. Si au*tem* iusu moriet*ur*.

P*ro*nuntians aute*m* etia*m* & de p*re*liatorib*us* sic facies a*m*pli*us* addis dieru*m* *ue*l horarum. id *est* q*ua* die congregabis. & partiris in .xxx. partem. & respiciens in spera. si susum remanserit: uincet. Si aute*m* iusu: uincetur.

⟨DIAGRAM⟩

Ite*m* unusquisq*ue* dies qualiter in augmentatione debeat co*m*putari. Si saturn*us* fuerit: ponis .xvii. `*ue*l xxvi´ Si solis: xiii. Si lunis: xviii. Si martis: xv. Si mercuri*us*: xxv. Si iuppit*er*: xi. Si ueneris: xv.

⟨DIAGRAM⟩

5 iusu] *read* iusum | **8** uincet] *read* uincit | iusu] *read* iusum | **9** ⟨DIAGRAM⟩ *this regular circular diagram is placed between the first and second paragraphs of explanatory text. The diagram has two rings around a central circle. No writing is placed in the outer ring. The central circle is divided into two parts by a solid horizontal line. The top part (N0) has seven rows (r) of numbers in three columns (c), and the bottom part (S0) has five rows in three columns (columns are separated by vertical lines): N0c1r1-7* i ii iii iiii vii ix x; *N0c2r1-6* xi xii* xiiii xvii xix xx; *N0c3r1-5* xxi xxiii xxiiii xxvi xxix; *S0c1r1-4* v vi viii xii; *S0c2r1-4* xv xvi xviii xxii; *S0c3r1-5* xxi xxiii xxiiii xxvii xxviii. *Ring 1 has a cross at the top, and contains the numerical letter values (from the top, clockwise):* **A** iii. **B** iii. **C** xxviii. **D** xxiiii. **E** xv. **F** iii. **G** vii. **H** vi. **I** xv. **K** vi. **L** xxi. **M** xxvi. **N** xv. **O** viii. **P** xiiii. **Q** xxi. **R** xiii. **S** ix. **T** viii. **V** v. **X** x. **Y** iii. **Z** ii.**:- | *xii] *read* xiii | **ii.] *read* iii. | **13** ⟨DIAGRAM⟩ *This regular circular diagram is placed underneath the second paragraph of explanatory text. The diagram has two rings around a central circle. No writing is placed in the outer ring. The central circle is divided into two parts by two sets of double horizontal lines. The top part (N0) has six rows (r) of numbers in three columns (c), and the bottom part (S0) has four rows in three columns (columns are separated by vertical lines): N0c1r1-7* i ii iii iiii vii ix; *N0c2r1-6* xi xiii xiiii xvi xvii xix; *N0c3r1-5* xx xxii xxiii xxvi `x´xvii* x; *S0c1r1-4* v vi viii xii; *S0c2r1-4* xv xviii xxi xxiiii; *S0c3r1-5* xxv xxviii xxix xxx. *Ring 1 has a cross at the top, and contains the numerical letter values (from the top, clockwise):* **A** iii. **B** iii. **C** xxviii. **D** xxiiii. **E** xv. **F** iii. **G** vii. **H** vi. **I** xv. **K** xv. **L** xxi. **M** xxiii. **N** xv. **O** viii.** **P** xiiii. **Q** xxi. **R** xii. **S** ix. **T** ix. **V** vi. **X** xvi. **Y** vi. **Z** iii. ⁝ | *`x´xvii] `x´x[`x´]vii | ** viii.] *read* viiii.

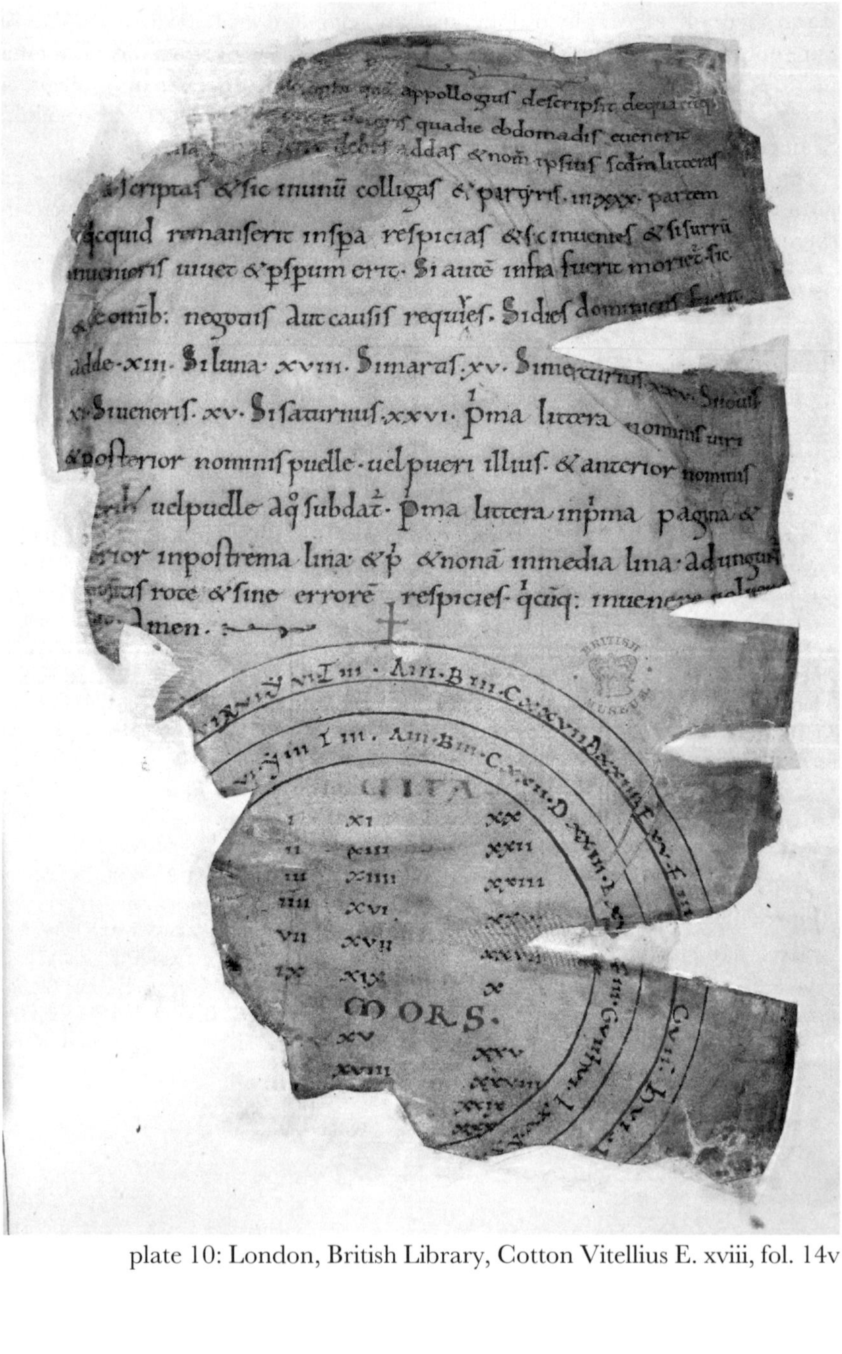

plate 10: London, British Library, Cotton Vitellius E. xviii, fol. 14v

2/6 London, British Library, Cotton Vitellius E. xviii, fol. 14v

(SP)ERE:–

(Ratio spere pythagori ph)ilosophi qua*m* appollogius descripsit de quacu*m*q*ue* (re scire uolueris consulere ut)puta de egris qua die ebdomadis euenerit (& ea die quota lu)na (fueri)t scire debes addas & nom*ine* ipsius *secundu*m litteras (infr)a scriptas & sic in unu*m* colligas & partyris. in .xxx. partem (&) q*ui*cquid remanserit in sp*e*ra respicias & sic inuenies & si surru*m* inuenieris uiuet & p*e*rsp*e*rum erit. **S**i aute*m* infra fuerit moriet*ur*. sic & de om*n*ib*us* negotiis aut causis requi`r´es. **S**i dies dominicus fuerit adde .xiii. **S**i luna .xviii. **S**i martis .xv. **S**i mercurius .xxv. **S**i iouis .xi. **S**i ueneris .xv. **S**i saturnus .xxvi.

P*ri*ma littera nominis uiri & posterior nominis puelle. uel pueri illius. & anterior nominis (pu)eri h*uius* uel puelle a q*uo* subdat*ur*. **P***ri*ma littera in p*ri*ma pagina & (ant)erior in postrema lina. & p*ri* & nona*m* in media lina. adiungunt*ur* (cum) positis rote & sine errore*m* respicies. q*ui*cu*m*q*ue* inuenere uolueris ···· nit. **A**men. **:–**

⟨DIAGRAM⟩

The margins of the page are damaged. The diagram is irreparably damaged at the left-hand and bottom margins | **2** appollogius] *read* apuleius *(though* apollonius *may have been intended)* | **6** surru*m*] *read* sursum | inuenieris] *read* inueneris | p*e*rsp*e*rum] *read* prosperum | **12** lina$_{1,2}$] *i.e.* linea | p*ri*] *read* prima | nona*m*] nonā; *read* nona | **13** errore*m*] errorē; *read* errore | q*ui*cu*m*q*ue*] *read* quidcumque | ···· nit] (discer)nit *Liuzza (2005)* | **15** ⟨DIAGRAM⟩ *this regular circular diagram is placed underneath the explanatory text. The diagram has three concentric rings around a central circle and a cross at the top outside the outer ring. The central circle is divided into two parts by headers: r1* **VITA.**; *r8* **MORS.** *Both parts consist of three columns (c) of numbers. The numbers under* **VITA.** *(N0) occupy 6 rows (r), those under* **MORS.** *(S0) take up 4 rows: N0c1r2-7* i ii iii iii vii ix; *N0c2r2-7* **xi xiii xiiii xvi xvii xix**; *N0c3r2-7* xx xxii xxiii xxvi xxvii x; *S0c1r9-12* (v vi vii)i (xii); *S0c2r9-12* **xv xviii** (**xxi xxiiii**); *S0c3r9-12* xxv xxviii xxix xxx. *Ring 2 (counting outwards from the central circle) is empty. Rings 1 and 3 both contain a list of numerical letter values. Ring 1 (from the top, clockwise):* **A** iii. **B** iii. **C** xxii. **D** xxiii. **E** xv. **F** iii. **G** vii. **H** vi. **I** xv. **K** xvi(.* **L** xxi. **M** xxvi. **N** xv. **O** ix. **P** xiii. **Q** xxi. **R** xiii. **S** ix. **T** viii. **V** v. **X**) vi. **Y** iii. **Z** iii. *Ring 3 (from the top, clockwise):* **A** iii. **B** iii. **C** xxvii.** **D** xxiiii. **E** xv. **F** iii. **G** vii. **H** vi. **I** (xv. **K** xv. **L** xxi. **M** xxiii. **N** xv. **O** ix. **P** xiiii. **Q** xxi. **R** xii. **S** ix. **T** ix. **V**) vi. **X** vi.*** **Y** vi. **Z** iii. | * xvi(.)] *read* xv(.) | ** xxvii.] *read* xxviii | *** vi.] *read* xvi.

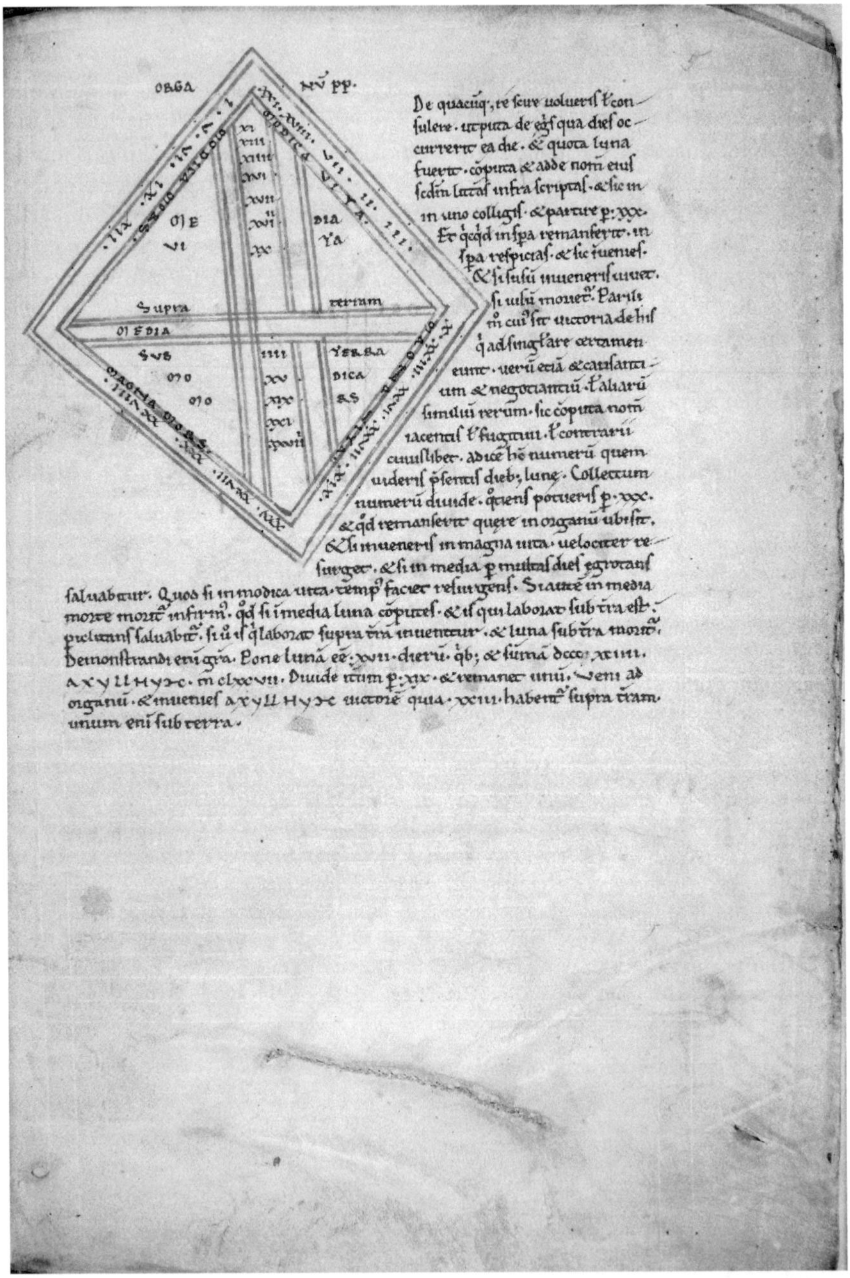

plate 11: London, British Library, Harley 3667, fol. 5r

2/8 London, British Library, Harley 3667, fol. 5r

ORGANV*M* PP.

⟨DIAGRAM⟩ De quacú*m*q*ue* ré scire uolueris *ue*l consulere. utputa de ęg*ri*s qua dies occurrerit ea die. & quota luna fuerit. co*m*puta & adde nom*en* eius s*ecundu*m litt*er*as infra scriptas. & sic in in uno colligis. & partire p*er* .xxx. Et q*ui*cq*ui*d in spe*ra* remanserit. in sp*er*a respicias. & sic i*n*uenies. & si susu*m* inueneris uiuet. si iusu*m* moriet*ur*.

Parili m*odo* cui*us* sit uictoria de his q*ui* ad sing*u*lare certamen eunt. ueru*m* etia*m* & causantium & negotiantiu*m*. *ue*l aliaru*m* similiu*m* rerum. sic co*m*puta nom*en* iacentis *ue*l fugitiui. *ue*l contraríí cuiuslibet. adice h*ui*c numeru*m* quem uideris p*re*sentis dieb*us* lunę. Collectum numeru*m* diuide. q*uo*tiens potu eris p*er* .xxx. & q*uo*d remanserit quęre in organu*m* ubi sit. & si inueneris in magna uita. uelociter resurget. & si in media p*er*multas dies ęgrotans saluabitur. Quod si in modica uita. temp*us* faciet resurgens. Si aute*m* in media morte morit*ur* infirm*us*. q*uo*d si i*n* media luna co*m*putes. & is qui laborat sub t*er*ra est: p*er*iclitans saluabit*ur*. si u*ero* is q*ui* laborat supra t*er*ra*m* inuenitur. & luna sub t*er*ra morit*ur*. Demonstrandi eni*m* gr*ati*a. Pone luna*m* e*ss*e .xvii. dieru*m*. q*ui*b*us* & su*m*ma*m* dcccxciiii. AXYLLHYM. mclxxvii. Diuide it*er*um p*er* .xix. & remanet unu*m*. Veni ad organu*m*. & inuenies AXYLLHYM uictore*m* quia .xxiii. habent*ur* supra t*er*ram. unum eni*m* sub terra.

1 PP.] *i.e. either* Pitagori Philosophi, *or* Pro Preliatoribus *(the Apuleian Sphere in Braekman (1988: 93) reads* pro preliatoribus*)* | **2** ⟨DIAGRAM⟩ *this rhomboid diagram is on the left-hand side of the page, the text is outlined to the right and underneath the diagram. The diagram is unusual in that the division between life and death is not from top to bottom, but from right to left. The diagram consists of a central area divided into two parts (N0 and S0) by two sets of double horizontal lines, in between is written:* MEDIA. *Around the central part are three rhomboid rings, the third (i.e. outermost) of which is empty. The central area (0) contains numbers and designations for the quality of life or death. The ring verging on the central area (1) contains designations for the quality of life or death, while the pertinent numbers are provided in ring 2. Overall, the diagram is compartmentalised into 8 parts (designated by the points of the compass): NW0, NE0* ME/DIA / VI/TA / Supra terram*; *N0* xi xiii xiiii xvi xvii xvi`ii´ xx; *NE1* MODICA VITA.; *NE2* xxi . xviii . vii . ii . iii.; *SE1* MAGNA VITA.; *SE2* x . xxiii . xxvi . xxvii . xix.; *SW0, SE0* SVB/TERRA** / MO/DICA / MO/RS; *S0* iiii xv xix xxi xxvi`i´i; *SW1* MAGNA MORS.; *SW2* xxv . xxvii . xxx . xxviii.; *NW1* MODICA MORS.; *NW2* i . v . vi . ix . xii. | * Supra terram] *this is strange because the division is right/left rather than top/bottom* | **SVB/TERRA] *Ibid.* | **4** in in] *read* in *(dittography)* | **7** Parili] -i < e | **9-10** uideris] *read* ~ adiacere | **16** dcccxciiii.] dccc[i]xciiii; *read* dcccxciii *(comparison with other Apuleian Spheres that calculate the outcome on the basis of arbitrary values for the days of the moon rather than the values of the days themselves reveals that this number is the value for the seventeenth day of the moon, see 2/7,10, Riess 1891-93: 383, Wickersheimer 1914: 166-67)* | **17** mclxxvii] *read* mcclxxvi *(see Riess and Wickersheimer); this number stands for the numerical value of the name Achilles (the sum for Achilles's name in the accusative in this form makes no sense but since the reading 1276 is supported by the published Spheres it must be correct. Note that Riess's and Wickersheimer's editions read* Achilles *and* Achillei. ΑΧΥΛΛΕΙC *would yield 1276 (1+600+400+30+30+5+10+200))* | .xix.] *read* .xxix. *(Spheres of the Peto-*

siris variety use 29 instead of 30 as the basis for calculations | **15-19** Demonstrandi... terra.] *this example motivates the outcome of a struggle between an unknown person (hereafter X, Hector in Riess and Wickersheimer) and Achilles. To do this, a calculation is needed in which the numerical value of the day of the moon is added to the letter values. A list of numerical letter values is not needed, because the example employs Greek letters, which have a fixed value. The value for the day of the moon is 893 (see above), to which the value of the name Achilles, 1276, (see above) is added. The outcome of this sum is omitted in this text, but the editions by Riess and Wickersheimer mention 2169. Factors of twenty-nine (not nineteen! or thirty, see above) are subtracted from the sum, which gives 23. If one consults the diagram, it transpires that Achilles is victorious over X.*

2/13 Oxford, St. John's College, MS 17, fol. 41rb/1-32

(DIAGRAM)

De quacumq*ue* re scire uolueris *ue*l consulere. utputa de ȩgris q*ua* dies occurrerit ea die. & q*uo*ta luna fuerit co*m*puta. & adde nom*en* ei*us* sec*un*d*u*m litt*er*as infra scriptas. & sic in uno colligis. & partire p*er* .xxx. Et q*ui*cq*ui*d in sp*er*a remanserit in sp*er*a respicias. & sic inuenies. Et si sursum ininueneris uiuet. si iussu*m* morietur.

Parili m*odo* cui*us* sit uictoria. de his qui ad sing*u*lare certamen eunt. ueru*m et*iam & causantiu*m* & negotiantiu*m*. *ue*l aliarum similiu*m* reru*m*. sic co*m*puta nom*en* iacentis. *ue*l fugitiui. *ue*l co*n*trarii cui*us*libet: adice h*ui*c numeru*m* que*m* uid*er*is adiacere p*re*sentis dieb*us* lunȩ. Collectu*m* numeru*m* diuide q*uo*ties potueris p*er* .xxx. & q*uo*d remanserit quȩre in organu*m* ubi sit. Et si inueneris in magna uita ueloc*it*er resurgat. & si in media p*er*multas dies egrotans saluabit*ur*. Quod si in modica uita. te*m*p*us* faciet resurgens. Si aut*em* in morte media morit*ur* infirm*us*. q*uo*d si in media luna co*m*pot*us* es. & is q*ui* laborat sub t*er*ra *est* p*er*iclitans saluabi*tur*. si u*ero* is q*ui* laborat sup*ra* t*er*ra*m* inuenit*ur*. & luna sub t*er*ra morit*ur*. demonstrandi eni*m* gr*ati*a. Pone luna*m*. e*ss*e .xvii. dieru*m*. quibus & su*m*ma*m* dccxciii. AXYLLHYM. mclxxvi. Diuide iteru*m* per .xix. & remanet unum. Veni ad organum & inuenies AXYLLHYM uictore*m* quia .xxiii. habenTVR super terram unum autem sub terra.

The diagram, which is placed above the text, has been excised in or after the sixteenth century (see pl. 9, p. 214; see also p. 543). Since 2/8,13 have a common exemplar, it stands to reason that the diagram must have been a rhomboid | **4** scriptas] -r- < [·] | **5** ininueneris] *read* inueneris *(dittography of* in*)* | iussu*m*] -s$_1$- < [·] | **10** q*uo*ties] *read* quotiens | **14** co*m*pot*us* es] *read* computes | **15-19** demonstrandi... terra.] *see 2/8, n. to ll. 15-19* | **16** dccxciii.] *read* dcccxciii.*; see 2/8, n. to l. 16* | mclxxvi.] *read* mcclxxvi.*; see 2/8, n. to l. 17* | .xix.] read .xxix.*; see 2/8, n. to l. 17.*

2/11 Oxford, St. John's College, MS 17, fol. 8rb

⟨DIAGRAM⟩

This Apuleian Sphere consists of a diagram only | **1** ⟨DIAGRAM⟩ *this compartmentalised circular diagram has three concentric rings around a central circle. The central circle (0) contains qualifications of life and death in Greek, and in Latin in the form of coded writing by vowel substitution. The ring verging on the central circle (1) contains numbers. Ring 2 contains designations for the quality of life and death in Greek. while ring 3 contains the same in secret writing. Overall, the diagram is compartmentalised into 8 parts (designated by the points of the compass), the top half for life and the bottom half for death. Outside the diagram are Greek glosses in a later hand. The numbers of the diagram are subdivided into groups designated by the Greek writing, as follows: W1-2* ΜΗCΟΘΙC*; W0-E0* ωΡωΙ ΖΟΗC ⁝ / ΚΡΟΘΑΝΑΘΟC.*; NW0, NE0, SW0, SE0 NW3* c ⋯ rc: :l ⋯ s u ⁝ /t: · ·c / m ⋯ r/t ·· s*; E1-2* ΜΗCΟΘΙC*; NW2* ΖΟΗ ΜΙCΡΑ*[*]; NW3* u ·· t · h ⋯ m ·· n ⁝ s*; NW1* i . ii . ii`i´ . iiii . vii . ix . x.*; N1-2* ΥΠΕΡΓΗΙω*; N0* ΜΕCΙ ΖΟΕ.*[**]; NE2* ΖΟΕ ΜΗΓΑΛΗ.*; NE3* u ⁝ t · c ·· t ;*; NE1* xx . xxii . xxii`i´ . xxvi . `xxvii.´*[***]; SE2* ΘΑΝΑΘΟC ΜΙCΡΟC.*[†]; SE3* m ⋯ rs h ⋯ m ·· n ·· s*; SE1* xxviii . xxix . xxx.*; S1-2* ΥΡωΓΗΥω*[††]; S0* ΜΕCΟC ΤΑΝΑΤΟC.*[†††]; SW2* ΘΑΝΑΘΟC ΜΗΓΑC*; SW3* m ⋯ rs c ·· t ;*; SW1* v . vi . viii . xii . xxv. *The following glosses have been added at a later date outside the diagram (ring 4 for ease of reference): NW4* ζωη. μικϱά*; N4* ὑπέϱγειον*; NE4* ζωὴ μεγάλη*; S4* ˙ υπόγειον | [*] ΜΙCΡΑ] *i.e.* ΜΙΚΡΑ | [**] ΖΟΕ.] *read* ~ xi xiii xiii xvi xvii xix | [***] `xxvii.´] *transposed from NE0* | [†] ΜΙCΡΟC] *i.e.* ΜΙΚΡΟC | [††] ΥΡωΓΗΥω] *i.e.* ΥΠωΓΗΥω | [†††] ΤΑΝΑΤΟC.] *read* ~ xv xviii xxi xxiiii.

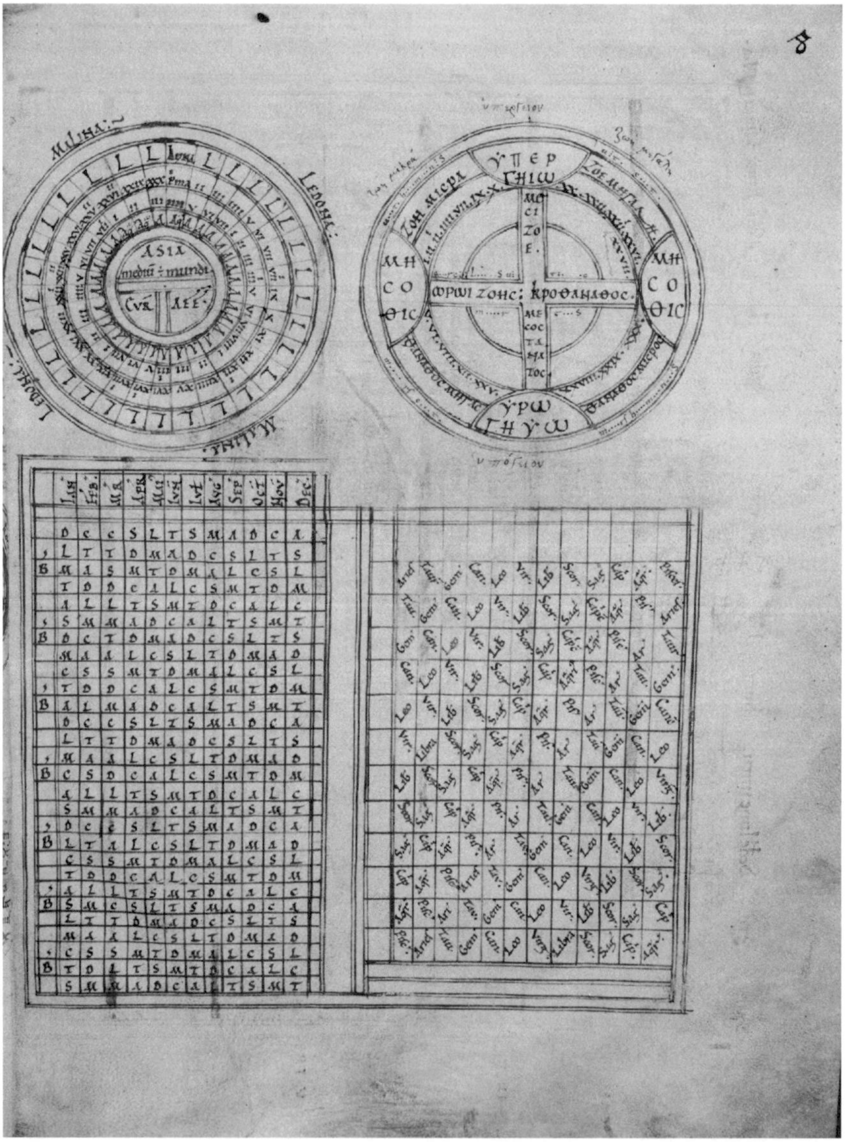

plate 12: Oxford, St. John's College, MS 17, fol. 8r

3 Birth Prognostics

Description

While some genre groupings share a common purpose (to report dangerous days for bloodletting, as Egyptian Days do) or structure (days of the moon, as lunaries do), birth prognostics are diverse texts which have in common that they have something to reveal about birth. The group comprises temporal and non-temporal prognostics, and within the temporal branch, texts pertaining to pre- and postnatal matters up to Judgement Day.[1] Birth prognostics address issues ranging from the development of the human foetus, the gender of an unborn child, the character and walk of life of a newborn child, and three miraculous days in the year on which only boys are born.[2]

3.1.1 Birth Prognostic, Temporal, Development of the Foetus

Literature

Wright (1841: 138-40); Rose (1894: 426-66); Förster (1903: 355, n. 1; 1908c: 36); Ferckel (1914); Singer (1961: I.xxiv); Hill (1961-63); Bonser (1963: 265); Talbot (1967: 19-20); Rubin (1974: 68); Cross and Hill (1982: 123-25); Deegan (1987: 22-24); Hollis and Wright (1992: 270); Cameron (1993: 183-84); Swanton (1993: 263); Mitchell (1998: 271-72); Chardonnens (2000); Hollis (2001: 197); Elsakkers (2004); Cilliers (2004, 2005)

Attributions

medieval: Augustine, Galen, Hippocrates; post-medieval: Octavius Horatianus, Soranus, Theodorus Priscianus

Author

Helvius Vindicianus

Branch of Superstition

observation of times: weekdays, months

Text

OE: 1. London, British Library, Cotton Tiberius A. iii, fols 40v-41r

[1] Not included are birth lunaries, which are discussed on pp. 426-28.

[2] Prognostics by the star sign at birth are not attested in Anglo-Saxon manuscripts, but they existed in Middle English (Taavitsainen 1988: 52-53). Classical birth prognostics by star signs and planets have been identified (Gundel 1927: 157-93).

Description

This text, the only one of its kind in an English manuscript, describes the development and growth of the human foetus in monthly stages.[1] If the text were to treat this matter solely, it would not be a prognostic. The last sentence of (1), however, tells us that if the baby has not yet been born in the tenth month, "in the mother it [the baby] becomes a fatality to her, most often on a Monday night".[2] This curious addition is likely to be original to the Anglo-Saxon text: no other redaction has been attested with this ending.

In the new introduction to the reprint of Cockayne's *Leechdoms*, Singer remarked: "pp. 144-147 are filled with two very curious passages [viz. 3.1.1/1 and 3.2/1] reminiscent of degenerate Greek medicine".[3] Singer did not elaborate upon the extent to which these two prognostics are degenerate and Greek, but it can be assumed that he had in mind texts "devoid of those living characteristics so honourably associated with ancient Greek medicine".[4] Talbot placed (1) and other birth prognostics and gynaecological texts in the context of the Hippocratic treatise *De mulierum affectibus*,[5] although the evidence does not warrant a direct association between the latter and (1). Consensus on how these birth prognostics should be interpreted has not been reached, but this may be due to the fact that modern scholars have failed to study them seriously. Rubin, for instance, claimed that "there is little of gynaecological value or knowledge in it [3.1.1/1]".[6] Mitchell commented: "it is not possible to say how widely they [3.1.1/1 and 3.2/1] were known or how seriously they were taken".[7]

Deegan is the only one so far who has discussed with integrity the knowledge portrayed in (1) with regard to the level of learning in classical and medieval times, and in the light of classical and modern embryology.[8] On the one hand, the development of the arterial system "into 365 shorter and longer" veins and arteries may have its foundation in sym-

[1] The text does not say so, but these months should probably be construed as lunar rather than solar. Galenic embryology uses a period of 280 days, which amounts to ten lunar months, forty weeks.

[2] Translation of text 3.1.1/1, ll. 18-19.

[3] Singer (1961: I.xxiv).

[4] Grattan and Singer (1952: 23).

[5] Talbot (1967: 19-20).

[6] Rubin (1974: 68).

[7] Mitchell (1998: 271).

[8] Deegan (1987: 23-24).

bolism or analogy rather than observation.[9] On the other hand, the comment that "In the third month it [the foetus] is human without a soul" cannot be dismissed as fiction so easily,[10] because the genesis and existence of the soul played a central role in Christian theology.[11] Even today, the entry of the soul into the human foetus is the subject of major controversies, for instance with regard to policies on abortion or the death of unborn children. In fact, the few other texts on the development of the foetus in the vernacular, in Old Frisian and Low Saxon manuscripts, are not encountered in a medical context, but in law codes. These text witnesses are found together with abortion laws, homicide laws and injury tariffs. Here, the information on the development of the foetus was employed to define the legal position of a pregnant woman and also that of the unborn child.[12]

In view of the Old Frisian and Low Saxon material, the gravity of the text is not in doubt. There are at least two more indications that it was quite an authoritative text. First, the text on the development of the foetus is encountered more than once in continental manuscripts. I have already referred to the Old Frisian and Low Saxon witnesses. To these may be added a Middle High German redaction, excerpts in the *Trotula* and works of Isidore and Vincent of Beauvais, a Middle English metrical redaction, and a Latin version in the Leiden manuscript Vossianus Lat. Q. 69, fol. 36v, recently identified by Bremmer.[13] The last item, particularly, may prove highly relevant to (1) since it is found in that part of the manuscript which betrays the influence of English learning, witness the presence of the Leiden Glossary (s. viii^{ex}, St. Gall).[14] In addition to texts on the development of the foetus, there are several continental manuscripts with texts of which the topic addressed in (1) is but an excerpt.[15]

[9] Translation of text 3.1.1/1, ll. 4-5.

[10] Translation of text 3.1.1/1, l. 7.

[11] Deegan (1987: 23-24), Elsakkers (2004: 128-29).

[12] On the Old Frisian (and Low Saxon) texts on the development of the foetus and their place in the Old Frisian legal system, see the outstanding study by Elsakkers (2004). See also Hill (1961-63).

[13] Ferckel (1914) printed the Middle High German redaction, Wright (1841: 138-40) the Middle English. Cilliers (2004: 345-46, n.10) referred to the *Trotula*, Isidore and Vincent of Beauvais. Bremmer will publish the Latin version in Vossianus Lat. Q. 69.

[14] Bremmer and Dekker (2006: 89-90, 91, 99 [157.2.7b]).

[15] Rose (1894: 426-66), Förster (1903: 355, n. 1), Wickersheimer (1966: 44 [XXIX. 7], 63 [LIII.1-2], 84 [LXVI.12-13], 101 [LXXVI.4], 120-21 [LXXVII.36], 141 [XCII. 4], 188 [CXVIII.14]), Cilliers (2005).See also Elsakkers (2004: 150-51, n. 75).

The second reason why the text on the development of the foetus is authoritative is that the Old Frisian and Low Saxon witnesses commonly refer to Augustine as the author of the text.[16] If the matter of the development of the foetus were not taken seriously, or were "reminiscent of degenerate Greek medicine", the attribution to Augustine would have been a considerable mistake. Elsakkers has argued that the ascription can be explained by the fact that Augustine wrote about early and late abortion, which equals a distinction preserved in the Old Frisian abortion laws.[17] Text (1) is not ascribed to any authority, but in his edition of a Middle High German redaction, Ferckel named Galen and Hippocrates as authorities to whom the text on the development of the foetus has been ascribed.[18] Post-medieval attributions include Octavius Horatianus, Soranus and Theodorus Priscianus.[19] The ascription to Augustine is not so far from the truth, particularly in view of Anglo-Saxon knowledge of embryology through Archbishop Theodore's *Laterculus Malalianus* 13, which deals with the formation of the foetus of Christ in terms of Augustinian embryology.[20] Authorship (1) cannot be traced back to Augustine himself, but to a contemporary of his: the late fourth century physician Vindicianus.[21] Bonser thought that the text on the development of the foetus originated with the Anglo-Saxons.[22] Cameron

[16] Hill (1961-63: 56). See also the discussion of this attribution by Elsakkers (2004: 125-26, 128-29).

[17] Elsakkers (2004: 128-29). Elsakkers saw another authenticating strategy in the deliberate reference to ensoulment, which she claimed was introduced by the Frisian translator. Text 3.1.1/1 already features a reference to the soul (that is, the absence of it), but the treatment of the topic in the Old Frisian material is new.

[18] Ferckel (1914: 306).

[19] Ferckel (1914: 306, n. 4). Hill (1961-63: 55) listed even more attributions, but he was under the mistaken impression that every name mentioned by Ferckel constitutes an attribution.

[20] Stevenson (1995: 54-55, 138, 196-200). The pseudo-Bedan treatise *De natiuitate infantium libellus* contains a section on foetal development. This section (Migne 1861-1904: I.959) is presumably a fragment, because it deals with the seventh to tenth months only. In contrast to 3.1.1/1, the pseudo-Bedan text differentiates between the growth of masculine and feminine foetuses. Bede was familiar with Theodore's medical opinions (see pp. 115-17), and it would be tempting to link the fragment on embryology in *De natiuitate infantium* with the *Laterculus* if it were not for the spurious attribution to Bede of the former treatise. *De natiuitate infantium* somehow escaped discussion in Jones's *Bedae Pseudepigrapha* (1939).

[21] On the link between Augustine and Vindicianus in view of the attribution in the Old Frisian texts, see Elsakkers (2004: 133-34).

[22] Bonser (1963: 265).

claimed to "know of no sources for either of these articles [viz. 3.1.1/1 and 3.2/1]",[23] which is remarkable because elsewhere he wrote that the works of Vindicianus were known in Anglo-Saxon England, and that Vindicianus "wrote on various subjects, chiefly gynaecology".[24]

Text (1), the excerpt in the *Trotula*, the Old Frisian and Low Saxon texts, and the witness in Vossianus Lat. Q. 69 represent a single chapter of Vindicianus' anatomical tract *Gynaecia*.[25] In this chapter, the growth of the foetus is described in monthly stages. The development outlined in (1) is as follows:

month	development
1	brain
2	membrane around the brain (week 6), arteries and veins, limbs
3	human without soul
4	firm in limbs
5	alive and growing, ribs, moving, mother in pain
6	skin, bones growing
7	toes and fingers growing
8	chest growing, heart and blood, firm body
9	birth (may be delayed)
10	birth, fatal on Monday night

table 17: growth of the human foetus

There is much variation in order and content between the Latin redactions published by Rose,[26] and it is hard to trace the vernacular texts to any particular Latin redaction. There is no consensus even as to the time of birth, which is sometimes placed in the tenth month.[27] In (1), the expecting mother lies witless because of the pain of the growing and moving foetus in the fifth month. In the hitherto published Latin redactions, the mother is merely nauseous, usually in the fourth or fifth month.[28] Four elements in (1) are absent in the *Gynaecia*: the creation of

[23] Cameron (1993: 184).

[24] Cameron (1993: 67).

[25] Rose (1894: 452-56). A characterisation of the *Gynaecia* is given by Cilliers (2005: 153-54).

[26] Rose (1894: 452-55, 465). See also Cilliers (2005: 222-26) and the table in Elsakkers (2004: 141).

[27] A detailed discussion of foetal development and the period of gestation in the *Gynaecia* is in Cilliers (2004: 353-64).

[28] See Cilliers (2004: 357-58).

365 veins and arteries;[29] the absence of the soul in the third month;[30] the pain caused by the growing and moving foetus; and finally, the fatality on Monday night if the baby is not born in time. (1) must have derived from a Latin original of Vindicianus' *Gynaecia* or a fragment containing chapter 20 of the work, possibly via an Irish route in view of the reference to the 365 veins and arteries. The Latin text identified by Bremmer contains all the attributes present in (1) but not in Rose's texts, except for the prognostic comment at the end of (1), which may well be original to the translation into Old English.

Vindicianus was well-known in both continental and insular medieval medicine for his *Epistula ad Pentadium nepotem suum de quattuor umoribus in corpore humano constitutis*.[31] This treatise is frequently represented in English and continental manuscripts alike. Vindicianus' *Gynaecia* is attested in continental manuscripts, but no (complete) Anglo-Saxon redaction of the text has as yet been brought to light. This may mean that the *Gynaecia* was considerably rarer in Anglo-Saxon England than the *Epistula ad Pentadium*. If this is indeed so, the survival of (1) is an extremely fortunate event, because in (1) we have not only the earliest text witness in the vernacular, but also one of the few pieces of evidence that Vindicianus' *Gynaecia*, at least in part, was known in early medieval England.[32]

---

[29] In discussing question 59 on the number of veins (answer: 365) in the *Prose Solomon and Saturn*, Cross and Hill (1982: 125) opined that the number 365 "derives from the Irish habit of using this figure to indicate totality in contexts where a precise or naturalistic figure cannot be obtained". If this is true, the addition may be restricted to the foetal texts of insular derivation, i.e. Vossianus Lat. Q. 69 and 3.1.1/1, which may explain the absence of the number symbolism in the (medieval continental) texts edited by Rose (1894) and Cilliers (2005).

[30] Some redactions of the *Gynaecia* refer to the beginning of movement in the foetus by using the term 'anima' (see Rose 1894: 454, 455). It is not unthinkable that the Anglo-Saxon translator somehow took 'anima' to refer to ensoulment rather than vivification.

[31] Cameron (1993: 53, 54, 67).

[32] But see also the introduction to the prognostic on gender prediction (pp. 241-44).

Edition

3.1.1/1 London, British Library, Cotton Tiberius A. iii, fols 40v/18-41r/11

Her onginð secgan ymbe mannes gecynde hu he on his modor innoþe to men gewyrðeð. ærest þæs mannes brægen bið geworden on his moder innoþe þonne biþ *þæt* brægen utan mid reaman bewefen on þære syxtan wucan.

On oðrum monðe þa ædran beoð geworden. on lxv. 7 þreo hundræd scytran 7 lengran in beoð todælede 7 *þæt* blod þonne floweð on þa fet 7 uppan þa handa. 7 he þonne byþ on limum todæled. 7 tosomne geawað.

On þam þriddan monþe he biþ man butan sawle.

On þam feorþan monþe he bið on limum staþolfæst.

On þam fiftan monþe he biþ cwicu. 7 weaxeð. 7 seo modur lið witleas. 7 þonne þa ribb beoð geworden. þonne gelimpð þæræ manigfeald sar þonne þæs byrþres lic on hire innoþe styrigende bið.

On þa*m* n þam syxtan monþe he byþ gehyd. 7 ban beoð weaxende.

On þam seofoþan monþe þa tan. 7 þa fingras. beoð weaxende.

On þam eahtoþan monþe him beoð þa breostþing wexende. 7 heorte. 7 blod. 7 he bið eall staþolfæstlice. geseted.

On þam nigoþan monþe witodlice wifum bið cuð hwæðer hi cennan magon.

On þam teoþam monþe *þæt* wif hit ne gedigð hyre feore. gif *þæt* bearn accenned ne biþ. forþam þe hit in þam magan wyrð hire to feorhadle oftost on tiwesniht.

Mitchell's claim (1995: 18) that he did not regularise the spelling of the Old English texts he cited is void in view of his editions of this text and 9.2.2/2 | **4** scytran] *read* scyrtran | **5** in] *read* hi | **6** geawað] *read* gearwað | **7** monþe] ~ ‖ ⟨*f. 41r*⟩ | **8** bið] biþ *Chardonnens (2000)* | **9** biþ] bið *Chardonnens* | **11** byrþres] *read* byrþnes | **12 On** þa*m* n þam] *dittography in which the second rubricated initial was left out* | **17** teoþam] *read* teoþan | gedigð] *Mitchell invoked the verb* geðicgan *(*to partake of*) with a transferred meaning* to escape with, *whereas this is unnecessary in view of the manuscript reading* gedigð, *from* gedigan *(*to survive, overcome, escape*)* | hit ne gedigð hyre feore] *an echo of this phrase is found in the text on the Dog Days in Vitellius E. xviii (6/1, ll. 6-7):* hit sume heora feore ne gedigað.

3.1.2 Birth Prognostic, Temporal, Three Miraculous Days

Literature

Migne (1861-1904: I.959-60); Birch (1878: 474; 1892: 253); Förster (1903: 354; 1929: 258-61); Thorndike (1923-58: I.688-89); Henel (1934-35: 346-47); Bonser (1963: 270); Thorndike and Kibre (1963: 1583); Taavitsainen (1988: 53); Hollis and Wright (1992: 268); Günzel (1993: 31); Epe (1995: 59); Liuzza (2001: 185)

Attribution

post-medieval: Bede

Branch of Superstition

observation of times: days

Texts

OE: 1. Cambridge, Corpus Christi College, MS 391, p. 718
2. London, British Library, Cotton Caligula A. xv, fol. 131r
3. London, British Library, Cotton Vitellius E. xviii, fol. 15r

L: 4. Cambridge, Corpus Christi College, MS 422, p. 49
5. London, British Library, Cotton Titus D. xxvi, fol. 4rv
6. Oxford, St. John's College, MS 17, fol. 3va

Description

The three miraculous birthdays is a brief text that lists three days on which boys only are born, whose bodies will not decay before Judgement Day. Of all temporal prognostics ordered by days, this is the only genre to report a number of propitious rather than unlucky days.[1] Texts on the three miraculous days are often attested side by side with those on the three Egyptian Days in the γ-sequence.[2] Scholarship on the miraculous birthdays has concentrated on text editions and explications of the purpose of this genre. The history and origin of the genre are not known.

As all Anglo-Saxon prognostics are Latinate in origin, this birth prognostic probably is as well, but no early Latin or Greek representatives can be pinpointed.[3] Several Latin redactions from the twelfth and thir-

[1] Thorndike (1923-58: I.688-89) cited a text which is the opposite of the one on the miraculous birthdays: "there are four other days and nights according to Bede on which no one is ever born or conceived, and if by chance a male is conceived or born, its body will never be freed from putridity". Unfortunately, Thorndike, who always referenced texts with meticulous care, did not include a source reference for these four unfortunate birthdays.

[2] See pp. 61-62.

[3] Förster (1929: 260), Henel (1934-35: 347).

teenth centuries have been identified,[4] but (5) is probably one of the earliest witnesses (s. xi[1]). A Latin representative of the three miraculous birthdays is incorporated in the pseudo-Bedan *De natiuitate infantium libellus*.[5] This treatise is spurious and contains several texts dealing with childbirth, including a fragmentary text on embryology and a weekday birth prognostic. Förster pointed out the existence of a Middle English text on the miraculous birthdays, and a German redaction dating from 1508 which is ascribed to Bede.[6] I have not found any medieval attributions to Bede, however. The Anglo-Saxon redactions range from the first half of the eleventh to the beginning of the twelfth centuries.

A clue as to the origin of the genre might be provided by the method of dating the three miraculous days. The English texts survive in three main redactions which can be distinguished as follows: redaction (a) refers to the months of the Roman calendar, (b) to dates in Roman calendar format, and (c) to the Hebrew calendar. Redaction (a) covers all texts in the vernacular (1-3): "that is one of the days at the end of December, and two at the beginning of January".[7] Redaction (b) is exemplified by (4): "that is the sixth kalends of April [27 March], the ides of August [13 August], and the third kalends of February [30 January]".[8] Redaction (c), finally, is as follows (5, 6): "that is the last [day] of Tebet and the first two of Sabat".[9] The use of the Roman calendar indicates a Latin origin for this genre, or a Latinate stage in its transmission. The reference to the Hebrew months might suggest that the texts on the three miraculous birthdays descended from a Hebrew source. This need not be the case, however, because knowledge of the names of the months in other languages, such as Latin, Greek, Egyptian and Hebrew, was common enough in computi and calendars, both in the early stages of the art of time reckoning, e.g. in Bede's *De temporum ratione*, and during its heyday in Benedictine Reform England.[10] For this reason, there is no basis for

[4] Henel (1934-35: 347), Thorndike and Kibre (1963: 1583, s.v. "Tres dies et noctes sunt in quibus si uir generatus fuerit", and "Tres dies pre aliis sunt obseruandi").

[5] Förster (1903: 354; 1929: 261). *De natiuitate infantium libellus* is printed in Migne (1861-1904: I.959-60).

[6] Förster (1903: 354; 1929: 261, n. 1).

[7] Translation of text 3.1.2/1, ll. 3-4.

[8] Translation of text 3.1.2/4, ll. 2-3.

[9] Translation of text 3.1.2/6, ll. 3-4. In the computus, Tebet and Sabat correspond to January and February.

[10] In his *De temporum ratione* XI-XV (Jones 1975-80: II.312-32), Bede treats of the months, their background and their names in various languages (cf. Wallis 1999: 281-84). The Hebrew names of the months and the Jewish lunar calendar are discussed ex-

positing a Hebrew origin for the prognostic on the three miraculous birthdays. Concerning a boy born on the three days, all redactions mention that "his body will not decay on earth before Judgement Day".[11] This reference to an event central to the Christian faith precludes a non- or pre-Christian genesis, or presupposes an intermediate Christian stage.[12]

The method of dating the three birthdays divides the redactions into two groups: those that date according to the months (a, c), and those that date with the Roman calendric system (b). If the relevant parts of (a) and (c) are set side by side, it would appear that the Old English is a translation of the Latin: (a) "þ*æt* is an þære daga on æftewardan decembre 7 ii. on forewardan Ianuaríí" (1), and (c) "id *est* nouissim*us* de thebeth. & duo p*ri*mi de sabath" (6). There is, however, a correspondence between (a) and (b) which does not occur in (c). Both (a) and (b) end with a phrase which testifies to the mysterious, hermetic nature of these days: (a) "there are few people who know these secrets", and (b) "it is an extraordinary mystery".[13] Within redaction (a), this comment is attested in two minor variants: (1, 3) "feawa manna syndon þe þas dagas cunnon" (there are few people who know of these days), and (2) "feawe synd þe þas geryne

tensively by Bede. He may have obtained this information from the *Laterculus* of Polemius Silvius: "an annotated Julian calendar; each month contains the names of the parallel Hebrew, Egyptian, Athenian and Greek months" (Wallis 1999: 42, n. 118). Later computi devote some attention to the names of the months as well. Byrhtferth's *Enchiridion* I.2 includes a list of names of the months in Hebrew, Egyptian, Greek and English (Baker and Lapidge 1995: 24). Baker and Lapidge (1995: 262) have argued that the names in Byrhtferth's table derive from the calendar in his computus, e.g. Vitellius E. iv, fols 35r-40v, St. John's College 17, fols 16r-21v (Baker and Lapidge 1995: 390-416). In addition to the computi mentioned just now, some Anglo-Saxon and post-Conquest calendars feature the names of the months in various languages, e.g. CTC R. 15. 32, pp. 15-26, CUL Kk. 5. 32, fols 50r-55v, Arundel 60, fols 2r-7v, Vitellius A. xii, fols 65v-71r, Vitellius E. xviii, fols 2r-7v, Bodley 579, fols 39r-44v (Wormald 1934: 128-39, 72-83, 142-53, 86-97, 156-67, 44-55, respectively). Finally, the names are included as glosses to Bede's *De temporum ratione* in St. John's College 17, fols 73v, 74v.

[11] Translation of text 3.1.2/1, ll. 2-3.

[12] Arguably, the genre may have been devised with a non-Christian setting of the end of times in mind, or the reference may have been added later, but as there is no evidence that this may have been the case, I reject this possibility.

[13] Translation of texts 3.1.2/2, l. 5 and 3.1.2/4, l. 3, respectively. Liuzza (2001: 185, 215) was not aware of the existence of 3.1.2/4, which is why he did not know that the comment in Old English on the hermetic nature has a Latin source. Förster (1929: 261) pointed out that the pseudo-Bedan *De natiuitate infantium libellus* (see above), contains the phrase "et suum mysterium mirabile est ualde" (Migne 1861-1904: I.960).

cunnan oþþe witan" (there are few who know of this secret).[14] Another minor variation between (1, 3) and (2) is in the reference that girls are not born on the three miraculous birthdays: where (1, 3) use "wif", (2) employs "wifmann".[15] This implies that redaction (a) should be divided into (a1) and (a2), i.e. texts (1, 3) and (2), respectively. The mention of baby girls is not found in (b), but is attested in (c). In speaking of the integrity of the body until Judgement Day, the vocabulary differs in all redactions: (a1) uses "ne forealdeð" (will not decay); (a2) "ne forrotað... ne fulað" (will not rot or corrupt); (b) "integru*m* manebit" (will remain intact); and (c) "nunq*uam*... putredine soluet*ur*. *sed* p*er*durabit" (will not end up in decay but will last).[16] Here, the phrasing of (a1, a2) resembles the negation of (c), rather than the affirmative statement of (b). On the basis of these findings, I conclude that there are two Latin redactions, both of which have influenced the Old English one. The variant readings (a1) and (a2) in the Old English redaction can be explained as representing two independent translations from a Latin source which resembled (c), but which had an important element from (b), to wit the comment on the hermetic knowledge of the birthdays.

Edition[17]

3.1.2/1 Cambridge, Corpus Christi College, MS 391, p. 718/2-8

ry dagas synd on .xii. monðum mid iii nihtum on ðam ne bið nan wif acenned 7 swa hwylc wæpman swa on ðam dagum accenned bið ne forealdeð his lichomo næfre on eorðan ær domesdæge þ*æt* is an þære daga on æftewardan decembre 7 ii. on forewardan Ianuarii feawe men synd þe þas cunan.

1 ry] *read* Ðry; *Förster (1929) suggested that the initial* 'Ð' *of the preceding line (i.e. the first letter of the last sentence of 9.2.5/1) properly belongs here, bur this is unlikely precisely because the* 'Ð' *is already in use* | ry... .xii.] *the remainder (about half) of the line is left blank in the manuscript* | **2** lichomo] *read* lichoma | **4** cunan] *read* dagas ~ *(see 3.1.2/3).*

[14] Texts 3.1.2/3, ll. 4-5, and 3.1.2/2, l. 5, respectively.

[15] Texts 3.1.2/1, l. 1, and 3.1.2/2, ll. 1-2, respectively.

[16] Texts 3.1.2/1, l. 2, 3.1.2/2, ll. 2-3, 3.1.2/4, l. 2, and 3.1.2/6, ll. 2-3, respectively.

[17] Order of the texts: 1, 3, 2, 4-6.

3.1.2/3 London, British Library, Cotton Vitellius E. xviii, fol. 15r/1-5

(**Ð**)ry dagas syndon on twelf monðum mid þrim ni(ht)um o(n þam ne bið) nan wif acenned ac swa hwilc wæpman swa on ðam dagum acen(ned bið ne) forealdað his lichama næfre on eorðan ær domesdæge. þ*æt* is an ðæra daga on æfteweardan decembre 7 tweigen on foreweardan ian(uarii); feawa manna syndon þe þas dagas cunnon:–

Margins damaged; text illegible on any medium except the manuscript itself | **2** ac] *read* 7 *(see 3.1.2/1,3).*

3.1.2/2 London, British Library, Cotton Caligula A. xv, fol. 131r/5-11

Ðreo dagas syndon on .xii. monðum mid þrim nihtum on þam ne bið nan wifmann akenned. 7 swa hwylc wæpnedmann on þa*m* dagum akenned bið ne forrotað his lichama næfre on eorðan ne he ne fulað ær domesdæge. nu is an þara daga on æftewyrdne dec*embre*. 7 þa twegen on foreweardan Ianuarie þam monðe. 7 feawe synd þe þas geryne cunnan oþþe witan.

3.1.2/4 Cambridge, Corpus Christi College 422, pp. 49/8-12

In anno sunt. tres dies & tres noctes. in quib*us* siquis. homo. genit*us*. fuerit sine dubio corp*us* eius. integru*m* manebit. usq*ue* in die*m*. iudicii: hoc e*st* vi kł apreli*s*. 7 idus. agustus 7 iii kł feb*ruarii*. 7 est mirabile. misterium:

3 agustus] *read* agusti.

3.1.2/5 London, British Library, Cotton Titus D. xxvi, fol. 4r/13-4v/1

Tres dies sunt in anno cu*m* totide*m* noctib*us* ut fertur in quib*us* mulier nu*n*qua*m* nascitur. & uir qui natus fuerit in ipsis. nu*n*qua*m* corp*us* illius putredine soluetur usq*ue* ad diem iudicii. id est nouissimus de theb*et*. & duo primi de sabath.

2 soluetur] *read* ~ sed perdurabit*(? see 3.1.2/6)* | **3** est] ~ ‖ ⟨*f. 4v*⟩.

3.1.2/6 Oxford, St. John's College, MS 17, fol. 3va/36-41

Tres dies *sunt* in q*uoque* anno cu*m* t*ri*b*us* noctib*us* ut ferunt in q*ui*b*us* mulieru*m* nunq*uam* nascit*ur*. & uir si nat*us* fuerit in ipsis nunq*uam* corp*us* ei*us* putredine soluet*ur*. s*ed* p*er*durabit usq*ue* ad die*m* iudicii. id *est* nouissim*us* de thebeth. & duo p*ri*mi de sabath;

1 ferunt] *read* fertur *(see 3.1.2/5).*

3.1.3 Birth Prognostic, Temporal, Day of the Week

Literature

Migne (1861-1904: I.960); Birch (1878: 477-78; 1892: 256); Meyer (1884: 207); Förster (1903: 354-55; 1908c: 39; 1912b: 296-308); Thorndike (1923-58: I.679); Gundel and Gundel (1959: 108-14); Hollis and Wright (1992: 264); Günzel (1993: 33); Epe (1995: 59); Liuzza (2001: 184)

Attribution

post-medieval: Bede

Branch of Superstition

observation of times: weekdays

Texts

OE: 1. Cambridge, Corpus Christi College, MS 391, p. 715
2. Oxford, Bodleian Library, Hatton 115, fols 148v-49r
L: 3. London, British Library, Cotton Tiberius A. iii, fol. 65r
4. London, British Library, Cotton Titus D. xxvi, fols 6v-7v
5. Oxford, St. John's College, MS 17, fol. 4ra

Description

The weekday birth prognostic foretells a child's character and walk of life depending on the day on which it is born. With regard to (4), Birch mentioned that this genre is "of great interest, no doubt, to the ancient soothsayer, and probably as trustworthy as those [auguries] we occasionally hear in these later times from doting mothers and maudlin nurses".[1] How ancient this soothsayer would have been, is not elucidated by Birch, unless he referred to the owner of Titus D. xxvi, xxvii, viz. Abbot Ælfwine.[2]

To my knowledge, no Latin witnesses antedating the eleventh century have been found. Förster wrote: "the diversity of the Latin texts may in part go back to diversity of the original Greek texts".[3] There are, however, no Greek ancestors attested for this genre, nor early Latin ones for that matter. The weekday birth prognostic is, like so many prognostics, a genre that just seems to exist from a certain period in the Middle Ages onwards. The obscurity of its beginnings is compensated for by the attention this genre received in post-medieval folklore—the "doting mothers

[1] Birch (1878: 478).
[2] See pp. 57-59.
[3] "Die Verschiedenheiten der Lateintexte mögen zum Teil schon auf Verschiedenheiten der zugrunde liegenden griechischen Texte zurückgehen" (Förster 1912b: 305).

and maudlin nurses" mentioned by Birch. Förster published several fifteenth- and sixteenth-century redactions in Latin as well as a number of analogues ranging from Old French to Modern English and Danish.[4] A weekday birth prognostic is incorporated in a condensed form in the pseudo-Bedan *De natiuitate infantium libellus*.[5] I have found no medieval birth prognostic of this type that is ascribed to Bede.

Förster's analysis of the Old English and Latin redactions of weekday birth prognostics is unsurpassed.[6] Rather than repeating his findings here, I present the most salient points. There is a peculiarity of the Latin weekday birth prognostics which might point to a link with lunaries. In the Latin texts (3-5), the phrase "the beginning of all things is good" is added to the entries for Monday, Tuesday, Thursday and Friday.[7] This phrase properly belongs to the prognostic genre of agenda lunaries, and so to the agenda part of collective lunaries.[8] Neither the Old English weekday birth prognostics nor the Latin analogues adduced by Förster include this phrase.[9] Text (1) states that a child will be "often ill and unhealthy" if born on Monday.[10] This phrase is not found in other witnesses of this genre, but it is encountered in an Old English redaction of the birth lunaries.[11] The similarities mentioned here indicate that the contents of lunaries must have influenced the weekday birth prognostics in some of the English redactions.

The contents of texts (1, 2) show overlap, but they differ in phrasing, e.g. "nafað he na mycle sorge" (he does not have many worries) versus "orsorglice leofæð he" (he lives without worry); and "he yfele cræftas leornað" (he learns evil crafts) versus "he bið disicreafti" (he is skilled in evil crafts).[12] There are similarities between (1) and (2), but the contents do not correspond closely enough to presume that they are independent

[4] Förster (1912b: 301-08).

[5] See p. 97-98, 231.

[6] Förster (1912b: 297-305).

[7] Translation of text 3.1.3/4, e.g. ll. 4-5.

[8] See Förster (1912b: 302, n. 3), and pp. 399-400, 422-23.

[9] See 3.1.3/1,2, and Förster (1912b: 301-03).

[10] Translation of text 3.1.3/1, l. 4.

[11] See texts 9.2.2/2,3. The link between "oft seoc 7 hunhal" (3.1.3/1, l. 4) and "a seoc 7 unhal" (9.2.2/2, l. 2) is remarkable in that the relevant Old English weekday birth prognostic is attested in CCCC 391, and the Old English birth lunaries in Caligula A. xv and Tiberius A. iii. The Old English birth lunary in CCCC 391, which would have been a more likely source of correspondence for 3.1.3/1, has the phrase "seoc 7 sicle" (9.2.2/1, l. 2).

[12] Texts 3.1.3/1, ll. 2, 12, and 3.1.3/2, ll. 1-2, 12, respectively.

translations of a common Latin exemplar. The entry for Monday, for instance, reads: "he will be greedy for the goods of men, and hateful, and often ill and unhealthy",[13] which does not at all resemble "he will be killed by people, whether he be a layman or a clergyman".[14] Latin (3-5) resemble each other to such an extent that they can be said to form one redaction. All three Latin texts perpetuate the erroneous reading "hora diuturna siue nocturna" for "hora diurna siue nocturna".[15] Likewise, the epithet "utilissimus" with reference to a Sunday child caused trouble in all instances: "uti illimus" (3), "uti [il]li" (4), and "utillimi" (5). In all three texts, the predictions match in spirit, but (5) differs from (3, 4): "qui nascentur. fortis erint [*sic*] & cupidi. & ferro p*er*ibunt. & uix ad ultimam p*er*uenient ętatem" versus "q*ui* nascent*ur* er*unt* fortes & cupidi. & ferro p*er*i*bunt*. & uix ad senile*m* ętate*m* p*er*uenient" (those who are born will be strong and beloved and die by the sword, and they will hardly reach old age).[16] Förster concluded that the Old English texts form two separate redactions, neither of which can be matched to any surviving Latin exemplars from Anglo-Saxon manuscripts. The Latin texts form two versions of one redaction: (3, 4) and (5). Text (5) was not known to Förster. He published three Latin redactions not featured in Anglo-Saxon manuscripts, one of which may be representative of the Latin text which was used as a basis for Old English (2).[17]

The diversity in text redactions of the weekday birth prognostic makes up for the lack of background information on this genre. In other words, five Anglo-Saxon attestations represent no fewer than three redactions of a prognostic genre of which I have not found any pre-eleventh-century instances. However, the variety between the vernacular redactions implies that the genesis of this genre must antedate the first attestations. Of all birth prognostics, this genre and the next seem to have stood the test of time most successfully because their message survives to this day.

[13] Translation of text 3.1.3/1, ll. 3-4.

[14] Translation of text 3.1.3/2, ll. 3-4.

[15] Thorndike (1923-58: I.679) thought that a distinction was being made between birth at night or during the day, but this is not the case: the text merely stresses the fact that a full day is composed of a day and a night.

[16] Texts 3.1.3/3, ll. 6-7, and 3.1.3/5, ll. 3-4, respectively.

[17] Förster (1912b: 301-05).

Edition

3.1.3/1 Cambridge, Corpus Christi College 391, p. 715/4-26

Gif mon bið acennen on sunnandæg oððe on nihte swa wer swa wif swa hweðer hit þonne bið nafað he na mycle sorge 7 he bið gesælig be his gebyrde.

Gif mon biþ acenned on mannandæg oððe on niht he bið manna góda gitsiende 7 lað 7 oft seoc 7 hunhal.

Gif on tiwesdæg oððe on niht bið accenned se bið æwfest 7 manþwære 7 gesibsum 7 manna leof.

Gif on wodnesdæg oððe on niht bið acenned se bið scearp on gewinne 7 wærwyrde 7 grimful.

Gif on þunresdæg oððe on niht se bið gesælig 7 wifmannum leof gif hit wær bið 7 wepnedmannum leof hit wif bið.

Gif mon bið acenned on frigedæg oððe on niht he bið awyried from mannum 7 he yfele cræftas leornað 7 he æfre bið yfelwyrde 7 oðra manna æhte srydeð 7 bið scort on wæstmum.

Gif mon bið acenned on sæternesdæg oððe on niht se gelimp dæda 7 biþ ealdorman be his gebyrdum 7 him beoþ men æfestgendre ac se þeahhweðre þa costunge þera æfestgendra manna he oferswiðeð.

1 acennen] *read* acenned | **3** mannandæg] *read* monandæg | **7** scearp] -p < o | **10** hit] *read* gif ~ | **12** srydeð] *i.e.* strydeð | **15** æfestgendre] *read* æfestgende.

3.1.3/2 Oxford, Bodleian Library, Hatton 115, fols 148v/19-149r/11

SWA hwilc man swa on sunnandæg. oððe on niht acenned bið. orsorglice leofæð he. 7 bið fægger.

Gif he on monandæg. oðþe on niht acenned bið. he bið acweald fram mannu*m*. lewde swa clæroc sweþer he bið.

Gif he on tiwesdæg bið acenned. oþðe on ða niht. se bið æwerd on his life. 7 bið man 7 ðwære.

Gif he bið on wodnesdeig oþðe on da niht acenned. he bið scarp 7 biter. 7 swiðe wær on his wordum.

Gif he bið acenned on þurresdæg oþðe on þa niht. he bið swiðe gesibsum. 7 wæleði. 7 wel geweaxeþ. 7 he bið god lufiende. 7 eallis fram wifum.

6 man 7 ðwære] *read* manðwære *(see 3.1.3/1; for a similar misreading of* þeof 7 sceaðe *for* þeofsceaðe *and* latro & ingeniosus *for* latro ingeniosus, *see the birth lunaries 9.2.2/1,8)* | **7** da] *read* ða | **9** on$_1$] ~ ‖ ⟨*f. 149r*⟩.

Gif he bið acenned on frigendeg oðþe on ða niht. we bið awerget fam mannu*m*. 7 he bið disicreafti. 7 fam allum mannu*m* he bið laþ. 7 æfre ifel þenceþ on his heortan. 7 he bið ðeof. 7 swide ondredende. 7 he lengne leofað: þon*ne* on midre ilde.

Gif he bið acenned on saternesdæg. oþðe on ða niht. his dæde beoð franlica. 7 he bið ealdorman swa wewer swa wif. swa wære he bið. tæla him gelimpeþ. 7 lange he leofaþ:-

11 we] *read* he | fam] *read* fram | **12** disicreafti] *Cockayne (1864-66) read* disi creafti *and translated this with* silly, and crafty, *but see Förster (1912b: 300, n. 3)* | fam] *read* fram | **13** swide] *read* swiðe | lengne] *read* leng ne | **15** franlica] *read* framlica | **16** wewer] *read* weþer | wære] *read* wær.

3.1.3/3 London, British Library, Cotton Tiberius A. iii, fol. 65r/11-22

DE NATIVITATE INFANTVM.

Die dominico. hora diuturna siue nocturna uti illimus erit qui nascetur magnusq*ue* & spendid*us*.

Die .ii. hora diuturna siue nocturna qui nascetur fortis erit omnib*us* reb*us* incipiendum bonum est.

Die .iii. feria. hora diuturna siue nocturna qui nascentur. fortis erint & cupidi. & ferro p*er*ibunt. & uix ad ultimam p*er*uenient ętatem omnib*us* reb*us* incipiendum bonu*m* est.

Die .iiii. f*eria*. hora diuturna siue nocturna q*ui* nascentur ad uerba dicenda plurimu*m*. faciles erunt.

Die .v. f*eria*. hora diuturna siue nocturna q*ui* nascentur. affabiles & honorifici erunt. omnib*us* reb*us* incipiendu*m*. optimum est.

Die .vi. f*eria*. hora diuturna siue nocturna nascentes uitales erunt. & luxuriosi. om*n*ib*us* reb*us* incipiendu*m* bonu*m* est.

Die sabbato. hora diuturna siue nocturna q*ui* nascentur rare utiles erunt nisi cursus lune contulerit.

1 INFANTVM] *read* Infantium | **2 D**ie dominico] **D**ie d- *on erasure* | diuturna] *read* diurna *in all instances (the error was widespread, see 3.1.3/4,5)* | uti illimus] *read* utilissimus *(this word caused problems more often, see 3.1.3/4,5)* | **3** spendid*us*] *read* splendidus | **4** .ii.] *read* ~ feria | **6** fortis erint] *read* fortes erunt *(confusion between singular and plural is also apparent in 3.1.3/4,5)* | **13** nascentes] *read* qui nascentur.

3.1.3/4 London, British Library, Cotton Titus D. xxvi, fols 6v/10-7v/1

De natiuitate Infantium

Die dominico hora diuturna. **S**iue nocturna uti li erit q*ui* nasc*etur* magnusq*ue* & splendidus.

Die .ii. f*eria* hora diuturna siue no q*ui* nasc*etur* fortis erit om*n*ib*us* rebus incipiendu*m* bonum est.

Die .iii. f*eria* hora diuturna siue noct*ur*na qui nasc*entur* fortis erunt & cupidi. & ferro p*er*ibunt & uix ad ultima*m*. p*er*uenient aetatem om*n*ib*us* rebus incipiendum bonum est.

Die .iiii. fr hora diuturna siue noct*ur*na siue qui nascentur ad uerba dicenda plurimu*m* faciles erunt.

Die .v. f*eria* hora diuturna siue nocturna qui nascentur affabiles & honorifici erunt om*n*ib*us* incipiendum rebus optimu*m* est.

Die .vi. f*eria* hora diuturna siue nocturna qui nascent*ur* uitales erunt. & luxuosi omnib*us* reb*us* incipiendum bonum est.

Die. Sabbato hora diuturna. siue nocturna qui nascent*ur* rare utiles erunt nisi cursus lune contulerit.

1 natiuitate] **nati[f]uitate** | **2** diuturna] *read* diurna *in all instances (the error was widespread, see 3.1.3/3,5)* | uti li] uti [il]li; *read* utilissimus *(this word caused problems more often, see 3.1.3/3,5)* | **4** no] no[···]; *read* nocturna | erit] -it < [··] | **6** noct*ur*na] ~ ‖ ⟨*f. 7r*⟩ | fortis] *read* fortes *(confusion between singular and plural is also apparent in 3.1.3/3,5)* | **9** fr] *read* feria | siue noct*ur*na siue] *delete* siue$_2$ | **12** incipiendum rebus] *the inverse order is more usual (see 3.1.3/3,5, 9.1/1)* | **13** luxuosi] luxu[··]osi; *read* luxuriosi *(see 3.1.3/3)* | **15** utiles] ~ ‖ ⟨*f. 7v*⟩.

3.1.3/5 Oxford, St. John's College, MS 17, fol. 4ra/31-45

Die d*omi*nico hora diut*ur*na siue noct*ur*na q*ui* nascent*ur* utillimi er*unt* & magni;

Die .ii. f*eria* q*ui* nascent*ur* fortes er*unt*. o*mn*ib*us* reb*us* incipiendis bonu*m* *est*;

Die .iii. f*eria*. q*ui* nascent*ur* er*unt* fortes & cupidi. & ferro p*er*ib*un*t. & uix ad senile*m* ętate*m* p*er*uenient o*mn*ib*us* reb*us* incipiendis bonu*m* *est*.

Die .iiii. f*eria* q*ui* nascent*ur* ad u*er*ba dicenda multu*m* faciles er*unt*;

Die .v. f*eria* q*ui* nascent*ur* affabiles er*unt* & honorifici o*mn*ib*us* reb*us* incipiendis bonu*m* *est*;

Die .vi. f*eria*. q*ui* nascent*ur* uitales er*unt* & lu`xuriosi;´

Die sabb*a*to q*ui* nascent*ur* raro utiles er*unt* n*isi* curs*us* lunę co*n*tulerit;

Each entry starts on a new line | **1** diut*ur*na] *read* diurna *(the error was widespread, see 3.1.3/3,4)* | utillimi] *read* utilissimi *(this word caused problems more often, see 3.1.3/3,4)* | **8** lu`xuriosi;´] -`xuriosi;´ *written three lines above for lack of space, transposition indicated.*

3.2 Birth Prognostic, Non-Temporal, Gender Prediction

Literature

Hoops (1889: 67); Förster (1908c: 37); Singer (1961: I.xxiv); Bonser (1963: 265); Talbot (1967: 20); Rubin (1974: 68); Deegan (1987: 22); Hollis and Wright (1992: 266); Cameron (1993: 183-84); Swanton (1993: 263-64); Epe (1995: 60); Mitchell (1998: 218); Hollis (2001: 197); Hanson (2004); Cilliers (2004, 2005)

Branch of Superstition

observation of signs: behaviour of the expectant mother

Text

OE: 1. London, British Library, Cotton Tiberius A. iii, fols 42v-43r

Description

This non-temporal prognostic helps predict the gender of a child prenatally with the help of observations of the behaviour of the expectant mother and her physique. Within the group of birth prognostics, the text which foretells the gender of an unborn child is unique in that, to my knowledge, it is the only non-temporal birth prognostic and one of the rare codified representatives of gender prediction in the early Middle Ages. The somewhat esoteric knowledge of (1) and its proximity in the manuscript to the text on the development of the foetus (3.1.1/1) have caused these texts to be studied together: whenever (1) is mentioned 3.1.1/1 is as well, and vice versa. I have pointed out that Singer saw evidence of "degenerate Greek medicine" in (1) and 3.1.1/1,[1] while Mitchell was not able to establish "how seriously they [3.1.1/1 and 3.2/1] were taken".[2] It will become apparent that a link between 3.1.1./1 and (1) is warranted, but not for the reasons noted above.

Text (1) offers a number of observations and tests with which to predict the gender of a child:

boy	girl
mother walks slowly	mother walks quickly
mother has hollow eyes	mother has swollen eyes
mother prefers lily	mother prefers rose
mother walks on her heels	mother walks on her toes
mother's belly is carried high	mother's belly is sunk down

table 18: predicting the gender of an unborn child

[1] Singer (1961: I.xxiv). See p. 224.

[2] Mitchell (1998: 271).

After these predictions, (1) continues with a dietary section which cautions the expectant mother to abstain from certain foodstuffs. In the fourth or fifth month, if the mother eats nuts or fruit "the child will be stupid".[3] Moreover, consumption of the meat of male animals will make the child "hump-backed and hydrocele".[4] The combination of gender predictions and dietary guidelines is unusual,[5] but there are no indications whatsoever which imply that (1) should be split into two separate texts. In fact, the wording of (1) is such that the text must have been considered as a close-knit unit: all entries for both the predictions and the dietary rules are introduced with the phrase "again, there is another way".[6] Even the first entry is introduced in this manner, which suggests that the source text will probably have been longer than (1).

No direct sources for (1) have been identified, nor have any analogues or variant redactions been established up to now. These facts set (1) aside from the other prognostics, all of which have analogues at least. Deegan wrote that "as far back as the Hippocratic writings, in the fifth and fourth century BC, signs were looked for which might help determine the sex of a child".[7] She referred to Hippocrates' *Aphorisms*,[8] but this text provides us with two predictions only: "if a woman is going to have a male child she is of a good complexion; if a female, of a bad complexion" (V.42); and "the male embryo is usually on the right, the female on the left" (V.48).[9] Incidentally, neither of these predictions are found in (1). Talbot mentioned texts such as (1), 3.1.1/1 and other birth prognostics as "material available in the fragments that surround" the Hippocratic medical text *De mulierum affectibus*.[10]

Even if Hippocratic gynacology served as the origin of gender predictions, this does not explain how the gap of fifteen hundred years between Hippocrates and (1) is bridged, the more so because no English manuscript containing Hippocratic medicine has been discovered. The prob-

[3] Translation of text 3.2/1, l. 15.

[4] Translation of text 3.2/1, l. 18. Swanton (1993: 264) translated Old English "healede" with "bent".

[5] Both topics are addressed, however, in Vindicianus' *Gynaecia* but not in the same place.

[6] Translation of text 3.2/1, l. 1.

[7] Deegan (1987: 22).

[8] Deegan (1987: 25, n. 49).

[9] Jones (1931: 169, 171). On the gender predictions in the *Corpus Hippocraticum*, see Hanson (2004: 285, 291-92, 298).

[10] Talbot (1967: 20).

lem is aggravated by the fact that scholars are quick to point out the link with Hippocratic medicine, but so far no one has evidenced this link by giving concrete examples. Arguably, Deegan's reference to Hippocrates' *Aphorisms* is in aid of comparison rather than evidence, but Talbot's statement lacks foundation. Rubin referred to (1) and 3.1.1/1 as "deriving from Hippocrates", as did Swanton.[11] In the case of 3.1.1/1, this ascription is incorrect, and in the case of (1), misguided. Cameron stated that he knew "of no sources for either of these articles".[12] Although 3.1.1/1 can be traced back to Vindicianus' *Gynaecia*,[13] Cameron is justly cautious in not identifying a source for (1).[14]

Nevertheless, a redaction of the *Gynaecia* possibly forms the link between 3.1.1/1 and (1). Chapter 21 of some redactions of the *Gynaecia* records the Hippocratic observations on gender prediction by means of the location of the foetus and the complexion of the mother.[15] Moreover, the same chapter of Vindicianus' *Gynaecia* preserves a number of other gender predictions , including one on the sluggish gait of the mother in the case of a baby girl,[16] a prediction that is also present (but reversed) in (1). This chapter also contains a section on the etymological link between the Latin words "genae" and "genua", in which the eyes of a foetus are said to be located on its knees, because the knees are convex, the eye sockets concave.[17] In some redactions of the *Gynaecia*, this account has become garbled and mixed with the section on gender prediction to such an extent that, if the eyes of the mother appear convex, a baby girl will be born, and if they appear concave, a baby boy.[18] This is precisely what (1) reveals as well. In conclusion, the translator of (1) may have made use of Vindicianus' *Gynaecia* for the first few predictions at least. The recent discovery of a Latin source for the text on the development of the foetus in the late eight-century section of the continental manuscript Vossianus Lat. Q. 69,[19] which has ties with Anglo-Saxon England, makes it likely

---

[11] Rubin (1974: 68), Swanton (1993: 263).

[12] Cameron (1993: 184).

[13] See pp. 223-28.

[14] Hoops (1889: 67) already pointed out that there are no classical writers whose works could have served as a basis for the contents of 3.2/1.

[15] Rose (1894: 456, 457), Cilliers (2004: 350-53; 2005: 184, 186). I use Rose's chapter numbers.

[16] Rose (1894: 456), Cilliers (2005: 186).

[17] Rose (1894: 456, 457). "quia genua sunt tumentia, oculi autem sunt cavi" (Cilliers 2005: 186).

[18] Rose (1894: 456, 457).

[19] See p. 225.

that Vindicianus' *Gynaecia* was known in England at least as early as the eighth century. This, together with the attestation of (1) and 3.1.1/1 in close vicinity in the same manuscript, may mean that a source for (part of) the Old English text on gender prediction has finally been identified.

We are unfortunate in having no close analogues to (1), particularly in view of the fact that we may have had one if we are to rely on Bald's *Leechbook*. In the list of contents of book II, chapter 60 is introduced as a group of gynaecological matters and treatments (on topics also treated by Vindicianus!), among others dealing with "many signs by which one can understand whether it will be a male or female child".[20] However, the treatments themselves—no less than "forty-one items"—,[21] are absent in the manuscript.

Edition

3.2/1 London, British Library, Cotton Tiberius A. iii, fols 42v/9-43r/2

Eft is oðer wise be þissum þingum þ*æt* þu meht witan on bearneacenum wife hwæþeres cynnes bearn heo cennan sceal. gif heo gæð late 7 hæfþ hole eagan heo cenneð cniht. gif heo hraðe gæþ 7 hafað aþundene eagan heo cenneð mædencild.

Eft oþer wise genim þa twa wyrta on hand þ*æt* is lilie. 7 rose. ber to bearneacenum wife hat niman þæra wyrta swa hwæþeræ swa heo wille gif heo nimð lilian he cenð cnyht gif heo nimð rosan heo cænð mæden.

Eft is oþer cræft be þon gif þ*æt* wif mid þam helum stæpeð swiðor on þa eorðan heo cenneð cnyht gif heo mid þam tan stæpeð swiðor on þa eorþan heo cænneð mæden.

Eft is oþer wise. gif þam wife bið þ*æt* hrif upastigen heo cenneð cnyht. gif hit byþ nyþer asigen heo cenneþ mæden.

Eft oþer wise gif wif biþ bearneacen feower monoð oþþe fife 7 heo þonne gelome eteð hnyte oþþe æceran oþþe ænige niwe bleda þonne gelimpeð hit hwilum þurh þ*æt* þæt þ*æt* cild biþ disig.

Eft is oþer wise be þon gef eteð fearres flæsc oððe ra*m*mes oþþe buccan oþþe bæres oþþe hanan oþþe ganran oþþe æniges þara neata þe strynan mæg þonne gelimpeð hit hwilum þurh þæt þ*æt* þ*æt* cild bið hoforode 7 healede.

7 he] *read* heo | nimð$_2$] ni- < m | mæden] m- < a | **9** tan] [s]tan | **16** eteð] *read* heo ~ | oððe] -e < a | **17** þara] ~ ‖ ⟨*f. 43r*⟩.

[20] "manigfeald tacn þ*æt* mon mæge *on*gitan hwæþer hit hysecild þe mædencild beon wille" (Royal 12. D. xvii, fol. 64r/6-7).

[21] "an7feowertig cræfta" (Royal 12. D. xvii, fol. 64r/13).

4 Bloodletting Prognostic, Day of the Week

Literature

Thorndike (1923-58: I.679); Liuzza (2001: 187, n. 41)

Branch of Superstition

observation of times: weekdays

Text

L: 1. London, British Library, Sloane 475, fol. 135v

Description

The part of the composite manuscript Sloane 475 containing (1) may have an English origin, which is why this uniquely attested prognostic is included here.[1] The weekday bloodletting prognostic lists two or three hours on each weekday on which bloodletting is recommended.

Scholarship on this type of prognostic has remained close to the facts. Thorndike stated that the user is "informed of the various hours of the days of the week when it is advisable to perform bloodletting", and he referred the reader to (1).[2] Liuzza observed that (1) is "a list of favourable hours in each day for bloodletting".[3] These two observations represent all the research that has been conducted on this bloodletting prognostic since Thorndike and Liuzza are two of the few scholars so far to have discussed the manuscript in which (1) is attested, and (1) has no known analogues or sources at all. Neither Förster nor Henel, who both wrote extensively on prognostics of lucky and unlucky times, were aware of the existence of a prognostic like this.

Bloodletting prognostics are not rare in medieval manuscripts. Frequently encountered genres are bloodletting lunaries (ten witnesses), Dog Days (twenty-eight witnesses), and Egyptian Days (forty-five witnesses).[4] Including (1), bloodletting prognostics make up nearly fifty percent of the Anglo-Saxon prognostic corpus, which, partly at least, can be accounted for by the importance bestowed on well-timed bloodletting in medieval medicine.[5]

Within the group of bloodletting prognostics, (1) stands out in that it gives a list of auspicious times for bloodletting, e.g. "on Tuesday, the

[1] But see pp. 42-43.

[2] Thorndike (1923-58: I.679).

[3] Liuzza (2001: 187, n. 41).

[4] Regimens are another genre which describe appropriate times for bloodletting, among others, but the genre is rare in Anglo-Saxon manuscripts (see pp. 31-33, 44-45).

[5] See pp. 142-47.

third, seventh and tenth hour is good".[6] This positivistic approach is unique to (1). The Dog Days outline a period in which bloodletting should be avoided on account of attendant complications. Egyptian Days assign days on which bloodletting will prove fatal. Bloodletting lunaries, finally, tell the enquirer whether bloodletting is good or bad on a given day of the moon. With the exception of (1), none of the above prognostic genres reports auspicious times only.

The subject matter of (1) is shared by other bloodletting prognostics, but the structure must have come from elsewhere. The weekday approach is similar to month and year prognoses and to weekday brontologies: the day of the week determines what will happen or when something should be undertaken. The focus in month and year prognoses and in weekday brontologies is different from (1), however. The latter narrows its scope to particular hours of a specific day, while the former give a forecast of the future beyond the weekday, sometimes predicting a sequence of events for an entire year. The combination of a weekday structure with a further specification by hours is encountered only in (1). Some texts on the twenty-four Egyptian Days specify hours, but such texts are rare, and the hours assigned are dangerous for bloodletting rather than beneficial.

Edition

4/1 London, British Library, Sloane 475, fols 135v/4-13

Incipiunt ora se quod. sanguin*em* minuare debes.
in primis die dominico hora .ii. S vi. S nona. bonum est.
Die lunis h*ora* .iiii. S .primis. S .xi. bonum est.
Die martius. h*ora* .iii. S .vii. S x. bonum est.
Die mercur. iii. h*ora* .iiii. S vii. x bona e*st*.
Die iaius. h*ora* .iii. S octaua. S .x. bonu*m* e*st*.
Die ueteris. h*ora* .v. S .octaua bonum est.
Die sabato. h*ora* .ii. viii. bonum est
quod omitenpore. obseruam dissunt;

The entries for Tuesday to Saturday start on new lines. The scribe uses a symbol resembling 'S' *for* '&' | **3** lunis] *read* lunae | **4 martius**] *read* martis | **5 mercur. iii.**] *read* mercurii. *(see pp. 170-71)* | **6 iaius**] *read* iouis | **7 ueteris**] *read* ueneris | **9** omitenpore. obseruam dissunt] *read* omni tempore obseruandi sunt.

[6] Translation of text 4/1, l. 4.

5 Brontologies

Alias

thunderbook, thunder prognostic

Description

Thunder was often used to predict the future in the Middle Ages.[1] Förster stated that the genre of prognostics most widely disseminated in Anglo-Saxon England was the brontology.[2] This claim should be modified when the number of attested brontologies (ten) is compared to text witnesses of the Egyptian Days (forty-five), for instance. However, there are no less than six brontological genres known from Anglo-Saxon manuscripts, all of which make use of a different structural set-up. In comparison to lunaries, for example, which comprise seven genres that all employ the days of the moon as a structural device, the brontologies display an unparalleled richness of temporal and non-temporal structures in the form of hours, weekdays, months and compass directions, equalled only by the structural diversity of birth prognostics.[3]

According to Liuzza, who wrote a perceptive article on the Anglo-Saxon brontologies, "divination by thunder was practised in the ancient world and continued into Christian culture as part of a larger interest in forecasting events by means of signs and portents".[4] Likewise, Förster remarked that predicting the future by thunder can be traced back to Babylonian origins.[5] Although a direct link between medieval brontologies and ancient practices is not immediately apparent, both are conceivably exponents of the desire to interpret the awe-inspiring event of a thunderstorm.

---

[1] Thorndike (1923-58: I.679), Harmening (1979: 118-20), Braswell (1984: 347), Kieckhefer (1989: 86), Liuzza (2004: 6-7).

[2] Förster (1912b: 285).

[3] Two structures not known in Anglo-Saxon England are the day brontology listing predictions for each day in the year (Hellmann 1896a: 237-38) and the zodiacal brontology (Egerton 821, fols 2v-5r; Förster 1908a: 52; Svenberg 1936: 7; Eriksson 1956: 9-10). Beccaria (1956: 213) mentioned, but did not identify, several brontologies.

[4] Liuzza (2004: 7).

[5] Förster (1903: 352; 1912b: 291; 1920: 55). Cf. Hellmann (1896a: 237-38), who made the first case for an ancient genesis of thunder prognostics, and Auty *et al.* (1980-99: III.1251). Babylonian brontologies are discussed in Jastrow (1905-12: II.705-48).

5.1.1.1 Brontology, Temporal, Canonical Hours (Night Office) and 5.1.1.2 Brontology, Temporal, Canonical Hours (Day Office)

Literature

Jastrow (1905-12: II.705-48); Förster (1908a: 45, 47, 48-49); Einarsson (1939: 183); Harmening (1979: 118-20); Auty *et al.* (1980-99: III.1251); Hollis and Wright (1992: 263); Epe (1995: 57); Liuzza (2001: 184; 2004: 18-20)

Branches of Superstition

observation of signs: thunder; observation of times: canonical hours

Texts

5.1.1.1

OE: 1. Cambridge, Corpus Christi College, MS 391, p. 714

5.1.1.2

OE: 1. Cambridge, Corpus Christi College, MS 391, pp. 714-15

Description

These thunder prognostics are structured by the canonical hours of the night and day office, respectively. In CCCC 391, the manuscript which contains both texts, an uninterrupted sequence of brontologies occurs on pages 713-15. These brontologies deal with weekdays, the hours of the night office, the compass direction from which thunder is heard, and the hours of the day office.[1] The last three texts as a group are comparable to, but not to be equated with, the hour brontology (5.1.2). Research on the sequence of thunderbooks in CCCC 391 has focussed on the absence of sources and on the issue whether the final three texts should be regarded as one unit.[2]

The canonical hour brontologies predict the course of certain events based on the time on which thunder is heard. In contrast to the other brontological genres, which focus on the weather to come and on the condition of crops and livestock, 5.1.1.1 and 5.1.1.2 specifically address human concerns and the spiritual state of mankind.[3] Of the eight predictions in the brontologies (three in 5.1.1.1/1, five in 5.1.1.2/1), seven deal with the following topics: the birth of a king or a bishop, the persecution

[1] Texts 5.1.3/1, 5.1.1.1/1, 5.2/1, and 5.1.1.2/1, respectively.

[2] Förster (1908a: 45), Liuzza (2004: 18-20).

[3] Both Auty *et al.* (1980-99: III.1251) and Epe (1995: 57) stated that brontologies focus primarily on human affairs, yet this is not correct. The canonical hour brontologies display an interest in the human situation, but the other brontologies have a wider scope, including meteorological phenomena and agricultural concerns.

of Christians, a visit by the Holy Ghost, peace, friendship and dread. The last prediction of 5.1.1.2/1 is the only one not primarily concerned with mankind: "If thunder comes at nocturns, it signifies rough weather and storms".[4] It is perhaps fitting that prognostics which bridge the gap between superstition and religion in the form of using both thunder and canonical hours, attend to the human situation, and do so more than any other prognostic genre.

The brontologies under discussion distinguish themselves from the other hour brontologies (5.1.2) in their focus on the canonical hours of the Benedictine night and day office:[5]

	Old English	canonical hours
5.1.1.1/1	on forantniht (at dusk)	compline
	on middeniht (at midnight)	nocturns
	on dæg (at daybreak)	matins
5.1.1.2/1	æt þære þriddan tide dæges (on the third hour of day)	terce
	æt þære vi tide dæges (in the sixth hour of day)	sext
	æt þære ix tide dæges (in the ninth hour of day)	nones
	æt þære x tide dæges (in the tenth hour of day)	vespers
	æt þære .xii tide dæges (in the twelfth hour of day)	nocturns

table 19: canonical hours in brontologies 5.1.1.1/1 and 5.1.1.2/1

The entries for nocturns are duplicated, but the predictions are not identical: 5.1.1.1/1 announces "holy souls travelling over the world",[6] whereas 5.1.1.2/1 predicts "rough weather and storms".[7] Förster noted the absence of the hour of prime and explained this by pointing out the ambiguity of the Old English word "dæg" in 5.1.1.1/1.[8] He took this word to represent an erroneously conflated reading of two entries, one for matins ("on dægræd"), and one for prime ("æt þære forman tide dæges"), leading to "on dæg" in the text.[9] The preferred reading according

[4] Translation of text 5.1.1.2/1, l. 7.

[5] On the hours, see Hampson (1841: II.201, s.v. *hours*, and *hours, canonical*), Knowles (1951: xvi-xvii), Symons (1953: xlii-xliv).

[6] Translation of text 5.1.1.1/1, l. 2.

[7] Translation of text 5.1.1.2/1, l. 7. Förster (1908a: 48) ignored the tenth hour in 5.1.1.2/1, and identified the twelfth hour as vespers. I follow Liuzza (2004: 20), who assigned the order noted above.

[8] Förster (1908a: 49). Cf. Liuzza (2004: 19).

[9] Förster (1908a: 49).

to Förster and Liuzza is "dægræd" for "dæg", i.e. matins.[10] Einarsson, however, pointed out that "dæg" can mean matins without it having to be a reduced form of "dægræd".[11]

Nearly a century ago, Förster observed that no Latin analogues had been identified for 5.1.1.1/1 and 5.1.1.2/1.[12] Förster's observation is still valid as no sources or close analogues have appeared in the meantime. The canonical hour brontologies do not exist in a vacuum, however, and similarities with other hour brontologies (5.1.2) are acknowledged:[13]

> (5.1.1.1/1) If thunder comes at dusk, it announces some deadliness impending.[14]
>
> (5.1.2/1) If [there is thunder] in the first hour of night, it signifies death.[15]

and

> (5.1.1.1/1) If it [i.e. thunder] comes at daybreak, it announces the birth of a king or a bishop.[16]
>
> (5.1.2/1) If [there is thunder] at daybreak, it signifies the birth of a king.[17]

The two examples above reveal correspondences in phrasing. In addition, both 5.1.1.1 and 5.1.1.2, and 5.1.2 are structured by hours. 5.1.1.1 and 5.1.1.2 list eight hours altogether, and 5.1.2 fourteen. Most of these hours correspond, but next to every third hour, 5.1.2 lists hours such as the seventh and eighth, which are not present in 5.1.1.2. Moreover, the sequence of night and day hours is interrupted by a group of predictions dealing with the direction from which thunder is heard.[18] In 5.1.2, these predictions are integrated with those for the hours, e.g. "If it has thun-

[10] Förster (1908a: 49), Liuzza (2004: 19). In text 5.1.2/1, "hora matutina" (matins) is glossed as "on tide dægræd" (ll. 13, 14).

[11] Einarsson (1937: 183).

[12] Förster (1908a: 45).

[13] Cf. Liuzza (2004: 19).

[14] Translation of text 5.1.1.1/1, l. 1.

[15] Translation of text 5.1.2/1, l. 4.

[16] Translation of text 5.1.1.1/1, l. 3.

[17] Translation of text 5.1.2/1, l. 14.

[18] Liuzza (2004: 20) commented that "knowing which direction was which" was essential to medieval time reckoning. Therefore, a text on the directions from which thunder is heard is not out of place in the brontological sequence in CCCC 391. Although I do not disagree with Liuzza, I would like to point out that neither hour nor directional brontologies are attested in a computistical context. Rather, they are without exception found in prognostic sections.

dered in the eighth hour from the south, it signifies an abundance of bread and oil, and pestilence among herds and quadrupeds".[19] In the case of 5.1.1.1 and 5.1.1.2, the texts are separated by an independent directional brontology (5.2), e.g. "if it [thunder] is heard in the south, it signifies the death of the king's wife".[20] Liuzza presented the sequence of brontologies in CCCC 391 as one unit, "clearly a single work", but "the text may be an aggregate of several related but different and originally separate texts".[21] Indications for the separate nature of these texts in CCCC 391 can be seen in the fact that the directional brontology is not fully integrated into the canonical hour brontologies: the subject boundaries are clearly perceived. Moreover, there is a subtle difference in phrasing of the hours in 5.1.1.1 and 5.1.1.2. The first uses the preposition "on" (as in "on middeniht"), the second employs "æt" (as in "æt þære þriddan tide dæges"). Both 5.1.1.1 and 5.1.1.2 use various verbs for the significance of the predictions: the first uses "cyðeð" and "becnað", the second "tacnoð" and "becnað".[22] This variety gives the impression of the canonical hour and directional brontologies in CCCC 391 not being a single text. The other hour brontologies, in contrast, display complete integration of the directional brontology, an absence of clear subject boundaries, and a uniformity in phrasing. The latter is evident from a consistent use of the preposition "on" (e.g. "on tide seofoðan"), and the verb "getacnað" for Latin "significat".[23]

The preceding remarks illustrate the similarities and differences between canonical and other hour brontologies. To try and establish textual precedence among these is impossible in view of the scant survivals and the absence of sources which share the features outlined above. Liuzza concluded that the canonical and other hour brontologies were not derived from each other: "they can be described in the terms of traditional source study only as 'analogues'".[24]

---

[19] Translation of text 5.1.2/2, ll. 14, 15.

[20] Translation of text 5.2/1, l. 3.

[21] Liuzza (2004: 18, 20, respectively).

[22] In 5.1.1.1/1, l. 2, for instance, the thunder of midnight "*becnað* halie saule ofer worulde farende" (signifies holy souls travelling over the world [my emphasis]).

[23] Text 5.1.2/1, ll. 23, 25.

[24] Liuzza (2004: 20).

Edition

5.1.1.1/1 Cambridge, Corpus Christi College 391, p. 714/5-10

Gif þunor cumeð on forantniht se cyðeð hwylcehwugu deaðlicnesse towearde

Gif he cymð on middeniht sé becnað halie saule ofer worulde farende

Gif he on dæg cumð sé kyðeð kininges gebyrd oððe b*iscopes*

1 cyðeð] c[·]yðeð | towearde] towea[·]rde | **2 G**if] **G**if[·].

5.1.1.2/1 Cambridge, Corpus Christi College 391, pp. 714/19-715/3

Gif ðunor æt þære þriddan tide dæges he tacnoð godes gast cumende þis middaneard to neosianne 7 to blisianne.

Gif þunor cumð æt þære vi tide dæges he becnað æhtnesse cri*st*es folces

Gif ðunor cumð æt þære ix tide dæges se becnað gesib 7 genihtsumnesse

Gif þunor cumð æt þære x tide dæges from gode. oððe from mannu*m* sé becnað ege in þam folce

Gif þunor cymð æt þære .xii tide dæges hreohnessa 7 stormas se becnað.

1 ðunor] *read* ~ cumð | **3** þunor] þunor[·] | **5** mannu*m*] ~ ‖ ⟨*p. 715*⟩.

5.1.2 Brontology, Temporal, Hours

Literature

Jastrow (1905-12: II.705-48); Förster (1908a: 45, 50-52; 1908c: 34-35; 1920: 55); Harmening (1979: 118-20); Auty *et al.* (1980-99: III.1251); Kieckhefer (1989: 86); Hollis and Wright (1992: 263); Günzel (1993: 33); Epe (1995: 57); Liuzza (2001: 184; 2004: 16-20)

Branches of Superstition

observation of signs: thunder, compass directions; observation of times: hours

Texts

L/OE: 1. London, British Library, Cotton Tiberius A. iii, fol. 37rv
L: 2. London, British Library, Cotton Titus D. xxvi, fols 9v-10v

Description

The hour brontology predicts the future with the help of the hours of day and night, and, for a limited number of hours, the direction from which thunder is heard. The subject matter and structure of canonical and other hour brontologies show some overlap. A comparison between the two brontological genres has already been made.[1] The origin of 5.1.2 is not known, but later analogues have been attested.[2]

The structure of the hour brontology is comparable to that of the canonical hour brontologies: predictions are made according to the hour on which it thunders. The entries in 5.1.2 represent fourteen out of the twenty-four hours in a day.[3] In addition, the seventh to tenth hours of day specify the direction from which thunder hails as follows: "from any part of the sky", "from the southern part", "from the north", and "from the east", respectively.[4] The integration of three discrete texts into one, i.e. brontologies for the hours of night, the compass directions, and the

[1] See pp. 248-51.

[2] Förster (1920: 55), Liuzza (2004: 17, n. 56).

[3] On the possibly mistaken order of some of the entries, see text 5.1.2/2. Identifying the hours is not straightforward. The hours most easily tagged are those which are numbered: the first, third, fifth hour of night, and the sixth, seventh, eighth, ninth, and tenth hour of day. "media nocte" may be equated with midnight (i.e. the sixth hour of night), and "hora nouissima diei" with the first hour of day. This leaves us with "hora uespertina" (either first vespers = tenth hour of day, or second vespers = twelfth hour of day or first hour of night), and the sequence of "gallicantu", "hora matutina" and "hora ortus solis". The latter group is troublesome because they all take place around sunrise, yet they must represent separate hours. Since they all precede the first hour of day, I take them to mean the tenth to twelfth hours of night.

[4] Translation of text 5.1.2/2, ll. 12, 14, 16, 18.

hours of day, is carried off more successfully in 5.1.2 than in the brontological sequence in CCCC 391. Nevertheless, Liuzza was able to identify traces of the originally separate nature of the genres in 5.1.2.[5]

The Old English of (1) is a direct gloss of the Latin text of (1). Aside from some small mistakes in (2) not present in (1) (e.g. metathesis of "notauerit" for "tonauerit") and vice versa (e.g. "ruias" for "ruinas"), the Latin texts (1) and (2) closely agree in content and phrasing. In view of the similarities, the texts are probably derived from a common source.[6]

Edition

5.1.2/1 London, British Library, Cotton Tiberius A. iii, fol. 37r/12-37v/4

gif hit þunrað on tide æfen hit getacnað acennednysse sumes miceles
Si tonitruauerit hora uespertina. significat natiuitatem cuiusdam magni.
gif on forman nihte tide hit getacnad cwealm
Si prima noctis hora: sign*ificat* mortalitatem.
gif on tide þriddan nihte *getacnað* yrre drihten oððe dom his on middanearde
Si hora tertia noctis. significat iram d*omi*ni uel iudicium eius in mundo.
gif on tide þriddan midre nihte hit *getacnað* sumne sweg utgangende of wurulde
Si hora quinta mediȩ noctis: significat aliquem sonum egredientem. de s*ecu*lo
oððe wrace on middangearde
*ue*l undictam in mundo.
gif on angræde hit *getacnað* gefeoht 7 gete blodes
Si gallicantu significat bellum & effusionem sanguinis.
gif on tide dægræd hit *getacnað* gebyrdtide cyniniges
Si hora matutina significat natiuitatem regis.
gif on tide upganges sunnan ge*tacnað* þeode sume togædere cumenne to geleafan
Si hora ortus solis significat gentem aliquam conuenient*em* ad fidem
cristes
chr*isti*.
gif on tide þære syxtan *getacnað* gydwildu arisende on middanerde 7 ehtnysse
Si hora .vi diei significat hereses surgentes in mundo & persecutionem
cristenra fra*m* gode geþafod
chr*isti*anorum a deo permissam.

3 getacnad] -n- <a; *read* getacnað | **7** þriddan] *read* fiftan *(Latin* quinta*)* | **10** undictam] *read* uindictam | **13** cyniniges] *read* cyninges | **19** syxtan] *read* ~ dæges *(Latin* diei *is not glossed because* þære syxtan *is over it).*

[5] Liuzza (2004: 18).
[6] Cf. Liuzza (2004: 17).

gif on tide seofoðan þunrað of gewylcum dæle heofonas wæstm 7
Si hora .vii. tonitruauerit de quacumq*ue* parte cęli fructum &
genihtsumnysse micele towerde *getacnað*
ubertatem magna*m* futuram significat.
gif on tide þære ehtoþa þunrað fra*m* dæle middæges *getacnað* genihtsumnysse
Si hora .viii. tonitruauerit a parte meridiane significat habundantiam
laf 7 eles 7 cwyld on heordum 7 fyþerfetu*m*
panis & olei & cladem in armentis & quadrupedibus.
gif on tide non þunrað fra*m* norðdæle awendiicge þeoda 7 wæpna
Si hora .ix. tonitruauerit ab aquilone mutationes genti*u*m & armorum
geruxlu 7 niwe torynas folca *getacnað*
strepidus & nouos concursus populorum significat.
gif on tide þunrað fra*m* eastdæle ryras buruga *getacnað*
Si hora .x. tonitruauerit ab orietate ruias urbium significat.
gif on tide æftemystan dæges reohnysse on se 7 bodung gefeohtes *getacnað*
Si hora nouissima diei. tempestatem in mari. & nuntium belli significat.
gif on midre nihte þunorrad gedon bið ungor micelne getacnað
Si media nocte tonitruum factum fuerit famem magna*m* significat.

27 middæges] ~ *seems to wrongly gloss Latin* meridiane, *but see Korhammer (1985: 258)* | **31** norðdæle] -l- < n | awendiicge] *i.e.* awendicge *(on doubling of* 'i', *see 7/4, l.2); read* awendincge *(on loss of* 'n', *see l. 36, and 7/4, l. 66)* | **32** genti*u*m] ~ ‖ ⟨*f. 37v*⟩ | **35** tide] *read* ~ teoþa *(Latin* .x.*)* | **36** orietate] *read* oriente *(see 5.1.2/2)* | ruias] *read* ruinas *(see l. 31)* | **40** magna*m*] -a_2- < u.

5.1.2/2 London, British Library, Cotton Titus D. xxvi, fols 9v/14-10v/9

De tonitruis dierum uel trium

Si notauerit hora uesp*er*tina significat natiuitatem cuiusda*m* magni.
i prima. noctis hora significat mortalitatem.
Si hora .iii. noctis sign*ificat* iram d*omi*ni. *ue*l iudicium ei*us* in mundo.
Si hora .v. medie noctis. sign*ificat* aliquem sonus ęgredientem de s*ecu*lo. *ue*l uindicta*m* in mundo.
Si gallicantu. sign*ificat* bellu*m* & effusione*m* sanguinis.
Si hora matutina. sig*nificat* natiuitate*m* regis.
Si hora ortu solis. sign*ificat* gente*m* aliqua*m* conueniente*m* ad fidem chr*ist*i.
Si hora vi. diei. sign*ificat* hereses surgentes in mundo & p*er*secutione*m* chr*ist*ianorum a deo permissam.

1 trium] *read* noctium | **2** notauerit] *for* tonauerit*(?); read* tonitruauerit *(see 5.1.2/1)* | **3** i] *read* Si | significat] ~ ‖ ⟨*f. 10r*⟩ | **5** sonus] *read* sonum *(see 5.1.2/1)* | **9** ortu] *read* ortus.

Si hora .vii. ton*itruauerit* de q*uacumque* parte celi fructum & ubertate*m* magna*m* futuram sig*nificat.*

Si hora .viii. ton*itruauerit* a parte meridiane. sig*nificat* habundantia*m* panis & olei & cladem in arm*en*tis & quadrupedib*us.*

Si hora ix. ton*itruauerit* ab aquilone mutationes gentium & armoru*m* strepitus & nouos concursus populor*um* sig*nificat.*

Si hora x. ton*itruauerit* ab oriente ruinas urbium sig*nificat:*

Si hora nouissima diei. tempestate*m* in mari. & nuntiu*m* belli sig*nificat.*

Si media nocte tonitruu*m* factum fuerit. famem magnum sig*nificat.*

15 cladem] ~ ‖ ⟨*f. 10v*⟩ | **20** nocte] -o- < e | magnum] *read* magnam | *Günzel (1993: 33) remarked that the last two entries of the text probably are misplaced (but see text 5.1.2/1): the* media nocte *entry should have been positioned after* hora .v. medie noctis *(i.e. the midnight hour after the fifth hour of night), and* hora nouissima diei *after* hora ortu solis *(i.e. the first hour of day after sunrise), but the texts that I know are structured as 5.1.2/1,2 are (see also Liuzza 2004: 17, n. 56).*

5.1.3 Brontology, Temporal, Day of the Week

Literature

Brand (1849-55: III.245); Migne (1861-1904: I.609-14); Hellmann (1896a: 237; 1896b: 61); Förster (1903: 350-52; 1908a: 45, 46-47, 52; 1908c: 35-36; 1912b: 290); Jastrow (1905-12: II.705-48); Bezold and Boll (1911: 7-8); Thorndike (1923-58: I.679); Jones (1939: 45-47); Harmening (1979: 118-20); Auty *et al.* (1980-99: III.1251); Hollis and Wright (1992: 263); Epe (1995: 57); Liuzza (2001: 184; 2004: 14-16, 18-19)

Attribution

post-medieval: Bede

Branches of Superstition

observation of signs: thunder; observation of times: weekdays

Texts

OE: 1. Cambridge, Corpus Christi College, MS 391, pp. 713-14
2. London, British Library, Cotton Tiberius A. iii, fol. 40rv
3. Oxford, Bodleian Library, Hatton 115, fol. 150v

Description

The weekday brontology aims to foretell the future depending on the weekday on which thunder is heard first in the year.[1] Like the year prognosis, which is structured along similar lines,[2] the predictions pertain to human affairs (e.g. the death of a king or judge), with some attention to agricultural concerns, such as the condition of crops and livestock. No Latin analogues or sources for the weekday brontology have been found in Anglo-Saxon manuscripts.

A redaction of the weekday brontology, together with a month brontology, a directional brontology and a prefixed introduction, makes up the pseudo-Bedan *De tonitruis libellus ad Herefridum*.[3] This book about thunder is presumably addressed to Herefrid (d. 909), bishop of Auxerre.[4] The thunderbook is the only prognostic to be included in the section *Didascalia genuina* in Migne's edition of Bede's works. This may be the reason why Jones is nowhere more stern in his rejection of Bede's

[1] Text 5.1.3/1, l. 1, states "gif hit þunreð ærest" (if it thunders first), 5.1.3/2, l. 1, "**G**if se forma þunor cymð" (if the first thunder comes), whereas 5.1.3/3, l. 1, simply relates "gyf hyt þunrie" (if it thunders). The scribe of the latter probably overlooked the reference to the first thunder of the year.

[2] Instead of thunder, the year prognosis uses the weekday on which New Year's Day or Christmas falls to predict the future.

[3] Printed in Migne (1861-1904: I.609-14).

[4] Jones (1939: 45-47).

pseudo-oeuvre than in his denunciation of *De tonitruis*. *De tonitruis* was once considered an adaptation of a passage in the Greek treatise on thunder *De ostentis*, by the seventh-century Laurentius Lydus.[5] As with more pseudo-Bedan prognostics, *De tonitruis* is first associated with Bede's writings in the sixteenth century.[6] Towards the end of the nineteenth century, the attribution was discredited, but not entirely successfully: Thorndike still called *De tonitruis* "Bede's translation of some work on divination from thunder".[7] Jones remarked that *De tonitruis*, probably written in the Cologne area, is uniquely preserved in a tenth-/eleventh-century manuscript, which he regarded as the first instance of the tract.[8] Liuzza called this observation into question on the basis of an early fourteenth-century manuscript in which a sequence appears comparable to the one in *De tonitruis*.[9] It is hard to see what influence *De tonitruis* or a text like it could have had on the Anglo-Saxon brontologies in view of its rare witnesses. Moreover, Jones's example hails from the continent, while Liuzza's dates from the fourteenth century. The only brontological sequence in the English manuscript CCCC 391 is not at all similar to *De tonitruis*. Therefore, there is no evidence that *De tonitruis* was known in Anglo-Saxon England.

Thorndike stated that "divination from thunder is another form of judicial astrology, if it may so be called, found in these early manuscripts".[10] Thorndike's 'early manuscripts' are those from the ninth century onwards containing computistical tracts,[11] but this is neither the context nor the era in which brontologies are encountered in English

---

[5] Migne (1861-1904: I.609, n. a), Hellmann (1896a: 237-38), Förster (1903: 352), Bezold and Boll (1911: 7-8), Jones (1939: 45). *De ostentis* contains, among others, a day brontology, listing entries for each day in the year. Liuzza (2004: 9) remarked that "the work [viz. *De tonitruis*] bears no more than a structural resemblance to Lydus' work". There are no signs that the Anglo-Saxons were familiar with the day brontology which lists predictions for each day of the year.

[6] Jones (1939: 45). Nevertheless, Noviomagus voiced reservations with regard to the status of *De tonitruis* as a Bedan tract, but these were excluded in later collections of Bede's works (Jones 1939: 46).

[7] Thorndike (1923-58: I.635, 679). Cf. Hellmann (1896a: 236-37; 1896b: 61).

[8] Jones (1939: 46). The attribution to Bede is not incomprehensible, because in the manuscript, *De tonitruis* is placed in Bede's *De temporum ratione*, between chapters LXV and LXVI (cf. Jones 1939: 46).

[9] Liuzza (2004: 16, n. 52).

[10] Thorndike (1923-58: I.679).

[11] Cf. Thorndike (1923-58: I.676).

manuscripts.[12] Several weekday brontologies in both Latin and the vernacular have been identified.[13] To my knowledge, no weekday brontologies are in existence from before the eleventh century.

The three Old English texts do not derive from a common exemplar, nor is there a Latin analogue close enough to be representative of a source text.[14] There may have been one Latin source for these texts,[15] but the Old English brontologies seem to be, or to have been copied from, independent translations.[16] The predictions show overall agreement across the texts, yet the phrasing differs to such an extent that the texts cannot have been copied from each other. The entry for Tuesday, for instance, reads:

(1) If it [viz. thunder] is heard on a Tuesday, crops will dwindle.[17]

(2) If it thunders on a Tuesday, it signifies the failure of crops.[18]

(3) If it thunders on a Tuesday, then it signifies the failure of crops.[19]

These three entries all predict a bad harvest, but the way this is described is not identical. The variation is partly due to small differences in phrasing, such as "þ*æt* tacnað" (2) versus "þonne tacneð þ*æt*" (3). However, the choice of vocabulary reveals that these texts are not copies from each other: the Latin phrase which may have been the source text, "fructus terra periclitabunt",[20] is variously translated as "wæstmas beoð gewanode" (1), "wæstma geswefrunge" (2), and "westmas geswidunge" (3). (1)

[12] The Anglo-Saxon brontologies date from the eleventh and twelfth centuries, and are found in prognostic sections. On this manuscript context, see pp. 49-59.

[13] Migne (1861-1904: I.609-14), Förster (1908a: 46-47, 52; 1908c: 36; 1912b: 290), Thorndike (1923-58: I.679, n. 1), Liuzza (2004: 16, n. 52). Förster (1903: 351) referred to several vernacular and Latin redactions, but he did not differentiate between the weekday and the month brontology, so his references should be used with care.

[14] The predictions of the Latin text published by Förster (1908a: 47) coincide to a large extent with those of the Old English texts, but not enough for this Latin text to be representative of the source text.

[15] Förster (1908c: 36).

[16] There are indications that the texts are not original translations. E.g. the predictions for Sunday and Monday have erroneously changed places in 5.1.3/3, ll. 1-3; 5.1.3/2, l. 2, reads "cyme bearna" for "cynnebearna", a typical minim problem, and the scribe of 5.1.3/1, l. 5, garbles "becnað landbegengena"' into "becland begena". These examples seem to imply that the texts were copied from earlier translations.

[17] Translation of text 5.1.3/1, l. 4.

[18] Translation of text 5.1.3/2, l. 5.

[19] Translation of text 5.1.3/3, l. 4.

[20] From a Latin analogue cited by Förster (1908a: 47).

employs a verb phrase, while (2) and (3) use noun phrases which do not feature identical nouns. It is possible to see many such differences in phrasing and grammar throughout the texts. There are, nevertheless, similarities between (2) and (3) which are not shared with (1). The prediction for Sunday, for example, is more detailed in (1), than in (2) or (3): "it means the death of kings or bishops, or many ealdormen will die in that year", versus "then it signifies the death of royal children".[21] In the entry for Friday, (2) and (3) predict the death of "sædeora" or "seodeora", whereas (1) predicts the death of "nytena". A Latin analogue has "oues & pecora peribunt",[22] so (1) is likely to have preserved the correct reading (Old English "nytena" means cattle). The nouns used in (2) and (3) on the other hand, seem to refer to sea-beasts, which does not make much sense.[23] In view of the differences between the texts, none of the English weekday brontologies will have been copied from the other. The similar predictions in (2) and (3) seem to indicate that these two texts represent minor variants of one redaction, (1) being an entirely different redaction.[24]

Edition

5.1.3/1 Cambridge, Corpus Christi College 391, pp. 713/20-714/5

On anweardne gear gif hit þunreð ærest on sunnandæg sé becnað kyninges oððe b*iscopes* deað oððe mænige ealdermen on þam geare sweltað.

Gif þunor bið gehered on monandæg sé becnað blodesgyte on sume ðeade.

[21] Translation of texts 5.1.3/1, ll. 1-2, and 5.1.3/2, ll. 1-2, respectively. The entries for Sunday and Monday (ll. 1-3) were exchanged by the scribe of 5.1.3/3. In view of the Old English texts 5.1.3/1 and 5.1.3/2, and the Latin analogue cited by Förster (1908a: 47), I assume that the exchange of predictions in 5.1.3/3 is a scribal error.

[22] Förster (1908a: 47).

[23] The standard translation is "sea-monster" or "sea-animal" (cf. Cockayne 1864-66: III.169; Bosworth and Toller 1898: 809, s.v. *sǽ-deór*; Liuzza 2004: 15, n. 50), yet I find this unsatisfactory. How is it possible that a reference in Latin to cattle ("pecus") changes into sea-beasts ("seodeora") in Old English? A possible answer is that "sædeora" and "seodeora" are corrupted readings of the otherwise unrecorded compound *"seamdeora", where "seam" means burden, or "the furniture of a beast of burden" (Bosworth and Toller (1898: 852, s.v. *seám*). Compounds with "seam-" have been attested, as the words "seamere" (beast of burden) and "seamhors" (pack-horse) illustrate, cf. Bosworth and Toller (1898: 852, s.v. *seámere*, *seám-hors*).

[24] The relationship between the texts was summarily discussed by Förster (1908c: 36), and in more detail by Liuzza (2004: 15-16, 19).

Gif on tiwesdæg hyered hered wæstmas beoð gewanode.
Gif on wodnesdæg biþ gehyred sé becland begena cwealm
6 **G**if on þunresdæg bið gehyred becnað wifa hryre.
Gif on frigedæg geþunrað þonne getacnað *þæt* nytena cwealm.
Gif on sæternesdæg geðunrað *þæt* tacnað demena 7 gerefena cwealm.

4 hyered hered] *read* bið gehered | **5** gehyred] gehy[e]red | becland begena] *read* becnað landbegengena *(see 5.1.3/2,3)*; ~ ‖ ⟨*p. 714*⟩.

5.1.3/2 London, British Library, Cotton Tiberius A. iii, fol. 40r/22-40v/5

On anweardan geare. **G**if se forma þunor cymð on sunnandæge. þonne tacnað *þæt* cyme bearna cwealm.
3 **G**if hit on monandæige þunrige þonne tacnað *þæt* micelne blodgyte on sumre þeade.
Gif hit on tiwesdæig þunrige. *þæt* tacnað wæstma geswefrunge.
6 **G**if hit on wodnesdæig þunrige. *þæt* tacnað landbigencgena cwealm. 7 cræftigra.
Gif hit on þunresdæig þunrað. *þæt* tacnað wifmanna cwealm.
Gif hit on frigedæig þunrige. *þæt* tacnað sædeora cwealm.
9 **G**if hit on sæternesdæig þunrige. *þæt* tacnað demena 7 gerefena cwealm.

1 anweardan] -a_3- < e | **2** cyme bearna] *read* cynnebearna *(see 5.1.3/3)* | **4** þeade.] ~ ‖ ⟨*f. 40v*⟩ | **8** sædeora] *see p. 260* | **9** þunrige] -g- < e.

5.1.3/3 Oxford, Bodleian Library, Hatton 115, fol. 150v/1-9

ON anwardne ger gyf hyt þunrie on sunandæg. þon*ne* tacnað *þæt* micelne blodesgyte in sumere þeode.
3 7 on oðerne: þon*ne* tacnað *þæt* weder cynebearn acwealð byð.
Gyf on tiwesdeg þunrieð. þonne tacneð *þæt* westmas geswidunge.
Gyf on wodnesdæg geþunrie. þon*ne* tacneð *þæt* lanð bigengene cwælm.
6 Gyf on þunresdæg þunrað. *þæt* tacnað wifmanna cwealm.
Gyf on frigedæg þunrað. þon*ne* tacnað *þæt* seodeora cwealm.
Gyf on sæternesdæg þunrað. þon*ne* tacnað *þæt* demena 7 gerestena cwealm:-

1 þunrie] *read* ~ ærest *(see 5.1.3/1)* | **1-3** micelne... þeode *and* weder... byð] *the predictions for Sunday and Monday should probably be exchanged (see 5.1.3/1,2)* | **3** acwealð] *read* acweald | **5** wodnesdæg geþunrie] wodnes dægge þunrie *Cockayne (1864-66)* | lanð bigengene] *read* landbigengene *(see 5.1.3/2)* | **8** gerestena] *read* gerefena *(see 5.1.3/1,2)*.

5.1.4 Brontology, Temporal, Month of the Year

Literature

Migne (1861-1904: I.609-14); Waitz (1879: 585-86); Hellmann (1896a); Förster (1903: 350-52; 1908a: 45, 52; 1912b: 285-91; 1920: 55); Jastrow (1905-12: II.705-48); Holthausen (1908); Perry (1914: 114); Thorndike (1923-58: I.679); Jones (1939: 45-47); Harmening (1979: 118-20); Auty *et al.* (1980-99: III.1251); Hunt (1987: 170); Taavitsainen (1988: 52-53); Kieckhefer (1989: 86-87); Hollis and Wright (1992: 263); Epe (1995: 57); Liuzza (2001: 184; 2004: 8-14)

Attribution

post-medieval: Bede

Branches of Superstition

observation of signs: thunder; observation of times: months

Texts

OE: 1. London, British Library, Cotton Vespasian D. xiv, fol. 103v
L: 2. London, British Library, Royal 2. B. v, fol. 190rv

Description

The month brontology foretells the future with regard to human affairs, agricultural concerns and meteorological circumstances, depending on the month in which it thunders first. This is one of the few prognostic genres centred around calendar months. Kieckhefer remarked that the month brontology may have been particularly useful "in regions where thunderstorms are relatively rare", but I am not convinced that this applies to England.[1] As mentioned before, the month brontology is part of the pseudo-Bedan *De tonitruis libellus ad Herefridum*.[2]

The *Handwörterbuch des deutschen Aberglaubens* states: "The month itself does not play a big role in superstition, just as nowadays simple folks rarely use it in the calculation of time".[3] This statement is somewhat ambiguous as to the identity of the "simple folks", but the observation that months play only a minor role in superstition is accurate as far as prognostics are concerned. Of the thirty-two genres studied in this chapter, just two prognostics are structured by months, three make use of months as an additional structuring element, and in one the events in each

[1] Kieckhefer (1989: 86).

[2] See pp. 257-58. The month brontology in *De tonitruis* is more elaborate than those under discussion here, but the predictions largely tend to agree (cf. Liuzza 2004: 11).

[3] "Der M[onat] selbst spielt im Aberglauben keine grosse Rolle, zumal ihn der einfache Mensch auch heute noch selten als Zeitbestimmung gebraucht" (Hoffmann-Krayer, Bächtold-Stäubli *et al.* 1927-42: VI.469, s.v. *Monat*).

month are predicted.[4] The calendar months, in contrast to weeks (which are fourths of the lunar sidereal month) or the thirty days of the moon of lunaries (which represent the lunar synodic month), had become an arbitrary, theoretical system of time-keeping which no longer bore any relationship with observable temporal phenomena by the time Augustus had finished changing the Roman calendar.[5] The limited use in prognostics of calendar months instead of days of the moon or weekdays may be occasioned by this arbitrariness of the calendar months.[6]

Several month brontologies have been identified in Latin, Greek and the vernacular, dating from medieval to modern times.[7] All of these analogues date from the twelfth century onwards. Liuzza is the first to edit (2),[8] which is an important text because it was added to the Regius Psalter at the end of the tenth century. This makes it the oldest month brontology attested so far. Förster assumed (1) to be a translation from the Latin on the basis of close similarities with a Latin text he printed.[9] Liuzza identified another analogue, and he concluded that "only a thorough commitment to the unidirectionality of Latin to English translation would lead anyone to speak of it as a 'source'".[10] I see no reason, however, to expect the genre of the month brontology to have been conceived in Old English and translated into Latin, especially in view of the fact that most prognostic genres I have studied are primarily transmitted in Latin rather than in the vernacular. Liuzza, moreover, found an older, Latin redaction which may be representative of the source text.[11]

[4] Two genres which are structured by months are the month brontology and the regimen. Months are used as an aid in structuring the twelve and twenty-four Egyptian Days, and the unlucky days. The month prognosis predicts the events in each month.

[5] On time reckoning and prognostics, see pp. 26-35.

[6] Calendar months were much used in the computus, so their hold on medieval time-keeping was considerable. The influence of calendar months is evident in regimens, which changed their structure from seasonal to monthly (see pp. 31-32).

[7] References are in Hellmann (1896a: 236-37), Förster (1903: 351-52; 1908a: 45, 52; 1912b: 288-89), Thorndike (1923-58: I.679, n.2), Liuzza (2004: 13, 14, n. 47); editions in Migne (1861-1904: I.609-14), Waitz (1879: 585-86), Förster (1903: 351; 1912b: 285-88, 291), Holthausen (1908), Perry (1914), Liuzza (2004: 10, 13-14). A facsimile of an illustrated month brontology is in Kieckhefer (1989: 87, fig. 8). The reference in Thorndike (1923-58: I.679, n.2) to Egerton 821, fols 2v-5r, pertains to a zodiacal brontology, which uses the twelve constellations rather than the calendar months and is therefore not a month brontology. Förster (1908a: 52) listed another zodiacal brontology.

[8] Liuzza (2004: 8).

[9] Förster (1903: 351).

[10] Liuzza (2004: 13-14).

[11] Cf. Liuzza (2004: 14, n. 47).

(1) and (2) are not related; they form different redactions as the following example illustrates:

> (1) In April, it [viz. thunder] announces a blissful year, and the death of evil men.[12]
>
> (2) If thunder occurs in the month of April, seeds are endangered, or ships.[13]

The examples illustrate that (1) and (2) differ considerably in content. The analogues printed by Liuzza and Förster agree with (1) more closely:

> If thunder is heard in the month of April, it signifies a happy and fruitful year, and the death of wicked people.[14]
>
> If in April, it will be a good year and fertile, and thieves will die.[15]

Förster's text shows more overlap with (1) than Liuzza's. Liuzza's analogue repeats the phrase "si tonitruus sonuerit" in every entry, whereas Förster's has the phrase "si tonat" for January only, and (1) the phrase "gyf hit þunreð" in the entries for January and February. Furthermore, the phrase "gyf hit þunreð" is a translation of "si tonat" (if it thunders), not of "si tonitruus sonuerit" (if thunder is heard). It is not unlikely that (1) is translated from a source text resembling the one printed by Förster.

Edition

5.1.4/1 London, British Library, Cotton Vespasian D. xiv, fol. 103v/9-25

Emb þunre

On Ianuari*us* monðe gyf hit þunreð: hit bodeð toweard mycele windes. 7 wel gewænde eorðe wæstme. 7 gefiht.

On febr*uarius* monðe: gyf hit þunreð: hit bodeð manegra manna cwealm. 7 mæst þære ricen.

A marginal note in a post-medieval hand (Talbot's?) reads: (pr)ognosticon tonitru. *A post-medieval hand (Nowell's?) has underlined several words (see also 17/2)* | **1 Emb þunre**] ~ *outlined to the end of fol. 103v/9-10.*

[12] Translation of text 5.1.4/1, l. 8.

[13] Translation of text 5.1.4/2, l. 8.

[14] "Si tonitruus sonuerit mense Aprilis, iocunditatiam et fructiferium annum et iniquorum mortem significat" (Liuzza 2004: 13).

[15] "Si in Aprili, annus bonus erit et fertilis et fures peribunt" (Förster 1903: 351).

On mærces monðe: hit bodeð mycele windes. 7 wæstmes wel gewænde. 7 folc unsehte.

On april: hit bodeð blisful gear. 7 yfelre manna deað.

On **M**ai hit bodeð hunger gear.

On Iuni*us* monðe: hit bodeð mycele windes. 7 wulfene wodnysse: 7 leona.

On **I**vli*us* monðe: hit bodeð wæstme wel gewænde. 7 oref forfærð.

On hærfest. hit bodeð god gear. 7 mæn sicelið.

On **S**et*em*bre: hit bodeð god gear. 7 riccere manna slege.

On **O**ctobre. hit bodeð mycelne wind 7 wæstme toweard 7 treowena wæstme gæsne.

On **N**ouembre. hit bodeð blisfull gear. 7 wæstme toweard.

On decembre: hit bodeð god gear on tilðe. 7 sibb. 7 sehte.

13 7] `ac´ ~ *(the scribe probably wanted* ac *to replace* 7, *but* 7 *was not expunged or erased; note that the Latin analogues printed by Förster (1903) and Liuzza (2004) use* et *in summing up, while 5.1.4/2 employs* uel*).*

5.1.4/2 London, British Library, Royal 2. B. v, fol. 190r/10-190v/7

Si tonitruu*m* fuerit i*n* m*en*se ianuario multe conuentiones *sunt* una de ouib*us* alia de homibus .iii. de peccorib*us* .iiii. de lignis .v. de eq*ui*s tim*en*du*m est* h*oc* tonitruu*m*.

Si tonitruu*m* fuerit i*n* m*ense* feb*ruario* ad aure*m* p*er*tinet *ue*l ad alia q*ue* referunt*ur* i*n* alia*m* areas 7 sem*en* p*er*ten*et*.

Sii tonitruu*m* f*uerit* i*n* m*en*se mar*tio* tim*en*du*m est* q*ui* ab eo exspectat*ur* mortalitas *ue*l iudiciu*m*.

Si tonitruu*m* erit i*n* m*en*se apr*i*l*i* semina p*er*iclitant*ur* *ue*l nabes.

Si ton*itruum* f*uerit* i*n* m*ense* mai*n*o pluuie magne er*unt* *ue*l erba *ue*l semina pullulab*unt*.

Si ton*itruum* f*uerit* i*n* m*en*se iuni*o* homines perecletant*ur* *ue*l ligna.

Si toni*truum* f*uerit* i*n* m*en*se iul*io* pisces pericletant*ur*.

Si toni*truum* er*i*t i*n* m*ense* agus*to* bilue *ue*l reptilia perecletantur.

Si toni*truum* er*it* in m*ense* sept*embri* uituli mori`e´ntur.

Sii ton*itruum* er*it* in m*ense* oct*o*b*ri* motantur aure.

Sii toni*truum* er*it* in mensis. no*uembri* obes crescunt.

2 homibus] *read* hominibus | **5** alia*m*] aliā; *read* alias | p*er*ten*et*] *read* pertinet *(*'e' *for* 'i' *and vice versa is common for this scribe, e.g.* bilue *(l. 13, for* belue*), and* perecletantur *(ll. 11, 13) vs.* periclitantur *(l. 8) vs.* pericletantur *(l. 12))* | **6** Sii] *the scribe uses a monogram for* Si, *which would explain this mistake (see also ll. 15, 16)* | q*ui*] *read* quia *(the mistake is probably occasioned by the* 'a' *of the word* ab *following)* | **8** nabes] *the scribe uses* 'b' *for* 'u' *more often, viz.* obes *(l. 16)* | **9** mai*n*o] maīo; *read* maio | **11** f*uerit*] ~ ‖ ⟨*f. 190v*⟩ | **14** mori`e´ntur] `e´ < u *(not expunged!)* | **15, 16** Sii] *see l. 6* | **16** mensis] *read* mense.

5.2 Brontology, Non-Temporal, Compass Directions

Literature

Migne (1861-1904: I.609-14); Jastrow (1905-12: II.705-48); Förster (1908a: 45, 47-48; 1912a: 63-64); Thorndike (1923-58: I.679); Jones (1939: 45-47); Harmening (1979: 118-20); Auty *et al.* (1980-99: III. 1251); Kieckhefer (1989: 86); Hollis and Wright (1992: 263); Epe (1995: 57); Liuzza (2001: 184; 2004: 19-20)

Attribution

post-medieval: Bede

Branch of Superstition

observation of signs: thunder, compass directions

Text

OE: 1. Cambridge, Corpus Christi College, MS 391, p. 714

Description

The directional brontology predicts future events based on the compass directions from which thunder is heard. This genre appears in the pseudo-Bedan *De tonitruis libellus ad Herefridum*, in the hour brontology, and as an independent text in a sequence of brontologies in CCCC 391.[1] No source has been identified for (1). I suspect that (1) and the other brontologies in CCCC 391 were collected from various older Old English exemplars in view of the differences in vocabulary in and phrasing of the texts. As with all brontologies, the predictions in (1) pertain to human affairs and agricultural concerns.

With regard to (1), Liuzza astutely observed that "time-keeping, whether by the sundial or the stars, depended on knowing which direction was which".[2] Despite the importance of directions in the computus, however, they played a minor role in structuring prognostics, even though these texts are often found in computi. Moreover, none of the English brontologies appears in a computistical context. Förster edited a modern directional wind prognostic, a genre I have not found in medieval manuscripts, but which has a long history according to Förster.[3]

Not many directional brontologies have been attested, so it is hard to find material that can be compared to (1). Förster printed a directional brontology which constitutes an independent text, like (1) does.[4] Other

[1] See the hour and weekday brontologies on pp. 253-54, 257-60.

[2] Liuzza (2004: 20).

[3] Förster (1912a: 64). The directional wind prognostic is based on the direction from which the wind blows on New Year's Eve.

[4] Förster (1908a: 48).

references are to texts incorporating directional brontologies, such as the hour brontology and *De tonitruis*.[5] A comparison between (1) and the analogues reveals that none of the latter is representative of the Latin source of (1). The compass directions they list are as follows:[6]

(1)	5.1.2/1	*De tonitruis*	Förster's analogue
	of gewylcum dæle heofonas de quacumq*ue* parte cęli		
of eastdæle	fra*m* eastdæle ab oriente	ab orientali	ab oriente
suð	fra*m* dæle middæges a parte meridiane	meridiana	ab austro
west oððe norð			
		ab occidentali	ab occidente
norðþunor	fra*m* norðdæle ab aquilone	boreæ	ab aquilone
mycel east oððe norðeast			

table 20: compass directions in directional brontologies

Förster's analogue and *De tonitruis* make use of all the cardinal points of the compass, but these are not uniformly designated. In 5.1.2/1, the west is omitted, but an unspecified "de quacumq*ue* parte cęli" is added, which may seem to lack discriminating value in view of the fact that thunder always comes from some direction, but which may indicate thunder overhead.[7] (1) makes use of all cardinal directions, but either the entry for "west oððe norð" was conflated from two originally separate entries, or the scribe specifically intended to employ two directions in one entry.[8] In addition to the cardinal points, (1) features an entry for "mycel east oððe norðeast", which is not found in the other directional brontologies.

The compass directions are not the only factor in which directional brontologies differ from each other. The level of textual independence and the direct prognostic context varies. Both (1) and the directional

[5] Migne (1861-1904: I.609-14), Thorndike (1923-58: I.679, n.3).

[6] From texts 5.2/1 and 5.1.2/1, Migne (1861-1904: I.610-11) and Förster (1908a: 48), respectively.

[7] Interestingly, a Babylonian text exists which also mentions lightning from all four cardinal directions at the same time as a possibility, cf. Jastrow (1905-12: II.725).

[8] On the compass and orientation in Old English and Anglo-Saxon England, see Derolez (1971), Brown (1978), Korhammer (1985).

brontology in *De tonitruis* can be read as independent texts, while the directional component in 5.1.2 is embedded in an hour brontology.[9] In *De tonitruis*, the directional brontology is followed by weekday and month brontologies. (1), on the other hand, is flanked by two canonical hour brontologies.[10] (1) and the directional brontology in 5.1.2 are attested in similar contexts, but whereas (1) may be read as a text in its own right, the directional brontology in 5.1.2 is fully integrated into the surrounding hour brontology to such an extent that it cannot be read independently, for instance:

> (1) Thunder from the north signifies the death of sheep and calves and youths.[11]
>
> (5.1.2/2) If it has thundered in the ninth hour from the north, it signifies changes in nations [migrations?] and the clash of arms and new concourses of people.[12]

The entry in 5.1.2/1 cannot be split up into a temporal and directional component: both are meaningful and necessary parts of the prognostic. The entries of (1) and 5.1.2/1 have little in common beyond the fact that they pertain to thunder from the north. The prediction in the entry of 5.1.2/1 is not a combination of the entry for nones in a canonical hour brontology plus that for the north in a directional brontology. This means that independent directional brontologies developed separately from integrated ones. If (1) and 5.1.2/1 are dissimilar, how do the predictions of (1) relate to *De tonitruis* and Förster's analogue? North thunder in *De tonitruis* predicts deaths and the wrongful behaviour of Christians.[13] Förster's analogue reports "the killing of a king and discord among relatives".[14] These predictions concern human affairs rather than the agricultural misfortunes related in (1). In conclusion, there are considerable differences between the directional brontologies discussed above. These differences manifest themselves on a structural level in the variation of the compass directions and the integration into a larger brontological context, and in the content of the predictions.

[9] See pp. 253-54.
[10] See pp. 248-51.
[11] Translation of text 5.2/1, l. 6.
[12] Translation of text 5.1.2/2, ll. 16-17.
[13] Cf. Migne (1861-1904: I.611).
[14] "iugulac*io*nem regis & discordiam int*er* p*ro*ximis" (Förster 1908a: 48).

The use of compass directions in the directional brontology is a unique enrichment of the structural features available for prognostics. The search for sources and analogues has not yet yielded a brontology that shows enough correspondences in either structure or content to be related to (1).

Edition

5.2/1 Cambridge, Corpus Christi College 391, p. 714/10-19

Gif þunorrade bið hlynende of eastdæle sé becnað cyninges deað oððe b*iscopes* oððe mycel gefeoht.

Gif he bið suð gehered sé becnað cininges wifes cwealm.

Þonne þunor cumeð west oððe norð ma bið mædena þonne cnihta þy geate ácenned

Se norðþunor becnað scepa deað 7 cealfra 7 geogoðe.

Gif þunor bið mycel east oððe norðeast mycel wæstm bið 7 god on riptid

4 geate] *read* geare | **5** ácenned] -d *partly illegible through hole.*

6 Dog Days

Literature

Hampson (1841: II.73-74); Migne (1861-1904: I.959-62); Payne (1904: 16-20); Jastrow (1905-12: II.584); Gundel (1907: 125-39); Singer (1917: 110); Rohde (1922: 245-46); Thorndike (1923-58: I.728); Gundel (1927: 146-57); Henel (1934-35: 331-33); Jones (1939: 88-89); Gundel and Gundel (1959: 14, 71-72); Bonser (1963: 296-99); Taavitsainen (1988: 55); Hollis and Wright (1992: 269); Cameron (1993: 161-62); Günzel (1993: 31); Epe (1995: 59); Voigts and Kurtz (2000: s.v. *dies caniculares*); Liuzza (2001: 186)

Attribution

post-medieval: Bede

Alias

hare dagas, *Dies Caniculares*

Branch of Superstition

observation of signs: Dog-star, astrometeorology

Texts

OE: 1. London, British Library, Cotton Vitellius E. xviii, fol. 13r
2. London, British Library, Harley 6258B, fol. 52rv
3. London, British Library, Royal 12. D. xvii, fols 5v-6r, 54v-55v

L/OE: 4. Cambridge, Corpus Christi College, MS 422, pp. 29-40

L: 5. Cambridge, Corpus Christi College, MS 9, pp. 3-14
6. Cambridge, Trinity College, O. 7. 41, fols 1v-7r
7. Cambridge, Trinity College, R. 15. 32, pp. 15-26
8. Cambridge, University Library, Kk. 5. 32, fols 50r-55v
9. London, British Library, Additional 37517, fols 2r-3r
10. London, British Library, Arundel 60, fols 2r-7v
11. London, British Library, Cotton Nero A. ii, fols 3r-8v
12. London, British Library, Cotton Titus D. xxvi, fol. 4v
13. London, British Library, Cotton Titus D. xxvii, fols 3r-8v
14. London, British Library, Cotton Titus D. xxvii, fols 22v-23r
15. London, British Library, Cotton Vitellius A. xii, fols 65v-71r
16. London, British Library, Cotton Vitellius A. xviii, fols 3r-8v
17. London, British Library, Cotton Vitellius E. xviii, fols 2r-7v

18. London, British Library, Egerton 3314, fols 18v-30r
19. London, British Library, Harley 3271, fols 120v-21r
20. London, British Library, Harley 3271, fol. 122v
21. London, British Library, Harley 3271, fols 123v-24r
22. Oxford, Bodleian Library, Bodley 579, fols 39r-44v
23. Oxford, Bodleian Library, Douce 296, fols 1r-6v
24. Oxford, Bodleian Library, Hatton 113, fols iii recto-viii verso
25. Oxford, St.John's College, MS 17, fol. 1va-1vb
26. Oxford, St.John's College, MS 17, fol. 1vb
27. Rome, Vatican City, Bibliotheca Apostolica Vaticana, Reg. lat. 12, fols 7r-12v
28. Rouen, Bibliothèque municipale, MS 274, fols 6r-11v

Description

It is remarkable that a genre such as the Dog Days, which is represented abundantly in Anglo-Saxon manuscripts, has received relatively little attention.[1] Förster, who laid the foundations for the study of almost every prognostic genre known in Anglo-Saxon England, referred not once to the Dog Days.[2] By the eleventh century, Dog Days had become a standard ingredient of Anglo-Saxon calendars,[3] as the many witnesses in the list above indicate, so that the neglect of this genre in studies on prognostics is undeserved.

The Dog Days signify the period in which the Dog-star is visible on the horizon. In classical and medieval sources, the Dog-star may refer both to Sirius in the constellation Canis Major and to Procyon in Canis Minor,[4] but the observance of Dog Days in Anglo-Saxon England was linked with the appearance of Sirius rather than Procyon, as an entry in the Harley glossary attests: "Canis or canicula, the star which is called Sirius".[5] An annotated version of Cicero's *Aratea* on the constellations

[1] Thorndike (1923-58: I.728), who discussed many prognostic genres, only briefly referred to the existence of moonbooks and Dog Days, for instance.

[2] Günzel (1993: 31, n. 4) claimed that Förster discussed moonbooks and Dog Days in his important article "Die altenglischen Verzeichnisse von Glücks- und Unglückstagen" (1929), but these are precisely the dangerous days he did not discuss.

[3] See pp. 26-29.

[4] Cf. Gundel (1907: 127).

[5] "Canis . *ue*l canicula . stella q*uae* sirius uocatur" (Oliphant 1966: 50/241). Texts 6/12,21 link the appearance of the Dog-star with Arcturus, the brightest star in the constellation Bootes: "Incipiente ortu canis u*el* ar`c´turi atq*ue* siri stellæ" (at the beginning of the appearance of the Dog-star, or the stars Arcturus and Sirius; 6/21, l. 2). The role

popular in late Anglo-Saxon England, studies the features of Sirius and Canis Major and includes a portrait of the constellation.[6] Knowledge of the Dog Days was transmitted through texts dealing with the Days and their import; texts discussing the medical aspects; and entries in the calendar. Texts on the Dog Days are sometimes followed by a moonbook, i.e. a paragraph enumerating a series of days of the moon on which bloodletting is particularly dangerous. Moonbooks should not be confused with lunaries.[7]

In Old English, the Dog Days are called "hare dagas", "dies caniculares" in Latin.[8] The Dog-star is called "hara steorra" in Old English, "canis" or "canicula" in Latin.[9] The meaning of the word "hara" is not clear. It has been interpreted as a form of the adjective "har" (hoary, grey).[10] Meritt, however, concluded that the element "canis" of the Canicular Days relates to "canus", which was in turn etymologically linked with Latin "candor" (brightness, heat), on the basis of Isidore's *Etymologiae*.[11] If Isidore's account of the Dog-star is compared with that of the Harley gloss, it is clear that the gloss must have derived from the description in the *Etymologiae*: "Canis . *ue*l canicula . stella q*uae* sirius uocatur . se hara steorra" (Harley), and "Canicula stella, quae et Sirius dicitur" (Isidore).[12] If Meritt is correct, therefore, "hara" must be interpreted as "bright" rather than "grey". In other words, the adjective pertains both

of Arcturus in this passage is unclear to me since Canis Major and Bootes rise in different parts of the sky and at different times. Gundel (1907: 140-50) did not mention the existence of a link between Arcturus and Sirius in classical sources.

[6] In the manuscripts Tiberius B. v, fol. 39v, Tiberius C. i, fol. 28r, Harley 647, fol. 8v, Harley 2506, fol. 41r. For illustrations, see McGurck, Dumville, Godden and Knock (1983: pl. XIV, fig. 114-16, p. 106). A study of Cicero's *Aratea* in Anglo-Saxon manuscripts is in McGurck, Dumville, Godden and Knock (1983: 67-78). See also the twelfth-century manuscripts Digby 83, fol. 63r (facsimile: http://image.ox.ac.uk/show?collection=bodleian&manuscript=msdigby83), and Durham, Cathedral Library, Hunter 100, fol. 63r (facsimile Mynors 1939: pl. 36b). Mynors (1939: 50) mentions the manuscripts Royal 13. A. xi and CTC R. 15. 32 in connection with Hunter 100.

[7] On the use of the terms 'moonbook' and 'lunary', see pp. 393-98.

[8] The entry for the start of the Dog Days in the calendar in 6/4, l. 1, reads: "**DIES CANICVLARES**" with the gloss "hare dagas".

[9] The gloss in Harley 3376 reads in full: "Canis . *ue*l canicula . stella q*uae* sirius uocatur . se hara steorra" (Oliphant 1966: 50/241).

[10] Bosworth and Toller (1882-98: 510, s.v. *hár*).

[11] Meritt (1954: 138 [4, A, 11]). Cf. Toller (1908-21: 508-09, s.v. *hár*), Henel; (1934-35: 332, n. 2), Meritt (1945: 56, note to l. 17), Campbell (1972: 39, s.v. *hár*). Isidore wrote "canus dictus a candido; et candidus quasi candor datus" (Lindsay 1911: I, X.59).

[12] Oliphant (1966: 50/241), Lindsay (1911: I, III.lxxi.14).

to the intense brightness of the Dog-star, and to its heat-intensifying properties, with "flammae candorem" as Isidore and Hyginus wrote.[13] The Isidorean etymology of "canis" and its Old English translation must have been common knowledge, because the glossators of the calendar in CCCC 422 (4) and the gloss in Harley 3376, and the scribe of (1) all employ the translations "hára steorra" or "hare dagas". The post-Conquest *Peri didaxeon* states: "therefore the days are called "cinotici", that is the canicular days".[14] The translation "caniculares" for "cinotici" (from Greek κύων, i.e. "dog") shows knowledge of the Days being Dog Days (canis), an alternative to the aforementioned Dazzling Days (canus).[15]

The period in which the Dog Days fall, was in Anglo-Saxon England set to 14 July-5 September.[16] In (1), for instance, the Dog Days number fifty-three days which commence "eighteen days before Lammas [1 August] and end thirty-five days after Lammas".[17] Calendars occasionally report the appearance of the Dog-star in addition to the Dog Days themselves, e.g. "**DIES CANICVLARES**" [14 July]; "**ORT*VS* CANICVLE**" [17 July]; "**FINIVNT DIES CANICVLARES**" [5 September] (4). The latitude of the monastery in which the texts were copied was not taken into account, despite the fact that Anglo-Saxon computists were aware of the influence of the latitude of the observer on observations on earth: witness the frequent inclusion in calendars and computi of the length of shadows at given times, and comments on the amount of daylight and latitude, in Bede's *Ecclesiastical History* (I.1), for instance.

The Dog-star Sirius was already observed in ancient times.[18] In Egypt, Sirius appeared with the flooding of the Nile, and its presence was considered a providential sign of fertility.[19] From the classical period onwards, the Dog-star was renowned for its nefarious influence on life on earth, particularly for its disease-bringing capabilities.[20] This notoriety may be explained in two ways. First, Sirius is the brightest star in the sky

[13] Lindsay (1911: I, III.lxxi.15), Viré (1992: 84, II.35). The Dog-star's heat-bringing qualities are discussed below.

[14] Translation of text 6/2, ll. 20-21.

[15] On the etymology of "canicula", "canis" and Sirius, see also Gundel (1907: 126-31).

[16] For a list of dates mentioned in the Anglo-Saxon texts, see table 33.

[17] Translation of text 6/1, ll. 8-9.

[18] Wissowa *et al.* (1894-1978: 2nd III.1.322-26, s.v. *Sirius*), *Reallexikon* (1950-: XVI. 797-98).

[19] Wissowa *et al.* (1894-1978: 2nd III.1.335-36, s.v. *Sirius*).

[20] Wissowa *et al.* (1894-1978: 2nd III.1.316, 343, s.v. *Sirius*).

and it was thought to reinforce the heat from the sun.[21] Isidore wrote of the Dog-star that "in conjunction with the sun its heat is doubled and bodies are dissolved and vaporised".[22] In the Corpus glossary, Sirius is called "the most fiery constellation".[23] (1) describes the Dog-star as follows: "[the Dog-star] is of a fiery and raging nature. It is through the sun's and the star's heat doubled to such an extent that it shines as strongly at midnight as at noon".[24] The second reason why Sirius was feared, is that the star rises when the summer is hottest, i.e. when hygiene is at its lowest. The account in Bald's *Leechbook* illustrates this:

> The wisest doctors taught that in this period [i.e. the Dog Days] no one should drink any [medicinal] potion or bleed his body in any place, except when it is necessary, and then one should remain inside at noon, because the air is most mixed [i.e. impure].
>
> Therefore, the Romans and all southern nations made themselves earth houses, because of the boiling heat and the venomousness of the air.[25]

The composer of Bald's *Leechbook* took great care in making his account of the Dog Days interesting for an Anglo-Saxon audience by not only revealing a precedent in the teachings of the wisest doctors, but also explaining the customs of the Mediterranean peoples. To us, this insight is particularly interesting because it links the visible presence of the Dog-star and its heat with an awareness of its influence on hygiene. The above examples elucidate that the factors of heat and lowered hygiene account for the dreaded appearance of the Dog-star.

In classical times, the Dog-star was used for a great variety of predictions, including weather, birth and illness prognostication.[26] The Dog Days in medieval texts had only one function: to caution people, especially the weak and those stricken with illness, not to undergo surgical procedures, such as bloodletting, or to take medication. The passage from Bald's *Leechbook* given above testifies to the belief in the harmful effects of medicine and bleeding. (1) also stresses the dangerous aspects of bloodletting:

[21] Cf. Gundel (1907: 131-39).

[22] "coniuncta cum sole duplicatur calor ipsius. et dissolvuntur corpora et vaporantur" (Lindsay 1911: I, III.lxxi.14).

[23] "sidus . ardentissimus" (Hessels 1890: 108/S323).

[24] Translation of text 6/1, ll. 2-4.

[25] Translation of text 6/3, ll. 12-17.

[26] Wissowa *et al.* (1894-1978: 2nd III.1.346-51, s.v. *Sirius*).

> therefore every man will be the weaker who is bled on these days, and some will not escape with their lives. And let no one who knows the truth bleed anyone in that period. And bloodletting is forbidden to all Christians in that period.[27]

The rationale behind these injunctions against bloodletting is that bleeding might lead to wound infections. The closing of a vein which has been bled might pose problems as well. After the account of the Dog Days, Bald's *Leechbook* gives advice on the best times for bleeding, and on remedying some of the dangers attendant upon bloodletting:

> If someone's bleeding wound grows bad, take then mallow, boil in water and bathe with it, and pound the lower part and apply.
>
> If you want to stop the bleeding in an incision, take kettle soot, rub it to dust, put on the wound....
>
> If you cannot stop a bleeding wound, take a fresh horse turd, dry in the sun or by a fire, rub it to dust very well, put the dust very thick on a linen cloth, tie up the bleeding wound with it during the night.[28]

In this quotation, the complications of bloodletting are revealed and remedies are provided. Presumably, complications could arise at any time, but they must have been especially feared during the season of the Dog Days, when heat and bad hygiene provided ideal situations for infections resulting from bloodletting. It is to be noted that the ingestion of medicinal potions is expressly forbidden during the Dog Days, but the application of external medication such as powders and compresses is not. The influence of the Dog Days on the balance of the humours is not yet an issue in Anglo-Saxon England, even though the theory of the humours was known.[29] Texts incorporating the Dog Days in medical tracts which also deal with the humours are either continental, or date to the post-Conquest period.[30]

There are twenty-eight attestations of the genre of Dog Days in Anglo-Saxon and early post-Conquest manuscripts. The occurrence of texts on the Dog Days in other medieval manuscripts has hardly been docum-

---

[27] Translation of text 6/1, ll. 5-8. On authenticating strategies and appeals to authority, see pp. 95-101.

[28] Translation of text 6/3, ll. 26-32.

[29] See pp. 32-33.

[30] E.g. Sloane 475, fols 7v-8r (continent, s. xii), *Peri didaxeon* (England, s. xii$^{4/4}$), St. John's College 17, fols 1-2 (Thorney, 1110-11), and CUL Gg. 5. 35, fols 425v-427v (Canterbury, *c.* 1100), Sloane 2839, fols107r-10v (England(?), *c.* 1100).

ented.[31] Dog Days are transmitted in three different formats:[32] (1) as part of a larger medical tract which deals with bloodletting, hygienic and dietary rules or the humours; (2) as a stand-alone text, i.e. not in a larger medical tract; and (3) as a bare set of dates in the calendar. Formats (2) and (3) developed out of (1), which resulted in a move of the Dog Days from an originally medical context into the computus, and in the case of the stand-alone format, into prognostic sections as well.

Moonbooks are sometimes attached to Dog Days of formats (1) and (2). A moonbook lists a series of days of the moon inappropriate for bloodletting and occasionally a number of good times as well:

> How one should avoid bloodletting on each of the six fives in a month, and when it is best. Doctors teach also that no one should let blood on the five nights' old moon, and again on the ten nights', and fifteen, and twenty, and twenty-five, and thirty nights' old moon, but between each of the six fives.[33]

Moonbooks assign a regular series of days of the moon. The bad ones are series of five and multiplications thereof.[34] Appropriate times are those in between bad days of the moon, or they form another regular sequence, as the following excerpt attests:

> How a vein is to be opened at the right time. The fourth moon is good, and fourteen, and twenty-four. On moon five, or ten, or fifteen, or twenty, or twenty-five, or thirty, it is dangerous to accept a potion or to let blood according to [the opinion of] doctors of old.[35]

Here, the sequence of good times comprises days of the moon with a four in it. As with the Dog Days, moonbooks prohibit bloodletting and medicinal potions. Not all medical tracts and stand-alone texts incorporate moonbooks.

The number of attestations of Dog Days per text format is as follows: four in medical tracts (2, 3, 25, 26); six as stand-alone texts (1, 12, 14, 19-21); and eighteen in calendar entries (4-11, 13, 15-18, 22-24, 27, 28).

[31] Some redactions in Middle English are listed by Voigts and Kurtz (2000: s.v. *dies caniculares*). Wickersheimer (1966: 51 [XXXVII.3], 157 [CIV.2]) mentioned only a few texts on the Dog Days, Beccaria a few more (1956: 122 [8.19], 204 [51.7], 206 [52.6], 211 [55.9], 392 [139.4]).

[32] The relationship between the formats and their contextual development is studied on pp. 153-57.

[33] Translation of text 6/3, ll. 19-22.

[34] For a list of days, see table 34.

[35] Translation of text 6/12, ll. 7-9.

The formats are discussed in turn. First, Dog Days in medical tracts are always part of a larger medical context.[36] (3) appears in Bald's *Leechbook*, (2) in the *Peri didaxeon*, (25, 26) in the first medical section of St. John's College 17. Within this medical context, the Dog Days are embedded in tracts addressing issues such as bloodletting, dietary and hygienic guidelines, or the humours. In addition to the Dog Days these tracts may include moonbooks (3, 26). In the manuscript, (25, 26) are sequenced, but they nevertheless form separate texts as the rubric of (26) seems to introduce a new text.[37] The period in which the Dog Days fall according to these texts varies. (3) and (26) have acceptable dates: 17 July to 5 September (3) and 18 July to 5 September (26). (2, 25), however, only mention the period in which the humours are active: the Dog Days are encapsulated by the period in which "yellow bile is growing inside".[38] In view of the many differences between the four texts, I conclude that they are unrelated to each other. Nevertheless, (3, 26) share certain features, as do (2, 25). The former two include a moonbook and are concerned mainly with bloodletting. (2, 25), on the other hand, have no moonbooks and deal with the humours, devoting space only cursorily to the Dog Days.

The second format, that of the stand-alone texts, is attested six times (1, 12, 14, 19-21), only one of which is in Old English (1). The texts are found in three manuscripts: Vitellius E. xviii (1), Titus D. xxvi, xxvii (12, 14), and Harley 3271 (19-21). These manuscripts probably all hail from New Minster, Winchester.[39] Except for (1), which dates to 1062, the stand-alone texts were copied in the early 1030s. In view of the date and place of origin, the stand-alone texts form a close-knit group. Such texts developed out of the medical format by shifting the focus to the effects of the Dog Days on people's health, and the prohibition of bloodletting and medication. As a rule, moonbooks accompany the Dog Days in the stand-alone format because they fit in with the injunctions against bleeding. (1) is the sole stand-alone text which lacks a moonbook, but Henel suspected that the moonbook of (1) was lost due to extensive fire damage in the manuscript.[40] The Latin stand-alone texts all feature a moonbook. The shift from a medical to a stand-alone format of the Dog Days en-

---

[36] See pp. 39-44.

[37] Cf. Wallis (1985: I.167-70; 1995: 122).

[38] Translation of text 6/2, ll. 19-20.

[39] Titus D. xxvi, xxvii and Vitellius E. xviii are from New Minster, Winchester. On the place of origin of Harley 3271, see Chardonnens (2007b).

[40] Henel (1934-35: 333).

abled these texts to move to other manuscript contexts. In Anglo-Saxon manuscripts, this meant that the stand-alone texts migrated to computi (1, 14) and, more frequently, to prognostic sections (12, 19-21).

The dates assigned by the stand-alone texts are 14 July to 5 September (1), and 18 July to 5 September (12, 14, 19-21). Both variants claim to measure the Dog Days from the appearance of the Dog-star, but in the case of (1) the first date pertains to the calendric start of the Dog Days.[41] (12, 21) introduce the Dog-star as follows: "Incipiente ortu canis".[42] (14, 19, 20) state that the Dog Days start "ab exortu caniculę".[43]

Concerns with bloodletting and dangerous days as main themes are evident from the immediate surroundings of some Dog Days texts. (14, 19, 20) are encountered in the β-sequence, with texts on the three and twenty-four Egyptian Days.[44] (12) is followed by a text on the twenty-four Egyptian Days and preceded by a γ-sequence, which contains texts on the three Egyptian Days and the three miraculous birthdays.[45]

In the pseudo-Bedan treatise *De minutione sanguinis, siue de phlebotomia*, a number of bloodletting prognostics are collected in a way I have not encountered in Anglo-Saxon manuscripts. *De minutione* boasts a tract on the humours with a moonbook and the Dog Days, texts on the three and twenty-four Egyptian Days, a bloodletting lunary, and yet another tract on the humours with a moonbook and the Dog Days.[46] Bloodletting lunaries, in particular, are not found in such a context in Anglo-Saxon manuscripts: they are most commonly attested either in a collection of lunaries (the α-sequence) or preceding the calendar.[47] Jones identified several witnesses of *De minutione*.[48] He did not find any pre-eleventh-century analogues for *De minutione*, which is not to say individual texts did not exist by then.[49] Singer thought that the Anglo-Saxon bloodletting

[41] As I have already pointed out, calendars sometimes distinguish between the start of the Dog Days and the appearance of the Dog-star several days later.

[42] Text 6/21, l. 2.

[43] Text 6/14, l. 2.

[44] See p. 61.

[45] See pp. 61-62.

[46] Migne (1861-1904: I.959-62). The contents of *De minutione* in the light of the prognostics known in Anglo-Saxon England are discussed by Förster (1929: 269).

[47] See pp. 60-61, 439-41.

[48] Jones (1939: 89).

[49] *Ibid.* However, the first part of *De minutione* is attested in the ninth-century manuscript Laon 426 bis (Beccaria 1956: 134 [15.3]; Wickersheimer 1966: 40 [XXVIII.3]). Payne (1904: 16-20) discussed the contents of *De minutione* and the spurious attribution to Bede, and reported a Middle English translation of the tract in Add. 5467. Bonser

prognostics were taken from *De minutione*.[50] On rational grounds, the Bedan attribution should be rejected on account of Bede's preference for Theodore's system of bloodletting rather than for the erratic weekdays and days of the moon assigned in prognostics.[51]

It is possible to distinguish three redactions of Anglo-Saxon stand-alone texts on the Dog Days: Old English (1), which contains information about the heat of the Dog-star not found in the Latin texts; Latin (12, 21), and Latin (14, 19, 20). A detailed comparison of the phrasing and content of the latter three texts is unnecessary, because even a quick look at the texts themselves suffices to reveal that they are almost identical. (12) and (21) are not entirely the same, but they show enough common features to be regarded as variants of one redaction. The phrasing of the good days of the moon in the moonbook differs, but the days assigned coincide: "day four is good, and fourteen and twenty-four", versus "day four will be very wholesome, and day fourteen will be good, and twenty-four is acceptable".[52] In the account of the Dog Days, (12) and (21) differ in phrasing but not in meaning. In view of the short time-span in which these stand-alone texts were transmitted, I conclude that this format enjoyed a sudden burst of popularity in eleventh-century Winchester.

The third and final format of the Dog Days are the entries in the calendar (4-11, 13, 15-18, 22-24, 27, 28). A considerable amount of research into Anglo-Saxon calendars has been carried out to discover which saints were venerated where, for instance, or to find out where calendars were copied and for whom.[53] Besides saints and festivals, calendars harbour a wealth of interesting meteorological, seasonal and prognostic knowledge. Dog Days as calendar entries are a terminal stage in the development of the genre, because it is impossible to reconstitute a body of medical knowledge from such entries if one is not already familiar with the dangers of these Dog Days. Therefore, the user of a calendar must be aware of the meaning of the Dog Days if the pertinent entries are to be of any value to him.[54]

Like so many texts, calendar entries on the Dog Days show some variation, depending on how the entries are phrased and where they are

(1963: 296-99) wrote a rambling account of bloodletting prognostics.

[50] Singer (1917: 110).

[51] See pp. 115-17.

[52] Translation of texts 6/12, l. 7, 6/21, ll. 8-9, respectively.

[53] E.g. Piper (1862), Atkins (1928), Henel (1934a), Wormald (1934), Baker and Lapidge (1995: xxxiv-lx).

[54] See pp. 147-48, 155.

placed. The most complete set of entries is one listing the beginning and end of the Dog Days and the appearance of Sirius, which two calendars have. Nine calendars list the beginning and end, two the beginning only. Four calendars feature the beginning and the appearance of the Dog-star, one the appearance of the Dog-star and the end of the Dog Days. The beginning of the Dog Days is variously entered on 11 July (which must be a mistake), 17 or 18 July (which are acceptable dates when the appearance of the Dog-star is not mentioned separately), and, most frequently attested, 14 July. The appearance of the Dog-star is placed on either 17, 18 or 19 July. The end is on 5 September, sporadically on 4 September.

The variation displayed in the dates is mirrored in the phrasing of the entries. Most regular, because rare, is the appearance of Sirius, which is entered as "ortus canicule", or "canicula oritur". The beginning of the Dog Days is listed as "dies caniculares (incipiunt(ur))", once as "dies caniculares hic incipiunt", and once as "dies caniculares .I.". The end is entered as "finiunt dies caniculares", "dies caniculares finiunt(ur)", "hic est finis dierum canicularum" or "hic finiunt dies caniculares". If the above range in entries is combined with the relevant dates, one arrives at a large number of possible configurations, many of which have actually been attested.[55]

The Dog Days probably are the prognostic genre most widely known in Western Europe from the classical period up to the present day. It is strange, therefore, to discover that Anglo-Saxon texts on the Dog Days have been neglected to such an extent that even Förster is silent on the topic. The Dog Days are supported by a long tradition by the time they are introduced into English manuscripts. In some cultures, the appearance of Sirius is interpreted favourably, but in medieval society, Dog Days were synonymous with heat, ill health and bad hygiene. The Dog Days are attested in three formats: in medical tracts on bloodletting, diet, hygiene or the humours; as stand-alone texts; and as entries in the calendar. Anglo-Saxon manuscripts feature all formats, with a decided preference for calendar entries.

[55] Texts 6/9,15,22 and 6/7,10 seem to form two redactions because they agree in the dates and part of the phrasing. The other Dog Day entries are exceedingly hard to analyse despite the fact that the calendars containing some of them are related (e.g. CCCC 422, Arundel 60, Titus D. xxvii, Vitellius E. xviii, cf. Henel 1934a; 1934-35: 335).

Edition[56]

6/1 London, British Library, Cotton Vitellius E. xviii, fol. 13r/27-37

Eahtatina nihtu*m* ær hlafmæssan gangeð se styrra up (se is gehaten) canes. þ*æt* is se hára steorra bið firenre gecynde 7 weallend(e. hi beoð þurh) þære sunnan hǽtu 7 þæs steorran to þa*m* swiþe getwifealded(e þæt hi scinað) swa swiðe on middeniht swa on midne dǽg. **A**nd hira li(chaman weaxað) 7 swellað. 7 hwilon berstað þæra daga beoð þreo 7 fif(tig þæt se steorra) biþ uppe. forþam byþ æghwilc man þe unhalre þe him (blod læte on þissum) dagum 7 hit sume heora feore ne gedigað. **A**nd nele nan man (æt nanre) tide þe riht cann in þa tid mannu*m* blod lætan. **A**nd eallu*m* criste(n)mannu*m* on þa tid is blodlætincg forboden. eahtatina nihtu*m* (ær hlaf)mæssan 7 (fi)f 7 þrittig nihta ofer hlafmæssan. dagas dies ca ······ g···i···eð ·····þa hwi(le) ·····

Margins damaged; text at right-hand and bottom margin illegible because lost. Text supplied is based on Henel (1934-35) | **2** bið] *read* he ~ | **6-7** hit sume heora feore ne gedigað] *an echo of this phrase is found in the text 3.1.1/1, l. 17:* hit ne gedigð hyre feore | **9-10** dagas dies ca ······ g···i···eð ····· þa hwi(le) ·····] *the bottom line is extensively damaged. It is impossible to reconstruct the original reading. Henel suspected that the lost passage was a moonbook.*

6/2 London, British Library, Harley 6258B, fols 51v/25-52v/9

Incipit lib*er* qui dicit*ur* p*er*i didaxeon.

er onginþ seo boc p*er*i didax`e´on. þ*æt* ys seo swytelung hu fela gera wæs behuded se læcecræft. 7 be his gewisnesse þa gelæredus læce gewíslíce smeadon. Þ*æt* wat se ærusta apollo. 7 his suna esculapfius 7 asclepius: 7 asclepius was ypocrates y`e´m. þeos .iiii.^{or} gemetu*m* ærest þa getymbru*n*ga þare læcecrafte. after noes flode. ymba a þusund wíntra. 7 fif hund wintra. on artaxis dæge. se was p*er*sa cingí hy aluste þa leoht þæra læcecræfte. Giwislica se apollon ærest he gemetta meþodicam. þ*æt* syndon sa ysene þa mann. mid cnifun hæle menn. 7 sculafius: empitrica*m*. þ*æt* is ilæcnunga of læcecrafte. 7 asclepíus: loícam. þ*æt* ys seo gehealdenysse þære æ. 7 þæs lifæs. 7 ypocras t`h´eoricam. þ*æt* ys foresceawunga þara seocnesse.

Margins damaged. For the Epistola peri hereseon, *which served as the source, see Glaze (2007)* | **2** er] *read* Her | boc] *the remainder of the line is left blank, probably for a rubric* | wæs] ~ ‖ ⟨*f. 52r*⟩ | **3** gewisnesse] *read* gewitnesse | gelæredus] *read* gelæredusþan | **4** wat] *read* was | esculapfius] *read* esculafius *(i.e. Scolafius)* | **6** a] ~ [sun] *(expunged)* | ymba a þusund wíntra] *in the margin:* circa m*ille* an*n*os | artaxis] *i.e.* Artaxerxes | **7** cingí] *read* cingc | **7** gemetta] ge[me`t´ta] metta *(expunged)* | **9** empitrica*m*] *read* empiricam | **10** t`h´eoricam] *read* teopericam.

[56] Order of the texts: 1-3, 12, 21, 14, 19, 20, 25, 26, 4-11, 13, 15-18, 22-24, 27, 28.

Þannu*m* plato 7 aristotiles þa gelæredusþan alwytyna. Þas æfterfylígdun: þas forecwedenan. læcu*m*. 7 hi gesæðdu*n*. þ*æt* feower wætu*n* syndon on þan manniscen lichama. forþam byð wylyd. ealswa middangeardes boga. þat ys þa wæte: on þan heafode. 7 þ*æt* blod: on þara breosta. 7 se ruwa gealla: on þan innoþe. 7 se swerta gealle ínnan ðare blædran And hyra angehylce rixaþ ðra monþas. þ*æt* ys fram .xviii. kł. Ian*uarii* usq*ue* in .viii. kł ap*ri*l*is* þ*æt* on ðan heafde se wate byð wexende Anð fram .xviii. kł ap*ri*l*is* usq*ue* ín viii. kł. Iulíí. þ*æt* ð*æt* blod biþ wexínde on þan breosten. Ab xviii. kł Iulíí usq*ue* i*n* octaua kł octobris. þ*æt* sa ruwa gealle byð wexenda. on þan innoþe. forþan synd þa dages genemnede. cínotici. þ*æt* sindan þa dæges caniculares 7 þara byd fif 7 feowertig. dæga. 7 on þam dage 7 on þan dagen ne mæg nan læce wel don fultu*m* ænigen seoce manne. Anð þe feorðan gescornesse ys ab .xviii. kł octobris. usq*ue* in .viii. kł Ian*uarii* þat se blace gealle wixt. on þara bladre. Þis gescead ys hæfter þam feorwer heorren. heofenes. 7 eorðan. 7 þara lyfte. 7 þara dupnesse. Þa wæs ealswa drihte licede. ealswa was se man geset. Þ*æt* þur þara smeagunga. 7 þarre endbirnesse. Vtan nu mymen æryst gewislice þane fruman of þan heafde.

12 æfterfylígdun] *in the margin:* secuti s*unt* | þas] *read* þan | **13** gesæðdu*n*] *read* gesæddun | **16** angehylce] *read* anra gehwylce | **17** .xviii.] ~ *glossed by* octodecimo | .viii.] ~ *glossed by* octo | **18** Anð] *read* And | .xviii.] ~ *glossed by* octodecimo*; Cockayne (1864-66: III.84) observed that "there is no such day as xviii. kal. Aprilis"* | **19** octaua] *read* octauam | octobris] o- < · | **20** genemnede] -n$_2$- < · | **21** byd] *read* byð | **21-22** 7 on þam dage 7 on þan dagen] 7 on þam dage ‖ 7 on þan dagen ⟨*f. 52v*⟩*; read* 7 on þan dagen *(dittography)* | **22** Anð] *read* And | **24** feorwer] *read* feowrer | **26** þarre] ~ [ed] *(expunged); read* þare | **26-27** mymen] *read* nymen.

6/3 London, British Library, Royal 12. D. xvii, fols 5v/20-6r/13 (in table of contents), 54v/19-55v/19 (text)

.lxxii **L**æcedomas on hwilce tid blod sie to forganne on hwilce to forlætenne 7 hu sie attres ful sio lýft on hlafmæsse tid. 7 be drencúm 7 utforúm on þam monþe 7 þ*æt*te wyrta on þam monðe sind to wy`r´canne.

Romane 7 eall suðfolc worhton hím eorþhus wið þære unlyfte. 7 hu món scyle blodlæse on þæra sex fifa ælcon on þæs monan eldo forgan on þritigúm nihta 7 hwonne betst to lætanne. 7 gif bloddolg yfelige. 7 gif þu wille ón snide blod forlætan oþþe ón ædre. oððe gif þu ne mæge bloddolg áwriþan. oþþe gif þu ne mæge geotend ǽdre awriðan oððe gif mon on sinwe beslea æt blodlætan

1 .lxxii] *entry in table of contents* | **2** sie] ~ ‖ ⟨*f. 6r*⟩.

.LXXII.

On hwilce tid blod sie to forganne *on* hwilce to lætenne. Blodlæs is to forganne fiftyne nihtu*m* ær hlafmæsse 7 æfter fif 7 þritig nihtu*m* forþon þon*ne* ealle æterno þing fleogaþ 7 mannum swiðe deriað. Læcas lærdon þa þe wisoste wæron þ*æt* nan man on þam monþe ne drenc ne drunce ne ahwær his lichoman wanige butan hís nydþearf wære: 7 þon*ne* *on* middeldagúm inne gewunode forþon þe sio lyft biþ þon*ne* swiþost gemenged.//

Romane him forþon 7 ealle suðfolc worhton eorþhus for þære lyfte wylme 7 æternesse. Eác secgeað læcas þ*æt*te geblowene wyrta þon*ne* sien betste to wyrcenne ge to drencu*m* ge to sealfu*m* ge to duste.

Hu món scule blodlæse ón þara six fifa ælcúm on monðe forgan 7 hwonne hit betst sie. Læcas lærað eác þ*æt* nan mán on þone fif nihta ealdne monan 7 eft .x. nihta 7 fiftyne 7 twentiges 7 fif 7 twentiges 7 þritiges nihta ealdne monan ne læte blod ac betweox þara sex fifa ælcúm. 7 nis nan blodlæstid swa god swa on foreweardne lencten þon*ne* þa yfelan wætan beoþ g*e*gaderode þe on wintra gedruncene beoð 7 on kalendas ap*ri*lis ealra selest þon*ne* treow 7 wyrta ærest úp sprytta ð þon*ne* weaxeð sio yfele gillestre 7 þ*æt* yfele blod on þa*m* holcu*m* þæs lichoman.

Gíf monnes bloddolh yfelige gením þon*ne* geormenleaf awylle on wætre 7 beþe mid. 7 gecnua nioþowearde lege ón.

Gif þu wille on snide blod forlætan. ním ceteles hru*m* gegnid to duste scead ón þa wunde. Gením rigenhealm eft 7 beren gebærn to duste.

Gif þu ne mæge bloddolh awriþan gením horses tord niwe adrige ón sunnan oððe be fyre gegnid to duste swiþe wel lege þ*æt* dust swiþe þicce on linenne clað wriþ mid þy þ*æt* bloddolh neahterne.//

Gif þu geotend ædre ne mæge awriþan genim þ*æt* selfe blod þe ofyrnð gebærn ón hatu*m* stane 7 gegnid to duste lege *on* þa ædre þ*æt* dust `7´ awrið swiðe.//

Gíf món æt blodlætan ón sinwe beslea meng tosomne weax 7 píc 7 sceapen smera lege on clað 7 on þ*æt* dolh.//

At three points 'nota' signs have been added in the margins in the section dealing with bloodletting (see pp. 141, 144) | **9** .LXXII.] *start of text proper* | **10** forganne] ~ ‖ ⟨*f. 55r*⟩ | **23** gegaderode] ~ ‖ ⟨*f. 55v*⟩ | **28** Gif] *a 'nota' sign has been entered into the margin, running from ~ to the end of the paragraph* | **33** Gif] *a 'nota' sign has been entered into the margin, running from ~ to the end of the paragraph* | **35** món] *a sign over ~ is linked to one next to a 'nota' sign in the margin.*

6/12 London, British Library, Cotton Titus D. xxvi, fol. 4v/2-17

Quali tempora ap*er*ienda s*it* uena

Incipiente artucanis. uel arcturi adq*ue* siria stella q*uo*d te*m*pus. Incipit a xv. kł agusti. usq*ue* nōn septe*m*b*ris*. & sunt dies numero .l. unde om*nes* q*ui* hoc te*m*pore sanguine detraxerint insaniores. redduntur. **M**ultos p*er*iculosa mors sequit*ur*. **D**e hoc aute*m* ideo medici tacuerunt quia causam dieru*m* istor*um* ignorauerunt. **S**ed nos cunctis chr*ist*ianis int*er*dicim*us*.

Quodo ap*er*ienda sit uena in te*m*pore .iiii. **L**una bona xiiii. xxiiii. In .v. luna. uel .x. uel .xv. u*el* .xx. u*el* xxv. u*el* xxx. **S***ecundu*m antiquor*um* medicoru*m* catarticu*m* accip*er*e. u*el* fleouotomu*m* facere p*er*iculosum est.

1 tempora] *read* tempore | **2** artucanis] *read* ortu canis *(see 6/21)* | siria] *read* sirii | **3** usq*ue*] usq*ue* in *6/21* | hoc] *read* in ~ | **4** sanguine] *read* sanguinem | **7 Q**uodo] *read* Quando | **8** antiquor*um*] *read* dictum ~ *(see 6/21).*

6/21 London, British Library, Harley 3271, fols 123v/25-124r/9

DE FLEBOTOMAT`I´TIONE. MENSIS. AGVSTI.

Incipiente ortu canis u*el* ar`c´turi atq*ue* siri stellæ. q*uo*d te*mpus* incipit `a´ .xv. ꝁ ag*us*`t´i usq*ue* in nona sept*embris*. Et sunt dies numero .l. Vnde om*nes* qui in hoc tempore sanguine*m* detraxerint: insaniores reddunt*ur*. multis periculosa mors sectat*ur*: eo q*uo*d medici inscior*um* causam tamen adtendentes ratione*m* `ignorantes´ q*ui*a hoc cunctis int*er*di`ci´mus chr*ist*ianis.

QVALI TE*M*PORE APERIENDA SIT VENA.

Quando uena aperienda sit .iii. luna erit saluberrima. & xiiii. luna erit bona. 7 xxiiii. accipienda est. Caue tibi .v. luna. 7 x. & xv. & xx. & xxv. necnon. 7 xxx. Caute secundu*m* dictu*m* antiquoru*m* medicoru*m* catarticu*m*. uel. f l´eb`o´tomu*m* periculosu*m* est accipere.

1 FLEBOTOMAT`I´TIONE] FLEBOTOMAT[A]TIONE -A- < I, -`I´- < [A] (*expunged*)*; read* FLEBOTOMATIONE | **2** Incipiente] I[I]ncipiente | ar`c´turi] -i < [·] | siri] *read* sirii | **3** ag*us*`t´i] -i < s | nona] *read* nonas | **4** multis] -i- < o*; read* multos | **5** sectat*ur*:] ~ ‖ ⟨*f. 124r*⟩ | inscior*um*] ~ *on erasure* | **5-6** `ignorantes´] *in left margin, transposition indicated* | **7** TE*M*PORE] -PO < E[·] | **8** .iii.] *read* .iiii. *(a moonbook on a series of fours is clearly intended, see also 6/12)* | **10** Caute] *this word makes no sense here; it may have been inserted erroneously in analogy to* Caue *(l. 9)* | catarticu*m*] *glossed by Old English* spiwdrenc*; the medical term* catarticum *(i.e.* καθάρτικον*) features in the Harley glossary as well:* Catartica . nom*en* medicine *(Oliphant 1966: 60/524), which is a gloss for Isidore's* Etymologiae*:* Catartica Graece, Latine purgatoria dicuntur *(Lindsay 1911: I, IV.ix.8)* | **10-11** f l´eb`o´tomu*m*] -`o´- < e (*expunged*).

6/14 London, British Library, Cotton Titus D. xxvii, fols 22v/16-23r/8

Est etiam istorum temporum obseruanda ratio. ne forte a quopiam heędem suprascriptę cause *ue*l medicine incautius exerceantur. hoc e*st* ab exortu caniculę qui est a xv. kł augusti. usq*ue* in nonas septembris dies quinquaginta numero. **S**ol*et* namque id sepissime contingere. ut in his flebotomati infirmitates non minuant. sed eas grauissimis doloribus augeant. adeo ut plerosq*ue* periculosa mors per hec subsequatur.

Sunt etiam hae lunationes summa cum diligentia adtendendę. ne in eis suprascriptę causę exerceantur. id e*st* quarta quintaq*ue* luna necne decima ac quinta decima. uigessima quoq*ue* necnon uigessima quinta tricessimaq*ue* **A**utenticorum in his medicorum cohibentur diuersorum potionum dictione. seu flebotomatum usus adhibenda.

1 quopiam] -q- < u | **1-2** suprascriptę] -c- < · | suprascriptę cause *ue*l medicine] *delete* cause *uel (see 6/19,20); probably a slip of the eye (see ll. 7-8:* suprascriptę causę*)* | **4** infirmitates] ~ ‖ ⟨*f. 23r*⟩ | **11** adhibenda] *read* adhibendi *(the sentence caused other scribes difficulty as well, see 6/19,20 and p. 170).*

6/19 London, British Library, Harley 3271, fols 120v/20-121r/4

Est etiam istor*um* tempor*um* obseruanda ratio. Ne forte a quopiam eędem suprascriptę medicine incautiu*s* exerceant*ur*. hoc est ab exortu canicule q*ui* e*st* a .xv. kł augusti. usq*ue* in nonas septembris. dies .l. numero. Sol*et* namq*ue* id sepissime contingere ut in his flebotomati infirmitates n*on* minuant. sed eas grauissimis dolorib*us* augeant adeo ut plerosq*ue* periculosa mors p*er* hęc subsequat*ur*.

Sunt etiam hę lunationes summa cu*m* diligentia adtendende. ne in eis sup*ra*scriptę cause exerceantur. id e*st* quarta quintaq*ue* luna. Necne decima ac quinta decima .xx. q*uo*q*ue* Necn*on* xxv. tricessimaq*ue*. Autenticoru*m* in hís medicor*um* cohibent*ur* diuersor*um* potionu*m* dictione. Seu flebotomatu*m* usus adhibendi

A line in the right margin indicates that the text on the three Egyptian Days (fol. 121r/21-30) should have followed instead of the intervening mass (see p. 530). The second copy of the β*-sequence, on fol. 122rv, is in consecutive order* | **7** exerceantur.] ~ ‖ ⟨*f. 121r*⟩.

6/20 London, British Library, Harley 3271, fol. 122v/7-19

DE DIEB*VS* CANICVLARIBVS.

Est etia*m* istorum te*m*poru*m* obseruanda ratio: ne forte a quópia*m* eęde*m* sup*ra*scriptę medicinę incautius exercean*tur*. hoc *est* ab exortu caniculę. q*ui est* a xv. kł agusti. usq*ue* in. NŌN septembr*is*. dies .l. numero. Solet namq*ue* `id´ sepissime contingere. ut in his flebotomati infirmitates non minuant: sed eas grauissimis doloribus a`u´gea`n´t: adeo ut plerosq*ue* p*er*iculosa mors p*er* hec subsequat*ur*;

1 eęde*m*] [h · ·]eęde*m*.

Sunt etia*m* he lunationes summa cum diligentia adtendendę: Ne in eis sup*ra*scripte cause exerceant*ur*. id *est* q*ua*rta q*ui*ntaq*ue* luna. necne. decima. uigessima q*uo*q*ue* necn*on* .xx^{ma}v.^{ta} tricessimaq*ue* Autentico*rum* in his medico*rum* cohibent*ur* diuersoru*m* potionu*m* dictione. seu flebotómatu*m* usus adibenda.

8 decima.] *read* ~ ac quinta decima | **10** adibenda] -a < i; *read adhibendi (the sentence caused other scribes difficulty as well, see 6/14,19 and p. 170).*

6/25 Oxford, St. John's College, MS 17, fol. 1va-1vb/16

Hi q*ua*ttuor humores d*omi*nant*ur* in suis locis. Sangu*is* d*omi*nat*ur* in dextro lat*ere*: in epate q*uo*d ictur uocam*us*. Al*iter* in corde. Colera rubea i*n* eode*m* lat*ere* ubi uesica plena *est* felle h*oc est* in dextro: Nigra i*n* sinistro q*uę* s*un*t plene. Fleuma au*tem* in capite scilicet una pars. alt*era* i*n* uesica.

Sangu*is* eni*m* feruens humid*us* 7 dulcis. Colera rubea: amara. uiridis. Nigra: acida. 7 frigida. Fleuma: frigida. salsa. 7 humida.

Hęc o*mn*ia *igitur* e*ss*e suis t*em*po*r*ib*us*. Sangu*is* uere. Colera rubea. ęstate. Colera nig*ra*: autumo. Fleuma: hieme.

Hi u*ero* humor*es* h*abe*nt respiratio*n*es p*er* singu*l*as partes corporis. Sangu*is* p*er* nares. Colera rubea. p*er* aures. Colera nig*ra*: p*er* oculos. Fleuma: p*er* os.

Quattuor hi humores. mores tales faciunt. Sangu*is* fac*it* ho*minem*. bonę uolu*n*tatis. si*m*plice*m*. mod*er*atu*m*. so*m*no plenu*m* 7 crassu*m*. Colera rubea fac*it* irac*un*du*m*. auaru*m*. tumidu*m*. t*r*iste*m*. inuidiosu*m*. sepe h*abe*nte*m* in pedib*us*: cicat*r*ice*m*. Fleuma. fac*it* co*m*positu*m* corpore. uigilante*m*. in se infra cogitante*m*. canes cito p*r*oduc*en*te*m*.

Corp*us* .iiii. h*abe*t i*n* se q*ua*litates. 7 .iiii. reb*us* co*n*sistit. ossib*us*. neruis. uenis. carne. Continet in se frigidu*m*. calidu*m*. humidu*m*. 7 siccu*m*. & eni*m* .iiii. h*abe*nt diu*er*sitates. Esurit. sitit. co*n*cupiscit. soporat*ur*. & .iiii. s*un*t us*us* nat*u*rę. manducare. bib*ere*. generare. dormire.

Itaq*ue* iubem*us* eos q*ui*b*us* colera d*omi*nat*ur*. ue*r*no. t*em*po*re* flebotomare. 7 autu*m*no corp*us* purgare. Nulla eni*m* res meli*us est* q*uam* purgatori*us* bon*us* 7 optim*us*. Talib*us* purgari expedit. Dagridii silis .iii. turis masc*u*li sil*is* .ii. aloene petro sil*is* .iii. Euforbii sil*is* .ii. H*ęc* o*mn*ia *tr*itis 7 *cum* aq*ua* calida dab*is* ieiuno bib*ere* hora matutina p*r*opt*er* humor*es* noxios depon*en*dos. Fit h*ęc* de albis rubeisq*ue* colorib*us*.

Nig*ra* u*ero* ex q*ui*b*us* melancolia nascunt*ur*. q*uę* uarietate*m* faciunt in corpore. uulnera int*r*insec*us* nut*r*iunt. & indigestio*n*es faciunt. His nulla res melior *est* q*uam* ut abstineant. 7 h*ęc* talia comedant suis t*em*po*r*ib*us*. Carnes berbecinas. de

The right margin is darkened and deformed which makes the end of the lines on fol. 1vb difficult to read. I am heavily indebted to Singer's edition of this text (1917) | **2** ictur] *read* ictus*(?)* | **3** Nigra] *i.e.* Colera nigra | plene] *read* splene | **6** acida] -c- < i | **8** autumo] *read* autumno | **12** Colera rubea] *read* ~ facit hominem imperterritum. an iustum. malicentum. bene manducantem et cito digerentem. Colera nigra *(see Singer 1917)* | **15** canes] *read* canos | **20** colera] *read* ~ rubea | flebotomare] -b- < o | **21** meli*us*] *read* melior | **22** Talib*us*] Tałib*us*.

sale. Iubemus non comedere caprinas. non leporinas. non porcinas. quia melancoliam nutriunt. insuper porcina caro uenenum melancolicis est. 7 stomachum graue facit. Bouinam carnem expedit sumere. Purgatur melancolicis. Dagridii silis .ix. agarici silis .ix. cassie 7 fistule silis .vi. reopontici silis .iiii. Hęc omnia teris 7 cum aqua calida ut supra.

Sanguis est calidus. humidus. 7 dulcis. Fleuma: salsa. acida. 7 sicca. Sicca maligna humoribus. Inter humores 7 sanguinem .xii. librę sunt in copore hominis. medietas sanguinis. & medietas humoris. Si sanguis superfluus humori fuerit facit elefantiosum. Porro quando hoc sentit inęquali corpori debes. succurere. At si humor. supererit sanguini: ydropicum facit. Oportet igitur ut adhibeat purgatorium corpori. aut flebotomum. ideo ut inęqualitas corporis compositionem salubritatis. (restitu)at. Quod si non fecerit. languoribus grauissimis laborabit.

Oportet medicum medicinam corpori adhibere. tam ····· (fleboto)mate. Nam id est caniculares dies. Quos non iubemus ullam (man)sionem. neque curam corpori adhibere. nisi infirmitas ·· aduenere in initium febricitanti uel pleorities (iu)bemus ut medicus omnem curam flebotomię uel expectationem quam explorauit a magistro suo faciat. ceteras ····res presumat. quia dies sunt caniculares.

Porro aperien ····· ingrediuntur. usque in id augusti que sunt dies .xxx. ··(ues)·· 7 subsolanus uentus id est uulturnus dominatur. Addi(untur) ·· dies. qui faciunt in unum dies .xlix: a quinquagesim ····· omnem curam corporis expedit medicum curare. Mul ····· medicorum fuere. qui non aspexere .xix. dies. neque par(ti) ····· neque per ingenium. morti haud potuere resistere. Ab autem septembri usque primo k decembris medicus cautelam habere debet.

30-31 graue] *read* grauem | **39** ideo] ~ ‖ ⟨*f. 1vb*⟩ | **44** flebotomię] f- < l.

6/26 Oxford, St. John's College, MS 17, fol. 1vb/17-32

DE FLEBOTOMIA.

Si necessitas fuerit omni tempore adhibendus est flebotomus. tamen precipue ab .viiii. k aprilis usque in viii k iulii. Tunc est utilitas detrahendi sanguinem. quia tunc sanguis augmentum habet. Sed postea obseruationes sunt temporum 7 qualitates. cursusque lunę obseruandę. hoc est .v. Lunam .x. (.xv. .xx.) .xxv. & .xxx. In his non oportet flebotomum imponere quia in his diebus quos medici quinnones uocant. hęc fieri haud oportet. & quia multi medicorum affirmant quod inf(initus) numerus ob negligentiam non obseruantium qualitates temporum & cursus lunę mortui sunt.

Nam tamen super omnia obseruandum est. ut a xv. k augusti usque .Ñ. septembris quos caniculares dies. pro stella quę canicula uocatur dicti. neque potionem neque flebotomum. debet aliquis habere infra dium. quia hi humores mixtis. Solum si ictus peruenerat quod non oportet nisi ut aperiantur. uene 7 uastitas. iniquitas q(uidem) sanguinum. Euaporetur esset ut nullomodo hic facere oportet.

I am heavily indebted to Singer's edition of this text (1917) | **5** obseruandę] -ę < a | Lunam] *read* Luna | **11** dium] *read* diem | mixtis] *read* mixti sunt(?).

6/4 Cambridge, Corpus Christi College, MS 422, pp. 29-40

⟨14 July⟩ **DIES CANICVLARES.** hare dagas
⟨17 July⟩ **ORT*VS* CANICVLE.**
⟨5 Sept⟩ **FINIVNT DIES CANICVLARES.** her geendioð þa hare dagas

1 ⟨*p. 35*⟩ | **3** ⟨*p. 37*⟩.

6/5 Cambridge, Corpus Christi College, MS 9, pp. 3-14

⟨14 July⟩ **Dies caniculares.**

1 ⟨*p. 9*⟩.

6/6 Cambridge, Trinity College, O. 7. 41, fols 1v-7r

⟨14 July⟩ Dies caniculares.
⟨5 Sept⟩ Dies cani*cu*lares finiunt.

1 ⟨*f. 4v*⟩ | **2** ⟨*f. 5v*⟩.

6/7 Cambridge, Trinity College, R. 15. 32, pp. 15-26

⟨14 July⟩ **Dies caniculares incipiunt*ur*.**
⟨5 Sept⟩ **Dies caniculares finiunt*ur*.**

1 ⟨*p. 21*⟩ | **3** ⟨*p. 23*⟩.

6/8 Cambridge, University Library, Kk. 5. 32, fols 50r-55v

⟨14 July⟩ **Dies caniculares.** *hic* in*cipiunt*
⟨19 July⟩ *Ort*us *canicule.*
⟨5 Sept⟩ *Hic* est *finis dierum* *canicula*rum.

1 ⟨*f. 53r*⟩ | **4** ⟨*f. 54r*⟩.

6/9 London, British Library, Add. 37517, fols 2r-3r

⟨14 July⟩ **DIES CANICVLARES INCIPIVNT.**
⟨17 July⟩ **ORTVS CANICVLAE.**

1 ⟨*f. 2vb*⟩.

6/10 London, British Library, Arundel 60, fols 2r-7v

⟨14 July⟩ **Dies caniculares incipiunt**
⟨5 Sept⟩ **Dies canicul*ares* finiuntur.**

1 ⟨*f. 5r*⟩ | **3** ⟨*f. 6r*⟩.

6/11 London, British Library, Cotton Nero A. ii, fols 3r-8v

⟨14 July⟩ Dies canculares .l.
⟨5 Sept⟩ hic finiunt d*ies* c(ani)`cula*res*´

1 ⟨*f. 6r*⟩ | canculares] *read* caniculares | **2** ⟨*f. 7r*⟩ | **2-3** c(ani)`cula*res*´] *right margin is trimmed so* -(ani)- *was lost;* `cula*res*´ *over the line.*

6/13 London, British Library, Cotton Titus D. xxvii, fols 3r-8v

⟨17 July⟩ **Dies caniculares incipiunt.**
3 ⟨5 Sept⟩ **Dies caniculares finiunt.**

1 ⟨*f. 6r*⟩ | **3** ⟨*f. 7r*⟩.

6/15 London, British Library, Cotton Vitellius A. xii, fols 65v-71r

⟨14 July⟩ **DIES CANICVLARES.**
3 ⟨17 July⟩ **ORTVS CANICVLĘ.**

1 ⟨*f. 68v*⟩.

6/16 London, British Library, Cotton Vitellius A. xviii, fols 3r-8v

⟨18 July⟩ **Incipiunt d*ies* caniculares.**
3 ⟨5 Sept⟩ **Finiunt d*ies* canicul*ares*.**

1 ⟨*f. 6r*⟩ | **3** ⟨*f. 7r*⟩.

6/17 London, British Library, Cotton Vitellius E. xviii, fols 2r-7v

⟨14 July⟩ **Dies kaniculares** `*hic incipiu(nt.)*´
3 ⟨5 Sept⟩ **Dies caniculares hic fini(unt.)**

1 ⟨*f. 5r*⟩ | **3** ⟨*f. 6r*⟩.

6/18 London, British Library, Egerton 3314, fols 18v-30r

⟨14 July⟩ **Dies caniculares.**

1 ⟨*f. 24v*⟩.

6/22 Oxford, Bodleian Library, Bodley 579, fols 39r-44v

⟨14 July⟩ **DIES CANICVLARES.**
3 ⟨17 July⟩ **ORTVS CANICVLAE.**

1 ⟨*f. 42r*⟩.

6/23 Oxford, Bodleian Library, Douce 296, fols 1r-6v

⟨14 July⟩ **Dies canicul*ares* incipiunt.**
3 ⟨4 Sept⟩ **Finiunt dies caniculares.**

1 ⟨*f. 4r*⟩ | **3** ⟨*f. 5r*⟩.

6/24 Oxford, Bodleian Library, Hatton 113, fols iii recto-viii verso

⟨14 July⟩ **DIES CANICVLARES INCIPIVNT.**
3 ⟨18 July⟩ **CANICVLA ORIT*VR*.**

1 ⟨*f. vi recto*⟩.

6/27 Rome, Vatican City, Bibliotheca Apostolica Vaticana, Reg. lat. 12, fols 7r-12v

⟨11 July⟩ **Dies caniculares.**
⟨5 Sept⟩ **Dies caniculares fini-**
3 **untur.**

1 ⟨*f. 10r*⟩ | **2** ⟨*f. 11r*⟩.

6/28 Rouen, Bibliothèque municipale, MS 274, fols 6r-11v

⟨14 July⟩ Dies caniculares.
⟨5 Sept⟩ Dies caniculares finiunt.

1 ⟨*f. 9r*⟩ | **2** ⟨*f. 10r*⟩.

7 Dreambook

Literature

Schindler (1858: 245-48); Steinschneider (1863); Cockayne (1864-66: III.ix-xiv); Büchsenschütz (1868); Birch (1878: 481-83; 1892: 258-59); Meyer (1884: 144-45); Graffunder (1906); Förster (1903: 356-57; 1908b: 302-05; 1908c: 32, 35, 36-37; 1910; 1911; 1916; 1921; 1925-26: 60-62, 64-65); Stoop (1909); Diepgen (1912); Drexl (1921; 1922; 1923; 1925; 1926); Thorndike (1923-58: II.290-302); Hélin (1925); Gardiner (1935: I.7-23); Svenberg (1936: 142-43); Best (1940); Blum (1943); Oppenheim (1956); Suchier (1957); Önnerfors (1960; 1977: 32-57); Bühler (1962); Pack (1963); Pongracz and Santner (1963); Kaiser and Krauss (1965); Schmitt (1965; 1966); Turville-Petre (1968); Kurland (1972); Lewis (1976); Martin (1977; 1979; 1981); Harmening (1979: 95-117); Oberhelman (1981, 1986, 1991); Fischer (1982a; 1982b; 1983; 1989); Tolles (1983); Braswell (1984: 348); Grub (1984); Hunt (1987: 180, n. 127); Taavitsainen (1988: 57); Berriot (1989); Kieckhefer (1989: 85-86); Klopfer and Lackner (1989); Hahn (1992); Hollis and Wright (1992: 264-65); Günzel (1993: 33-34); Miller (1994); Epe (1995); Hermes (1996); Penot (1998); Liuzza (2001: 188-89); Holowchack (2002); Wit (2002); Mavroudi (2002); Haag (2003: 44-45); Mooij-Valk (2003); Näf (2004); Pick and Roper (2004); DiTommaso (2005: 231-59, 378-402); Brodersen (2006)

Alias

Somniale Danielis

Attribution

medieval: Daniel

Branch of Superstition

observation of signs: dreams, oneiromancy, *somnimancy

Texts

OE:	1. London, British Library, Cotton Tiberius A. iii, fols 38r-39v
	2. London, British Library, Cotton Tiberius A. iii, fol. 42rv
	3. Oxford, Bodleian Library, Hatton 115, fols 150v-52v
L/OE:	4. London, British Library, Cotton Tiberius A. iii, fols 27v-32v
L:	5. London, British Library, Cotton Titus D. xxvi, fols 11v-16r
	6. London, British Library, Sloane 475, fols 217v-18r

Description

Dreambooks pertain to dreams of revelatory content, i.e. dreams which carry meaning with regard to events in the future of the dreamer's life.[1] Dream interpretation with the help of such dreambooks has been the subject of many studies. In this respect, it is strange to see that dream interpretation is only cursorily treated in the *Handwörterbuch des deutschen Aberglaubens*, under the contrived designation 'somnimancy'.[2] The *Lexikon des Mittelalters* refers the reader to lunaries without devoting even one word to dreambooks.[3] The entry for lunaries relates the existence of specific lunaries, including dream lunaries,[4] but dream lunaries and dreambooks are two different prognostic genres altogether. Rather than repeating a considerable body of scholarship, I refer the reader to existing works for a detailed discussion of dreambooks.[5]

Alphabetical dreambooks, the only type of dreambooks known in Anglo-Saxon England, are lists of dream subjects with interpretations.[6]

[1] Since I discuss medieval alphabetical dreambooks only, the psychology and place of dreams in a wider historical and cultural perspective are not studied here, but see Büchsenschütz (1868), Diepgen (1912), Lewis (1976), Hahn (1992), Miller (1994), Hermes (1996), Holowchack (2002), Näf (2004), Pick and Roper (2004).

[2] Hoffmann-Krayer, Bächtold-Stäubli *et al.* (1927-42: VIII.31, s.v. *Somnimantie*). The nonce-word 'somnimancy' is used instead of the accepted 'oneiromancy'.

[3] Auty *et al.* (1980-99: VIII.964, s.v. *Traumbücher*).

[4] Auty *et al.* (1980-99: VI.5, s.v. *Lunar*).

[5] Of particular relevance are Förster (1908b: 302-05; 1908c: 32, 35, 36-37; 1910; 1911; 1916; 1921), Thorndike (1923-58: II.290-302), Önnerfors (1960; 1977: 32-57), Pongracz and Santner (1963), Schmitt (1966: 181-200), Martin (1977; 1979; 1981), Grub (1984: xxi-xxxvii) and Epe (1995). Fischer (1982a) deserves separate mention as he has benefited extensively from the work of Schmitt (1966), so much so that Fischer translated almost literally many notes from Schmitt's work without acknowledgement. Two instances will illustrate this. (1) "Die Astrologie zählte man zusammen mit der nicht scharf von ihr geschiedenen Astronomie zu den 'Freien Künsten', sofern sie nicht, wie es sehr häufig der Fall war, mit magischen oder mantischen Vorstellungen in Verbindung trat" (Schmitt 1966: 182, n. 3) versus "Astrology, which figured together with astronomy in the *artes liberales*, was censured only when dealing with forbidden topics or processes, such as magic or soothsaying" (Fischer 1982a: 163, n. 2). (2) "Im Zuge des im Spätmittelalter epidemisch wachsenden Hexenwahns wurden Zauberei und Hexerei von kirchlicher Inquisition und weltlicher Gerichtsbarkeit als Ketzerei verfolgt" (Schmitt 1966: 182, n. 4) versus "During the judicial secularization of the Church in the later Middle Ages, magic and witchcraft were branded as heresy by both ecclesiastical and lay courts" (Fischer 1982a: 163, n. 3).

[6] Byzantine dreambooks are the first to order the entries alphabetically, an arrangement which has been retained in medieval dreambooks. Dreambooks ordered by topic have been attested, also in Byzantine texts, but the Greek 'Danielis' tradition followed

The entries in a dreambook are simple sentences introducing the dream subject and its significance, e.g. "to catch birds in a dream signifies gain".[7] Sometimes entries take the form of "if you see/it seems that... then" constructions: "if you see a dragon flying over you, it signifies treasure", and "if it seems that he is bathing or washing himself in the sea, it means happiness".[8] Entries may also be phrased as "if you dream... then" constructions: "if you dream that you see two moons, it means joy and happiness".[9]

The dream *topoi* in most medieval dreambooks are presented in alphabetical order, though this order rarely extends beyond the first letter. The order of the entries for the letter 'a' in the glossed dreambook (4), for instance, is: "Aues", "Aues", "Aues", "Asinos", "Arma", "Asinos", "Asinos", "Aquas", "Arbores", "Arbores", "Aerem", "A bestiis", "Arcum", "Anullum", "Anullum", "Anullum", "Aurum", "Absinthium", "Acetum", "Agrimoniam", "Alba", "Arare". It is immediately apparent that the alphabetical order is restricted to the initial letter, which, in turn, gives rise to a sequence with only a limited attempt at gathering entries on the same *topos*: the "Asinos" dreams have been put together, but not without an "Arma" dream slipping in. The "A bestiis" dream would not be in its place in the 'a' sequence of the dreambook, if it had been made by a modern compiler.[10] It would have been more appropriate with the "Bestias" dreams under the letter 'b'. However, medieval dreambooks rely on a strict alphabetical order of the first letter, as a dream with the subject "Cum mortuo loqui" appears under 'c' rather than under the letter 'm' with the "Mortuum" dreams.[11] Likewise, entries starting with the preposition 'in' are listed under 'i', and not under the first letter of the dream subject. While the Latin dreambooks, which are translations from the Greek, are ordered alphabetically, translations in the vernacular are not. Thus, the first seven entries in (1) pertain to "earn" (eagle),

by medieval compilers presented the entries in alphabetical order. For an example of dreambooks following other structures than the alphabet, see that of Achmet ben Sirin (Drexl 1925; Klopfer and Lackner 1989; Oberhelman 1991; Penot 1998) and the late medieval text of Hans Lobenzweig (Schmitt 1966).

[7] Translation of text 7/5, l. 2.

[8] Translation of texts 7/4, l. 573, and 7/1, l. 19, respectively.

[9] Translation of text 7/4, l. 567.

[10] Fischer (1982a) arranged entries from more than twenty medieval dreambooks according to their dream subjects in alphabetical order. This is useful for finding correspondences between the interpretation of dreams on the same *topos*, but the resulting edition is far removed from the order in the manuscripts.

[11] Text 7/4, l. 167.

"beon" (bees), and "fugelas" (birds), which reflects the Latin 'a' sequence "aquilam", "apes", "aues".

Aside from the order, the entries for the letter 'a' reveal a tendency for dreambooks to include series of dreams on one *topos*. If it is possible to see a ring in a dream, for example, it is equally possible to receive one or to give someone a ring.[12] Many dream subjects feature this kind of diversity: one can ride a horse which is white, black, yellow, bay or brown.[13] The colour of the horse determines the meaning of the dream. The variety in dream *topoi* can be quite extensive: water dreams consist of the following building blocks: (a) to see/drink from/wash oneself/swim/fall into (b) a bath/fish pond/well/sea/river/flood, while the water is (c) cold/hot/clean/dirty. Each combination leads to another dream interpretation. The range of *topoi* introduced in dreambooks is huge.[14] Pongracz and Santner made a useful division into the human body, people, actions, animals, the outside world, nature and the cosmos.[15] Comprehensive lists of dream subjects have been published.[16]

Dreambooks have existed in many cultures from the third millennium BC onwards. Mesopotamian clay tablets form the oldest written evidence of dream interpretation, followed by Egyptian, Greek, Arabic and Latin dreambooks, and those in the European vernaculars in the Middle Ages.[17] Even today, dreambooks are published for an eager public of DIY dream interpreters in the long wake of Freudian and Jungian dream explication for psychoanalytical purposes.[18] It is hard to find a direct link between Assyrian and Anglo-Saxon dreambooks, but strikingly they have some dream *topoi* in common, thereby bridging a period of

[12] See text 7/4, ll. 33-38.

[13] See text 7/4, ll. 190-201.

[14] Part of the range is the result of variation introduced like that in dreams about water and horses, i.e. based upon an existing subject. Martin (1977: 153-65; 1981: 79-85) and Fischer (1982a: 11-13) distinguished a number of mechanisms which account for some of the variation, including instances of sloppy copy, substitution, and simplification.

[15] Pongracz and Santner (1963: 115-219). Cf. Martin (1977: 74-76).

[16] Fischer (1982a: 16-20), Epe (1995: 268-77). A list of dreams and interpretations allowing comparison between Egyptian, Assyrian, Greek, Jewish, medieval and modern dreambooks is in Pongracz and Santner (1963: 227-388).

[17] Thorndike (1923-58: II.290-302) and Pongracz and Santner (1963: 13-102) provided a survey of dreambooks throughout the ages. Oppenheim (1956) studied dream interpretation of the ancient Near East, and published and translated an Assyrian dreambook. An Egyptian dreambook is edited in Gardiner (1935: I.7-23).

[18] Pongracz and Santner (1963: 103-13).

several millennia. Thus, dreams of animals, blindness, incest, water, the dead and kissing are attested in both dream traditions.[19] This seems to indicate that such dream *topoi* are either part of the Jungian collective subconscious, or that the knowledge preserved in dreambooks was somehow transmitted from one era and culture to the next. Förster perceptively remarked: "how else should an alphabetical dreambook in Welsh, printed in 1910, take into account that a twentieth-century Welsh farmer's wife was capable of dreaming of sleeping with an Ethiopian, the typical eunuch of the Byzantine court?"[20] It may be difficult to demonstrate the transition from Assyrian to Anglo-Saxon dreambooks, but an analogous process is evident in the transition from Arabic and Greek to Latin to vernacular dreambooks.

Arabic and Greek dreambooks, which represent the art of dream interpretation of the late classical and Byzantine period, comprise a number of distinct texts attributed to various authorities, including Achmet ben Sirin, Artemidoros, Astrampsychos, Daniel, Germanos and Nikephoros.[21] These dreambooks are thought to have come into existence between the second and tenth centuries.[22] The manuscript evidence for some dreambooks however, is of a much later date. The oldest Greek dreambook of Daniel, for instance, dates from the fifteenth century, but it is assumed that this type was developed in an earlier period. The dreambooks that gained an audience in the Middle Ages represent the *Somniale Danielis* tradition. This is confirmed by the correspondences in dream *topoi* between the Greek 'Danielis' dreambooks and the Latin texts, and the rubrics of medieval dreambooks, which are often attributed to Daniel, e.g. "**De somnior*um* diuersiitate** [*sic*] **sec*und*um**

[19] See the dreams on these *topoi* in 7/4, for instance, and Oppenheim (1956: 258-59, 275, 280, 283, 287). Remarkably, the variety in water dreams in Anglo-Saxon dreambooks is paralleled in the Assyrian dreambook.

[20] "Wie sollte sonst z.B. ein um 1910 gedrucktes neukymrisches Traumbuch noch mit der Möglichkeit rechnen, daß eine wallische Bauernfrau des 20. Jahrhunderts träumen könne, mit einem 'Äthiopier', dem typischen Haremseunuchen des byzantinischen Hofmilieus, im Bette zu liegen?" (Förster, 1925-26: 61-62).

[21] See Thorndike (1923-58: II.290-94), Martin (1977: 2-11), Grub (1984: xxiv-xxvii). Oberhelman (1981) studied and translated many of the Greek dreambooks. Editions of individual texts are in Stoop (1909), Drexl (1921; 1922; 1923; 1925; 1926), Pack (1963), Kaiser and Krauss (1965), Oberhelman (1991), Penot (1998), Mavroudi (2002), Mooij-Valk (2003), Broderson (2006). A Latin translation of various Greek dreambooks has appeared in 1603 in *Artemidori Daldiani et Achmetis Sereimi F. oneirocritica, Astrampsychi et Nicephori versus etiam oneirocritici*.

[22] Cf. Önnerfors (1977: 33-42), Grub (1984: xxv-xxvii).

ordinem abcharii [*sic*] **danielis proph*ete*"** (1). Such attributions have led scholars to name this type of prognostic *Somniale Danielis*.[23]

Alphabetical dreambooks were tremendously popular in the Middle Ages, witness the many attestations from the ninth century onwards, but no Latin dreambooks prior to the ninth century have been found. The oldest Latin dreambooks are incorporated in Uppsala, Universitetsbibliotek C. 664, and Harley 3017.[24] The earliest Anglo-Saxon witnesses of dreambooks, in Tiberius A. iii and Titus D. xxvi, both eleventh-century (1, 2, 4, 5), are of different redactions than the Uppsala and Harley texts. Numerous dreambooks survived: DiTommaso has compiled a list of more than 150 witnesses, including early printed texts.[25] The six English dreambooks thus represent only a fraction of the attestations. Despite a majority in Latin, dreambooks are found in Old English, Middle English, Icelandic, German, French, Irish, and Welsh.[26] The Old English dreambooks are the earliest in the vernacular and date from the first half of the eleventh century and after.

The first taxonomy of medieval dreambooks was proposed by Martin,[27] who revealed that Förster's rudimentary classification of the Latin dreambooks into two groups was deficient.[28] Martin distinguished several redactions: distinct 'a' and 'b' redactions; several versions of a hybrid 'a/b'; the earliest redaction of Harley/Uppsala, which includes material not found in 'a' or 'b'; and the lengthy late medieval redaction in All Souls College 81.[29] Epe has recently reexamined the classification with an eye to the Old English dreambooks.[30] The earliest Latin redactions follow geographic boundaries in that the 'a' redaction is found in English and 'b' in continental manuscripts.[31] According to Martin, the 'b' redac-

[23] Cf. Martin (1977: 70-71), DiTommaso (2005: 247-58).

[24] The dreambook in Harley 3017 has been studied and edited by Martin (1977: 88-90, 260-63; 1979; 1981: 24-25, 169-72), the one in Uppsala C. 664, by Grub (1984).

[25] DiTommaso (2005: 379-97).

[26] Latin dreambooks have been published by Martin (1977; 1979; 1981), Grub (1984), among others. On texts in the vernacular, see Martin (1977: 148-49). Middle English dreambooks have been published by Förster (1911) and Bühler (1962); Icelandic by Turville-Petre (1968); German by Graffunder (1906) and Fischer (1982b); French by Hélin (1925), Suchier (1957) and Berriot (1989); Irish by Best (1940); Welsh by Förster (1921).

[27] Martin (1981: 4-12).

[28] Förster (1911: 51), Martin (1981: 3).

[29] Martin (1977: 50-66, 128-47; 1981: 4-12, 63-78).

[30] Epe (1995: 74-101).

[31] Martin (1977: 50; 1981: 4).

tion is thought to have arrived in England after the Conquest, but Epe classed the Old English dreambooks (1-3, the second supplement of 4) among the hybrids.[32] These texts antedate the Norman Conquest, which would suggest that a 'b' redaction already circulated in England in Anglo-Saxon times. The two main distinctions between 'a' and 'b' reside in differences in the predictions, and to entries attested in one redaction but not in the other.[33] Both 'a' and 'b' seem to have been based upon a single Latin translation of a Greek dreambook, 'a' probably being closer to the original than 'b'.[34]

The Latin dreambooks (5, 6) represent redaction 'a'. (4) consists of an extensive 'a' series of 249 entries (4a) and a first supplement of twenty-one entries (4b), and a second supplement of thirty-two entries of a hybrid showing close affinity with 'a' (4c).[35] Martin has shown that none of the texts of redaction 'a' can have served as an exemplar for any of the others.[36] Therefore, (4-6) have been transmitted independently and do not derive from a common exemplar. (4a-b) is the longest extant witness of redaction 'a': it comprises 270 entries.[37] There are indications for the scribe of the interlinear Old English gloss of (4) to have used an existing gloss. Förster adduced errors in which the glosses do not correspond to the Latin text and vice versa, and spelling mistakes.[38] The three dreambooks in Old English (1-3) are hybrids.[39] Although (1) and (2) are found in the same manuscript, they are fragmentary and not directly related. (3), which postdates the dreambooks in Tiberius A. iii by more than a century, shows close affinity with (1), despite the fact that (3) has fewer entries than (1), and that (3) has several entries not present in (1). It is likely that (1) and (3) share a common exemplar, the more so because the two manuscripts probably hail from the same foundation, viz. Christ Church, Canterbury and share more prognostics.

[32] Epe (1995: 94-101).

[33] Martin (1981: 4-6).

[34] Martin (1977: 52-53; 1981: 7-9). Martin did not wish to offer a definitive answer in the matter of Latin translations and originals of the 'a' and 'b' dreambooks, but he did provide a useful discussion of the matter, which seems to support the view that 'a' and 'b' derived from one translation.

[35] Martin (1977: 57-58; 1981: 10).

[36] Martin (1981: 65).

[37] Text 7/4 has 302 entries in all, but the second supplement is here not taken into account.

[38] Förster (1910: 45-47).

[39] The relationship between the Old English dreambooks has been studied extensively by Förster (1908b: 302; 1910: 39-47; 1916: 264-70) and Epe (1995: 94-101).

Edition[40]

7/1 London, British Library, Cotton Tiberius A. iii, fols 38r/2-39v/23

⟨1⟩ **G**if mann mæte þ*æt* he geseo earn on his heafad ufan. þ*æt* tacnað wurþmynt.

⟨2⟩ gif him þince þ*æt* he feala earna ætsomne geseo. þ*æt* byþ yfel nið. 7 manna sætunga 7 seara.

⟨3⟩ **G**if him þince þ*æt* he geseo beon hunig. beran þ*æt* biþ þ*æt* he on eadigum hadum feoh gestrynþ.

⟨4⟩ **G**if him þince þ*æt* hine beon stikian þ*æt* byþ þ*æt* his mod byþ astyred fram eltheodigum mannum.

⟨5⟩ **G**if him þince þ*æt* he geseo beon into his huse fleon þ*æt* byþ þæs huses ælednyss.

⟨6⟩ **G**if him þince þ*æt* he geseo feala fugela ætsomne þ*æt* byþ æfest. 7 geflit. 7 cyd.

⟨7⟩ **G**if he fugelas geseo betweonan heom winnan. þ*æt* biþ þ*æt* rice hadas heom betweonan winnan.

⟨8⟩ **G**if hin þince þ*æt* hine næddre tere. beorge him georne wið yfele wimmen.

⟨9⟩ **G**if him þince þ*æt* hine earn swyþe ete. þ*æt* byþ deaþ.

⟨10⟩ **G**if him þince þ*æt* he hine on hatum wætere baþige. oððe þwea. þ*æt* biþ þæs lichaman tiddernys.

⟨11⟩ **G**if him þince þ*æt* he on cealdum wætre baþige. þ*æt* byþ hys lichaman hælo. 7 gesynto.

⟨12⟩ **G**if him þince þ*æt* he hine on sæ baþige oþþe ðwea. þ*æt* biþ bliss.

⟨13⟩ **G**if him þince þ*æt* he fæger wæter geseo. oððe oferfare. þ*æt* byþ orsorhnyss.

⟨14⟩ **G**if him þince þ*æt* he drof wæter geseo. ne deah þæt.

⟨15⟩ **G**if him þince þ*æt* he go`l´d finde. þ*æt* biþ god. 7 yfel þamþe hit gecynde ne biþ.

⟨16⟩ **G**if him þince þ*æt* he feala penegas finde

⟨17⟩ 7 ne oþhrine. god þ*æt* byþ. gif he nymeþ ne deah þæt.

⟨18⟩ **G**if him þince þ*æt* he hæbbe ar oððe isen. þ*æt* byþ god swefem.

Entries 16 and 17, originally one entry, have been split up on the basis of 7/3. Comparison with 7/3 reveals that one entry has been omitted after 37. This redaction would, therefore, have had at least 97 entries | **1** ufan] *read* ~ gesettan *(see 7/3)* | wurþmynt] *read* micel ~ *(see 7/3)* | **6** astyred] *read* swyþe ~ *(see 7/3)* | **13** hin] *read* him | tere] ehte *7/3* | **14** ete] *read* ehte | **17** he] *read* ~ hine | wætre] -t- < [·] | **22** go`l´d] `l´ *added between* o *and* d, *so not over the line* | god] *read* ~ swefen *(see 7/3)* | **24-25** finde 7 ne oþhrine] *entries 16 and 17 are one in 7/1, but 7/3 makes clear that this is wrong. The ending of entry 16 should read* ...finde þæt biþ æfst; *the opening of entry 17* **G**if him þince þæt he penegas geseo 7 ne oþhrine.... | **25** he] *read* ~ hie | þæt] *read* ~ him *(see 7/3)* | **26** swefem] *read* swefen.

[40] Order of the texts: 1, 3, 2, 4-6.

⟨19⟩ **G**if him þince þ*æt* he lead hæbbe. sum unwyrd him byþ toweard.

⟨20⟩ **G**if him þince þ*æt* he æt forþgewitenum menn anlices onfo. of unwenum him cymð gestreon.

⟨21⟩ **G**if him þince þ*æt* he æt ricu*m* menn feos onfo. þ*æt* byþ alysednys hys brca.

⟨22⟩ **G**if him þince þ*æt* his hus byrnð. micel blæd him biþ toweard.

⟨23⟩ **G**if him þince þ*æt* hæ oft byrnan þ*æt* byþ mycel gestreon.

⟨24⟩ **G**if him þince þ*æt* he his hus timbrie þ*æt* byþ þ*æt* hys god byþ weaxende.

⟨25⟩ **G**if him þince þ*æt* his hus toworpen sy. sum ætlætnes him byþ toweard.

⟨26⟩ **G**if him þince þ*æt* he hwit hrægel geseo. þ*æt* byþ micel wurþmynt.

⟨27⟩ **G**if him þince þ*æt* he his beard scere. þonne biþ his brocc lytliende.

⟨28⟩ **G**if him þince þ*æt* his earm sy ofaslegen. þ*æt* byþ his goda alætnes.

⟨29⟩ **G**if him þince þ*æt* he miceles hrægeles geweald age. þ*æt* biþ þ*æt* he ofercymþ ealle his find.

⟨30⟩ **G**if him þince þ*æt* he aht beran geseo. þ*æt* biþ ungeradnys.

⟨31⟩ **G**if him þince þ*æt* he mid gerenedan gyrdle begyrd sy. biþ anmodnys.

⟨32⟩ **G**if him þince þ*æt* he hæbbe gyldene beah. þ*æt* byþ þ*æt* he geþyhþ healicne ealdordom.

⟨33⟩ **G**if him þince þ*æt* he hæbbe ruh lic. þ*æt* biþ hys goda wanung.

⟨34⟩ **G**if him þinge þ*æt* he ne mæge yrnan. mycel broc him byþ towerd.

⟨35⟩ **G**if him þince þ*æt* he blindne man geseo. geborenne. þ*æt* byþ forlætnys his goda.

⟨36⟩ **G**if him þince þ*æt* he spiwe. þ*æt* byþ swa hwæt swa he ana wat þ*æt* wyrþ geypped.

⟨37⟩ if him þince þ*æt* he wiþ cyng sprece. him cymþ gefealic gifu to. 7 god.

⟨One entry missing⟩

⟨38⟩ **G**if him þince þ*æt* he stige on heanne munt. þ*æt* tacnaþ god.

⟨39⟩ **G**if him þince þ*æt* he of dune astige. he onfehþ broces dæl.

⟨40⟩ **G**if him þince þ*æt* he mid his freondes wife hæme. þ*æt* bið adl.

⟨41⟩ **G**if him þince þ*æt* he mid his agenum wife hæme. þ*æt* bið god swefen.

⟨42⟩ **G**if him þince þ*æt* he hine georne to gode gebidde. micel gefea him biþ toweard.

⟨43⟩ **G**if him þince þ*æt* he sy. ungyrd. broc þ*æt* biþ.

⟨44⟩ **G**if him þince þ*æt* he dracan geseo: god þ*æt* biþ.

⟨45⟩ **G**if him þince þ*æt* he deme dom. þ*æt* bið god.

⟨46⟩ **G**if him þince þ*æt* his heafod sy bescoren þ*æt* byþ broc.

⟨47⟩ **G**if him þince þ*æt* he hæbbe micel feah tiddernes him biþ towerd.

28 anlices] -ic- [··] | **30** brca] *read* broca *(see 7/3)* | **31** blæd] *read* ~ 7 torhtnys *(see 7/3)* | **32** hæ] -æ < i; *I follow Förster (1916) but the manuscript reading is unclear* | oft byrnan] *read* ofbyrne *(*ost byrnen *7/3); ~* ‖ *⟨f. 38v⟩* | **34** ætlætnes] *i.e.* alætnes | **41** biþ] *read* þæt ~ | **45** þinge] *read* þince | **50** if] *read* Gif | **58** ungyrd] *i.e.* ungyred.

⟨48⟩ **G**if him þince þ*æt* he hæbbe niwe sceos. mid broce him cymþ gestreon.

⟨49⟩ **G**if him þince þ*æt* he bec hæbbe þ*æt* biþ uncuð hlaford oððe ealdorman.

⟨50⟩ **G**if him þince þ*æt* he huntige beorge him georne wið his fynd.

⟨51⟩ **G**if him þince þ*æt* he hundas geseo. 7 hi hine gretan beorge him eac wið his fynd.

⟨52⟩ **G**if him þince þ*æt* he geseo hundas yrnan þ*æt* byþ micel god toweard.

⟨53⟩ **G**if him þince þ*æt* he fixas geseo. þ*æt* biþ ren.

⟨54⟩ **G**if him þince þ*æt* he bradne monan geseo. þ*æt* biþ. god swefen.

⟨55⟩ **G**if him þince þ*æt* he hwit hors geseo oððe on ride. þ*æt* biþ weorðmynt.

⟨56⟩ **G**if him þince þ*æt* he on blacan horse ride þ*æt* biþ his modes angnes.

⟨57⟩ **G**if him þince þ*æt* he on readum horse ride. þ*æt* biþ his goda wanung.

⟨58⟩ **G**if him þince þ*æt* he on fealewum horse. oððe on grægium ride. þ*æt* biþ god swefen.

⟨59⟩ **G**if him þince þ*æt* he wer slea. þ*æt* bið gecyd wiþ his freond.

⟨60⟩ **G**if him þince þ*æt* he his feond slea. beorge him georne wiþ frecne þing.

⟨61⟩ **G**if him þince þ*æt* he þeofas geseo. him byþ god towerd.

⟨62⟩ **G**if him þince þ*æt* he deadne mann cysse. þ*æt* biþ lang lif. 7 god.

⟨63⟩ **G**if him þince þ*æt* he geseo scyp yrnan. god ærende. him biþ towerd.

⟨64⟩ **G**if him þince þ*æt* he hnyte somnige. god þ*æt* bið gif he hi ne ytt. 7 yfel gyf he hy ytt.

⟨65⟩ **G**if him þince þ*æt* he oþerne cysse. god þ*æt* bið.

⟨66⟩ **G**if him þince þ*æt* he hunig ete. oððe geseo. þ*æt* bið angnys.

⟨67⟩ **G**if him þince þ*æt* he bellan geseo. oððe gehyre. weorðmynt him byþ towerd.

⟨68⟩ **G**if him þince þ*æt* he on circean singan gehyre mycel god þ*æt* tacnað.

⟨69⟩ **G**if him þince þ*æt* he mann geseo mid wæpne gewundod. ymbhydig sorh þ*æt* biþ.

⟨70⟩ **G**if him þince þ*æt* he wæpen wege. orsorhnys þ*æt* byþ.

⟨71⟩ **G**if him þince þ*æt* he wiþ his scrift sprece. þ*æt* tacnað his synna forgyfennysse.

⟨72⟩ **G**if him þince þ*æt* his wif si mid bearne. þ*æt* bið god swefen.

⟨73⟩ **G**if him þince þ*æt* he næddran geseo þ*æt* bið yfeles wifes niþ.

⟨74⟩ **G**if him þince þ*æt* he geseo lic beran. ne biþ. ne biþ þ*æt* nan laþ.

⟨75⟩ **G**if him þince þ*æt* he æt woruldgeflitum si. þ*æt* tacnað him adl towerd.

⟨76⟩ **G**if him þince þ*æt* he hæbbe hwit sceap. þ*æt* tacnað god.

⟨77⟩ **G**if him þince þ*æt* he hæbbe ferrhryðer. ne byþ þ*æt* naþor ne god ne yfel.

65 huntige] ~ ‖ *⟨f. 39r⟩* | **77** him$_2$] *read* he ~ | **78** þeofas] *read* þeowas (servants, *but 7/3 also has ~);* þeofas (thieves) *is unlikely because of the positive interpretation* | **82** hy] -y < i | **87** circean] cir.|cean | **90** þince] -c- < g | **95** ne biþ. ne biþ] *read* ne biþ *(dittography)* | **96** þ*æt*$_2$] ~ ‖ *⟨f. 39v⟩*.

⟨78⟩ **G**if him þince *þæt* he erige oððe sauwe. gestreon him biþ towerd.

⟨79⟩ **G**if him þince *þæt* he awiht on godcundum bocum ræde. oððe leornige. micel wurðmynt him byþ towerd æt gode.

⟨80⟩ **G**if him þince *þæt* he on hwylcere fægerre stowe si nið his modes him cymeð.

⟨81⟩ **G**if him þince *þæt* he geseon ne mæge. lære ic hine *þæt* he him beorge wið his ehtend.

⟨82⟩ **G**if men þince *þæt* he seoluc. oððe godewebb hæbbe. *þæt* bið god hwilum. 7 hwilum leasung.

⟨83⟩ **G**if him þince *þæt* he befyled si. god *þæt* bið.

⟨84⟩ if him þince *þæt* he wurðlic ref geseo. *þæt* biþ god.

⟨85⟩ **G**if him þince *þæt* he feala swyna ætsomne geseo. þonne mæig he wenan broces.

⟨86⟩ **G**if him þince *þæt* he feala henna geseo oððe. hæbbe. *þæt* biþ god.

⟨87⟩ **G**if him þince *þæt* he henne æiru hæbbe. oððe þicge. ne deah him þæt.

⟨88⟩ **G**if him þince *þæt* he gæt geseo. þonne mæg he wenan þæs laðwendan feondes him on neawyste.

⟨89⟩ **G**if him þince *þæt* he feala stodhorsa hæbbe oððe geseo awestnys hys goda *þæt* bið.

⟨90⟩ **G**if him þince *þæt* he feala gosa hæbbe. god *þæt* byð.

⟨91⟩ **G**if him þince *þæt* he sceap pullige. ne bið *þæt* god.

⟨92⟩ **G**if him þince *þæt* he piper ete. ne deah *þæt*.

⟨93⟩ **G**if him þince *þæt* he feala spera ætsomne geseo. þonne tacnað *þæt* þu ofercymst ealle þine fynd.

⟨94⟩ **G**if hine mæte *þæt* he win drince. *þæt* tacnað his lichaman hæle.

⟨95⟩ **G**if him þince *þæt* he byrnende candele geseo oððe on handa hæbbe. *þæt* bið god.

⟨96⟩ **G**if him þince *þæt* he ele hæbbe oþþe mid smyrige. micelne gefean *þæt* tacnað ægþer ge her on worulde ge æfter.

108 if] *read* Gif.

7/3 Oxford, Bodleian Library, Hatton 115, fols 150v/10-152v/3

⟨1⟩ **G**yf mon meteð þ*æt* he geseo earn on his heafod unfange settan. þ*æt* tacnað micel weorðmynd.
⟨2⟩ Gyf þe þince þ*æt* þu geseo feola earna ætsamne. þ*æt* byð yfel nið.
⟨3⟩ Gyf þe þince þ*æt* þu geseo beon hunig beran. þ*æt* byð þ*æt* he on eádegum handum feoh gestreonað.
⟨4⟩ Gyf hine beon stingen. þ*æt* byð þ*æt* his moð byð swiðe onstired fram ælþeodegum mannu*m*.
⟨5⟩ Gyf him þince þ*æt* he geseo beon into his huse fleogan. þ*æt* byð þes huses awestmas.
⟨6⟩ Gyf him þineg þ*æt* he geseo fela fugla ætsamne. þ*æt* byð æfest 7 gecid.
⟨7⟩ Gyf he fuglas geseog betwenan winnan. þ*æt* byð þ*æt* rice hades winnað heom beotweonan.
⟨8⟩ Gyf his nædre ehte. beorge him wyð ífle iwfmen.
⟨9⟩ Þon*ne* him wynce þ*æt* his earn ehte. þæt bið eað.
⟨10⟩ Gyf him þince þ*æt* he hine on hatu*m* wætere þwea. þ*æt* byð his lices tidernes.
⟨11⟩ Gyf him þince þ*æt* he hine on cealdum wéterum þwea. þ*æt* byð his lices hælo 7 gesynto.
⟨12⟩ Gyf him þince þ*æt* he hine on sæ baðige. oððe þwea: þ*æt* byð blisse.
⟨13⟩ Gyf he fæger weter geseo. odde oferfæreþ. þ*æt* byð orsorgnesse.
⟨14⟩ Gyf hine meteð þ*æt* he drof wæt*er* geseo. ne deah þæt.
⟨15⟩ Gyf he gold findeð. god swefn þ*æt* bið. 7 yfel þemþe hit cynde ne bið.
⟨16⟩ Gyf he mancas oððe penigas findæg. þ*æt* bið æfst.
⟨17⟩ Gyf him þince þ*æt* he penigas gesio. 7 ne oðrine: god þæt bið. Gyf he hie nimeð: ne deahg þ*æt* him.
⟨18⟩ Ðon*ne* him þince ár oððe isen þ*æt* he habbe. þ*æt* bið god.
⟨19⟩ Gyf him þince þ*æt* he læd habbe. sum unwird him byð toweard.
⟨20⟩ Gyf him þince þ*æt* he æt forðgewitenu*m* men ahtes onfo. of unwenu*m* him cymeð gestreon.

Comparison with 7/1 reveals that entries have been omitted as follows: one entry each after 27, 65, 69 and 73, ten entries each after 42 and 60 | **1** unfange settan] *read* ufan gesettan | **3** nið] *read* ~ 7 manna sætunga 7 seara *(see 7/1)* | **6** Gyf] *read* ~ him þince þæt *(see 7/1); the omission is repeated, see ll. 13,19,21,22,31* | moð] *read* mod | **9** awestmas] *read* awestnes | **10** þineg] *read* þince | gecid] *read* geflit 7 cid *(see 7/1)* | **11** betwenan] *read* ~ heom | **13** Gyf] *read* ~ him þince þæt *(see 7/1)* | his] *read* hine | him] *read* ~ georne *(see 7/1)* | iwfmen] *read* wifmen | **14** him] [·]him, -im < n | wynce] *read* þynce | his] *read* hine | ehte] *read* swiðe ~ *(see 7/1)* | eað] *read* deað | **15** þwea] *read* baðige oððe ~ *(see 7/1)* | **19** Gyf] *read* ~ him þince þæt *(see 7/1)* | odde] *read* oððe | **20** þæt.] ~ ‖ ⟨*f. 151r*⟩ | **21** Gyf] *read* ~ him þince þæt *(see 7/1)* | **22** Gyf] *read* ~ him þince þæt *(see 7/1)* | **25** god] *read* ~ swefn *(see 7/1)*.

⟨21⟩ Gyf him þince þ*æt* he æt ricumen feos onfo. alysse dæt byð broca.

⟨22⟩ Gyf him þince þ*æt* his hus burnat. micel bled 7 torhtnes him byð towæard.

⟨23⟩ Gyf he ost byrnen. þ*æt* bið micellicu gestreon.

⟨24⟩ Gyf man meteg þ*æt* he his hus timbrie. þ*æt* byð his weaxnes.

⟨25⟩ Gyf him þinceg þ*æt* his hus sí toworpen. sum æfwela him bið toweard.

⟨26⟩ Gyf him þinceg þ*æt* he hwit hrægl gesio. þ*æt* byð micel wurðmind.

⟨27⟩ Gyf him þince þ*æt* he his bearn scire. þon*ne* byð his broc litligende.

⟨One entry missing⟩

⟨28⟩ Þon*ne* him þinceg þ*æt* he micles heres gewald age. þanne ofercymeð he ælle hise feond.

⟨29⟩ Gyf hine meteg þ*æt* he awiht beran geseo. þ*æt* byð ungerades.

⟨30⟩ Gyf him þinceg þ*æt* he seo mid gerenode gyrdel sio gyrded. ðæt byð anmodnes.

⟨31⟩ Gyf hine mæte þ*æt* he hebbe beag. þ*æt* byð þ*æt* he geþihð healic ealdordom.

⟨32⟩ Gyf him þince þ*æt* he habbe ruh lic. þon*ne* byð his goda waniend.

⟨33⟩ Gyf hine mete þ*æt* he ne mæge yrnan. miccel broc him byd toweard.

⟨34⟩ Þonne him þince þ*æt* he spiwe. þ*æt* byð swa hwæt swa he ana wiste þ*æt* hit wéorðæð yppe.

⟨35⟩ Gyf hine mete þ*æt* he geseo blindne man geborenne. þ*æt* byð forlætnesse his gode.

⟨36⟩ Gyf him þince þ*æt* he mid cyninge sprece. him cumeð gefealucu tide 7 god.

⟨37⟩ Gyf hine mete þ*æt* he gebunden si. lære ic hine þæt he him beorge wyð frecno þing.

⟨38⟩ Gyf him þince þ*æt* he stige on heah clif. þ*æt* tacnað god.

⟨39⟩ Gyf him þince þ*æt* he of dune astige. broces del he onfehþ.

⟨40⟩ Gyf hine mete þ*æt* he mid his freondes wyfe hæme. þæt byð adle.

⟨41⟩ Gyf him þince þ*æt* he mid his agene wife heme. þ*æt* byð god swefn.

⟨42⟩ Gyf hine mete þ*æt* he hine to gode gebidde. micel gyfe him byð toweard.

⟨Ten entries missing⟩

⟨43⟩ Þonne him þince þ*æt* he fiscas geseo. þ*æt* byð regn.

29 ricumen] *read* ricum men | alysse] *read* alyssednes *(see 7/1)* | dæt] *read* ðæt | broca] *read* his ~ *(see 7/1)* | **31** Gyf] *read* ~ him þince þæt *(see 7/1)* | ost byrnen] *read* ofbyrne *(*oft byrnan*7/1)* | micellicu] mycel *7/1* | **33** toweard] *read* toweard | **35** bearn] *read* beard *(see 7/1); this is a translation of a Latin* barba *dream, so* beard *is the correct reading* | **37** heres] *Förster (1916) read* heses, *but the scribe has used a continental* 'r' *repeatedly, not an insular* 's'*; the scribe used a long* 's' *throughout, which makes it unlikely that he wrote* heses *here; read* hrægeles *(Förster has argued that this represents a Latin* uestimenta *dream, which makes the* hrægeles *reading is 7/1 the preferred one)* | **39** ungerades] *read* ungeradnes | **40** he seo] *read* he *(*seo *is redundant in view of* sio *later on)* | **42** beag] *read* gyldene ~ *(see 7/1)* | þ*æt*$_3$] þ*æt*[·] | healic] *read* healicne | **44** byd] *read* byð | **49** gefealucu tide 7 god.] -lucu tide 7 god. *on erasure;* ~ ‖ ⟨*f. 151v*⟩ | **54** adle] *read* adl | **56** hine$_2$] *read* ~ georne *(see 7/1).*

⟨44⟩ Gyf him þince þ*æt* he bradne monan geseo. þ*æt* byð god swefn.

⟨45⟩ Gyf mon mete þ*æt* he hwit hors hæbbe. oððe on ride. þ*æt* byð weorðmind.

⟨46⟩ Gyf him þince þ*æt* he on blacum horse ride. þ*æt* byð his goda modes eagnes.

⟨47⟩ Gyf him þince þ*æt* he on redum horse ride. þ*æt* byð his goda wanigend.

⟨48⟩ Gyf him þince þ*æt* he on fealawan horse ride þæt byð god. oððe grægan. þ*æt* byð god swefn.

⟨49⟩ Gyf man meteð þ*æt* he wær slea. þ*æt* byð gecid wyð his freond.

⟨50⟩ Gyf him þince þ*æt* he oððerne slea. beorge he him georne wyf fræcno þing.

⟨51⟩ Gyf him þince þæt he þeofas geseo. him byd toward.

⟨52⟩ Gyf hine mete deadne man ancysse. þ*æt* byð lang lyf.

⟨53⟩ Þon*ne* him þince þ*æt* he geseo scyp yrnan. god ærende him byð towerd.

⟨54⟩ Gyf hine mete hnyte somnie. god þ*æt* byð.

⟨55⟩ Gyf him þince þ*æt* he oððerne cysse. god þ*æt* bioð.

⟨56⟩ Gyf hine mete þ*æt* he hunig æte. oððe geseo. þ*æt* byð ængnes.

⟨57⟩ Gif him þinceð þ*æt* he bellan geseo. oððe gehire. weorðmind him byð toweard.

⟨58⟩ Gyf hine mete þ*æt* he cirican geseo oððe singan gehire: micel god þ*æt* tacnað.

⟨59⟩ Gif him þince þæt he iseo man mid wæpnan gewundodne. ymbhidig forg þ*æt* byð.

⟨60⟩ Gyf him þince þæt he wæpen wege. þ*æt* byð orsorh.

⟨Ten entries missing⟩

⟨61⟩ Gyf man mæte þ*æt* he seon ne mæge. læric hine þ*æt* he him his eahtent beorge.

⟨62⟩ Gyf man mæte þ*æt* he seolac. oððe godweb `h´æbbe. god hit byð. 7 hwilum læasung.

⟨63⟩ Gyf mon meæ þ*æt* he filed sy. god þ*æt* byð.

⟨64⟩ Gyf man mete þ*æt* he weorðlice gerestod sio. goð þ*æt* byð.

⟨65⟩ Gyf man mæte þ*æt* he feola swysa ætsamne geseo. þonne mæg he hine wenen broces.

61 goda] *delete ~ (see 7/1); probably an eye slip (see l. 62)* | eagnes] *i.e.* angnes | **63** þæt byð god] *delete ~ (see 7/1)* | **66** wyf] *read* wyð | **67** þeofas] *read* þeowas *(*servants, *but 7/1 also has ~);* þeofas *(*thieves*) is unlikely because of the positive interpretation* | byd] *read* byð | toward] *read* god *~ (see 7/1)* | **68** mete] *read ~* þæt he *(see 7/1)* | ancysse] *read* cysse *(*an- *probably carried over from* man*)* | lyf] *read ~* 7 god *(see 7/1)* | **70** mete] *read ~* þæt he *(see 7/1)* | byð] *read ~* gyf he hi ne ytt 7 yfel gyf he hi ytt *(see 7/1); the scribe probably skipped an entire line* | **72** ængnes.] ~ ‖ *⟨f. 152r⟩* | **75** cirican geseo oððe] *read* on cirican *(see 7/1);* geseo oððe *is probably an eye slip (see l. 73)* | **77** forg] *read* sorg | **79** orsorh] *read* orsorhnes *(see 7/1)* | **81** læric] *i.e.* lære ic | him] *read ~* wyð *(see 7/1)* | **83** byð] *read ~* hwilum *(see 7/1)* | **85** meæ] *read* mete | **86** weorðlice gerestod] *this makes no sense (see Förster 1916, 291, n. 3);* wurðlic ref *7/1* | goð] *read* god | **87** swysa] *read* swyna | hine] *delete ~ (see 7/1).*

⟨One entry missing⟩

⟨66⟩ Gyf man mæte þ*æt* he henne ægeru hæbbe. oðð þicge ne deah hym þ*æt*.

⟨67⟩ Gyf mon mete þ*æt* he gæt geseo. þon*ne* mæg he wenan þæs laðwendan feondes him on æweste.

⟨68⟩ Gyf mon mæte þ*æt* he feola stodhorsa habbe. oððe geseo. awestnesse his goda ðæt tacneð

⟨69⟩ Gyf man mete þ*æt* he fela gosa hæbbe. god þ*æt* byð.

⟨One entry missing⟩

⟨70⟩ Gyf man mæte þ*æt* he pip*er* ete. ne deah þ*æt*.

⟨71⟩ Gyf mon mete þ*æt* he fyled spǽren geseo ætsamne. þ*en*no byð þ*æt* þæt he on his feondu*m* his willan gewryhð.

⟨72⟩ Gyf mon mete þ*æt* he win drince. hele hym byð toweard.

⟨73⟩ Gyf man mæte þ*æt* he byrnende candele on handa habbe. god þ*æt* byð;-

⟨One entry missing⟩

90 oðð] *read* oððe | **92** æweste] *read* næweste *(the* 'n' *was probably dropped because of preceding* on*)* | **98** fyled spǽren] *read* feala spera *(see 7/1)* | þ*en*no] þn̄o; *read* þonne | **99** feondu*m*] ~ ‖ ⟨*f. 152v*⟩ | gewryhð] -r- < w.

7/2 London, British Library, Cotton Tiberius A. iii, fol. 42r/5-42v/8

⟨1⟩ **G**if man mæte þ*æt* his mon ehte. yfel þ*æt* bið.

⟨2⟩ **G**if him mæte þ*æt* his onsyne fæger si god þ*æt* bið. 7 him bið wurðmynt toweard. 7 gif him þince unfæger. yfel þ*æt* bið.

⟨3⟩ **G**if him mæte þ*æt* he si mid æniges cynnes irene slægen. ymbhydu þ*æt* beoð. 7 sorge þ*æt* tacnað.

⟨4⟩ **G**if him mæte þ*æt* he sweord wege. orsorhness yfela þ*æt* bioþ.

⟨5⟩ if him þince þ*æt* he gimmas sceawige. þ*æt* bioð mænigfeald. 7 uncuðlic þing.

⟨6⟩ **G**if man mæte þ*æt* he micel rice hæbbe þ*æt* byð wurðmynt.

⟨7⟩ **G**if man mæte þ*æt* he on wyllan þwean þ*æt* byð gestreon.

⟨8⟩ **G**if man mæte þ*æt* he fela hunda ætsomne geseo. þonne scilde he hine wið his fynd ful georne.

⟨9⟩ **G**if man mæte þ*æt* he deadne mann cysse. langsum lif 7 gesæliglic him biþ towerd.

⟨10⟩ **G**if man mæte þ*æt* he penegas *oððe* mancsas finde. þ*æt* tacnað æfæste.

⟨11⟩ **G**if man mæte þ*æt* he finde. 7 ne grete. þ*æt* tacnað bliðes mannes onsion. gif he nimþ. ne deah him þ*æt*.

⟨12⟩ **G**if hi*m* þince þ*æt* his earn swyþe eahte. þ*æt* byþ mycel gefea.

1 Gif... bið] ~ *not in Förster (1908b), corrected (1908c)* | **4** si] -i < e | **7** if] *read* Gif | **9** þwean] *read* þwea.

⟨13⟩ **G**if he geseo twegen monan. þ*æt* byþ micel gefea.

⟨14⟩ **G**if he geseo þ*æt* man oþerne man slea. beorge him wiþ broc.

⟨15⟩ **G**if him mæte þ*æt* he geseo hwitne ocsan. oððe onufan sitte. þ*æt* bið wurðmynt.

⟨16⟩ **G**if him þince blæc *oððe* red. yfel þ*æt* byþ 7 broc.

⟨17⟩ **G**if man mæte þ*æt* he geseo hwitne oxan 7 micelne. þ*æt* biþ gefea.

⟨18⟩ **G**if he hornleasne oxan geseo. þonne ofercymð he his find.

⟨19⟩ **G**if him mæte þ*æt* his earmas beon fægere gegerede. þ*æt* bið freodscype.

⟨20⟩ **G**if man mæte þ*æt* he micles þinges geweald age. þ*æt* bið þ*æt* he him his fynd to gewealde getihð.

⟨21⟩ **G**if him þince þ*æt* he yrne swyþe. þonne byð him broc towerd.

⟨22⟩ **G**if him þince þ*æt* he micel god hæbbe. þ*æt* bið his goda wanung.

⟨23⟩ **G**if him mæte þ*æt* he stele þ*æt* þe wurð underne 7 cuð. þ*æt* he ær ana witan sceolde.

⟨24⟩ **G**if man mæte þ*æt* him si his swura gebunden. beorge him þonne georne wið ealle frecne þing.

⟨25⟩ **G**if man mæte þ*æt* he of heahre dune fealle. god þ*æt* bið þearfan. 7 þam weligan yfel.

⟨26⟩ **G**if man mæte þ*æt* he si uppahafen. god þ*æt* tacnað.

24 he$_2$] -e < t | **25** fægere] ~ ‖ ⟨*f. 42v*⟩ | **30** þ*æt* þe] *delete* þe | þ*æt*$_3$] *read* ~ þe *(confusion about when to write* þe *and when not to write it is evident)* | **32** beorge] -ge < n.

7/4 London, British Library, Cotton Tiberius A. iii, fols 27v/12-32v/16

be swefena mistlicnesse æft*er* endebyrdnessæ abecedes danielis
De somnior*um* diuersiitate s*ecun*d*um* ordinem abcharii danielis
þ*æt* witegan.
proph*ete*.

fugelas on swefenu*m* se þe gesyhð 7 mid him winn*eð* saca sume hit getacnað
⟨1⟩ **A**ues in somnis qui uiderit & cum ipsis pugnauerit lites aliquas significat.
fugelas on swefnum gefon gestreon hit getacnað
⟨2⟩ **A**ues in somnis capere. lucru*m* significat.
fugelas sum þincg fra*m* hi*m* gegripan hearpan hit getacnað.
⟨3⟩ **A**ues aliquid a se rapuisse damnum significat.
assan oððe hecenu gesihð gylt ceapes hit getacnað.
⟨4⟩ **A**sinos uel edos uiderit. crimen negotii significat.

2 diuersiitate] *i.e.* diuersitate *(doubling of* 'i' *is frequent with this scribe and that of the Latin, see ll. 224,265,316,370,602, 5.1.2/1, 9.1/1, 17/4 and Förster 1910: 55, n. 5)* | **abcharii**] *read* abcdarii | **3** þ*æt*] *read* þæs | **5** winn*eð*] winn& | **7** swefnum] -w- < · | **9** hearpan] *read* hearm.

wæpnu on swæfnum beran bewerunge hit getacnað
⟨5⟩ **A**rma in somnis portare. tutamentum significat.
assan etan geswinc hit getacnað.
⟨6⟩ **A**sinos edere laborem. significat.
assan clipiende oððe untiende yrnan sume sace wyðerwyrdnysse
⟨7⟩ **A**sinos clamantes aut solutos currere aliquam litem aduersarię
hit getacnað.
Significat.
fugeles sceottende gesihð feonda yfele sprece hit getacnað.
⟨8⟩ **A**ues bullientes uiderit. inimicorum malam locutionem. significat.
treow. mid wæstme gesihð. gestreon gewilnode hit getacnað.
⟨9⟩ **A**rbores cum fructu uiderit. lucrum exsperatum. significat.
treow uppastigan sumne wyrðscype he begyt
⟨10⟩ **A**rbores ascendere. aliquam dignitatem optinebit.
weder hlutter gesihð ceapes ferðrunge hit getacnað.
⟨11⟩ erem limpidem uiderit negotii expeditionem significat.
fram wyldeoru*m* se þe hine gesihð ehtan fra*m* feondu*m* he byð oferswiðe(d)
⟨12⟩ **A** bestiis qui se uiderit infestare ab inimicis superabitur
bogan bendan oððe flan asendan geswinc oððe angsumnysse ge*tacnað*.
⟨13⟩ rcum tendere uel sagittas mittere. laborem u*el* anxietatem. signific*at*.
ring on swefnum gesihð stowe gewilnode hit ge*tacnað*.
⟨14⟩ **A**nullum in somnis uiderit. locum exsperatum significat.
ring on swefnum underfon carleaste ge*tacnað*
⟨15⟩ nullu*m* in somnis accipere. securitatem significat.
ring syllan hearm ge*tacnað*.
⟨16⟩ **A**nullum dare dampnu*m* Significat.
gold on swefnum handlian forðunge ceapes ge*tacnað*.
⟨17⟩ **A**urum in somnis trectare. expeditionem negotii. significat.
wermod drincan. sace hefige hit ge*tacnað*
⟨18⟩ **A**bsinthium bibere. litem grauem. Significat.
eced drincan on swefnu*m* untru*m*nysse ge*tacnað*
⟨19⟩ **A**cetum bibere in somnis. infirmitatem. significat.
garclifan etan ærende fullic ge*tacnað*
⟨20⟩ grimoniam edere. nuntium fedum. significat.
hwite oððe beorhte hine gescrydan wynsumnysse ge*tacnað*
⟨21⟩ **A**lba aut splendida se uestire. iocunditate*m*. Significat.

15,16 edere] sedere *will have been intended (see Martin 1981: 98), but the gloss* etan *agrees with the Latin* | **17** clipiende] -e- < [·] | untiende] *read* untiede *(see l. 222 and Förster 1910: 48, n. 4)* | **21,22** fugeles, **A**ues] *the gloss agrees with the Latin but this reading makes no sense though it attested more often (see 7/5 and Martin 1981: 99); the correct reading is* aquas *(see 7/6)* | **28** erem] *read* Aerem | **29** oferswiðe(d)] -s- < w | **30** superabitur] ~ ‖ *⟨f. 28r⟩* | **32** rcum] *read* Arcum | **34** exsperatum] -sp- *on erasure* | **35** swefnum] -f- < · | carleaste] -te *on erasure* | **36** nullu*m*] *read* Anullum | **37** ring] [·]ring | **46** grimoniam] *read* Agrimoniam.

erian se þe hine gesihð swincu mæste him ongean cumað.
⟨22⟩ **A**rare qui se uiderit. labores maximas ei obueniunt.
beard hi*m* beon bescoren heorm hit ge*tacnað*.
⟨23⟩ **B**arba sibi tondi dampnum. significat.
braccas on swefnum gesihð earleaste ge*tacnað*.
⟨24⟩ **B**racas in somnis uiderit. securitatem. significat.
on folan sittan swicunge ceapes hit ge*tacnað*.
⟨25⟩ **B**ordore sedere. deceptionem negotii. significat.
wilde hine gesihð untrumnysse. ge*tacnað*
⟨26⟩ **B**rutum se uiderit. infirmitate*m*. Sig*nificat*.
eormas strange habban wexinge hit ge*tacnað*.
⟨27⟩ rachia ualida habere. incrementum. Significat.
wildedeor temian se þe hine gesihð gyfe oððe þanc wiðerwinnena ge*tacnað*.
⟨28⟩ **B**estias domare qui se uiderit: gratiam aduersariorum. significat.
wildedeor yrnende. gesihð sume gedræfednysse ge*tacnað*.
⟨29⟩ **B**estias currentes uiderit. aliqua*m* turbationem. significat.
on beþe hine þwean anxsu*m*nesse ge*tacnað*.
⟨30⟩ **B**alneo se lauare. axietatem. significat.
gebyrdne hine gesihð glæncge getacnað
⟨31⟩ **B**arbatum se uiderit. ornamentum. Significat.
oferslop hwit haban blisse ge*tacnað*.
⟨32⟩ **B**yrrum album habere. letitiam. Significat.
oferslop bleofah habban ærende fullic ge*tacnað*
⟨33⟩ **B**yrrum coloreum habere nuntium fedum significat.
gefeohtu oððe heþene gesihð blisse on openum hit openað.
⟨34⟩ ella uel barbaros uiderit. letitiam in publico pat*et*.
buteran etan hærende god ge*tacnað*
⟨35⟩ **B**utirum edere. nuntium bonum. Significat.
oxan grasiende gesihð sige ceapas ge*tacnað*.
⟨36⟩ **B**oues pascentes uiderit. agonia*m* negotii significat.
oxan slapende gesihð yfelnysse ceapes ge*tacnað*
⟨37⟩ **B**oues dormientes uiderit. malitiam negotii significat.
wildedeor. sprecende gesihð teonan hefige ge*tacnað*.
⟨38⟩ **B**estias loquentes uiderit molestias graues. significat.
mid rocce beon gescrid orsorhnysse ge*tacnað*
⟨39⟩ **C**lamide uestri. Securitatem. Significat.

53 earleaste] *read* carleaste | **60** rachia] *read* Brachia | **63** gedræfednysse] -d_2- < · | **66** axietatem] *i.e.* anxietatem *(loss of* 'n' *is more frequent with this scribe and that of the Latin, see ll. 150,246,248,258,322,348,516, 9.2.2/5, 9.2.4/5 and Förster 1910: 56, n. 3; 63-64, n. 8)* | **71** bleofah] bleofa[·]h | **74** ella] -a < o; *read* Bella | letitiam] -i_1- < t | **76** Significat] -f- < · | **83** beon] ~ *on erasure* | **84** uestri] uest- *on erasure; read* uestiri.

cynehelm gewilces þinges onfon blisse hit getacnað.
⟨40⟩ **C**oronam cuiusq*ue* rei accipere lętitiam. Significat.
blindne se þe hine gesihð lettincge ge*tacnað*
⟨41⟩ **C**ecum qui se uiderit inpeditione*m*. S*ignificat*.
heofen ligenne gesihð sume unrihtwisnysse on eallu*m* embhwyrfte
⟨42⟩ **C**ęlum flammeum uiderit. aliquas iniquitates in toto orbe
ongean cuma(ð)
obueniunt.
hwerhwettan oððe cyrfet gesihð on swefnum untrumnysse ge*tacnað*.
⟨43⟩ ucumeres aut cucurbitas uiderit in somnis. infirmitate*m* significat.
wex drige etan saca mid ungecoplicu*m* ge*tacnað*.
⟨44⟩ eram aridam edere. lites cum inportunis. Significat.
culfran gesihð sume unrotnysse ge*tacnað*.
⟨45⟩ **C**olumbas uiderit. aliqua*m* tristitia*m*. Significat.
on cwearterne se þe hine gesihð sume carfulnesse oððe teonan
⟨46⟩ **C**arcere qui se uiderit. aliquam sollicitudinem uel calumpniam
ge*tacnað*
significat.
heofod wit habban gestreon ge*tacnað*
⟨47⟩ **C**aput albu*m* habere. lucrum. Significat.
heafod him beon gescoren hearm ge*tacnað*
⟨48⟩ **C**aput sibi tondi. dampnum signific*at*.
mid gescy niwum beon gescod gestreon of ungewenedu*m* ge*tacnað*.
⟨49⟩ **C**alciamento nouo calciari lucrum ex insperato. Significat.
mid gescy ealdum beon gescod swicunge ge*tacnað*
⟨50⟩ **C**alciamento ueteri calciari: deceptionem. significat.
swicyngas gadirian oððe wyrcean geswinc hit getacnað.
⟨51⟩ **C**lauos colligere uel facere laborem. Significat:
hundas beorcynde gesihð oððe hi*m* laðhetan fynd þine þe oferswiðan secað
⟨52⟩ **C**anes latrantes uiderit. uel eis infestare. inimici. tui te superare querunt.
S*ignificat*.
hundas blegan gesihð þanc hit getacnað.
⟨53⟩ **C**anes ludere uiderit. gra*tia*m. Significat.
heofod þwean fram ælcu*m* ege 7 ælcere fræcennysse he bið alesed.
⟨54⟩ **C**aput lauare. ab omni metu & omni periculo liberabitur.
cyse geongne onfon gestreon ge*tacnað*.
⟨55⟩ **C**aseum recentem accipere. lucru*m*. Signific*at*.

85 cynehelm] cyne[l ·]helm | **90** flammeum] flamineum *Förster (this scribe's minims are difficult at times, but other dreambooks support* flammeum*)* | **92** obueniunt] -b- < o; ~ ‖ ⟨*f. 28v*⟩ | **94** ucumeres] *read* Cucumeres | **96** eram] *read* Ceram | **98** uiderit] ~ [uiderit] *(crossed out)* | **107** gescy] -y < i | **111** swicyngas] *read* spicyngas *(*'wyn'/'p' *confusion is more frequent with this scribe, see ll. 134,542)* | **113** secað] *read* ~ getacnað *(Significat not glossed)* | **114** latrantes] -ra- < nt | **116** blegan] *i.e.* plegan *(see l. 308)*.

sealt gif he bið sace hit getacnað.
⟨56⟩ **S**alsum si fuerit. litem. Significat.
olfendas geseon 7 fram hi*m* gesihð laðhetan sace hit ge*tacnað*.
⟨57⟩ **C**amelos uidere & ab eis se uiderit infestare. litem significat.
gleda se þe hine gesihð etan fynd þine be þe yfela sprecað
⟨58⟩ **C**arbones qui se uiderit edere inimici tui de te mala loquuntur.
eahþyrlu gesihð oððe on him hine belocene geseo on sumum teonan oððe
⟨59⟩ **C**ancellos uiderit aut in eis se reclusum uideat. in aliqua calumpnia uel
on hæftnoðe bið gehæfd
custodia detinetur.
cartan wirtan oððe rædan ærende fullic hit getac*nað*
⟨60⟩ artam scribere aut legere nuntium fedum significat.
mete swiwan hearm hit getacnað
⟨61⟩ **C**ibum uomere. dampnu*m*. Significat.
spiwan saca hit ge*tacnað*
⟨62⟩ **C**eroma uomere. lites. significat.
yrnan se þe hine gesihþ 7 he ne mæg lettinge hit getacnað
⟨63⟩ urrere qui se uiderit & non potest inpeditionem. Significat.
on cræte sittan sace hefyge hit getacnað
⟨64⟩ **C**urru sedere. litem grauem. Significat.
wex oððe taperas gesihð blisse hit getacnat
⟨65⟩ **C**eram uel cereos uiderit. gaudium. Significat.
mid deadu*m* spellian gestrion hit ge*tacnað*
⟨66⟩ **C**um mortico fabulare. lucrum. Significat.
mid his swuster gelicgan hearm hit ge*tacnað*.
⟨67⟩ **C**um sorore concumbere. dampnu*m*. Significat.
mid his meder orsorhnysse hit ge*tacnað*
⟨68⟩ **C**um matre. securitem. Significat.
mid medene gelicgan agsumnesse hit
⟨69⟩ **C**um uirgine concumbere anxietate*m*. Signific*at*.
mid his gemacan gelicge angsumnysse hit.
⟨70⟩ **C**um coniuge sua concumbere anxietate*m*. Significat.
bec gewilces þinges onfon oððe rædan oððe rædende lestan
⟨71⟩ **C**odicellos cuiusq*ue* rei accipere. uel legere. aut legente audire
geselþe timam hit getacnað.
felicitatem temporis significat.

122 sace] -ce *on erasure* | **124** olfendas] -l- < i | hi*m*] ~ *over* se; *read* ~ hine (se *not glossed)* | **125** infestare] -f- < i | **128** him] h- < l | **132** wirtan] *read* writan | **133** artam] *read* Cartam | **134** swiwan] *read* spiwan *(see l. 111)* | **137** spiwan] *read* wex ~ (**C**eroma *not glossed)* | **139** urrere] *read* Currere | Significat] -f- < i | **142** getacnat] *read* getacnað | **145** mortico] *read* mortuo | **149** securitem] *read* securitatem | **150** agsumnesse] *i.e.* angsumnesse *(see l. 66)* | hit] *read* ~ getacnað | **152** gelicge] *read* gelicgan | hit] *read* ~ getacnað | **154,155** gewilces] ~ *over* **C**odicellos | **155** legente] *read* legentem | **156** timam] *read* timan | **157** felicitatem] ~ ‖ ⟨*f. 29r*⟩.

þonne man hine gesihð sumne teonan hefine hit
⟨72⟩ **C**um plures se uiderit. aliquam calumniam grauem. Significat.
heordredena se þe gesihð swicunge hit getacnað
⟨73⟩ **C**ustodias. qui uiderit. deceptione*m*. Significat.
cimbalan oððe psalteras oððe strengas ætrinan saca hit
⟨74⟩ **C**imbala aut salteria aut corda tangere lites significat.
hearpan gesihð orsorhnesse ceapes hit ge*tacnað*
⟨75⟩ **C**ithara*m* uiderit. securitatem negotii. Significat.
mid deadu*m* sprecan micel gestrion hit
⟨76⟩ **C**um mortuo loqui. grande lucrum. Significat.
ligræsceas gesihð orsorhnesse hit ge*tacnað*
⟨77⟩ **C**oruscationes uiderit. lucrum. Significat.
teð his feallan sum of h`i´s magu*m* swylt.
⟨78⟩ **D**entes suos cadere. aliquis de parentibus suis morietur.
teð neoðeran oððe tuxas þana afeallað gif mid blode oððe butan
⟨79⟩ **D**entes inferiores aut maxillares cui ceciderint si cum sanguine aut sine
sare fræmde he bið fra*m* magu*m*;
dolore. alienus erit a parentibus.
on huse his offrian wexincge oððe blisse hit ge*tacnað*.
⟨80⟩ **D**omo sua sacrificare incrementu*m* letitię significat.
hus his feallan hearm mid manegum hit getacnað
⟨81⟩ **D**omum suam cecidisse. dampnum cum pluribus significat.
hus feallan 7 towyrpan hearm hit ge*tacnað*.
⟨82⟩ **D**omum cecidisse & destruere. dampnum. Significat.
hus his byrnan gesyhð fræcenysse lifes ge*tacnað*
⟨83⟩ **D**omum suam ardere uiderit. periculum uitę significat.
swete etan on manegum leahtrum bið ofsett hit ge*tacnað*
⟨84⟩ **D**ulcia edere. in multis criminibus opprimitur. significat.
mid biscoprocce scrydan him gestreon getacnað of cynne.
⟨85⟩ **D**almatica uestire. sibi lucrum significat ex semine.
dracan gesihð sumne wyrðscipe hit g*etacnað*
⟨86⟩ **D**racones uiderit. aliqua*m* dignitatem. Significat.
on horse hwitu*m* sittan belimp god *getacnað*
⟨87⟩ **E**quo albo sedere. euentu*m* bonu*m* Significo.
on horse sweartan sittan anxsumnesse *getacnað*
⟨88⟩ **E**quo nigro sedere anxietatem significo.
on horse gelewum sittan hynðe *getacnað*
⟨89⟩ **E**quo flauo sedere detrimentum. significo.

158 man] *read* ma | **158,162,166** hit] *read* ~ getacnað | **168** orsorhnesse] gestrion *may be more appropriate since* ~ *glosses* securitatem *throughout this dreambook, while* gestrion *glosses* lucrum *(see Förster 1910: 53, n. 4)* | **171** cadere] -r- < · | **172** þana] *read* þam | **176** wexincge oððe blisse] *the glossator probably thought* incrementu*m* letitię *meant* growth or joy, *not* growth of joy | **191** Significo] *the text reads* significo *repeatedly for the* 'e' *dreams*.

on horse dunnan sittan ferðrunge *getacnað*
⟨90⟩ **E**quo baio sedere expeditione*m* S*ignifico.*
on horse brunum sittan ceap fulne *getacnað*
⟨91⟩ **E**quo castaneo sedere. negotiu*m* fedum. Significo.
hors wilde yrnan oððe fram hi*m* hearmian hearm *getacnað*
⟨92⟩ **E**quos solutos currere aut ab eis. infestare. dampnum significat.
dru`n´cenne hine gesihð untrumnesse *getacnað*
⟨93⟩ **E**briosum se uiderit. infirmitate*m*. Significo.
belysnode gesihð hearm hit *getacnað*
⟨94⟩ **E**unuchos uiderit. dampnu Significo.
ylp gesihð laðne oððe `gramne´ sume wrohte hit getacnað.
⟨95⟩ **E**lephantum uiderit infestum. aliqua*m* accusatione*m* significat.
ylpesban handlian lettincge *getacnað*
⟨96⟩ **E**borum trectare. inpeditione*m*. Significo.
ylpesban becgan oððe beceapan unrotnyssa mæste *getacnað*
⟨97⟩ **E**boru*m* emere aut uendere tristitias maximas Significat.
melu on swefnum handlian eacan ceapas ge*tacnað*
⟨98⟩ **F**arinam in somnis trectare. incrementum negotii. Significat.
mid isene geslægene gesihð carfulnysse ge*tacnað*
⟨99⟩ **F**erro percussum uiderit. sollicitudinem. significat.
isen gewylces þinges handlian sume untrumnyssa hit *getacnað*
⟨100⟩ **F**errum cuiusq*ue* rei trectare. aliquas infirmitates significat.
ansine his on swa wilcu*m* þinge gesihð lif lang hi*m* bid geseald.
⟨101⟩ **F**aciem suam in quacumq*ue* re uiderit uita longa ei datur.
ansine hiwlice hine habban fultum 7 wyrðmynt rumran *getacnað*
⟨102⟩ **F**aciem formosa*m* se habere. auxilium & honorem ampliorem. Significat.
ansine fullice habban mid manegum bið ofþryccend.
⟨103⟩ **F**acie*m* turpem habere. multis criminibus subprimitur.
flod drof gesihð æbyliigða hit *getacnað.*
⟨104⟩ **F**lumen turbulentum uiderit. offensiones. significat.
hwætas sume andlian untrumnysse *getacnað*
⟨105⟩ **F**rumenta aliqua trectare. infirmitatem Significat.
broðer oððe swuster gesihð fra*m* wyrstu*m* wundum bið geswenct
⟨106⟩ **F**ratrem uel sororem uiderit. a pessimis ulceribus fatigatur.
pitt gesihð 7 on þane befealð sume teonan hit ge*tacnað.*
⟨107⟩ **F**ossam uiderit & in ea ceciderit. aliquam calumpniam significat.
wylspring on huse his gesihð beon geopenad eacan oððe blisse
⟨108⟩ **F**ontem in domo sua uiderit aperiri. incrementum uel letitiam.
getacnað
Significat.

205 dampnu] *read* dampnum | **215 F**erro] ~ ‖ ⟨*f. 29v*⟩ | **218** bid] *read* bið | **222** manegum] ~ *halfway over* criminibus; *read* ~ sacum (criminibus *not glossed*) | ofþryccend] *read* ofþrycced *(see l. 17 and Förster 1910: 48, n. 4)* | **224** æbyliigða] *i.e.* æbyligða *(see l. 2).*

æmyttan swa wilce gesihð saca þa mæstan ge*tacnað*
⟨109⟩ **F**ormicas quascumq*ue* uiderit. lites maximas. significat.
flod on huse his infaran fræcendnesse he þolað
⟨110⟩ **F**lumen in domo sua introire. periculu*m* ipse patietur.
scinlacu gesihð gestreon of ungewendum hit *getacnað*
⟨111⟩ antasmas uiderit. lucrum ex insperato. Significat.
fictreow gesihð saca mid ungedafenlicum *getacnað*
⟨112⟩ **F**icum uiderit. lites cum inportunis. Significat.
fictreow sweart onfon unrotnyssa *getacnað*
⟨113⟩ icum nigrum accipere. tristitiam S*ignificat.*
lof mid wine onfon 7 drican untrumnysse ge*tacnað*
⟨114⟩ **F**olium cum uiuo accipere. & bibere. infirmitatem significat.
leaf mid niwan wine niman 7 drican geselðe timan *getacnað*
⟨115⟩ **F**olia cum recente uino accipere & bibere. felicitate*m* temporis significat.
uðwitan gesihð twysehtan henðe *getacnað*
⟨116⟩ **F**ilosophos uiderit disiungi. dampnu*m*. Significat.
suna oððe dohtra beon acennede gesihð eacum getacnað
⟨117⟩ **F**ilios aut filias nasci uiderit. incrementum. Significat.
swurdboran hine gewordene gesihð hearm fullic *getacnað*
⟨118⟩ ladiatorum se factu*m* uiderit. dampnum fedum significat.
swurd beran 7 be him plegean unheaðnysse *getacnað*
⟨119⟩ **G**ladium ferre & de ipso ludere anxietatem significat.
swurdwegede anbidian gehende saca mæste *getacnað*
⟨120⟩ **G**ladiantes expectare uicinas. litas maximas. S*ignificat.*
gimm of ringe forleosan sum þinc forlæt
⟨121⟩ **G**emmam de anulo perdidisse. aliquid admittit.
henne ægru lecgan gestreon mid carfulnysse *getacnað*
⟨122⟩ **G**allinam oua parere lucrum cum sollicitudine significat.
henne mid cicenum gesihð ceapas eacan *getacnað*
⟨123⟩ **G**allinam cum pulcinis uiderit. negotiii incrementu*m* significat.
hæþene feohtende gesihð 7 fram him cidan saca mid fræcednysse
⟨124⟩ **G**entiles pugnantes uiderit. & ab eis infestare. lites cum periculo.
getacnað
Significat.
geblissian on swefnu*m* unrotnysse *getacnað*
⟨125⟩ **G**audere in somnis. tristitiam significat.
hagol on swefnum unrotuysse *getacnað*
⟨126⟩ **G**randinem in somnis. tristitiam significat.

241 antasmas] *read* Fantasmas | **245** icum] *read* Ficum | **246,248** drican] *i.e.* drincan *(see l. 66)* | **247** uiuo] *read* uino | **254** fullic] *read* fullicne | **255** ladiatorum] *read* Gladiatorum | **258** swurdwegede] *i.e.* swurdwegende *(see l. 66)* | **265** negotiii] *i.e.* negotii *(see l. 2)* | **266** fram] f[·]ram | cidan] laðhetan *may be more appropriate for Latin* infestare | **267** lites] ~ ‖ ⟨*f. 30r*⟩ | **272** unrotuysse] *read* unrotnysse.

hagol on swefnu*m* gesihð hearm welreowne ge*tacnað*
⟨127⟩ **G**randinem in somnis uiderit. dampnu*m* crudele significat.
buccan oððe get gesihð ferðrunge *getacnað*
⟨128⟩ **H**ircos uel capras uiderit. expeditionem. Significat.
cuman habban andan get*acnað*
⟨129⟩ **H**ospites habere. inuidiam. Significa.
gesihð freodscipe fegð
⟨130⟩ **H**erculem uiderit amicitiam iungit.
mann ofslean bewerunge ge*tacnað*
⟨131⟩ **H**ominem occidere. tuntamentum. Significa.
casere hine beon gewordene wyrðscype *getacnað*
⟨132⟩ **I**mperatorem se factum aliquem honore*m* Significa.
on strete oððe on palentan abutangan uneaðnysse *getacnað*
⟨133⟩ **I**n platea uel palatio deambulare. anxietatem. S*ignificat.*
brynas on gewilcre stowe gesihð sume fræcednysse *getacnað*
⟨134⟩ **I**ncendia in quocumq*ue* loco uiderit aliquod periculum significat.
on flod swymman anxsumnesse ge*tacnað*
⟨135⟩ **I**n flumen notare. anxietatem. Significat.
on wille hine þwean gesreon *getacnað*
⟨136⟩ **I**n fonte se lauare. lucrum. Significat.
on se hine þwean blisse getacnað.
⟨137⟩ **I**n mare se lauare. letitiam. Significat.
on wæle fulum þwean sume wrohte *getacnað*
⟨138⟩ **I**n gurgite sordido lauare. aliquam accusationem significat.
on sæ feallan gestreon *getacnað*
⟨139⟩ **I**n mare cecidisse. lucrum significat.
on mere feallan blisse
⟨140⟩ **I**n piscina cecidisse. gaudiu*m* S*ignificat.*
on wæle fulan feallan sumne teonan ge*tacnað*
⟨141⟩ **I**n gurgite sordido cecidisse. aliqua*m* calumpnia*m*. Significat.
cildru gesihð 7 mid him plegað gesælðe timan ge*tacnað*
⟨142⟩ **I**nfantes uiderit & cum ipsis luderit felicitatem temporis. significat.
on tru*m*nyssa sume gesihð carfulnysse *getacnað*
⟨143⟩ **I**nfirmitates aliquas uiderit. sollicitudinem significat.
on blegstowe oððe on wafungstowe *and*bidian hine gesihð styrunge
⟨144⟩ **I**n thearum u*el* in amphitheatrum exspectare se uiderit. tumultum

279 Significa] *read* significat | **283** tuntamentum] *read* tutamentum | Significa] *read* significat | **284** gewordene] ~ *over* aliquem*; read* ~ sume *(*aliquem *not glossed)* | **285** Significa] *read* significat | **290** ge*tacnað*] ḡe *instead of* gē | **291** notare] *read* natare | **292** gesreon] *i.e.* gestreon *(see ll. 358,370, 9.1/1)* | **296** wrohte] -r- < w | **300** blisse] *read* ~ getacnað *(Significat not glossed)* | **305** temporis] -ris < [· ·] | **306** on tru*m*nyssa] *read* untru*m*nyssa*; the scribe probably read* in firmitates *and glossed this with* ~ *(see Förster 1910: 58, n. 5)* | **308** blegstowe] *i.e.* plegstowe *(see l. 106)* | **309** thearum] *read* theatrum.

sume *getacnað*
aliquem. S*ignificat.*
on æppeltune gan anxsumnysse hefige *getacnað*
⟨145⟩ **I**n pomerio ambulare. anxietatem grauem significat.
on brede hine beon gemetne lif lang hi*m* bið geseald
⟨146⟩ **I**n tabula se pingi uiderit. uita longa ei datur.
beon gegyrd trymniige
⟨147⟩ **L**una cingi. tutamento. S*ignificat.*
forleosan geleafan tolysinge *getacnað*
⟨148⟩ **L**una p*er*dere. fidei salutationem. Significat.
gyldenne bygyrdan. andan *getacnað*
⟨149⟩ **L**una aurea cingere. inuidiam. Significat.
stragnysse ge*tacnað*
⟨150⟩ **L**una pertica cingi. ualitudines. Significat.
monan beorhtne gesihð blisse. ge*tacnað*
⟨151⟩ **L**unam claram uiderit. inuidiam. Significat.
monan twegen gesihð andan ge*tacnað*
⟨152⟩ **L**unas duas uiderit. inuidiam. Significat.
monan blodigne gesihð. hearm *getacnað*
⟨153⟩ **L**unam sanguinem uiderit. damnum. Significat.
monan of heofene feallan oððe upastigan gesihð geswinc *getacnað*
⟨154⟩ **L**unam de cęlo cecidisse. u*el* ascendere uiderit. laborem. significat.
monan wittne gesihð gestreon ge*tacnað.*
⟨155⟩ **L**unam albam uiderit. lucrum. Significat.
monan bleoh habban hynðe *getacnað*
⟨156⟩ **L**unam colores habere. damnum. Significat.
spic handlian sum of his magum swylt
⟨157⟩ **L**ardum trectare aliquis de parentibus eius morietur.
linene claðas waxan gesihð hearm *getacnað*
⟨158⟩ **L**inea uestimenta lauare uiderit. dampnum Significat.
linen reaf scredan sume seocnysse *getacnað*
⟨159⟩ **L**ineam uestem uestire. aliquam egritudine*m* Significat.

314 gemetne] ~ *over* uiderit*; read* ~ gesihð *(*uiderit *not glossed)* | **316** trymniige] *i.e.* trymnige, *or does it read* trymmige*(?, see l. 2 and Förster 1910: 59, n. 1); read* ~ getacnað *(*S*ignificat not glossed)* | **317 L**una] *here and in the next three entries ~ means* girdle. *The glossator probably did not know what to do with ~. Martin (1981: 140, n. a162) has argued that these are displaced* zona *dreams (but see Cockayne 1864-66: III.207, n. a)* | **319** salutationem] *the gloss reads* tolysinge, *so Latin* solutionem *would be better* | **322** stragnysse] *i.e.* strangnysse *(see l. 66); read* mid gyrdle gerenedan beon gegyrd ~ *(***L**una pertica cingi *not glossed)* | **323** pertica] *Cockayne translated ~ as* peach-coloured, *but* partica/partita *(Old English* gerenedan*) is a more frequently attested reading (see 7/1 and Martin 1981: 168)* | ualitudines] -n- < t | **325** inuidiam] *the gloss reads* blisse*; so Latin* gaudium *would be a better reading (*gaudium *is more frequently attested, see Martin 1981: 140)* | **329** sanguinem] *read* sanguineam | **331** uiderit] -t < · | significat.] ~ ‖ ⟨*f. 30v*⟩.

leon yrnende gesihð ferðrunge ceapas *getacnað*
⟨160⟩ **L**eonem currentem uiderit. expeditionem negotii Signific*at*.
leon slæpende gesihð awyrigende cep *getacnað*
⟨161⟩ **L**eonem dormientem uiderit. malignum negotium. Significat.
leon wedan fe`o´ndes gestric *getacnað*
⟨162⟩ **L**eonem infestare. inimici seditione*m* Significat.
ærendraca gesihð lettige *getacnað*
⟨163⟩ **L**egatum se uiderit. inpeditionem. Significat.
leohtfatu handlian untrumnysse *getacnað*
⟨164⟩ **L**uminaria trectare. infirmitate*m*. Signific*at*.
leohtfatu hine gesihð orsorhnysse *getacnað*
⟨165⟩ **L**uminaria se uiderit. securitatem. Significat.
stanes asendan seocnesse *getacnað*
⟨166⟩ **L**apides mittere. egritudinem. Significat.
cidan on swefnu*m* ceapes eacan *getacnað*
⟨167⟩ **L**itigare in somnis. negotii incrementu*m*. Signific*at*.
bet him gestreht 7 wel gesreht gesihð beorhtnysse *getacnað*
⟨168⟩ **L**ectum sibi stratum & bene stratum uiderit. claritatem. Significat.
sæ smylte gesihð ceapas fyrðrunge ge*tacnað*
⟨169⟩ **M**are placidum uiderit. negotii expeditione*m* significat.
sæfixas gesihð anxsumnysse hefige *getacnað*
⟨170⟩ **M**aris pisces uiderit. anxietatem graue*m*. Significat.
handa hi*m* befylde gesihð weorca unrihte *getacnað*
⟨171⟩ **M**anus sibi inquinatas uiderit. opera iniqua significat.
modes his deade oððe cucu gesihð blisse ge*tacnað*
⟨172⟩ **M**atrem suam mortuam aut uiuam uiderit. gaudium. Significat.
maran hine gesihð bliss læsse hit his 7 hynðe *getacnað*
⟨173⟩ **M**aiorem se uiderit. gaudium minus est. 7 detrimentum. Significat.
wif tospræddu*m* loccum hine gesihð. gesriicg *getacnað*
⟨174⟩ **M**ulierem sparsis crinibus se uiderit. seditionem significat.
mus 7 leo on swefnum orsorhrysse ge*tacnað*
⟨175⟩ **M**us & leo in somnis. securitatem. Significat.
faran bigswicæ ge*tacnað*
⟨176⟩ igrare. deceptionem. Significat.
deade gesihð blisse *getacnað*
⟨177⟩ **M**ortuum uiderit gaudiu*m*. Significat.

344 awyrigende] *read* awyrigedne | **348,349** ærendraca, **L**egatum] -r_2- < a; *the gloss fits Latin* legatum *but see ll. 548,549 (see Martin 1981: 142)* | **348** lettige] *i.e.* lettinge *(see l. 66)* | gesihð] *read* hine ~ *(*se *not glossed)* | **358** bet] *read* bed | gesreht] *i.e.* gestreht *(see l. 292)* | **366** modes] *read* moder | **368** maran] *read* ~ lytlian *(see l. 369)* | bliss] *read* blisse | **369 M**aiorem] *read* ~ minorare *in accordance with other dreambooks (see Martin 1981: 144)* | **370** gesriicg] *i.e.* gestricg *(see ll. 2,292), Cockayne's* gestriicg *and Förster's* gespriicg *are spurious* | **372** orsorhrysse] *read* orsorhnysse | **375** igrare] *read* Migrare.

deadne cyssan lif tolibbenne *getacnað*
⟨178⟩ ortuum osculari. uitam uiuendi. Significat.
cnihtas gesihð blisse ge*tacnað*
⟨179⟩ **M**ilites uiderit. letitiam S*ignificat.*
handa þwean teonan hefige *getacnað*
⟨180⟩ **M**anus lauare malestias graues. Significat.
ripu gaderian blisse *getacnað*
⟨181⟩ **M**esses colligere. letitiam Significat.
hunig niman hine gesihð warnige þ*æt* he na fra*m* oðru*m* si beswicen
⟨182⟩ **M**el accipere se uiderit. caueat ne ab alio seducatur. S*ignificat.*
scipu gesihð god ærende *getacnað*
⟨183⟩ **N**aues uiderit. bonum nuntium. Significat.
hnyte gaderian saca ge*tacnað*
⟨184⟩ **N**uces colligere. lites S*ignificat.*
nest fugela gesihð sige ceapas *getacnað*
⟨185⟩ **N**idus auium uiderit. agonia*m* negotii Significat.
swawas gesihð blisse
⟨186⟩ iues uiderit. letitia*m* S*ignificat.*
mist ofer eorþan nan god *getacnað*
⟨187⟩ **N**ebula super terram. nullum bonum. Significat.
gifta don hearm *getacnað*
⟨188⟩ **N**uptias facere. dampnum. Significat.
baru*m* fotum gan hearm *getacnað*
⟨189⟩ **N**udis pedibus ambulare dampnum. Significat.
pipdram singan gehyreð gehende blisse
⟨190⟩ **O**rgana cantare audierit. uicinas letitias.
gebed don geseligran timan *getacnað*
⟨191⟩ **O**rationem facere. feliciora tempora. Significat.
banu sume handlian hatunge *getacnað*
⟨192⟩ **O**ssa aliqua trectare. odium significat.
weorcu handlian lættinge *getacnað*
⟨193⟩ **O**pera trectare. inpeditionem. Significat.
elebeamus handlian gestreon *getacnað.*
⟨194⟩ **O**liuas trectare. lucrum significat.
sc`e´ap gesihð gescorene hynðe *getacnað*
⟨195⟩ **O**ues uiderit tonsas. dampnum. Significat.

379 ortuum] *read* Mortuum | **383** malestias] *read* molestias | **386** beswicen] *read* ~ getacnað *(Significat not glossed)* | **393 N**idus] *read* Nidos *(see Martin 1981: 148)* | **394** swawas] *read* snawas | blisse] *read* ~ getacnað *(Significat not glossed)* | **395** iues] *read* Niues | **397 N**ebula] *read* Nebulam *(*mist *is acc. sg.)* | **401** Significat.] ~ ‖ ⟨*f. 31r*⟩ | **403** uicinas] ~ [letitias] | **410** elebeamus] *read* elebeamas.

cossas syllan hearm
⟨196⟩ **O**sculum dare. dampnum S*ignificat*.
ren gesihð blisse *getacnað*
⟨197⟩ **P**luuiam uiderit. letitiam significat.
mædenu niman on þeawe godne timan *getacnað*
⟨198⟩ **P**uellas accipere more. bonum tempus Significat.
rihne hine gesihð gewordenne fræcednysse eacan *getacnað*
⟨199⟩ **P**ilososum se uiderit factum periculi incrementu*m*. significat.
pytt gesihð 7 on hine befealð teonan *getacnað*
⟨200⟩ **P**uteum uiderit & in eum ceciderit calumpniam Significat.
feoh underfon sace
⟨201⟩ **P**ecuniam accipere. litem Significat.
wepan on swefnu*m* blisse ge*tacnað*.
⟨202⟩ **P**lorare in somnis gaudium Significat.
palman underfon wyrðment *getacnað*
⟨203⟩ **P**almam accipere. honorem Significat.
laf wexenne niman freodscipas *getacnað*
⟨204⟩ **P**anem candidum accipere accusationem. Significat.
hlaf wexenne niman freodscipas niwe gefegð
⟨205⟩ **P**anem cerarium accipere. amicitias. nouas iungit.
laf berenne niman blisse *getacnað*
⟨206⟩ **P**anem ordeacium accipere letitiam. Significat.
gerwigan wife hus wexincge *getacnað*
⟨207⟩ **P**arare mulieri domum. incrementum. Significat.
briwas niman gestreon mid carfulnysse *getacnað*
⟨208⟩ **P**ultes accipere lucrum cu*m* sollicitudine. Significat.
bricge gesihð carleaste *getacnað*
⟨209⟩ **P**ontem uiderit. securitatem. Significat.
swin gesihð untrumnysse *getacnað*
⟨210⟩ **P**orcos uiderit. infirmitate*m*. Significat.
fet þwean anxsumnysse *getacnað*
⟨211⟩ **P**edes lauare. anxietatem significat.
lead handlian untrumnysse *getacnað*
⟨212⟩ **P**lumbum trectare. infirmitatem. Significat.
crætu hwite gesihð oððe sittan ceapas lettincge ge*tacnað*
⟨213⟩ **Q**uadrigas albas uiderit uel sedere. negotii inpeditionem Significat.

414 hearm] *read* ~ getacnað *(Significat not glossed)* | **420** rihne] *read* ruhne | **421 P**ilososum] *read* Pilosum | **424** sace] *read* ~ getacnað *(*Significat *not glossed)* | **425** Significat] -g- < · | **427 P**lorare] **P**lo[·]rare | **430** wexenne] ~ *wrongly glosses* candidum, *probably an eye slip (see l. 432); read* wittne | freodscipas] ~ *wrongly glosses* accusationem, *probably an eye slip (see l. 432); read* wrohte | **431** accusationem] *Förster (1910: 63, n. 3) wrongly claimed that Cockayne had misread* accusationem *for* accusatorem | **435** Significat] -i_1- < a.

fyþerfete swa wilc swa gesihð uneaðnysse *getacnað*
⟨214⟩ **Q**uadrupedem quicu*m*q*ue* uiderit. anxietatem. Significat.
crætu wite sittan wyrðment ge*tacnað*
⟨215⟩ **Q**uadrigas albas sedere. honorem Significat.
fyþerfete sprecan feondscipas cinigas *getacnað*
⟨216⟩ **Q**uadrupedem loqui inimicitias regis. Significat.
hlihhan oððe gnyrende gesihð unrotnyssa ge*tacnað*
⟨217⟩ **R**idere aut stridentes uiderit. tristitiam significat.
rosan gesihð strengþa *getacnað*
⟨218⟩ **R**osam uiderit ualitudines Significat.
ryselas oððe swefel gesihð hefige teonan *getacnað*
⟨219⟩ **R**esinas u*el* sulphur uiderit. grandes molestias Significat.
cyningas gesihð of wurlde gywitan *getacnað*
⟨220⟩ **R**eges uiderit. de s*ecu*lo migrare Significat.
cyninges bodan underfon micel hit his tagan.
⟨221⟩ **R**egis nuntium accipere. magnum est signum.
staþu astigan geswinc *getacnað*
⟨222⟩ **R**ipas ascendere laborem. Significat.
of staþe niþerstigan godne timan *getacnað*
⟨223⟩ **R**ipa descendere. bonum tempus. Significat.
froxas gesihð anxsumnesse ge*tacnað*
⟨224⟩ **R**anas uiderit anxionem Significat.
sunnan twa gesihð wyrðscip ge*tacnað*
⟨225⟩ **S**oles duas uiderit. honorem. Significat.
sunan beorhte gesihð blisse *getacnað*
⟨226⟩ **S**olem spendidum uiderit. gaudium Significat.
sunan oððe monan gesihð blisse domes *getacnað.*
⟨227⟩ **S**olem u*el* lunam uiderit. letitiam `iudicii´. Significat.
sterran oððe feala gesihð blisse *getacnað*
⟨228⟩ **S**tellas cum plures uiderit. letitiam. Significat.
blod of his sidan dropian hearm ge*tacnað*
⟨229⟩ **S**anguinem de suo latere distillare. dampnum. Significat.
on læddran sittan swicuncge *getacnað*
⟨230⟩ **S**cola sedere deceptionem. Significat.
fra*m* næddran laðre þolian feondes gesihðe *getacnað*
⟨231⟩ **S**erpente infesto pati. inimici uisionem Significat.
sittan on swefnum untrumnysse *getacnað*
⟨232⟩ **S**edere in somnis infirmitatem. Significat.

454 cinigas] *Cockayne's* cyngas *and Förster's* cincgas *are spurious* | **460** ryselas] ~ *wrongly glosses* resinas*; read* glær *(Cockayne suggested* hluttor pic*)* | **461** sulphur] -r < l | **464** tagan] -g- < t; *read* tacen | **471** anxionem] *read* anxietatem | **472** wyrðscip] *read* wyrðscipe | **475** spendidum] ~ ‖ *⟨f. 31v⟩; read* splendidum | **478** oððe] *delete ~ (see l. 479)* | **479** **S**tellas cum plures] *read* Stellas plures *(see Martin 1981: 159)* | **483** **S**cola] *read* Scala.

þunor gehyran oððe geseon ærende god *getacnað*
⟨233⟩ **T**onitruam audire u*el* uidere. nuntium bonum. Significat.
ungewyderu gesihð gestrion *getacnað*
⟨234⟩ **T**empestates uiderit. lucrum significat.
þystru gesihð untrumnysse *getacnað*
⟨235⟩ **T**enebras uiderit. infirmitatem Significat.
webbu swa wilc swa wyfð 7 blisse oððe unrotnysse gesihð god ærende
⟨236⟩ **T**ela quicumq*ue* texerit & letitiam siue tristitiam uiderit bonum nuntium
getacnað
Significat.
cwydas don trimnige *getacnað*
⟨237⟩ **T**estamenta facere tutamentum Significat.
eorðan styrunge gesihð. sum þine he forlæt
⟨238⟩ **T**erre motum uiderit. aliquid admittit.
mearcian se þe hine gesihð anxsumnese ge*tacnað*
⟨239⟩ **T**ricare qui se uiderit. anxietatem. Significat.
windeardes ripe fulle gesihð blisse ge*tacnað*
⟨240⟩ **V**ites maturas plenas uiderit letitiam significat.
wineard wyrcen bliðnysse lif *getacnað*
⟨241⟩ **V**indemiare. hilaritate*m* uite significat.
swingon on swefnum god æfterfiligð
⟨242⟩ **V**apulare in somnis bonum prosequitur.
huntað don gestreon ge*tacnað*
⟨243⟩ **V**enationem facere. lucrum. Significat.
soridan se þe hine gesihð winsumnysse *getacnað*
⟨244⟩ **V**estire qui se uiderit. iocunditate*m* Significat.
beran to hi*m* gewræþan gesihð feondes styrunge ge*tacnað*
⟨245⟩ **V**rbum ad se infestare uiderit inimici seditionem Signific*at*.
win drican untrumnysse *getacnað*
⟨246⟩ **V**inum bibere. infirmitatem. Significat.
reaf hiwlic habban blisse *getacnað*
⟨247⟩ **V**estem formosam habere. letitia*m* Significat.
on wege fennigum lædan oððe gan teonan hefige *getacnað.*
⟨248⟩ **V**ia lutosa ducere *ue*l ambulare molestias graues significat.
wif lædan hearm *getacnað*
⟨249⟩ **V**xorem ducere. dampnum significat.
loc hine geseon corcið *getacnað*
⟨250⟩ **C**apillum se uidere incrementum. Significat.

489 Tonitruam] *read* Tonitruum | **495** nuntium] nu[·]ntium | **497** Significat] Signi-[·]ficat | **500** þine] *read* þinc | **502** anxsumnese] *read* anxsumnesse | **504** windeardes] *read* wingeardas | **506** lif] *read* lifes | **512** soridan] *read* scridan | **513 V**estire] *read* Vestiri | **515 V**rbum] *read* Vrsum | **516** drican] *i.e.* drincan *(see l. 66)* | **525** *first supplement starts here.*

mid oðrum cynehelm deað *getacnað*
⟨251⟩ um ceteris corona. mortem Significat.
mid wepnem þwean geteorung *getacnað*
⟨252⟩ **C**um masculo lauare. defectionem Significat.
untrumnysse
⟨253⟩ **C**um altio peccare infirmitatem. Significat.
mid his yldran sprecan oððe gan fyrðrunge.
⟨254⟩ **C**um altiore loqui aut ambulare expeditione*m*. S*ignificat.*
enneleac geseon eagena sar hit getacnað
⟨255⟩ **C**epas uidere. oculorum. dolorum. Significat.
beheafdian hine gestreon ge*tacnað*
⟨256⟩ **D**ecollare se uidere. lucrum Significat.
on beþe hine þwean anxsumnesse *getacnað*
⟨257⟩ **I**n balneo se lauare. anxietatem. Significat.
on cwearterne geseon hearm *getacnað*
⟨258⟩ **I**n carcere se uidere dampnum Significat.
on fiscwole þweon winsumnyse
⟨259⟩ **I**n piscario lauare. iocunditatem. Significat.
on slode þwean blisse ge*tacnað*
⟨260⟩ **I**n flumine lauare gaudium. Significat.
on wyll feallan sume wrohte hit getacnað
⟨261⟩ **I**n fontem cecidisse aliquam accusationem Significat.
gebundenne hine gesihð hearm hit getacnað
⟨262⟩ **L**igatum se uidere dampnum. Significat.
swimma*n*n hine geseon hear*m* *getacnað*
⟨263⟩ **N**atare se uidere dampnum. Significat.
ele geseon blisse *getacnað*
⟨264⟩ **O**leum uidere. letitiam Significat.
orcyrd geseon hearm *getacnað*
⟨265⟩ **O**rtum uidere dampnum SignificaT.
æppla gaderian gramam *getacnað*
⟨266⟩ **P**oma colligere molestiam significat.
se þe hine fleon gesiht stowe awendan
⟨267⟩ **Q**ui se uolare uiderit locu*m* mutare S*ignificat.*

527 um] *read* Cum | **528** wepnem] *read* wepmen | **530** *This entry not translated in Cockayne* | untrumnysse] *read* mid oðrum syngian ~ getacnað | **531** altio] *read* alio | **532** fyrðrunge] *read* ~ getacnað *(the scribe probably overlooked a* -ge ge *sequence in the exemplar)* | **536** hine] ~ *over* uidere*; read* ~ geseon *(*uidere *not glossed)* | **539** anxietatem] -e$_1$- < a | **540** cwearterne] ~ *over* carcare se*; read* ~ hine *(*se *not glossed)* | **542** fiscwole] *read* fiscpole *(see l. 111)* | þweon] *read* þwean | winsumnyse] *read* winsumnysse getacnað *(*Significat *not glossed)* | **543** Significat] S̄ignificat | **544** slode] *read* flode | **547 In**] ~ ‖ ⟨*f. 32r*⟩ | **550** swimma*n*n] swimmān*; read* swimman | **556** gramam] *read* graman | **558** awendan] *read* ~ getacnað *(*S*ignificat not glossed).*

se þe on wræcsit gesihð mid micelu*m* gyltum heo*m* ofsett *getacnað*
⟨268⟩ **Q**ui in exill`i´o se uiderit magnis criminibus opprimi significat.
winberian sure geseon sace *getacnað*
⟨269⟩ **V**uas acerbas uidere litem significat.
nægelas geseon anxsumnysse *getacnað*
⟨270⟩ **V**ngulas uidere. angustiam Signific*at*.
gif þu swefnast þe twege monan geseon gefean 7 blisse *getacnað*
⟨271⟩ **S**i somniaueris te duas lunas uidere. gaudium & lętitiam significat.
gif þu gesihst þ*æt* of hehstu*m* þu fealst niþer to þearfan godan 7 to
⟨272⟩ **S**i uideris quod de altissimo cadas de subtus. ad pauperem bonum & ad
weligan yfelan *getacnað*
diuitem malum significat.
gif þu gesihst dracan ofer þe fleogende goldhord *getacnað*
⟨273⟩ **S**i uideris draconem super te uolante*m* thesaurum significat.
gif þu gesihst ansine þine fægere blisse *getacnað.*
⟨274⟩ **S**i uideris faciem tuam pulchram gaudium S*ignificat.*
gif þu gesihst þ*æt* þu on wætere fægere inga oððe oferga
⟨275⟩ **S**i uideris quod in aqua pulcra intres aut ultra ambulaueris.
sorhseaste *getacnað*
Securitate*m*. S*ignificat.*
gif þu gesihst þ*æt* þu on wætere fægru*m* inga oððe oferga nan
⟨276⟩ **S**i uideris quod in aqua pulcra intres aut ambulaueris. nullu*m*
god *getacnað*
bonu*m* S*ignificat.*
gif þu gesihst þ*æt* þu mid swurde bist begyrd sorhleaste hit getacnað.
⟨277⟩ **S**i uideris quod gladio eris cunctus securitatem. Significat.
gif þu gesihst gimmas deorwyrða findan spellu *getacnað*
⟨278⟩ **S**i uideris gemmas pretiosas inuenire parabolas. Significat.
gif þu gesihst manega get ydel *getacnað*
⟨279⟩ **S**i uideris multas capras. uanitatem. significat.
gif þu gesihst þ*æt* þu demst folc god oððe wyrðscipe *getacnað*
⟨280⟩ **S**i uideris quod iudicas populum. bonum uel honorem significat.
gif þu gesihst fela hunda of feondu*m* þinu*m* þe warnian *getacnað*
⟨281⟩ **S**i uideris multos canes. de inimicis tuis te cauere. Significat.

560 wræcsit] *read* wræcsið hine *(*se *not glossed); Förster (1910: 67, n. 5) read* wræc, *placed* sit *after* exil`i´o *and claimed that it was added by the scribe of the Latin. I have three objections: (1)* wræcsit *is written in Anglo-Saxon minuscule as one word by the glossator; (2) the supposed transposition is not indicated while others are; (3)* sit *makes more sense in the gloss (*wræc *means* misery, wræcsið *means* exile*)* | **561** criminibus] $-i_3-$ < e | **567** *second supplement starts here* | **578** sorhseaste] *read* sorhleaste | **580,582** *entry not in Cockayne* | **580** fægru*m*] ~ *agrees with Latin* pulcra, *but read* fulan *(see l. 581), probably an eye slip (see l. 576)* | **581** pulcra] ~ *is an unlikely reading in view of the interpretation of the dream (probably an eye slip, see l. 577); read* sordido | ambulaueris] *read* ultra ~ | **585** cunctus] *read* cinctus.

gif þu gesihst coss þe syllan nehstan god *getacnað*
⟨282⟩ **Si** uideris osculum te dare proximo. bonu*m*. S*ignificat*.
gif þu gesihst manega hlafas blisse *getacnað*
⟨283⟩ **Si** uideris plurimos panes letitiam. Significat.
gif þu gesihst beon þe beswican oððe derian lif þin beon ascyrud fra*m*
⟨284⟩ **Si** uideris apes te illudere u*el* nocere. uitam tuam moueri de
mannum *getacnað*
hominibus. Significat.
gif þu gesihst beon fleon on huse þiinum forlætincge *getacnað*
⟨285⟩ **Si** uideris apes uolare in domo tua. desertionem significat.
gef þu gesihst snacan ongean þe cuman ongean hyfele wyfmen þe bewerian
⟨286⟩ **Si** uideris colubrum contra te uenire. contra malas feminas te defendere
mynegað
ammon*et*;
gif þu gesihst earn fleon wif þin gegripan deað *getacnað*
⟨287⟩ **Si** uideris aquilam uolantem. uxorem tuam rapere morte*m* significat.
gif þu gesihst þe on wearmu*m* watere þwean hynðe lichaman ge*tacnað*
⟨288⟩ **Si** uideris te in calida aqua lauare. dampnum corporis. Significat.
gif þu gesihst þe on wætere cealdan þwan hælðe lichaman *getacnað*
⟨289⟩ **Si** uideris te in aqua frigida lauare: sanitatem corporis significat.
gif þu gesihst fæla penega oððe findast bigspllu oððe tælincga oððe
⟨290⟩ **Si** uideris plures denarios aut inuenies parabolas uel irrisiones. u*el*
wærginga *getacnað*
maledictiones significat.
gif þu gesihst of handu deades su*m* þincg niman be suman dæle þe
⟨291⟩ **Si** uideris de manu mortui aliquid accipere. de aliqua parte tibi
cuman feoh *getacnað*
uenire pecuniam significat.
gif þu gesihst hus þin byrnende findan þe feoh *getacnað*
⟨292⟩ **Si** uideris domum tuam ardentem. inuenire te pecuniam. Significat.
gif þu gesihst hearmas þine bemancude god *getacnað*
⟨293⟩ **Si** uideris brachia tua truncata: bonum significat.
gif þu gesihst feala claða habban feond þine on andwealde þinu*m*
⟨294⟩ **Si** uideris multa uestimenta habere. inimicum tuum in potestate tua
habban *getacnað*
hab*ere* Signifi*cat*.
gif þu gesihst hring gyldenne habban wyrðscipe ge*tacnað*
⟨295⟩ **Si** uideris anulum aureum habere. honorem. Significat.

598 ascyrud] *read* astyrud | **602** þiinum] *i.e.* þinum *(see l. 2)* | **608** wif] w- < f | **610** ge-*tacnað*] ḡe | **613** significat.] ~ ‖ ⟨*f. 32v*⟩ | **614** bigspllu] *read* bigspellu | **622,623** *there must be confusion between the interpretation of a dream on building a house (which is a good sign and leads to money) and the topos of a dream on a burning house (which is a bad sign and leads to mortal danger), see ll. 183,655, 7/1, 7/3.*

gif þu gesihst þe spiweþan don geþancu 7 geþeahtu þine tostredde 7 to
⟨296⟩ **Si** uideris te uomitum facere. cogitationes & consilia tua dispersa & ad
nahte getealde beon *getacnað*
nichilata esse. significat.
gif þu gesihst swiran þine gewriþene wærne þe beon *þæt* þu naht unrihtnes ne
⟨297⟩ **Si** ui`d´eris collum tuum ligatum. cautu*m* te esse. ne quid iniquum
do *getacnað*
facias. Significat
gif þu gesihst of hehre stowe nyþer on þystrum þe fealla*nn* anxsumnyssa oððe
⟨298⟩ **Si** uideris de alto l oco subtus in obscuro te cadere angustias uel
teonan *getacnað*
iniurias significat
gif þu gesihst *þæt* þu gewilnige wif nexstan þines yfel sar on
⟨299⟩ **Si** uideris quod concupiscas uxorem proximi tui. malum dolorem in
lichaman *getacnað*
corpus. Significat.
gif þu gesihst mid wife þinu*m* licgan god *getacnað*
⟨300⟩ **Si** uideris cum uxore tua accumbere: bonu*m* Significat.
gif þu gesihst þe gebiddan to drih`t´ne micel blisse þe tocumon
⟨301⟩ **Si** uideris te orare ad d*ominu*m: grande gaudium tibi aduenisse
hit getacnað.
significat.
gif þu gesihst timbrian hus þin feoh þin wexan hit getacnað.
⟨302⟩ **Si** uideris fabricare domum tuam. pecunia*m* tuam crescere significata.

640 fealla*nn*] feallā̄n; *read* feallan | **655** significata] *read* significat.

7/5 London, British Library, Cotton Titus D. xxvi, fols 11v/8-16r

⟨1⟩ **A**ues in somnis uidere. & cu*m* illis pugnare. lite*m* significat.
⟨2⟩ **A**ues in somno capere. lucrum sig*nificat.*
⟨3⟩ **A**ues ebullientes. inimicor*um* locutione*m* sig*nificat.*
⟨4⟩ **A**rma in so*m*no portare. fortitudine*m* sig*nificat.*
⟨5⟩ **A**uem alique*m* rapuisse. dampnum sig*nificat.*
⟨6⟩ **A**sinu*m* uidere. laborem sign*ificat.*
⟨7⟩ **A**rbores confractos uidere. lucru*m* sig*nificat.*
⟨8⟩ **A** bestiis infestare. inimicor*um* locutione*m* sig*nificat.*
⟨9⟩ **A**rcumittere `*&*´ sagitta*m* tendere. anxietatem sig*nificat:*

Post-medieval title: Alphabetum somniale excerptum ex Daniel*is* libro. *Entries 64 and 65, originally one, have been split up on the basis of 7/4. Changes to the text have been carried out by another scribe* | **3 A**ues] *read* Aquas *(see 7/4)* | ebullientes] *read* ~ uidere | **5** rapuisse] *read* a se ~ | **6** uidere] ~ *on erasure* | **7** confractos] *read* cum fructu *(see 7/4)* | **9 A**rcumittere] *read* Arcum mittere | **A**rcumittere `*&*´ sagitta*m* tendere] arcum tendere uel sagittam mittere *is more usual (see 7/4)* | anxietatem] anxi‖etatem ⟨*f. 12r*⟩.

⟨10⟩ **A**nulu*m* in somnis accip*ere*. securitate*m* sig*nificat*.
⟨11⟩ **A**nulum dare. dampnum sig.
⟨12⟩ **A**urum tractare. expectatione negosii sig*nificat*.
⟨13⟩ **A**bsente*m* bibere. litem sig*nificat*.
⟨14⟩ **A**cetu*m* bibere. infirmitatem sig*nificat*.
⟨15⟩ **A**lba ut splendida uestire. infirmitate*m* sig*nificat*.
⟨16⟩ **A**rare uidere labore*m* sig*nificat*.
⟨17⟩ **B**arba sibi tundi dampnum sig*nificat*.
⟨18⟩ **B**estias curres uidere. p*er*turbatione*m* sig*nificat*.
⟨19⟩ **B**arbatu*m* se uidere. dampnum sig*nificat*.
⟨20⟩ **B**\`*i*´rru*m* album habere. laetitia*m* sig*nificat*.
⟨21⟩ **B**estias loquentes uidere. modestia*m* sig*nificat*.
⟨22⟩ **B**utru*m* uidere. nuntiu*m* bonu*m* sig*nificat*.
⟨23⟩ **C**lamide*m* uestiri. securitate*m* sig*nificat*
⟨24⟩ **C**orona*m* accipere. letitiam sig*nificat*.
⟨25⟩ **C**elu*m* fla*m*meu*m* uidere iniquitates in toto orbe ueniunt.
⟨26⟩ **C**olumbas uidere. aliqua*m* tristitiam sig*nificat*.
⟨27⟩ **C**apill\`*atu*m´ se uidere. crementu*m* sig*nificat*.
⟨28⟩ **C**apud albu*m* abere. lucrum sig*nificat*
⟨29⟩ **C**apud sibi mundi dampnu*m* sig*nificat*.
⟨30⟩ **C**alcimenta ueter\`*a*´ calciare. da*m*pnu*m* sig*nificat*
⟨31⟩ **C**anes la\`*c*´rantes uidere. & eis infestare. inimici tui te sup*er*are quer*unt*.
⟨32⟩ **C**anes ludere. uidere gra*tia*m aduersarii.
⟨33⟩ **C**apud lauare. gaudium sig*nificat*.
⟨34⟩ **C**aseum recente*m* accip*ere*. lucrum s*ignificat*.
⟨35⟩ **C**oruscationes uidere. lucrum sig*nificat*.
⟨36⟩ **C**artas scribere. aut legere: nuntiu*m* bonum sig*nificat*.
⟨37⟩ **C**arbones uidere. inimici tui te superabunt.
⟨38⟩ **C**ybum uomere. dampnum sig*nificat*.
⟨39⟩ **C**um ceteris corona*m*. mortem sig*nificat*.
⟨40⟩ **C**eras *ue*l cereos uidere. gaudium sig*nificat*.
⟨41⟩ **C**um mortuo loqui. lucrum s*ignificat*.

11 sig] *read* significat | **12** expectatione negosii] *read* expeditionem negotii *(see 7/4)* | **13 A**bsente*m*] *read* absinthium | **15** ut] *read* aut | infirmitate*m*] *topos and interpretation do not agree,* iocunditatem *(7/4) makes more sense* | **18** curres] *read* currentes | **21** modestia*m*] *read* molestiam | **22 B**utru*m*] *part of* -u_1- *and all of* -t- *are faded and may have been erased imperfectly, on the basis of which Günzel (1993) suggested* brutum*; this solution must be rejected because the interpretation coincides with the topos* butirum, *not with* brutum *(see 7/4)* | uidere] *read* edere *(see 7/4)* | **25** iniquitates] ~ ‖ *⟨f. 12v⟩* | ueniunt] *read* obueniunt | **27 C**apill\`*atum*´] -*a*- < [·] | crementu*m*] *read* incrementum | **29** mundi] *read* tundi | **30 C**alcimenta] *read* calciamenta | **31** la\`*c*´rantes] *read* latrantes | quer*unt*] *read* ~ significat *(see 7/4)* | **32** aduersarii] *read* ~ significat *(see 7/4)* | **33** lauare] -ar- < [··]; ~ [&] *(expunged by later hand)* | **35 C**oruscationes] -e- < i | **37** uidere] *read* edere *(see l. 134, 7/4)* | **39** ceteris] *glossed interpretatively by* \`scilicet *hominibus*´ | sig*nificat*.] ~ ‖ *⟨f. 13r⟩* | **41** loqui] -u- < i.

⟨42⟩ **C**um sorore recumbere. da*m*pnu*m* s*ignificat*.
⟨43⟩ **C**um matre. securitatem sig*nificat*.
⟨44⟩ **C**um uirgine. ancxiętate*m* sig*nificat*.
⟨45⟩ **C**um coniuge sua. ancxiętate*m* s*ignificat*.
⟨46⟩ **C**um masculo lauare. defectione*m* s*ignificat*.
⟨47⟩ **C**um altio peccare. infirmitate*m* s*ignificat*.
⟨48⟩ **C**u*m* altione loq*ui*. aut ambulare: expeditione s*ignificat*.
⟨49⟩ **C**epas uidere. oculor*um* dolo`*re*m´.
⟨50⟩ **D**ecoll`*atu*m´ se uidere. lucru*m* s*ignificat*.
⟨51⟩ **D**omu*m* sua*m* sacrificare. letitia est.
⟨52⟩ **D**omu*m* sua*m* destruer`*e*´ da*m*pnu*m* s*ignificat*
⟨53⟩ **D**omu*m* sua*m* ardere. p*er*iculum sig*nificat*.
⟨54⟩ **D**racones uidere. dignitatem s*ignificat*.
⟨55⟩ **D**entes sibi cadere. aliquem `*amicu*m *p*er*dere*´
⟨56⟩ **D**omu*m* sua*m* cadere uidere. da*m*pnu*m* s*ignificat*.
⟨57⟩ **D**almaticum indui. lucrum sig*nificat*.
⟨58⟩ **A**equu*m* albu*m* sedere. nuntiu*m* bonu*m* s*ignificat*
⟨59⟩ **E**briosu*m* se uidere. infirmitate*m* s*ignificat*.
⟨60⟩ eq*uo* nigro sedere. axietatem s*ignificat*.
⟨61⟩ **E**unuchos uidere. dampnum s*ignificat*.
⟨62⟩ **F**arinam tractare. dampnum s*ignificat*.
⟨63⟩ **F**aciem formosa*m* uidere. honore*m* s*ignificat*.
⟨64⟩ **F**aciem
⟨65⟩ turbulenta*m*. crimen s*ignificat*.
⟨66⟩ **F**ossam uidere & in ea*m* cadere: calu*m*nia*m* s*ignificat*.
⟨67⟩ **F**ilios aut filias nasci. da*m*pnu*m* s*ignificat*.
⟨68⟩ **G**ladiatore*m* se uidere. factu*m* da*m*pnu*m* s*ignificat*.
⟨69⟩ **F**emina*m* anuli p*er*didid isse. aliquot ammittere s*ignificat*.
⟨70⟩ **G**audere in somnis. tristitiam s*ignificat*.
⟨71⟩ **H**ospites habere. `*uiduitate*m´ sig*nificat*.
⟨72⟩ **I**n balneo lauare. ancxietate*m* s*ignificat*.
⟨73⟩ **I**n carcære se uidere. calu*m*niam s*ignificat*.
⟨74⟩ **I**nfantes uidere & cu*m* ipsis ludere. gaudium s*ignificat*.
⟨75⟩ **I**n pomeriu*m* ambulare. ancxiętate*m* s*ignificat*.

45 sua] -a < o | **47** altio] *read* alio *(but see 7/4)* | **48** altione] *read* altiore | expeditione] *read* expeditionem | **49** dolo`*re*m´] -`*re*m´ < [··]; *read* ~ significat *(see 7/4)* | **50 D**ecol-l`*atu*m´] -`*atu*m´ < c[··] | **52** destruer`*e*´] -`*e*´ < [·] | **55** `*perdere*´] *read* ~ significat *(see 7/4)* | **56** s*ignificat*.] ~ ‖ ⟨*f. 13v*⟩ | **60** eq*uo*] *read* Aequo | axietatem] *read* anxietatem | **62** dampnum] incrementum negotii *7/4* | **63** uidere] *read* se habere *(see 7/4)* | **64 F**aciem] *read* ~ turpem se habere multis criminibus supprimitur *(see 7/4)* | **65** turbulenta*m*] *read* Flumen ~ | **67** da*m*pnu*m*] incrementum *would fit the topos better (see 7/4)* | **69 F**emina*m* anuli] *read* gemmam de anulo *(see 7/4)* | perdididisse] *read* perdidisse | **71** `*uiduitate*m´] ~ *on erasure; read* inuidiam *(see 7/4)* | **73** s*ignificat*.] ~ ‖ ⟨*f. 14r*⟩.

⟨76⟩ **I**n flum*en* natare. ancxiętate*m* s*ignificat*.
⟨77⟩ **I**n tabula pictum se uidere. uitam longam s*ignificat*.
78 ⟨78⟩ **I**n mare lauare. letitiam s*ignificat*.
⟨79⟩ **I**np*er*ator se uidere. factu*m* honore*m* s*ignificat*.
⟨80⟩ **I**n palatio deambulare. ancxiętatem sig*nificat*.
81 ⟨81⟩ **I**n fonte*m* lauare. lucrum sig*nificat*.
⟨82⟩ **I**n gurgite solido lauare. accussatione*m* s*ignificat*
⟨83⟩ **I**n piscario lauare. iocunditate*m* s*ignificat*.
84 ⟨84⟩ **I**n flum*en* lauare. gaudium sig*nificat*.
⟨85⟩ **I**n fonte*m* ce`*ci*´disse. aliqua*m* accussatione*m* s*ignificat*
⟨86⟩ **I**n mare ce`*ci*´disse. lucrum s*ignificat*.
87 ⟨87⟩ **I**n piscina*m* ce`*ci*´disse gaudiu*m* s*ignificat*.
⟨88⟩ **L**una*m* claram uidere. gaudium s*ignificat*.
⟨89⟩ **L**una*m* sanguineam. gaudium s*ignificat*.
90 ⟨90⟩ **L**una*m* de cęlo descendere. uidere laborem sig*nificat*
⟨91⟩ **L**eone*m* infestare. inimici seditione*m* s*ignificat*.
⟨92⟩ **L**una*m* colorosam uidere. da*m*pnum s*ignificat*.
93 ⟨93⟩ **L**igatum se uidere. dampnum s*ignificat*.
⟨94⟩ **L**uminaria uidere. lucrum sig*nificat*.
⟨95⟩ **L**apides mittere. aegritudine*m* s*ignificat*.
96 ⟨96⟩ **L**ectum suu*m* bene stratu*m* uid*ere*. caritate*m* s*ignificat*.
⟨97⟩ **M**are pisces uidere. ancxiętate*m* s*ignificat*.
⟨98⟩ **M**anus inq*ui*natas habere. da*m*pnu*m* s*ignificat*.
99 ⟨99⟩ **M**atre*m* sua*m* mortua*m* aut uiduam uidere. gaudium s*ignificat*.
⟨100⟩ **M**aiorare `*&*´ minorare se uidere detrim*en*tu*m* sig*nificat*.
⟨101⟩ **M**uliere*m* sparsis crinib*us* uidere. da*m*pnu*m* s*ignificat*
102 ⟨102⟩ **M**igrare se uidere. da*m*nu*m* s*ignificat*.
⟨103⟩ **M**ortuu*m* uidere. gaudiu*m* s*ignificat*.
⟨104⟩ **M**ortuum osculari. uita uiuendi s*ignificat*.
105 ⟨105⟩ **M**anus lauari. molestiam s*ignificat*.
⟨106⟩ **M**esses colligere. letitiam s*ignificat*.
⟨107⟩ **M**el accipi. ab alio decipi s*ignificat*
108 ⟨108⟩ **N**aues uidere. bonu*m* nuntium s*ignificat*.
⟨109⟩ **N**uces colligere. lite*m* s*ignificat*.
⟨110⟩ **N**atare uidere. damnu*m* s*ignificat*.

77 pictum] p[un]ctum, -i- < [u] | **82** solido] *read* sordido *(see 7/4)* | **85** accussatione*m*] -ne*m* < [··] | **88** claram] -a_2- < · | **89** sanguineam] *read* ~ uidere *(see 7/4)* | gaudium] dampnum *would fit the topos better (see 7/4)* | **90** cęlo] ~ ‖ ⟨*f. 14v*⟩ | **96** caritate*m*] *read* claritatem | **99** mortua*m*] mor[ie]tua*m*; [ie] *erased by second hand (sublinear connecting line added between* mor- *and* -tua*m)* | uiduam] *read* uiuam | **100 M**aiorare `*&*´] *read* Maiorem *(see 7/4)* | **101** crinib*us*] cri[mi]nib*us*; [mi] *erased by second hand (sublinear connecting line added between* cri- *and* -nibu*s)* | uidere] uid[·]ere; ui- < in; [·] *erased by second hand (sublinear connecting line added between* uid- *and* -ere*)* | **106** colligere] ~ ‖ ⟨*f. 15r*⟩.

⟨111⟩ **N**iuem uidere. lętitia*m* *significat*.
⟨112⟩ **N**ebula*m* in terra uidere. bonum est.
⟨113⟩ **N**uptias facere. dampnum est.
⟨114⟩ **N**udos pedes ambulare. da*m*num est.
⟨115⟩ **O**rgana cantica uidere. uicinas laudes *significat*.
⟨116⟩ **O**leum uidere. letitiam *significat*.
⟨117⟩ **O**ratione*m* facere. letitiam *significat*.
⟨118⟩ **O**ssa tractare. odiu*m* *significat*.
⟨119⟩ **O**liuas uidere. lucru*m* *significat*.
⟨120⟩ **O**ues uidere. tonsas da*m*pnu*m* *significat*.
⟨121⟩ **O**sculu*m* dare. da*m*pn*um* *significat*.
⟨122⟩ **O**rtu*m* uidere. da*m*pnu*m* *significat*.
⟨123⟩ **P**luuia*m* uidere gaudiu*m* *significat*.
⟨124⟩ **P**ilosu*m* uidere. da*m*pn*um* *significat*.
⟨125⟩ **P**uteum uidere. & in eu*m* cadere: dampnu*m* *significat*.
⟨126⟩ **P**lorare in somnis. lętitia*m*.
⟨127⟩ **P**alma*m* accip*er*e. honore*m* *significat*.
⟨128⟩ **P**ane*m* candidu*m* accip*er*e. accussatione*m* *significat*.
⟨129⟩ **P**anem ordeaceu*m* accip*er*e. letitia*m* *significat*.
⟨130⟩ **P**ontem uidere. securitate*m* *significat*.
⟨131⟩ **P**orcos uidere. in infirmitate*m* \`*cadere*´ *significat*.
⟨132⟩ **P**edes lauare. ancxietate*m* *significat*.
⟨133⟩ **P**oma colligere. molestia*m* *significat*.
⟨134⟩ **Q**ui se uidit carbones uidere inimicor*um* *significat*.
⟨135⟩ **Q**ui se uolare uidit. locu*m* mutare *significat*.
⟨136⟩ **Q**ui \`*se*´ in exiliu*m* uid*it*. magnis criminib*us* opprimi *significat*.
⟨137⟩ **Q**ui \`*se*´ currere non posse uidit: inpedictione*m* *significat*.
⟨138⟩ **R**idere q*ui* se uidit. tristitia*m* *significat*.
⟨139⟩ **R**osa*m* uidere. ualitudine*m* *significat*.
⟨140⟩ **R**eges uidere. de s*e*c*u*lo migrare *significat*.
⟨141⟩ **R**ipas asscendere. labore*m*
⟨142⟩ ipas descendere. nuntiu*m* bonu*m* est.
⟨143⟩ **S**oles duos uidere. honorem *significat*.
⟨144⟩ **S**ole*m* splendidum uidere. gaudiu*m* *significat*.

112 bonum] *read* nullum ~ *(see 7/4)* | **115** cantica uidere] *read* cantare audire *(see 7/4)* | **120 O**ues uidere. tonsas] *over* **O**ues *and* tonsas *two marks are written in the second hand; Günzel has argued that this means the text was changed into* oues tonsas uidere. *However, most dreambooks read the text as it stands, so I discard the emendation (the marks are probably syntactical glosses)* | **126** lętitia*m*] *read* ~ significat *(see 7/4)* | **127 P**alma*m*] ~ ‖ *⟨f. 15v⟩* | **131** in infirmitate*m* \`*cadere*´] *read* infirmitatem; in in- *is most likely a dittography which led to the addition of* cadere *by the second hand as a verb was seemingly lacking* | **134** uidere] *read* edere *(see l. 37)* | **137** inpedictione*m*] *read* impeditionem *(see 7/4)* | **141** labore*m*] *read* ~ significat *(see 7/4)* | **142** ipas] *read* Ripas | **144** *significat*.] ~ ‖ *⟨f. 16r⟩*.

⟨145⟩ **S**olem *uel* luna*m* uidere. letitia*m* iudicii s*ignificat*.
⟨146⟩ **S**tellas plures uidere. letitiam s*ignificat*.
⟨147⟩ **S**anguine*m* de latere suo distillare. dampnu*m* s*ignificat*.
⟨148⟩ **S**cala*m* sedere. da*m*pnu*m* s*ignificat*.
⟨149⟩ **S**erpentem uidere. inimicu*m* s*ignificat*.
⟨150⟩ **T**onitruo audire. gaudium s*ignificat*.
⟨151⟩ **T**empestates uidere. lucru*m* s*ignificat*.
⟨152⟩ **T**enebras uidere. infirmitate*m* s*ignificat*.
⟨153⟩ **T**erre motu*m* uidere. aliq*uo*d a*m*mitti s*ignificat*.
⟨154⟩ **V**itres maturas plenas uidere. letitia*m* s*ignificat*.
⟨155⟩ **V**indemiare `ue*l uicdemias uid*ere´. hilaritate*m* s*ignificat*.
⟨156⟩ **V**uuas aceruas uid*ere*. lite*m* s*ignificat*.
⟨157⟩ **V**ngulas uid*ere* angustia*m* s*ignificat*.
⟨158⟩ **V**enatione*m* facere lucr*u*m s*ignificat*.
⟨159⟩ **V**estiri qui se uid*it*. Iocunditatem significat.

149 uidere] *the circumstance of just seeing a snake in a dream has not been recorded in any other dreambook before the fourteenth century; it is more likely that the dream follows the pattern of that of other predatory animals (so* infestari, *see 7/4)* | **150 T**onitruo] *read* tonitruum | **151 T**empestates] **T**empesta[·]tes | **153** a*m*mitti] *read* ammittit | **154 V**itres] *read* Vites | **155** `*uicdemias*´] *read* uindemias*; this addition is not recorded in any other dreambook* | **156 V**uuas] *read* Vuas.

7/6 London, British Library, Sloane 475, fols 217v/13-218r/19

⟨1⟩ **A**ues in somnis uidere cu*m* ipsis pugnarę lites signis;
⟨2⟩ Aues in sonnis cap*ere* lucru*m* signus.
⟨3⟩ Asinas. q*ui* uiderit crem*en*tis signus.
⟨4⟩ Arma i*n* so*m*nis portare tutam*en*tu*m*. signu*m*.
⟨5⟩ Aue*m* in so*m*nis a re rapta*m* q*ui* uiderit da*m*nu*m* significat.
⟨6⟩ Asinos edęrę labore*m* significat;
⟨7⟩ Aqúas bulięntes q*ui* derit inimicór*um* locutíonis significat.
⟨8⟩ Arbores cu*m* frúctu. uidere lucru*m* separatu*m* significat.
⟨9⟩ Are*m* scendere aliqua*m* dignitate*m* optinere sign*us*
⟨10⟩ Arcu*m* tendere. & sagittas. mitterę & anarietate `sign*us*´
⟨11⟩ Anulu*m* accip*ere* securitate*m* significat.
⟨12⟩ Anullu*m* dare da*m*nu*m*. signu*m*.
⟨13⟩ Auru*m* tractari. expedicione negocii significat.

Text ends at the bottom of fol. 218r, but the verso of this quire ending is empty | **1** cu*m*] *read* & ~ | **2** sonnis] *i.e.* somnis | **5** a] *read* aliquid ~ | re] *read* se | **6** edęrę] *read* sedere *(see 7/4)* | **7** derit] *read* uiderit | **8** frúctu] frúc‖tu ⟨*f. 218r*⟩ | **9** Are*m* scendere] *read* arbores ascendere *(see 7/4)* | **10** & anarietate] *read* laborem & anxietatem | `sign*us*´] *transposition from line below indicated* | **13** tractari] *read* tractare | expedicione] *read* expedicionem.

⟨14⟩ Absinciu*m* bib*ere*;
⟨15⟩ Acetu*m* u*e*l pusca*m* bib*ere* infirmitate*m* significat.
⟨16⟩ Agrimonia ederę.
⟨17⟩ Ad sacrificiu*m* *qui* se uiderit sacrificare letitia*m* sign*us*.
⟨18⟩ Alba aut spendida ueste indui iocu*n*ditate*m* signus
⟨19⟩ Aráre *qui* se uiderit laborę́s maxime obuenient ei signu*m*.
⟨20⟩ Alciore*m* se uiderit. grauit*er* languebit signis.
⟨21⟩ Barba*m* sibi tondi dandu*m* signu*m*.
⟨22⟩ Barba*m* sibi radi similit*er* dannu*m* significat;
⟨23⟩ Burdoné sedęre ctióne*m* negottię significat.
⟨24⟩ Bestias domare. *qui* uide derit gr*atiam* aduersarii significat;
⟨25⟩ Barbatu*m* se uidę́re crem*en*tu*m* significat.
⟨26⟩ Birro albo haberę letitia*m* significat.
⟨27⟩ Bellu*m* u*e*l barbarus. uidérę lę́titia*m* significat.
⟨28⟩ Butiru*m*. ederę nuntiu*m* bonu*m* sign*um*.
⟨29⟩ Boues pascentes uidę́re agonia negotie sign*um*.
⟨30⟩ Bestias. loquentes uidere

14 bib*ere*] *read* ~ litem grauem significat *(see 7/4)* | **16** Agrimonia] *read* Agrimoniam | ederę] *read* ~ nuntium fedum significat *(see 7/4)* | **17** sacrificiu*m*] sacrifici[fici]u*m*, u < i_5 | **18** spendida] *read* splendida | **21** dandu*m*] *read* damnum | **23** ctióne*m*] *read* deceptionem | **24** uide derit] *read* uiderit | **29** agonia negotie] *read* agoniam negotii.

8 Egyptian Days

Alias

Dies Egyptiaci, *Dies mali*

Description

The genre of Egyptian Days takes a prominent place among the prognostics on account of its enduring popularity from the early Middle Ages onwards.[1] There is no other genre of unlucky days that is so frequently attested in medieval manuscripts as is the Egyptian Days.[2] The collective designation 'Egyptian Days' comprises three genres that can be distinguished by the number of days they mention: either three, twelve or twenty-four days. Late classical and early medieval commentaries on the Egyptian Days usually focus on the twenty-four days, which gives the impression that the other two types were as yet unknown. The three days fall on three Mondays in the year, which means they do not fall on the same date every year. The twelve and twenty-four Egyptian Days are fixed dates in the calendar. Bloodletting, medication and the consumption of goose meat prove fatal on any of the Egyptian Days because of their malevolent properties. For this reason, the days are also known as *Dies mali*,[3] perpetuated in the English adjective 'dismal':

> Mentioned in 1256 as the English or Anglo-French name for Fr. *les mals jours*: whence it appears to be OF *dis mal* = L *dies mali* evil days, unlucky days. It was thus originally a substantive of collective meaning; when 'day' was added, making 'dismal days'... its attributive use passed into an adjective, and, its original application being obscured, it was finally before 1600 extended from *day*, *days*, to be a general attribute.[4]

---

[1] See pp. 336-92. *Paulys Realencyclopädie* (Wissowa *et al.* 1894-78: suppl. III.22-23, s.v. *Aegyptiaci, dies-*), remarkably, lacks any information but references to the work of Mommsen (1863: 374) and Schmitz (1877: 307-20). Other reference works do have substantial entries: DuCange *et al.* (1937-38: III.106-07, s.v. *Dies Aegyptiaci*); Hoffmann-Krayer, Bächtold-Stäubli *et al.* (1927-42: I.223-26, s.v. *Ägyptische Tage*; IV.928-29, s.v. *Kalendar* §3a; V.192, s.v. *Konzil*; VIII.564, s.v. *Stunde*; VIII.1436-37, s.v. *Unglückstage* §2); Granlund *et al.* (1956-82: XII.591-93, s.v. *Olycksdagar*); Simpson and Weiner (1992: s.v. *dismal* A.1, B.1; *Egyptian* A.1.b).

[2] Unlucky days are days on which various actions prove harmful or dangerous. They come in many guises, including Dog Days, Egyptian Days and the genre named the unlucky days. Several other genres are described by Worm (1626), Loiseleur (1872), Keil (1957), and Thorndike (1923-58: I.688-89).

[3] Daunou (1842-48: IV.32) mentioned that unlucky days in general are called "*infausti, atri, ominosi, jours funestes, noirs, de mauvais présage*".

[4] Simpson and Weiner (1992: s.v. *dismal*).

The twenty-four Egyptian Days are first attested in a Western source in the calendar *Fasti Philocaliani*, dated AD 354.[5] There is no trace of the Egyptian Days between 354 and their re-emergence in the ninth century.[6] The best introduction is Steele's "Dies Aegyptiaci"; the following brief overview of the reception and interpretation of the Egyptian Days is much indebted to this article.[7] The individual genres of Egyptian Days are discussed separately.

The lack of text witnesses of the Egyptian Days in the early Middle Ages is compensated for by the presence of historic sources that comment on the use of these Egyptian Days. It is a strange irony to observe that the year 354 not only occasioned the first written evidence of the Egyptian Days but also the birth of St. Augustine of Hippo, who wrote in his *Expositio ad Galatas*:

> Therefore, let the reader choose which of the two meanings he wishes, as long as he understand that the superstitious observation of times leads to such grave danger to the soul, that the apostle has remarked on this topic: "I am afraid of you, lest I have bestowed upon you labour in vain" [Gal 4:11]. Although these words are read with such renown and authority in churches all over the world, our congregations are still filled with people who accept from astrologers the times when to do things. So much so, that often even those who, as the saying goes, do not know where they are walking, do not hesitate to warn us not to start any building or work of that kind on days which they call Egyptian.[8]

---

[5] The list of Egyptian Days in this calendar is in Mommsen (1863: 374), a facsimile of the calendar in Mommsen (1863: 334-56). On the Egyptian Days in this calendar, see Salzman (1990: 13, 33, 242).

[6] Steele (1919: 110) mentioned 785 as the year in which the first text on the Egyptian Days reappears in a Western manuscript, to wit Karlsruhe, Hof- und Landesbibliothek, Reichenau 229. This manuscript, however, dates from s. ix^{in} (Holder and Preisendanz 1906-18: I.521-27). In addition, Steele (1919: 110, 115-16, 120-21) made a case for an early eighth-century emergence of both the three and twenty-four Egyptian Days on the basis of the pseudo-Bedan *De minutione sanguinis, siue de phlebotomia* (see pp. 278-79).

[7] Steele (1919).

[8] "Ergo eligat lector utram uolet sententiam, dummodo intelligat ad tantum periculum animae pertinere superstitiosas temporum obseruationes, ut huic loco subiecerit apostolus: 'Timeo uos, ne forte sine causa laborauerim in uobis'. Quod cum tanta celebritate atque auctoritate per orbem terrarum in ecclesiis legatur, plena sunt conuenticula nostra hominibus, qui tempora rerum agendarum a mathematicis accipiunt. Iam uero ne aliquid inchoetur aut aedificiorum aut huiusmodi quorumlibet operum, diebus quos aegyptiacos uocant saepe etiam nos monere non dubitant nescientes, ut dicitur, ubi ambulant" (*Expositio ad Galatas* 35.1-3; Divjak 1971: 103).

Of all the wrongs that can be perpetrated through observation of times, Augustine singled out the Egyptian Days.[9] In one of his letters, St. Ambrose—whose father, incidentally, died *c.* 354 AD—concerned himself with Gal 4:10-11 as well:

> But you will agree that it is a different thing to observe in a pagan fashion what things should be started at which moon, that the fifth day, for instance, should be avoided and nothing started on that day, and also that various lunar cycles recommend or advise against certain days for doing business, just as many are accustomed to shunning the unlucky or Egyptian Days.[10]

Despite the censorial attitude of these church fathers towards the Egyptian Days, it was at times considered noteworthy to stress that someone adhered to the days as Proclus Diadochus (411-85) is said to have done according to his biographer, Marinus of Neapolis (*c.* 450-*c.* 500):

> and he observed the unlucky days of the Egyptians more diligently than those peoples did [the Romans and Phrygians],and, moreover, he singularly gave himself to fasting on certain days because of some apparitions.[11]

From the commentaries of Augustine, Ambrose and Marinus, the Egyptian Days appear to be known under this name in early times. Moreover, the Egyptian Days are explicitly referred to as unlucky days on which not to undertake something new or to conduct business, but their health-impairing properties are not explicitly stated. There is a marked difference in attitude towards these days between Augustine and Ambrose on the one hand, who denounced the observation of Egyptian Days, and Proclus on the other, who is said to have observed the Egyptian Days diligently. The Egyptian Days, then, were initially considered a pagan custom.

Why the name 'Egyptian Days' was given to this prognostic genre has not been resolved. Augustine and Ambrose remain silent on this point.

[9] For a similar view, see Augustine's *Enchiridion* XXI.79 (Evans 1969: 93).

[10] "Sed aliud est obseruare gentilicio more ut qua luna quid adoriendum sit iudices, ut puta quintam esse fugiendam nihilque ea inchoandum, uarios quoque cursus lunae obeundis negotiis commendare uel cauere quosdam dies, quemadmodum plerique posteros dies uel Aegyptiacos declinare consuerunt" (*Epistulae extra collectionem traditae* 13.4; Zelzer 1982: 223-24).

[11] Translated from the Latin translation by Boissonade (1814: 46): "Aegyptiorum nefastos dies diligentius observabat, quam illi ipsi, ac insuper certis diebus peculiariter ieiuniis vacabat propter aliquas apparitiones". The original text in Greek is in Masullo (1985: 75-76).

Marinus called them "the unlucky days of the Egyptians", thereby implying that the Egyptians themselves invented them. Thorndike remarked that "there seems to be no doubt that these days were a relic of the unlucky days in the ancient Egyptian calendar".[12] Loiseleur even claimed that some specific days go back to Chaldean times, though evidence for this supposition is lacking.[13] The system of Egyptian Days does not correspond to the Egyptian system of lucky and unlucky days, which were much more prolific. The lucky and unlucky days of the Egyptians vary from seven to fifteen days per month in one Egyptian calendar.[14] It is easier for us to see how the genre of the three Egyptian Days came into being, because these days—three Mondays in April, August and December, respectively—correspond to seasonal changes in Egypt.

Texts on the Egyptian Days rarely attempt to explain the origin of the name. The texts on the twelve Egyptian Days, which are uniquely attested in two computistical manuscripts connected with Byrhtferth's computus, try to interpret the name of the genre: "these days, too, must be observed every month, on which the people of the Egyptians are cursed together with Pharaoh".[15] Some texts have a justification to the effect that Egypt is a term for darkness: "if darkness is called, with a Greek term, Egypt, then we rightly call the days of death dark".[16] In the twelfth and thirteenth centuries, the designation Egyptian Days was repeatedly etymologised and interpreted by the encyclopedists.[17] Bartholomaeus Anglicus (*c.* 1190-1250), for instance, claimed that the Egyptian Days commemorate the plagues sent upon the Egyptians:

> Of those days one is Egyptian, the other is not. That day is Egyptian on which God sent some kind of plague over Egypt. Hence, as there are twenty-four Egyptian Days, it is clear that God sent more plagues over the

[12] Thorndike (1923-58: I.686).

[13] Loiseleur (1872: 246).

[14] See Chabas (1865), Budge (1899: 224-28), Dawson (1926: 263). Papyri containing Egyptian calendars of lucky and unlucky days date back to *c.* 1500 BC. The days in these calendars were subdivided into three parts. Each part of the day is either good or bad, so a day can be entirely lucky or unlucky, or a combination thereof (see Thorndike 1923-58: I.686). Some texts on the twenty-four Egyptian Days feature hours which are especially dangerous, though such texts are not as frequently attested as hourless ones (see p. 362). There is also a twelfth-century Syriac version of the Egyptian Days, translated from the Greek, in which there are thirty-three unlucky days per year (cf. Budge 1913: II.557). Two Greek texts are in Salmasius (1648: 816-18).

[15] Translation of text 8.2/1, ll. 1-2.

[16] Translation of text 8.3/22, ll. 2-3.

[17] See Steele (1919: 118-19), Thorndike (1923-58: I.687).

> Egyptians than the ten which are more famous than the others. They are placed in the church calendar, not because something should be left undone on those days more than on others, but so that we be reminded of the miracles of God.[18]

Bartholomaeus' assertion that there were fourteen additional plagues which somehow did not make it into Exodus dispensed with the discrepancy between the ten plagues recorded in the Bible and the twenty-four Egyptian Days. Whereas Ambrose and Marinus called these days unlucky, and Augustine and Ambrose regarded them as pagan, Bartholomaeus asserted that they are a token of God's miracles. Bartholomaeus, however, does agree with Augustine and Ambrose in that one should not refrain from doing something on an Egyptian Day. It should also be noted that he explicitly referred to the twenty-four Egyptian Days, and the entry of these days in church calendars.[19]

Peter Comestor (died *c.* 1178) also noted the connection between the biblical plagues and the Egyptian Days:

> It should be noted that there were more plagues in Egypt than the ten which Exodus enumerates; but they happen not to have been so devastating and that is why no mention is made of them. Hence, some days are called Egyptian, because on those days Egypt suffered. We keep only two of them in every month in our memory, although there were actually more. It should not be believed that the Egyptians, experienced though they were in astronomy, considered those days as unlucky for starting a task, or a journey or bloodletting.[20]

[18] "Dierum autem alius est egyptiacus, alius non. Egyptiacus est dies ille in qua misit deus plagam aliquam in egyptum. Vnde cum sint uigintiquattuor dies egyptiaci, patet quod plures misit deus plagas super egyptios quam decem que inter ceteras magis sunt famose. Ponuntur autem in kalendario ecclesie, non quia aliquid sit in illis plus quam in aliis omittendum sed ut miracula dei ad memoriam reducantur" (*De rerum proprietatibus* IX.20; 1485).

[19] The majority of texts on the twenty-four Egyptian Days are attested in calendars (see pp. 359-61). Trevisa's translation of Bartholomeus' *De rerum proprietatibus* elaborates upon the calendar reference by giving the cognomen 'evil days' to the Egyptian Days: "Þe dayes *egipciaci* beþ iset in þe calendar of holy chirche and ben iclepid *dies mali* 'euel dayes'" (*De rerum proprietatibus* IX.21; Seymour 1975: I.535).

[20] "Notandum quia plures fuerunt in egipto plage quam decem, quas exodus enumerat, sed non fuerunt adeo graues forte, et ideo tacentur. Vnde quidam dies egiptiaci dicuntur, quia in his passa est egiptus, quorum duos tantum in singulis mensibus notamus ad memoriam, cum plures forte fuerunt. Nec est credendum, quod egiptii licet astrorum periti, deprehenderunt dies hos nefastos in inchoatione operis, uel itineris, uel minutionis" (*Historia scholastica* Liber Exodus 24; 1474).

Not only did Peter remark that the ten biblical plagues were more magnificent than the others, but also that there might have been even more than twenty-four plagues. Bartholomaeus, in contrast, was quite specific about the number. Furthermore, Peter Comestor negated the idea that the Egyptian Days were regarded unlucky by the Egyptians themselves.

Joannes de Sacrobosco (d. 1256), famed for his *Sphaera mundi*, wrote a treatise on the computus in which he expounded on the Egyptian Days:

> It should be noted that in every month there are two days which are called ill[-natured], evil and Egyptian. Ill[-natured] because of their effect, for according to the opinion of some people, if someone falls ill on these days, he will hardly recover or never at all. Evil because it is bad to start any task on these days, on account of their evil constellations. Egyptian because they were invented by the Egyptians.... Many evils [i.e. plagues] have befallen them [the Egyptians], whence twice in every month, as is noted in the calendar, some even sacrificed human blood to Pluto on these days. Therefore, it is forbidden that anyone let blood on these days lest he seem to sacrifice to a demon.[21]

To my knowledge, Joannes is the only author to have drawn attention to the various names of the Egyptian Days. The opinion that the Egyptian Days are in the calendar to warn people not to let blood in order not to raise the suspicion that they are sacrificing to a demon, is not encountered elsewhere either.

From the above survey of the Egyptian Days, it emerges that these days were widely known in the Middle Ages. The church fathers commented upon the days around the time of the first text witness of the genre; the encyclopedists interpreted their nature on the basis of texts that were copied from the ninth century onwards. One issue that requires further research is how the Egyptian Days earned their name and what they signified in the first place. All commentaries postdate the first calendar to contain Egyptian Days, so they are interpretative in hindsight. Moreover, all explanations seem to focus on the twenty-four Egyptian Days only.

---

[21] "Notandum etiam, quod in quolibet mense sunt duo dies, qui dicuntur aegri, mali, et aegyptiaci. Aegri ab effecto. Secundum enim opinionem quorundam, si quis in his aegrotaret diebus, uix uel nunquam euaderet. Mali quia malum erat incipere aliquod opus in his diebus, propter malas eorum constellationes. Aegyptiaci, quia ab Aegyptiis erant inuenti.... Contigerunt eis plurima mala, ita quod bis in mense quolibet, sicut in Calendario notatur, quidam etiam in his diebus humanum sanguinem Plutoni sacrificabant. Vnde prohibitum est, ne quis in his diebus sibi minuat, ne uideatur sacrificare daemoni" (*Libellus de anni ratione*, cap. Quid Calendae, Nonae, et Idus; 1566).

8.1 Egyptian Days, Three Days Per Year

Literature

Worm (1626: 59); Hampson (1841: II.107-09, s.v. *Egyptian Days*); Migne (1861-1904: I.955, 959-62); Birch (1878: 472-74; 1892: 252-53); Camus (1891: 211); Förster (1903: 352-54; 1929: 270-77); Payne (1904: 16-20); Steele (1919); Smith (1919-33: I.70); Thorndike (1923-59: I.685-88, I. 695-96); Henel (1934-35: 345); Jones (1939: 88-89); Grattan and Singer (1952: 43); Keil (1957: 50-58); Bonser (1963: 296-99); Rubin (1974: 64); Taavitsainen (1988: 53); Hollis and Wright (1992: 268-29); Cameron (1993: 165); Günzel (1993: 31); Epe (1995: 59); Wallis (1995: 121); Liuzza (2001: 185)

Alias

plihtlice dagas

Attribution

post-medieval: Bede

Branch of Superstition

observation of times: weekdays

Texts

OE: 1. Cambridge, Corpus Christi College, MS 391, p. 718
2. London, British Library, Cotton Vitellius C. viii, fol. 22rv
3. London, British Library, Cotton Vitellius E. xviii, fol. 15r
4. London, British Library, Harley 585, fol. 190rv
L: 5. Cambridge, Corpus Christi College, MS 422, p. 49
6. London, British Library, Cotton Titus D. xxvi, fols 3v-4r
7. London, British Library, Cotton Vitellius A. xii, fol. 44rv
8. London, British Library, Harley 3271, fol. 121r
9. London, British Library, Harley 3271, fol. 122v
10. Oxford, St. John's College, MS 17, fol. 3va
cont: 11. Oxford, Bodleian Library, Digby 63, fol. 36rv

Description

Of the three genres that constitute the Egyptian Days, that of the three Egyptian Days ranks second in popularity, with ten attestations in English manuscripts. This genre is rarely discussed independently. Henel, for instance, mentioned the three Egyptian Days in his study of the twenty-four Egyptian Days, while Loiseleur's "Les jours égyptiens" ignores the three days altogether.[1]

[1] Henel (1934-35: 335-46), Loiseleur (1872).

The earliest texts on the three Egyptian Days are from the continent and date from the ninth century, witness (11) and the text in Harley 3017.[2] The three Egyptian Days also form part of the pseudo-Bedan treatise *De minutione sanguinis, siue de phlebotomia*, which contains a number of bloodletting texts, and have been included in the Bedan corpus under the title *De tribus diebus periculosis*.[3] The spurious nature of the attribution of both treatises was pointed out by Jones,[4] but prior to this *De minutione* and *De tribus diebus* were sometimes taken to be Bede's. On this basis, the emergence of the genre of the three Egyptian Days was assigned to the seventh century.[5] Förster referred to Greek redactions of the three Egyptian Days, but he did not date the texts.[6] In a later article, he identified a Greek text from the fifteenth century.[7] Therefore, Förster placed the origin of the genre in Byzantium rather than in Rome.[8] Since the Greek text postdates the Latin ones by about six centuries, I am not convinced that Förster is right. The first Anglo-Saxon witnesses date from the beginning of the eleventh century. It is remarkable that there are no fewer than four texts in Old English, because translations of texts on the three Egyptian Days are not often encountered in other vernaculars.[9]

The designation 'Egyptian Days' was already known in Middle Ages, as rubrics indicate: "**hic noctantur** [*sic*] **dies egiptiaci qui obseruandi sunt per om*n*ia ne quis sanguine*m* audiat in eis minuere**" (6); "**DE DIEBVS ĘGYPTIACIS**" (7); and "DE TRIBVS DIEBVS AEGYPTIAC*IS*" (9). One Old English redaction even goes so far as to provide a explanatory gloss of the name 'Egyptian Days': "there

[2] Schmitz (1877: 313-15), Steele (1919: 120), Förster (1929: 275), Wickersheimer (1966: 31-32 [XXII.6], 33-34 [XXII[10], 52 [XXXVIII.1], 59 [XLVIII.6], 141 [XCII.3], 151-52 [XCIX.9], 175 [CXIV.2]) published some other Latin texts on the three Egyptian Days, but there are to my knowledge no other catalogues in which they are collected, except for Beccaria (1956: 216-17 [56.14], 232 [67.3], 329-30 [108.23]). An Old French version is published by Camus (1891: 211).

[3] Migne (1861-1904: I.959-62, 955).

[4] Jones (1939: 88-89). See also pp. 97-98, 278-79.

[5] Steele (1919: 108) already spoke of "pseudo-Bede", but Loiseleur (1872: 210), for instance, wrote "le plus ancien, du moins à ma conaissance, nous a été conservé par le célèbre historien anglais, Bède le Vénérable".

[6] Förster (1903: 353-54).

[7] Förster (1929: 276).

[8] Förster (1929: 275-76).

[9] Förster (1903: 354; 1929: 276-77), and the fragment copied by the Tremulous Worcester hand in CCCC 391, p.721.

are three days in the year that we call 'egiptiaci', which is in our language 'plihtlice dagas' [dangerous days]".[10]

The three Egyptian Days are Mondays near three dates in the calendar, on which it is dangerous to bleed a human being or cattle, as well as to take medicinal potions, because doing so will be lethal. The same injunction is found in texts on the Dog Days and the twenty-four Egyptian Days.[11] Death does not strike instantly. Bloodletting is fatal within three to seven days, whilst (11) promises death within fifteen days. Consumption of a medicinal potion leads to certain death within fifteen days. Some texts also report that people who are born on one of the three Egyptian Days will die an evil death.

Occasionally, the consumption of goose meat (Latin "auca") is prohibited: "whoever has eaten goose on these three days will die within forty days".[12] This prohibition is usually ignored or misrepresented in studies of the Egyptian Days. Thorndike, for instance, read "aqua" for "auca", and was consequently unable to shed light on this curious injunction and translated: "if one drinks water on those three days, he will die within forty days".[13] When Keil discussed the injunctions in texts on the Egyptian Days, he erroneously adduced Thorndike's mistranslation as evidence of the injunction against taking potions.[14] Grattan and Singer gave their imagination free rein:

> The latter [i.e. 8.1/4] is of interest because in the last sentence there is an odd warning against goose flesh after blood-letting. As goose taboo is Celtic it may well be that the A.S. lore of lucky and unlucky days for bleeding was introduced by Irish missionaries.[15]

Aside from Egyptian Days in the calendar of AD 354, the first witnesses are ninth-century and continental, not from Bede's England.[16] Lacking

[10] Translation of text 8.1/4, ll. 1-2.

[11] See pp. 274-76, 351-52.

[12] Translation of text 8.1/7, ll. 9-10.

[13] Thorndike (1932-58: I.685). This misreading is sometimes found in medieval times as well: "si de aqua in istis tribus diebus manducauerit ante xl dies morietur" (Wickersheimer 1966: 141 [XCII.3]). The reference to eating water is awkward.

[14] Keil (1957: 53).

[15] Grattan and Singer (1952: 43). The statement is accepted by Rubin (1974: 64). The goose taboo is mentioned in Caesar's *De bello Gallico* V.12. The issue of whether this taboo was known among all the Celtic tribes is wisely ignored by Grattan and Singer.

[16] Likewise, Bonser (1963: 298), a follower of Grattan and Singer, cited a text on the three Egyptian Days from the Welsh medical compendium *Meddygon Myddfai*. This text includes a reference to the consumption of goose meat, but the content of the text did

any evidence whatsoever, Grattan and Singer's bold assumption should be rejected. Steele claimed he had found the prohibition in English manuscripts only, yet this claim is wrong.[17] Birch attempted to interpret the injunction using English sources.[18] Förster commented that a Greek text on the three Egyptian Days mentions a swine rather than a goose.[19] For now, it is impossible to identify how and where the prohibition against goose meat came to be associated with the Egyptian Days, and what the rationale behind it is. I suspect the prohibition may derive from dietary and hygienic rules. Tracts on the humours, for instance, also appoint appropriate times for certain foods, including meat.[20]

The goose prohibition came to be incorporated in another form in texts on the twenty-four Egyptian Days. Here, some days in the year are mentioned on which the consumption of goose meat is very dangerous:

> Moreover, one should take heed not to consume goose meat on the last day of March, nor on the last day of December. Goose meat is always unhealthy for the weak, just as more other meats that we cannot list here.[21]

Latin texts make mention of the first day of August in addition to the two listed in the Old English goose prohibition.[22] Furthermore, the Latin texts speak of Mondays near these dates. Three Mondays linked to three dates in the year make the goose prohibitions in texts on the twenty-four Egyptian Days resemble abbreviated texts on the three Egyptian Days, in which everything but the dates and the injunction not to eat goose meat has been omitted. For this reason, Henel regarded the goose prohibition in texts on the twenty-four Egyptian Days as corrupted witnesses of the three Egyptian Days.[23] The other way around, i.e. that texts on the three Egyptian Days are amplified goose prohibitions with the addition of guidelines on bleeding and medication taken from the twenty-four Egyptian Days, is unlikely because the goose prohibition in texts on the three Egyptian Days occupies a marginal position at the end of the text,

---

not originate in Wales since it is a translation of a Latin text on the three Egyptian Days.

[17] Steele (1919: 120-21). For continental goose prohibitions, see Wickersheimer (1966: 33-34 [XXII.10], 59 [XLVIII.6]).

[18] Birch (1878: 473-74, n. 3).

[19] Förster (1903: 353). I have found a reference to swine and goose in Theodorus Priscianus's *Gynaecia* V.17 (Rose 1894: 235, l. 8-10).

[20] See, for instance, texts 6/25, 12/1.

[21] Translation of text 8.3/3, ll. 33-36.

[22] See, for instance, text 8.3/16, ll. 38-40.

[23] Henel (1934-35: 345). Cf. Günzel (1993: 31).

while it is sometimes not even present at all. It is, therefore, probable that Henel's supposition is correct, and that the goose prohibition in the text on the twenty-four Egyptian Days is an atrophied version of the three Egyptian Days.

The three Egyptian Days fall on three Mondays each year, related to three dates in the calendar.[24] The Latin texts show a high degree of agreement in that they all assign Mondays around the same dates: the Monday after 25 March, the first Monday of August and the last Monday of December (5-10). The Old English texts vary from the Latin, which may be due to a failure to interpret the Roman calendar date "viii kł aprilis" properly. (1, 3) read: "that is the last Monday of April before it ends, and the first Monday of August, and the last Monday of December, *before* it ends".[25] However, (2, 4) contain a small but significant variant reading: "the third is the first Monday *after* the end of the month December".[26] This variant is not encountered in the Latin texts on the three Egyptian Days, and is therefore likely to have come into existence in the process of translation.

It is possible to distinguish an indeterminate number of redactions in Latin and two in the vernacular. The Latin texts all exhibit variation to such an extent that it is hard to establish how many redactions there are. This difficulty is occasioned by the phrasing of the texts and the level of completeness of the information provided. (8, 9) are certainly related because they are found in the same manuscript and are based on one exemplar.[27] The two redactions in Old English are distinguished on account of the dates they contain, viz. (1, 3) and (2, 4). Moreover, the explanatory gloss "*þæt* is on ure geðeode plihtlice dagas" for 'Egyptian Days' is present in (2, 4) but not in (1, 3).[28] More variants in phrasing and vocabulary distinguish the two redactions, which suggests that the two redactions are independent translations from the Latin.

[24] The dates are listed in table 35.

[25] Translation of text 8.1/1, ll. 2-4.

[26] Translation of text 8.1/4, ll. 5-6.

[27] 8.1/9 is part of an improved copy of the β-sequence which contains 8.1/8 (see pp. 38-39, 61).

[28] Text 8.1/2, ll. 1-2.

Edition[29]

8.1/1 Cambridge, Corpus Christi College, MS 391, p. 718/9-22

Ðry dagas synd on xii monðum þa synd swiðe unhalwende monnum oððe nytenum blod on to forlætene oððe drenc to drincane þ*æt* is se æftemæste monandæg on Ap*ril*is ær he gange of tune 7 se forma monandæg on AGUS*TUS* monað 7 se æftemæste monandæg on decEM*BER* monað. ær he gange of tune

se ðe on ðam .iii. monandagum men o(ðð*e*) nytene blod forlæteð on þone ðridan dæg he sceal sweltan oððe he ne gebiðeð þæs seofðan dæges 7 gif he drinc drinceð to læcecrefte ær .xv. dagan he sceal sweltan 7 gif hwylc man acenned bið on þissum iii dagum he sceal sweltan yfele deaðe 7 Se ðe et goseflæsc on þisson .iii. dagan ær .xl. dæge he sceal sweltan.

The Tremulous Worcester hand probably used this Old English text for his version in CCCC 391, p. 721/12-15: þreo dawes beoþ ón tweolf moneþ. þ(et) beoþ swuþe unhalewende monne oþer nutene. blod un to forletene. oþer drnc to drínkene. þet is þe æftemeste monandai | **6** gebiðeð] *read* gebideð | seofðan] *read* seofoðan.

8.1/3 London, British Library, Cotton Vitellius E. xviii, fol. 15r/6-15

Find eft þry dagas on twelf monðum. þa syndon swiðe unhalwende (mon)num oððe nytenum blod to forlætenne. oððe drenc to drincanne. þ*æt* is se æftemesta monandæig on aprilis. ær he gange of tune. 7 se forma monandæg on agustus monðe. 7 se æftemesta monandæg on decembres monðe `ær he gange of tune.´

Se þe on þam þrim monandagum mannu*m* oððe nytenum blod forlæteð. ær feowerteoðan dæge he sceal swyltan. oððe he ne gebideð þæs seofeðan dæges. 7 gif he drenc drincð to læcecræfte. ær fiftyne dagan he sceal swyltan. 7 gif hwilc man ace(nned bið on) þysum þrim dagum. he sceal swyltan yfelan deaðe. 7 se ðe et(eð gose)flæsc on þysum þrim dagu*m*. he sceal swyltan ær feowertugu*m* dag(um)

Margins damaged; text legible with difficulty and sometimes lost altogether | **1 F**ind] *read* Sind | **F**ind eft þry dagas on] *the opening caused considerable difficulty:* Sindon þry dagas on *Förster (1929),* Find eft þry dagas be *Henel (1934-35),* Sindon þry dagas synd on *Liuzza (2001)* | **2** blod] ~ on *8.1/1* | **4** `ær he gange of tune.´] *transposition indicated* | **5-6** ær feowerteoðan] *read* on þone þridan.

[29] Order of the texts: 1, 3, 2, 4-10.

8.1/2 London, British Library, Cotton Vitellius C. viii, fol. 22r/12-22v/4

Þry dagas syndon on geare þe we egiptiace hatað þ*æt* is on ure geðeode plihtlice dagas on ðam nateþæshwon for nanre neode ne mannes ne neates blod þæm monðe þe we aprilis hatað Se nyxta monandæg. 7 þon*ne* is se oðer ingangende þe monð þe we agustus hatað Se æresta monandæg þon*ne* is se þridda. 7 se æresta monandæg æft*er* utgange þæs monðes decemb*ris*.

Se ðe on þisu*m* þrim dagu*m* his blod gewanað. sy hit man sy hit nyten. þæs ðe we secgan hyrdon þ*æt* sona on ða*m* forman dæge oððe on ða*m* feorðan his lif he geendoð oþþe gif his lif lengre bið þ*æt* he to ðam seofoðan dæge ne becymð. oððe gif he hwyle ne drenc drincð þa*m* þri*m* dagum his lif he geendað. 7 se ðe on þys ylcu*m* þrym dagu*m* goseflæsces onbyrgð binnan feowertiges daga fyrste his lif he geendað.

Punctuation of later date attested but not represented here | **2** blod] *read* ~ sy to wanienne þæt is þonne utgangendum *(see 8.1/4; the scribe probably overlooked a whole line)* | **4** 7 se] *read* se *(7 probably misplaced for* 7 þon*ne* is se þridda. se*)* | **7** feorðan] *read* ~ dæge *(see 8.1/4)* | **8** bið] ~ ‖ ⟨*f. 22v*⟩ | **9** hwyle ne] *read* hwylcne | geendað] *read* ~ binnan .xv. dagum gif hwa on þisum dagum acenned bið yfelum deaðe he his life geendað *(see 8.1/4; the scribe probably overlooked a whole line)* | þys] *read* þysum.

8.1/4 London, British Library, Harley 585, fol. 190r/7-190v/16

Þry dagas syndon on geare þe we egiptiaci hatað þ*æt* is on ure geþeode plihtlice dagas on þam natoþæshwon for nanre neode ne mannes ne neates blod sy to wanienne þ*æt* is þon*ne* utganggendu*m* þam monþe þe we aprelis hatað se nyhsta monandæg án. þon*ne* is oþer ingangendum þam monþe þe we agustus hatað se æresta monandæg. þon*ne* is se þridda se æresta monandæg æfter utgange þæs monþes decembris.

Se þe on þysum þrim dagum his blod gewanige sy hit man sy hit nyten þæs þe we secgan gehyrdan þ*æt* sona on þam forman dæge oþþe þam feorþan dæge his lif geændað oþþe gif his lif længre bið þ*æt* he to þam seofoþan dæge ne becymð oððe gif he hwilcne drænc drincð þa*m* þri*m* dagum his lif he geændað binnan .xv. dagum. gif hwa on þis dagu*m* acænned bið yfelu*m* deaðe he his lif geændað 7 se þe on þys ylcum þrim dagu*m* goseflæsces onbyrigeð binnan feowortiges daga fyrste he his lif geændað.

4 þon*ne*] 7 þon*ne* *8.1/2* | **5** þæs] ~ ‖ ⟨*f. 190v*⟩ | **9** lif$_1$] *read* ~ he | **11** þis] *read* þisum | **12** þys] *read* þysum.

8.1/5 Cambridge, Corpus Christi College, MS 422, pp. 49/4-8

Isti sunt. tres dies anni. p*re* aliis obiseruandi p*rimus est* .viii. kł ap*rilis*. & p*rimus* dies. agusti. & nouisim*us est* tertia kł dece*m*br*is*
qui in is dieb*us* homine*m*. *ue*l pec*us*. inciderit tertia die. morietur. Siquis. in p*re*dictis. dieb*us* nat*us* fuerit. mala morte. moriet*ur*

1 obiseruandi] *read* obseruandi | **2** nouisim*us est* tertia kł dece*m*br*is*] *read* tertia est exeunte decembre *or* tertia est nouisimus decembris.

8.1/6 London, British Library, Cotton Titus D. xxvi, fols 3v/9-4r/12

hic noctantur dies egiptiaci qui obseruandi sunt per om*n*ia ne quis sanguine*m* audiat in eis minuere

Dies enim aegyptiaci in quibus nulliusmodi nec p*er* ulla necessitate non lic*et* homine*m*. nec pecus sanguinem minuere. **I**sti tres dies p*er* om*n*ia cauende sunt. **I**d est viii kł apr*ilis* illo die lunis. intrante agusto illa dies lune similiter. exeunte dec*em*brio illa dies lunę cu*m* multa diligentia obseruande sunt quia om*n*ia uena plena sunt.

Qui istis trib*us* dieb*us* homine*m* inciderit aut pecus stati*m* aut die tertio moriturus erit. aut .vii.mu*m* diem non p*er*tingit. **E**t si potione*m* accep*er*it ante xv. dies morit*ur* & si masculus aut femina his dieb*us* nati fuerint mala morte morientur. & si de auca in ipsis dieb*us* manducauerit ante xv. dies moritur.

1 noctantur] *read* notantur | **3** p*er*] *read* pre | **5** apr*ilis*] ~ ‖ ⟨*f. 4r*⟩ | lunis] *read* lunae | **8 Q**ui] *read* ~ in.

8.1/7 London, British Library, Cotton Vitellius A. xii, fol. 44r/26-44v/1

DE DIEBVS ĘGYPTIACIS.

Hos dies maxime obseruare debemus. in quibus nullomodo. neq*ue* ulla necessitate lic*et* homini u*e*l pecori sanguine*m* minuere. nec inpendere. id *est* .viii. kł ap*ri*lis. illo die lunis. Et intrante augusto. illo die lunis. cu*m* omni diligentia obseruandu*m* est. quia tunc om*ne*s uenę plenę sunt. Eexeunte aut*em* dece*m*b*re* illo die lunis.

Qui in istis trib*us* dieb*us* homine*m* inciderit. aut pecus. aut stati*m*. aut die tercio moriet*ur*. aut ad septimu*m* n*on* p*er*ting*et*. Et si potione*m* acceperit. ante dies .xv. morietur. quisquis auca*m* in istis trib*us* dieb*us* manducauerit. ante .xl. dies morietur. sic aute*m* alii dies plurimi sic*ut* supra scriptu*m* est. s*ed* isti tres p*er* om*n*ia obseruandi sunt.

4,6 lunis] *read* lunae | **5** Eexeunte] *read* Exeunte | **10** sic*ut*] ~ ‖ ⟨*f. 44v*⟩.

8.1/8 London, British Library, Harley 3271, fol. 121r/21-30

P*ost* viii kł april*is*. illa dię lunę & intrante augusto illa dię lunę. & exeunte decembre illa dię lunę similiter obseruandu*m est* cu*m* om*n*i diligentia: ne flebotomatio exerceatur quia om*ne*s uene plene sunt;

Qui in his trib*us* dieb*us* ho*mine*m *ue*l quodcu*m*q*ue* animal inciderit: si ilico mortuum n*on* fuerit: die tertia mori*etu*r: aut certe septima die; Siquis u*ero* potione*m* biberit: ante xv.^{cim} dies mori*etu*r; & si quilib*et* masculus. *ue*l femina his supradictis dieb*us* nati fuerint. male morte morient*ur*; Et si de auca comederint: ad quindeci*m* dies non p*er*tingent;

A line in the right margin indicates that this text should have followed the one on the Dog Days instead of the intervening mass in the manuscript (see p. 530). Another copy of the β*-sequence on fol. 122rv is in consecutive order* | **7** male] *read* mala.

8.1/9 London, British Library, Harley 3271, fol. 122v/19-28

DE TRIBVS DIEBVS AEGYPTIAC*IS*.

P*ost* viii. kł apr*ilis* illa die lunę. & intrante agusto illa die lunae: & exeunte dece*m*bre illa die lunę. simili*ter* obseruandu*m est* cu*m* om*n*i diligentia ne flebotomatio exerceatur. quia om*ne*s uenę plenę sunt.

Qui in his trib*us* dieb*us* homine*m* inciderit uel q*uo*dcu*m*q*ue* animal: si ilico mortuu*m* non fuerit: die tertia morietur. aut certe septima die. Siq*uis* u*ero* potione*m* biberit: ante .xv. dies morietur. Et si quilibet masculus uel femina his supradictis diebus nati fuerint: mala morte morient*ur* Et si de auca comederint: ad xv. dies non p*er*tingent.

2 intrante] ~ *on erasure* | **3** flebotomatio] flebo to ma[·]tio, -to- *on erasure.*

8.1/10 Oxford, St. John's College, MS 17, fol. 3va/29-35

Hi tres dies pl*us* s*un*t obseruandi. Int*ra*nte augusto p*ri*mus dies lunę obseruand*us est*. & exeunte dec*em*b*ri* simili*ter* ille dies lunę: & .viii. kł apr*ilis* ille ęque dies lunę.

Qui in istis dieb*us* homine*m* incid*er*it. aut pec*us* mox moriet*ur*. aut die t*er*cio: q*uia* o*mn*is uena plena *est*. Et si infans in istis dieb*us* nat*us* fuerit. mala morte moriet*ur*;

1 lunę] -ę < · | **2** dec*em*b*ri*] *i.e.* decembre | **3** aut] *read* statim ~.

8.2 Egyptian days, Twelve Days per Year

Literature

Liuzza (2001: 186)

Branch of Superstition

observation of times: dates

Texts

L: 1. London, British Library, Cotton Tiberius C. i, fol. 7rb
2. Oxford, St. John's College, MS 17, fol. 40va

Description

Under the section on the twenty-four Egyptian Days, Liuzza listed the usual text witnesses, as well as the two texts on the twelve Egyptian Days.[1] Liuzza called the latter prognostic genre unusual, which it is, but it is even stranger that he listed it under the twenty-four Egyptian Days.

The twelve days can be identified as Egyptian Days through their introductory line: "these days, too, must be observed every month, on which the people of the Egyptians are cursed together with Pharaoh".[2] The text then proceeds to list one Egyptian Day per month. If the dates are compared to those of the twenty-four Egyptian Days, it is evident that they do not coincide even once.[3] Therefore, it is unlikely that the twelve Egyptian Days evolved out of the twenty-four Egyptian Days. Among the many types of unlucky days, no other genre uses the same one-day-per-month set-up as do the twelve Egyptian Days.[4]

As far as I know, (1, 2) are the only copies of the twelve Egyptian Days: no sources or analogues have been identified. These texts derive from a common exemplar, as many texts do in the manuscripts Tiberius C. i + Harley 3367 and St. John's College 17.[5] This exemplar is connected with material Byrhtferth used in compiling his computus. In view of the absence of any further witnesses of the twelve Egyptian Days, and their dissimilarity to any other type of unlucky days, it is hard to place the genre in its historical setting. The genre may have been conceived by the compiler of the exemplar of the manuscripts containing (1, 2), possibly Byrhtferth himself. On the other hand, it might also have originated on the continent and have been brought to England in the computistical

[1] Liuzza (2001: 185-86).

[2] Translation of text 8.2/1, ll. 1-2. See also pp. 332-35.

[3] See tables 36, 37.

[4] On the many types of unlucky days, see Loiseleur (1872), Keil (1957), Thorndike (1923-58: I.688-89).

[5] See pp. 35, 72, 85.

works that Abbo brought with him or with the influx of manuscripts in early Anglo-Norman England. It is impossible to decide which is the more likely possibility, but the unique appearance of the genre in two related English manuscripts would seem to favour an English genesis.

Edition

8.2/1 London, British Library, Cotton Tiberius C. i, fol. 7rb/1-15

Isti q*uo*q*ue* dies obseruandi s*un*t in sing*u*lis m*en*sib*us*. in q*ui*b*us* dieb*us* maledict*us* e*st* pop*u*l*us* ęgyptiorum cu*m* pharaone.
In m*en*se ian*uario* .iii. dies i*d est* p*ri*m*us*
In febr*uario* .ii.
In mar*tio* .vii.
In apr*ili* .v.
In maio .vii`i´. *ue*l vii.
In iun*io* .vii.
In iul*io* .v.
In aug*usto* .xiii.
In sept*embri* .ix.
In oct*obri* .ii.
In nou*embri* .ix.
In dec*embri* .xiii.

Entries for February-December are in columns.

8.2/2 Oxford, St. John's College, MS 17, fol. 40va/18-39

Isti dies obseruandi s*un*t in sing*u*lis m*en*sib*us*. in q*ui*b*us* dieb*us* maledict*us est* pop*u*l*us* egyptior*um* cu*m* pharaone.
In m*en*se ian*uario*: .iii. dies id *est* p*ri*m*us*:
In febr*uario*: .ii.[a]
In mart*io*: vii.
In apr*ili*: v.
In mai*o*: viii. *ue*l .vii.
In iun*io*: vii.
In iul*io*: v.
In aug*usto*: xiii.
In sept*em*b*ri*: ix.
In oct*o*b*ri*: ii.
In nou*em*b*ri*: ix.
In dec*em*b*ri*: xiii.

Each entry starts on a new line | **1** Isti] *read* ~ quoque.

8.3 EGYPTIAN DAYS, TWENTY-FOUR DAYS PER YEAR

Literature

Worm (1626: 54-64); Salmasius (1648: 814-20); Muratori (1723-58: II. 2.1023-41); Gebelin (1773-82: IV.186-93); Hampson (1841: II.76-77, 107-09, s.v. *Dies malæ* and *Egyptian Days*, respectively); Daunou (1842-48: IV.31-32); Brand (1849-55: II.44-51); Migne (1861-1904: I.759-86, 955-56, 959-62); Mommsen (1863: 374); Loiseleur (1872); Schmitz (1877: 307-20); Birch (1878: 475-76, 504-05; 1892: 253-55, 276-77); Cuissard (1882); Meyer (1884: 210); Skeat (1888: 2-3); Payne (1904: 16-20); Budge (1913: II.557-59); Sudhoff (1916); Singer (1917: 110); Steele (1919); Smith (1919-33: I.70); Wildhagen (1921: 97); Thorndike (1923-58: I.685-89, I.695-96); Förster (1929: 265-70); Henel (1934-35: 335-46); Svenberg (1936: 6, 141); Jones (1939: 73, 88-89); Grattan and Singer (1952: 42-43); Södergård (1954); Keil (1957); Bonser (1963: 296-99); Alauzier (1970-71); Martin (1977: 21, 25); Harmening (1979: 165-69); Stuart (1979); Taavitsainen (1988: 53); Kieckhefer (1989: 86-87); Salzman (1990: 13, 33, 242); Hollis and Wright (1992: 268); Cameron (1993: 163-64); Günzel (1993: 30, 31); Epe (1995: 58); Stevenson (1995: 51); Wallis (1995: 117-18, 120-21); Hirsh (1997); Liuzza (2001: 185-86); Cordoñer (2003: 234, 238)

Attributions

medieval: Hippocrates, Hucbald, Isidore;[1] post-medieval: Bede

Branch of Superstition

observation of times: dates

Texts

OE: 1. London, British Library, Cotton Caligula A. xv, fols 130v-31r
2. London, British Library, Cotton Vitellius E. xviii, fol. 15rv
3. London, British Library, Harley 3271, fols 90v-91r

L: 4. Cambridge, Corpus Christi College, MS 422, pp. 29-40
5. Cambridge, Trinity College, O. 7. 41, fols 1v-7r
6. Cambridge, Trinity College, R. 15. 32, pp. 15-26
7. Cambridge, Trinity College, R. 15. 32, p. 37
8. Cambridge, University Library, Kk. 5. 32, fols 50r-55v
9. London, British Library, Additional 37517, fols 2r-3r
10. London, British Library, Arundel 60, fols 2r-7v
11. London, British Library, Arundel 155, fols 2r-7v

[1] These attributions are not attested in Anglo-Saxon sources, but in continental manuscripts, see Beccaria (1956: 378 [133.30]), Wickersheimer (1966: 57 [XLVIII.4], 156 [CIV.1], 139-40 [XC]).

12. London, British Library, Cotton Caligula A. xv, fols 129v-30r
13. London, British Library, Cotton Tiberius C. vi, fol. 114r
14. London, British Library, Cotton Titus D. xxvi, fol. 5r
15. London, British Library, Cotton Titus D. xxvii, fols 3r-8v
16. London, British Library, Cotton Titus D. xxvii, fol. 22rv
17. London, British Library, Cotton Vitellius A. xii, fols 72v-77v
18. London, British Library, Cotton Vitellius A. xviii, fols 3r-8v
19. London, British Library, Cotton Vitellius E. xviii, fols 2r-7v
20. London, British Library, Egerton 3314, fol. 18r
21. London, British Library, Egerton 3314, fols 18v-30r
22. London, British Library, Egerton 3314, fol. 50rv
23. London, British Library, Harley 863, fols 1r-6v
24. London, British Library, Harley 3271, fol. 120v
25. London, British Library, Harley 3271, fol. 122rv
26. London, British Library, Sloane 475, fols 216v-17r
27. Oxford, Bodleian Library, Digby 63, fols 40r-45v
28. Oxford, Bodleian Library, Douce 296, fols 1r-6v
29. Oxford, Bodleian Library, Hatton 113, fols iii recto-viii verso
30. Oxford, St. John's College, MS 17, fols 16r-21v
31. Oxford, St. John's College, MS 17, fol. 40vb
32. Rome, Vatican City, Bibliotheca Apostolica Vaticana, Reg. lat. 12 , fols 7r-12v
33. Salisbury, Cathedral Library, MS 150, fols 3r-8v

cont: 34. Oxford, Bodleian Library, Digby 63, fol. 36r

Description

No system of unlucky days can compare to the twenty-four Egyptian Days, which were generally feared in medieval Western Europe. Nowadays, most people live in ignorance of these unlucky days, but ever since the fourth century, Egyptian Days have been subjected to commentary and study.[2] The first modern scholars who brought together information on the history of the Egyptian Days are from the seventeenth and eighteenth centuries, among whom Ole Worm—translator of Abdul al-Hazred's *Al Azif*—, Salmasius, Muratori and Gebelin.[3] The prognostic genre of Egyptian Days is the only one that can lay claim to such a long tradition of scholarship, going back to the encyclopedists and ultimately the works of Ss. Ambrose and Augustine.

[2] See pp. 330-35.

[3] Worm (1626: 54-64); Salmasius (1648: 814-20); Muratori (1723-58: II.2.1023-41); Gebelin (1773-82: IV.186-93).

The twenty-four Egyptian Days are first attested in a calendar of AD 354.[4] This date is considerably earlier than the first attestations of the three and twelve Egyptian Days, which are from the ninth and twelfth centuries, respectively.[5] Despite the unusually early attestation in the calendar,[6] the origins of the twenty-four Egyptian Days are unknown. The days do not resemble the system of lucky and unlucky days of Egyptian calendars.[7] The twenty-four Egyptian Days may have come into being in the Roman civil calendar, a supposition which is strengthened by the first attestation and by the fact that early commentaries upon the Egyptian Days discuss these days in the light of time reckoning. After the first witness, the genre disappear for over 500 years to emerge once more in the ninth century. The copies in Harley 3017, the Leiden fragment Vossianus Lat. F. 96A, fol. 2v (s. viii^ex or ix) and (34) are some of the earliest attestations.[8] The first English attestation (27) is a series of calendar entries from the fourth quarter of the ninth century, the immediate source for which may have been continental because the manuscript was partly composed on the continent before being taken to England.[9] The first translation into Old English dates from the first quarter of the eleventh century. Wickersheimer mentioned some more early witnesses in Laon 426 bis.[10] Incidentally, this manuscript also contains the first part of the pseudo-Bedan *De minutione sanguinis, siue de phlebotomia*, which contains a number of bloodletting prognostics.[11] In addition to the inclusion of the twenty-four Egyptian Days in *De minutione*, the genre was also represented in Bede's corpus as the independent text *De Ægyptiacis diebus* and in a calendar.[12] The spurious nature of the attributions to Bede is discussed elsewhere.[13]

In the eleventh century and after, texts on the twenty-four Egyptian Days are more frequently encountered in insular manuscripts. It is perhaps not entirely appropriate to speak of a vogue, but in the eleventh and

[4] See pp. 330-35.

[5] See pp. 335-346.

[6] There are not many prognostics which can be traced as far back as this. Exceptions are the twenty-four Egyptian Days, the Apuleian Sphere and the dreambook.

[7] See p. 333.

[8] The Harley and Digby texts will be published in the future. The Leiden text has been published by Stuart (1979); see also Bremmer and Dekker (2006: 85, 87 [156a.3]).

[9] See p. 536.

[10] Wickersheimer (1966: 39-40 [XXVIII.2, 6]).

[11] Migne (1861-1904: I.959-62).

[12] Migne (1861-1904: I.759-86, 955-56).

[13] See pp. 97-98, 278-79.

twelfth centuries, texts on the twenty-four Egyptian Days feature in surprisingly large numbers for a prognostic. This is confirmed by the text corpus: of thirty-three attestations, all but two are from the eleventh and twelfth centuries. This example illustrates that not only do the later texts far outnumber the earlier ones, but also that the texts on the twenty-four Egyptian Days from the eleventh and twelfth centuries contribute extensively to the total size of the prognostic corpus. The continental evidence provides a different picture: the number of texts listed by Beccaria and Wickersheimer from medieval medical manuscripts is fairly stable for the ninth, tenth and eleventh centuries.[14] This may indicate that the genre experienced a late start in English manuscripts.[15]

In speaking of the Egyptian Days, medieval commentators commonly referred to the genre of the twenty-four days rather than that of the three or twelve days.[16] This would suggest that the medieval designation 'dies egyptiaci' was a generic name which pertained mainly to the twenty-four-day genre, despite the fact that the three and twelve Egyptian Days were also known as Egyptian Days.[17] In calendars, Egyptian Days are entered as "dies egyptiacus", "dies mala", "dies" or abbreviations thereof. Texts dealing with the Egyptian Days rarely identify these days with a rubric, but (22, 25) do. The texts themselves sometimes state that they deal with the Egyptian Days, but more usually they present a set of injunctions comparable to that of the three Egyptian Days:

> About the Egyptian Days in the year which are cursed. On these days people should not bleed themselves, nor accept a [medicinal] potion, nor start any kind of work.[18]

and

> Do not kill nor be bled, nor let vineyards be planted, nor let the harvest be collected, nor let wine be bought or sold, nor animals be tamed, nor any-

[14] Beccaria (1956: 123 [8.20], 134 [15.6], 139 [18.2], 182-83 [43.6, 9], 194 [48.5], 213 [55.22], 216 [56.14], 218 [57.6], 270 [84.17], 287 [91.12], 311 [101.12], 378 [133.30], 392 [139.4], 394 [140.3]), Wickersheimer (1966: 13 [II.1], 31 [XXII.5,6], 40 [XXVIII.6], 51-52 [XXXVIII.1], 53 [XL], 56 [XLVI.2], 57-59 [XLVIII.4,6], 64 [LIV.1], 65 [LVII], 139 [LXXXIX], 139-40 [XC], 141 [XCII.3], 151 [XCIX.6], 155-56 [CII.1-3], 156 [CIV.1], 158 [CVIII.1,2], 174-75 [CXIV.2]).

[15] On the treatment of prognostics in continental and English manuscripts, see chapter two.

[16] See pp. 330-35.

[17] See pp. 337-38, 345.

[18] Translation of text 8.3/31, ll. 1-3.

> thing that shall pertain to progress be begun, because these days are cursed by the Lord.[19]

These quotations reveal that the twenty-four Egyptian Days were simply regarded unfavourably because they are cursed. In other words, despite the elaborate scholastic commentaries upon the name and nature of the Egyptian Days, the texts themselves commonly do not reveal what the days stand for beyond their cursed nature.[20]

In comparison with the three Egyptian Days, the number of prohibitions for the twenty-four days is larger. The first quotation illustrates that the customary injunctions against bleeding and medicinal potions apply, but the second quotation includes a series of prohibitions which are more reminiscent of agenda lunaries than of unlucky days.[21] Texts on the three Egyptian Days usually mention the period within which the breach of an injunction proves fatal, e.g. "if someone drinks a medicinal potion, he will die within fifteen days".[22] The twenty-four Egyptian Days merely report the prohibitions, not the consequences of ignoring them. As I discussed before, the twenty-four Egyptian Days sometimes also contain an injunction against eating goose meat.[23] This injunction is rare, because it only occurs in two types of texts, viz. the translation into Old English (1-3), and a specific Latin redaction (16, 21, 22). Steele has argued that the attachment of dietary and medical concerns to the Egyptian Days hailed from Greek texts on unlucky days.[24]

The Old English texts feature a warning resembling a moonbook, but lacking the regularity of the moonbook series:

> Now again about the moon: much is to be warned that one does not let blood on the fourth night of the old moon, or on the fifth night, as the books tell us, before the moon and the sea are in agreement.[25]

[19] Translation of text 8.3/13, ll. 1-3.
[20] See pp. 330-35.
[21] See pp. 422-23.
[22] Translation of text 8.1/3, l. 7.
[23] See pp. 338-40.
[24] Steele (1919: 112). His sources for this notion are texts on the three Egyptian Days, and a text on the unlucky days of the month in Budge's *Syriac Book of Medicines* (1913: II.557) which is thought to be of Greek descent. Although Steele is right in assuming a later attribution of medical consequences to the Egyptian Days—the early formats of calendar entries and hexameter verses lack injunctions—these attributions may have come from a variety of medical sources, particularly regimens, which sometimes also contain information on Dog Days and Egyptian Days (see Stuart 1979).
[25] Translation of text 8.3/1, ll. 23-25. On moonbooks, see pp. 276-77.

A moonbook is a regular series of days of the moon on which something is forbidden or encouraged. Standard moonbook series are sequences of the numbers four or five and multiplications thereof. In the quotation from the text on the twenty-four Egyptian Days, the basic numbers of the moonbook series are mentioned, but not the fact that these are iterative. The passage is given both a learned and a computistical twist by the phrases "as the book tells us" and "before the moon and the sea are in agreement". In fact, the reference to the relationship between the moon and the sea is decidedly Ælfrician. In both his homily *Octabas et circumcisio Domini* and the computistical tract *De temporibus anni*, Ælfric commented upon the influence of the moon upon the sublunar, but he was careful to distinguish between computistical knowledge and prognostic use of time reckoning.[26] The translator of the twenty-four Egyptian Days must have made use of Ælfric's homilies, while Ælfric was familiar with some prognostic genres. Therefore, it is not entirely unlikely that the translator also used Ælfric's works to justify the rudimentary moonbook in his text.[27]

The twenty-four Egyptian Days fall on fixed dates in the calendar, which is why they lend themselves well to inclusion in calendars. Each month has two Egyptian Days, but there is some variation in the dates on which they fall.[28] Gebelin thought that this variation was governed by the culture and climate of the place where the texts and calendars were copied.[29] Loiseleur refuted this notion, but he acknowledged that a variant set of dates may be adhered to in a location once this set had come into being.[30] It is obvious that Gebelin's claim does not hold if we look at the dates in the English texts, which show more variation than is warranted by the cultures and climates of the island:[31]

[26] See below and pp. 98-101, 117-21.

[27] An article of mine on this matter is forthcoming.

[28] The full list of dates per text is displayed in table 37.

[29] Gebelin (1773-82: IV.191).

[30] Loiseleur (1872: 244).

[31] Numbers in bold type represent the basic series which is attested most frequently. An 'x' in the list means that the date in question is lacking and cannot be extrapolated from known data. In this table I have regularised the findings, though it should be noted that some calendars have three dates for one particular month (8.3/8,15,18), which is, presumably, an error since there are only two Egyptian Days per month.

Jan	Feb	Mar	Apr	May	June	July	Aug	Sept	Oct	Nov	Dec
1,25	2,x	**1,28**	3,21	x,23	x,20	3,x	**1,30**	2,25	**3,22**	x,24	7,22
2,24	**4,26**	3,27	3,23	**3,25**	7,x	6,13	7,20	**3,21**	3,26	**5,28**	11,27
2,25	5,18	10,21	3,24	4,25	9,16	7,22		7,x	4,x		**12,15**
	6,x	12,23	4,11	6,17	**10,16**	**13,22**		13,20			13,x
	8,24		**10,20**		10,26	14,22					

table 21: Egyptian Days, dates

These dates are taken from English manuscripts. If continental texts are taken into consideration, the range is even bigger.[32] Examining the rationale behind all variant dates may prove impossible, but there is a logical and reasonable explanation underlying the variation of the set contained in the Old English texts (1, 2, 3).[33] These three texts follow the basic series for January to November, while the dates for December seem to differ per text:

(1)	(2)	(3)
7,22	*12,25	12,15

table 22: Egyptian Days, dates for December

The month December appears to contain as many variants dates of the Egyptian Days as there are Old English texts. This led Förster to remark: "that the numbers often do not coincide will not surprise those who are familiar with the mistakes of medieval scribes".[34] Furthermore, in his edition of (1), Förster noted for the first date for December (the seventh) that "the exemplar may well have read twelve".[35] Rather than dismiss variation as error, it is more fruitful to discover how the variants came into being in the first place.

The first observation is that Förster himself made an essential mistake in his edition of (2)—which will not surprise those who are familiar with the mistakes of modern scholars. (2) is found in Vitellius E. xviii, a manuscript extensively damaged by the Cottonian Fire of 1731. The fire has burnt the outer margins to a crisp, and it is, therefore, exceedingly hard to read the text in these places. When Förster edited (2) from photo-

[32] For lists, see Worm (1626: 55, 57, 61), Gebelin (1773-82: IV.191, 192), Loiseleur (1872: 214, 249), Schmitz (1877: 320), Steele (1919), Keil (1957: 46-47, 49), Stuart (1979: 240).

[33] My analysis of the dates in the Old English translations of the twenty-four Egyptian Days has appeared in Dutch in Chardonnens (2007a).

[34] "[daß] die Zahlen öfter nicht stimmen, wird den Kenner mittelalterlicher Kopistenfehler nicht weiter in Erstaunen setzen" (Förster 1929: 269).

[35] "die Vorlage las wohl .xii." (Förster 1929: 268).

graphs of the manuscript,[36] he copied the dates for December as follows: "On December se twelfta and ær his ende se seofe(ða)" (in December the twelfth and before its end the *seventh*).[37] The second date, written on the damaged right-hand side of the recto page, is barely legible, which explains Förster's conjecture. However, even on microfilm one can read with some effort: "On december se twelfta. 7 ær his ende se seofenteoða" (in December the twelfth and before its end the *seventeenth*). Inspection of the manuscript confirms my findings. This means that one of the variants, the spurious 12 and 25 December, has never existed, so we are left with the basic set 12 and 15 December (2, 3) and the variant set 7 and 22 December (1).

In addition to (1), seven texts feature the dates 7 and 22 December (5, 11-13, 20, 23, 31). If the variant set were aberrant, I would not expect it to show up so frequently. Text (1), which displays the variant set, is preceded in the manuscript by a Latin text on the twenty-four Egyptian Days which has not been noticed by previous editors, viz. (12).[38] In view of the vicinity of (12), on folios 129v-30r, one page before (1), on folios 130v-31r, there cannot be any doubt as to what influenced the variant set of dates for December in (1). The three Old English texts (1-3) derive from a single translation of the Latin which is not related to (12). It is thus impossible that (1) is was independently based upon the Latin text (12) preceding it. In isolation, (1) might have an example of Förster's "Kopistenfehler". This perspective, however, necessitates the conclusion that the supposed error in (1) is a continuation of a variant reading in (12), in which case we had better speak of a deliberate emendation on the part of the scribe.

The change from the basic set 12 and 15 December to the variant 7 and 22 December has up to now been unaccounted for. It seems puzzling how one set could have developed out of the other, yet there is a possible mechanism which might explain this development. The key to the shift in dates lies in the method of enumerating the dates and the format of some texts on the twenty-four Egyptian Days.[39] A number of texts list the dates formulaically: the first date is counted from the beginning of the

[36] Cf. Henel (1934-35: 336, n.1).

[37] Förster (1929: 268). Round brackets indicate Förster's reconstructed reading of the damaged text.

[38] Neither Henel (1934-35) nor Förster (1929) mention this Latin text. If Förster had seen it, he would most certainly not have made his remark about sloppy copies.

[39] Text formats and enumeration mechanisms are discussed in detail below.

month and the second date from the end of the month, as in "In the month of December, the seventh, and before it ends the tenth day".[40] The format of the hexameter verses makes use of this formula in a series of enigmatic verses. The verse for December typically reads: "Dat duodena cohors septem inde decemque decembri". Two sets of dates can be derived from this line, depending on how it is read: either "the twelfth cohort hence gives seventeen [from the end] to December", or "the twelfth cohort hence gives seven and ten [from the end] to December". The first yields the basic set 12 (duodena) December and 15 (septem... decemque)—seventeen days from the end of the month. Alternatively, the set is 7 and 22 December—ten days from the end of the month. This variant set can be arrived at as follows. Three numbers, instead of two, present themselves in the Latin verse: the distributive "duodena" (a distributive for metrical reasons but taken to mean an ordinal number) which modifies the feminine noun "cohors", and the numerals "septem" and "decem(que)" ambiguously split up by the adverb "inde". Rather than reading the phrase "septem... decemque" as one number (seventeen), it might be construed to consist of two (seven and ten). Since most numbers in the hexameter verses are numerals; the distributive is hardly used in these verses.[41] This might cause ambiguity in that "duodena" is not taken to be the first date but a modifier of "cohors". The adverbial split and the occurrence of a distributive could easily have given rise to the notion that the first date is "septem" and the second "decem(que)", i.e. 7 and 22 December. Once the variant reading was recognised by readers of the hexameter verses,[42] it may have been incorporated into other text formats, such as calendars, and stand-alone texts like (12). Subsequently, the variant set may have overruled the basic series of dates in the Old English translation of the twenty-four Egyptian Days of (1) because the scribe had just copied (12), which contained the variant set of dates.

This somewhat lengthy example provides an illustration of how texts on the twenty-four Egyptian Days may come to incorporate different

[40] Translation of text 8.3/12, l. 16.

[41] Distributives are found in four instances only: April (undeno), June (quindenum), September (denam) and December (duodena).

[42] That this has been actually happened is attested by a text on the Egyptian Days in London, British Library, Royal 15. B. xix (s. x, Rheims), fol. 126r, which has the verse lines flanked to left and right by columns of first and second dates per month. The line for December reads as follows: "**.vii. D**at duodena cohors septe*m* inde dece*mque* dece*m*bris **.x.**". Moreover, some calendars incorporating the hexameter verses have the variant set of dates for December (e.g. 8.3/5).

sets of dates. Moreover, I have shown how a variant set of dates can be extracted from the basic set. I am not suggesting that such processes underlie all variant dates, but I do think they provide a rational basis for variants that might otherwise be rejected as instances of sloppy copy.

To both the hexameter verses and some stand-alone texts certain constraints are said to apply that have become exceedingly academic in the sense that scholars have tried to fit the Egyptian Days into a spurious mathematical framework. Hexameter verses and some stand-alone texts mention the two dates per month for the Egyptian Days in a formulaic manner, in which the first date is counted from the beginning of the month, and the second from the end of the month.[43] The hexameter verse for January, for instance, reads: "Iani prima dies et septima fine timetur" (in January the first day, and the seventh from the end is feared). A stand-alone text may read: "mense ianuario i & antequam exeat die vii" (in the month of January, the first and before it ends the seventh day). Both give the following Egyptian Days: the first of January and the seventh before its end, i.e. the twenty-fifth. Working with a small text corpus, some scholars have assumed that the Egyptian Days must fall between certain fixed dates. Mommsen, for one, remarked: "of the Egyptian Days of any month, the first falls between the second and seventh, the last between the eighteenth and twenty-fifth of the month".[44] Mommsen's rule is premature as Schmitz has shown,[45] for it is founded solely on his knowledge of the Egyptian Days as presented by the calendar of AD 354. Table 21 illustrates that the Egyptian Days for August are 1 and 30, dates which fall outside Mommsen's range, but which occur in almost all texts on the Egyptian Days.

There are many more texts on the twenty-four Egyptian Days than the entries in the fourth-century calendar, and the variation in dates among these texts, though not immense, is considerable. Nevertheless, some scholars adhere to Mommsen's argument, or have slightly adjusted the formula, as Thorndike did:

---

[43] Steele (1919: 110) called this the "Bononian method". I have not been able to discover why he named it this way.

[44] "dies Aegyptiaci cuiusvis mensis priores cadunt inter secundum et septimum, posteriores fere inter decimum octavum et vigesimum quintum mensis dies" (Mommsen 1863: 374).

[45] Schmitz (1877: 308).

> Eleven days is the farthest removed that any Egyptian Day is from the first of the month and twelve the most from the close, so that they never fall in the middle of a month nor on the very first or last day.[46]

Likewise, Keil wrote:

> in every month there are two [days], of which the first unlucky day of the month is not removed further from the beginning of the month than the second one is from the end of the month. Therefore, the days cannot be close to each other in the middle of the month. It also does not occur that the days fall on the Kalends or the day "pridie kalendas", i.e. on the first or last day of the month.[47]

Again, these rules do not apply: the basic dates for February—the fourth, and the third from the end of the month—exemplify that the first date can be removed further from the beginning of the month than the second is from the end of the month. Moreover, whereas it is true, to my knowledge, that the second date never falls on the last day of the month, the first date has already been shown to be able to fall on the first day of the month. What Keil meant by the dates not being close together in the middle of the month is a matter of debate; 12 and 15 December are quite close to each other in my opinion. The previous example also disproves Thorndike's rule that the limit for the first date is eleven days from the beginning of the month, and for the second date twelve days from the end of the month.

Joannes de Sacrobosco mentioned that the Egyptian Days stem from the constellations known in Egyptian astronomy,[48] which implies that a system underlying the Egyptian Days was already sought for in the Middle Ages. William Durandus quelled any doubts about the systematic nature of the dates by stating: "however, it does not avail us to know the points of their constellations due to the error in our time reckoning".[49] The urge to justify the rationale behind the dates of the Egyptian Days is, therefore, not new to modern scholarship.

---

[46] Thorndike (1923-58: I.685).

[47] "auf jeden Monat fallen zwei [Tage], von denen der erste Unglückstag des Monats nicht weiter vom Monatsanfang entfernt ist als der letzte vom Monatsende. Es kommen also niemals die Tage in der Monatsmitte dicht nebeneinander zu liegen, auch kommt es nicht vor, daß sie auf die Kalenden oder den Tag *pridie Kalendas*, d. h. auf Monatsanfang oder Monatsende fallen" (Keil 1957: 27).

[48] See p. 335.

[49] "tamen illarum constellationum puncta scire propter errorem nostri computi non ualemus" (Davril, Thibodeau and Guyot 1995-2000: III.148).

The foregoing mathematical rules have probably come into existence through misinformation based on too small a corpus of texts. The variation in dates is extensive considering the large number of witnesses that have come down to us.[50] Nevertheless, some regularities can be observed. First, the rule that the first date is counted from the beginning of the month, and the second date from the end applies to hexameter verses and some stand-alone texts. Second, I have yet to encounter a text that has an Egyptian Day on the last day of the month. Third, there is no text in which the Egyptian Days for one month are on consecutive days. Fourth, there is a tendency for the Egyptian Days not to fall on immovable feasts.[51] Despite these regularities, it does not avail us to devise a mathematical formula that captures a system supposedly underlying the Egyptian Days.

I have already alluded to the existence of different text formats for the twenty-four Egyptian Days. There are three main formats:

> (I) Egyptian Days entered into the calendar on specific dates.
> (II) Egyptian Days listed in mnemonic verses. There are twelve- and twenty-four-line verses in which the dates are linked to symbols of violence stressing the evil nature of the Egyptian Days.[52] These verses may appear: (a) at the top of each month in the calendar; (b) in isolation (as stand-alone verses); or (c) with a short introduction.
> (III) Egyptian Days in stand-alone texts. These texts usually have an introduction to the subject matter of Egyptian Days and enumerate the days in various ways: (a) by listing them with the help of verses and an interlinear formulaic reiteration; (b) by listing them in the formulaic manner; (c) by listing them using Roman dates. Stand-alone texts may incorporate additional warnings, such as the rudimentary moonbook and the goose prohibition.

[50] In the course of nearly three centuries of research on the Egyptian Days, many texts have been found in medieval manuscripts, one of the most extensive reviews of this subject is Steele (1919). More texts, mainly continental, can be found in Muratori (1723-58: II.2.1023-41), Loiseleur (1872), Schmitz (1877: 307-20), Keil (1957), Wickersheimer (1966), Stuart (1979). A select index of manuscripts is in Thorndike (1923-58: I.695-96).

[51] I.e. major feasts such as Christmas, Epiphany and Assumption Day. It is impossible for the Egyptian Days not to fall on Saints' Days as these are omnipresent in the Christian calendar. 8.3/15 has three Egyptian Days for December, the last of which is 25 December. I dismiss this reading because there are only two Egyptian Days per month, and because Christmas Day is highly unlikely to be an unlucky day.

[52] Additionally, two- and four-line verses exist, but these have not been attested Anglo-Saxon or early Anglo-Norman manuscripts and seem to have been a scholastic invention.

The threefold format of texts on the twenty-four Egyptian Days outlined here may serve to provide a tentative reconstruction of the development of this genre. The twenty-four Egyptian Days started out as a calendric genre (I). To memorise the dates more easily, mnemonic verse were devised (II). Calendars sometimes use such verse headings to list the Egyptian Days (IIa). Some calendars contain either entries or verses, and some have both, which makes it unlikely that the verses were designed to replace calendar entries. With the development of verses, the Egyptian Days were able to exist independently from the calendar (IIb). Then these verses were elaborated upon with a short introduction (IIc). Moreover, by associative attraction additional items appeared, such as formulaic reiteration, or dietary guidelines (IIIa). With the focus on formulaic reiteration and additional items, the verses disappeared and what remains is the stand-alone text with formulas (IIIb). Alternatively, the disappearance of the verses gave the opportunity to reformulate the days using Roman dates, or these dates may have been extracted from the calendar (IIIc). I do not claim that any one of these formats gained in popularity over the others at any point in time. After all, calendar entries are found well after the first texts proper came into being. Nevertheless, the outline reveals a diachronic development—in the sense that one format may have developed out of another—, which implies that at a certain period in time there was a choice of formats, whereas in the beginning the genre was found in calendars only. The distribution of formats is as follows:

	attestations
calendar (I)	18 (4-6, 8-11, 15, 17-19, 23, 27-30, 32, 33)
verses in calendar (IIa)	9 (5, 10, 17-19, 21, 23, 28, 30)
verses in isolation (IIb)	2 (7, 20)
verses + intro (IIc)	2 (22, 26)
stand-alone + verses, formulaic reiteration and extras (IIIa)	3 (16, 24, 25)
stand-alone + intro and formulas (IIIb)	6 (1-3, 12, 13, 31)
stand-alone + intro and Roman dates (IIIc)	1 (14)

table 23: Egyptian Days, distribution of formats

It is immediately apparent that there is a marked preference for the inclusion of Egyptian Days in the calendar, both as entries on the days themselves, and as verses. This may be occasioned by the fact that Egyptian Days fall on fixed dates in the year, which makes the calendar a good vehicle for presenting them. Entries on the relevant days are listed as "dies egyptiacus", "dies mala", "dies", or abbreviations thereof. These entries are commonly outlined on the right-hand side of the page rather than written immediately after the date. An exception is the entry for 1 August, which is sometimes written in the left margin, i.e. preceding the date (6, 10, 23). Most Egyptian Day entries in the calendar are rubricated. Therefore, they are easily spotted by a trained eye, even though the entry is sometimes no more than a simple "D" (8-10, 15, 23). Scribes who inserted entries on the Egyptian Days must have been aware of what the days signified, as some calendars alternate between "dies egyptiacus" and "dies mala" (27-29), which is a sign that the Egyptian Days were associated with evil. Calendar (30) even glosses the entry for 25 January: "**D*ies* egyptiaca i*d est* mala**".

Among the nineteen calendars incorporating Egyptian Days, it is hard to find even two which are similar. This has at least five causes. First, it is possible that mistakes occur when scribes copy twenty-four entries. When the entry is not written immediately next to the appropriate date but in the margin, transpositions of one or more days can happen easily. The second date for October, for instance, is 22, but some calendars have 23 (29, 32). Second, many calendars do not contain a full set of Egyptian Days. Only six calendars feature the full set (5, 6, 15, 18, 23, 29). The completeness of the set of dates depends upon scribes not missing even one "D" or "D M" in the margin of their exemplar. In this respect, it is revealing that there are two calendars which lack, among others, the Egyptian Day entry for 1 August (4, 9). It is likely that the exemplar contained an entry for the Egyptian Day for 1 August in the left-hand margin, which is easily overlooked. Five calendars feature less than half the number of entries (8, 17, 27, 28, 30). Third, some calendars are over-complete in that they contain three instead of two entries for one particular month (8, 15, 18). Calendar (8) lists 1, 27 and 28 March as Egyptian Days. It is probable that the scribe made a mistake of the type mentioned above in that he erroneously entered the second date for March under 27 instead of the usual date 28, and corrected it without erasing or expunging the faulty reading. (18) has entries for 7, 12 and 15 December. The entry for 12 December was erased. A preference for 7 over 12 December may have arisen out of the ambiguity displayed by the hexameter verses, as discussed before. The most improbable triple sequence is in (15), viz. 12, 15 and 25 December. 12 and 15 December represent the basic set, while 25 December, Christmas Day, is impossible because Egyptian Days and church feasts do not coincide. Fourth, there are many ways in which Egyptian Days can be entered into a calendar: "dies egyptiacus", "dies mala", "dies", "d eg", "d m", "d", etc. The chance of finding two calendars which have identical phrasing is almost nil. Fifth, most calendars display the basic series of Egyptian Days, and some display incidental variations on the set. Others, however, differ significantly. Aside from mistakes and incompleteness, variation occurs of the type visible in the Old English texts explained above, i.e. 7 and 22 rather than 12 and 15 December (5, 11, 23). Such variation is attested more than once. Some calendars seem to make use of dates utterly unlike the basic series (4, 9, 27, 33). These calendars are uniquely attested and employ dates that do not resemble the basic or variant series. (27, 33) are the earliest witnesses of Egyptian Days in England, so these may be representative of a kind of continental usage which did not gain currency in England. (4, 9), however, are problematic because they are contemporary with calendars that feature the more regular series.

If these provisions are taken into account, it appears that four calendars exhibit sets which cannot be correlated to the basic or variant series (4, 9, 27, 33). Of the fifteen remaining calendars, three follow the variant set (5, 11, 23), eleven feature the basic series when errors and incompleteness are disregarded (6, 8, 10, 15, 17-19, 28-30, 32) and one has verses only (21). Of the three witnesses of the variant set (5, 11) list the dates as "dies egyptiacus" throughout, but no direct links between these calendars have been identified. Calendar (23) lists the dates as "dies mala" and "dies" and has no ties with (5, 11). The basic series is featured in eleven calendars, but incompleteness, overcompleteness and extensive variation in phrasing make it impossible to discover concrete relationships between them.

Verses on the twenty-four Egyptian Days are designed to function mnemonically through the use of metre or rhyme. These verses come in a variety of shapes, the most common in English manuscripts being twelve-line hexameter ones, which typically run as follows:

> Iani prima dies et septima fine timetur.
> Ast februi quarta est precedit tertia finem.
> Martis prima necat cuius sic cuspide quarta est.
> Aprilis decima est undena a fine minatur.
> Tertius est maio lupus est et septimus anguis.
> Iunius in decimo quindenum a fine salutat.
> Tredecimus iulii decimo innuit ante kalendas.
> Augusti nepa prima fugat de fine secundam.
> Tertia septembris uulpis ferit a pede denam.

Tertius octobris gladius decimo ordine nectit.
Quinta nouembris acus uix tertia mansit in urna.
Dat duodena cohors septem inde decemque decembri.

Hexameter verses have been attested from the ninth century onwards,[53] and have been wrongfully ascribed to Bede.[54] I have explained earlier that the hexameter verses make use of a formula in which the first date is counted from the beginning of the month and the second from the end of the month, e.g. "Iani prima dies et septima fine timetur" signifies 1 January and the seventh from the end, i.e. 25 January. In addition, hexameter verses mention the relevant month and usually include a reference to violence, death or danger. Remarkably, all instances but one of the hexameter verses are of the type I reproduced above, with some minor textual variation here and there (the exception is text 20). In continental medieval manuscripts, entirely different verses are attested next to the one discussed here.[55]

Some poems incorporate particularly dangerous hours on the Egyptian Days, the so-called Egyptian Hours, as text (20) does:

dies horam horam fine dies
Septima dat primam. sextam pede dena decembris

The interlinear gloss clarifies what the verse line conveys: the first hour on the seventh day and the sixth hour on the tenth day before the end of December are Egyptian Hours. This format is first attested in England in the early post-Conquest manuscript Caligula A. xv + Egerton 3314, and I have not been able to find any more examples in English manuscripts. All kinds of variants upon the Egyptian Day and Hour poems exist in continental manuscripts.[56] The Egyptian Hours are thought to have come into existence in the tenth century,[57] yet despite this early date and an influx of computistical and astronomical science in Benedictine Reform England, verses including hours are not found in pre-Conquest manuscripts.

An uncommon type of verse are twenty-four-line verses dealing with the twenty-four Egyptian Days and providing zodiacal information.

[53] Steele (1919: 113), Jones (1939: 73, 88).
[54] Migne (1861-1904: I.759-86, 955-56).
[55] Steele (1919: 112, 116, 117). Cf. Keil (1957: 36-37).
[56] See Muratori (1723-58: II.2.1023-41), Loiseleur (1872), Schmitz (1877: 307-20), Steele (1919).
[57] Steele (1919: 114).

These verses were not known to Steele. I have found only one instance of this type, heading the months in the calendar of Vitellius A. xviii: "*Vicenam* quin*tam iani* pri*mam*q*ue caueto. / Rorat aquarius hanc. manet alt*er*a sub capricorno*" (18). Here, end-rhyme is used, and the passage through the zodiac is mentioned. In addition, the representation of dates in a formulaic way has been abandoned, though not consistently, as the verse for March illustrates: "*Prima necat martis. quarta*m*q*ue *a fine timemus*".

Verses listing the twenty-four Egyptian Days are attested sixteen times in Anglo-Saxon manuscripts: nine in calendars (5, 10, 17-19, 21, 23, 28, 30), two in isolation (7, 20), two with introductions (22, 26), and three in stand-alone texts (16, 24, 25). Of these poems, all are twelve-line verses closely resembling the one introduced before, except for the twenty-four line zodiacal verse (18) and the glossed Egyptian Hours poem (20). The development of the verse format has already been discussed. It is striking that the verses proved very popular in calendars (format IIa) and as stand-alone texts (IIIa), whereas the number of verses in isolation (IIb) or with an introduction (IIc) is negligible. Apparently, the text required a context to exist in. The only twelve-line hexameter verses with an introduction are in the English part of the composite manuscript Sloane 475 (26),[58] and in the post-Conquest Caligula A. xv + Egerton 3314 (22). Here, the verses are enveloped by an introduction and a conclusion which explain the name of the Egyptian Days, how many there are, that one hour is particularly dangerous on each Egyptian Day, and that one should refrain from bloodletting and undertaking anything new. This redaction is often referred to as the 'Si tenebrae' poem after the opening lines "**S**i tenebre ęgyptiis [*sic*] greco sermone uocantur; / **I**nde dies mortis tenebrosos iure uocamus" (22). Migne included the 'Si tenebrae' in Bede's works under the title *De Ægyptiacis diebus*.[59]

Excluding (18, 20), the English twelve-line hexameter verses belong to several redactions. Textual variation limits itself to minor differences in vocabulary, none of which affects the meaning of the text. For instance, the verse for May "Tertius est maio lupus est et septimus anguis" may also be phrased as "Tertius in maio lupus est et septimus anguis" (5, 17, 30), or "Tertius a maio lupus est et septimus anguis" (21). The only instances where verse lines differ significantly are: "Ast februi quinta e*st* undenaque serui*et* umbris" (7) and "**AST FEBRVI QVARTA EST SED SEPTIMA SERVIET VMBRIS**" (30) for "Ast februi quarta est

[58] See pp. 42-43.

[59] Migne (1861-1904: I.955-56).

precedit tertia finem"; "**Prima necat iunii *qui*ndena a fine minat*ur***" (23) for "Iunius in decimo quindenum a fine salutat".[60] Despite these different readings, the fact that most witnesses achieve such agreement in phrasing is a sign that the mnemonic qualities of the text are indeed considerable.

Stand-alone texts on the twenty-four Egyptian Days are prose works which may contain an introduction on the nature of the days, and sometimes a metrical component in the form of hexameter verses (IIIa). These verses have an interlinear prose reiteration in the formulaic manner of counting the dates from the beginning and end of the month. If there are no verses, the introduction is followed by the formulas for each month (IIIb), or a straightforward list of Roman dates (IIIc). These formats have little in common besides the fact that they can exist as stand-alone texts, have a large prose component, and mostly include an introduction.

The rarest prose format are the Roman dates (IIIc). As far as I know, there is only one English witness, in the eleventh-century manuscript Titus D. xxvi (14). The introduction of (14) prohibits bloodletting, the planting of vineyards, harvesting and the undertaking of something new. Steele claimed a Greek origin for this introduction on the basis of two Greek texts printed by Salmasius.[61] However, Salmasius did not date the Greek texts, so it is impossible to determine which came first, the Latin or the Greek. The Latin texts emerged in the ninth century, as Steele's examples illustrate.[62] Birch exultantly took (14) for an English invention when he wrote that it was "proof of the existence of vineyards in England, which has been so often denied, so often explained away".[63] Unfortunately for Birch, the reference to vineyards must be "explained away" as part of the continental origin of the text. There is no reason to posit an English genesis for this format since ninth-century continental witnesses have been attested, including the *Epistola de diebus Ægyptiacis* attributed to Hippocrates.[64]

After the introduction, (14) continues with a long but incomplete list of Roman dates:

> .iiii. NŌN. Ian*uarii* .iii. NŌN apr*ilis*. ix. KŁ febr*uarii* .ix. KŁ. mai [*sic*] .vi. IĎ. FEBR*VARII* .ii. NŌN mai [*sic*] .vi. KŁ. mart*is* .xvi. KŁ. iun*ii* .v. NŌN

[60] "Prima" in text 8.3/23 may be a mistake for "Dena".

[61] Steele (1919: 109, 111), Salmasius (1648: 816-18).

[62] Steele (1919: 111).

[63] Birch (1878: 475, n. 5).

[64] Wickersheimer (1966: 57 [XLVIII.4], 156 [CIV.1]), Steele (1919: 111).

> mar*tis* .v. ID̄. iun*ii* .vi. KŁ apr*ilis* .xvi. KŁ iul*ii* NŌN iulii .xi. KŁ agusti .vii. ID̄ agustus. [*sic*] xiii. KŁ. Sept*embris* .iiii. NŌN. Sept*embris* .vii. KŁ. oct*o*-b*ris* .v. NŌN. oct*o*b*ris*. vii KŁ noue*mbris*.[65]

A list such as this offers numerous opportunities for mistakes. Indeed, the dates for November and December are missing. Of the twenty dates mentioned, only three coincide with the basic series. Comparison with copies of the Roman date prognostics in other manuscripts reveals that there are large differences between the lists.[66] An 'i', 'v' or 'x' is easily misplaced or overlooked, which makes this format an unreliable vehicle for the transmission of Egyptian Days.

Next are the stand-alone texts with verses and formulaic reiteration (IIIa), of which I have found three instances (16, 24, 25). This format is characterised by a hexameter poem in which each verse line is followed by a prose reiteration which uses formulas and which mentions the relevant Roman dates as well:

> **I**ANI PRIMA DIES. 7 SEPTIMA FINE TIMETVR.
> It is dangerous to be bled in the beginning of January on the first day, that is the kalends of January, and before its end the seventh day, that is the eighth kalends of February.[67]

After the last verse *raisonné*, the text ends with a goose prohibition.[68] The three texts of this format have much in common: they form part of the β-sequence; they probably all hail from New Minster, Winchester; and they were copied in the period 1023 x 1032, in the manuscripts Titus D. xxvii (16) and Harley 3271 (24, 25). Texts (16, 24, 25) represent one redaction, which is evident from the identical way of phrasing from beginning to end. The only differences of any significance are the presence of a rubric in (25); the inclusion of the phrase "**P**ericulosum est flebotomari" in the prose reiteration for January in (16); and the names of the months which preface the verse lines in (24, 25). (24, 25) are copies from the same exemplar.[69] The exemplar for the Harley copies will have been the same as, or very closely related to, the one for (16).

[65] Text 8.3/14, ll. 4-8.
[66] Cf. Schmitz (1877: 311), Wickersheimer (1966: 13 [II.1], 57 [XLVIII.4], 156 [CIV.1]), and Sloane 475, fol. 8r.
[67] Translation of text 8.3/16, ll. 1-3.
[68] See pp. 338-40.
[69] See pp. 38-39.

The final stand-alone format contains an introduction, a list of Egyptian Days in the formulaic manner, and sometimes a rudimentary moonbook (IIIb). The formulaic lists which mention the first date from the beginning of the month and the second date from the end proved quite popular. I have found six witnesses in English and about twenty in continental manuscripts.[70] In English sources, this format has appeared in three distinct redactions: one in Old English (1-3) and two in Latin (a: 12, 13; b: 31). Latin redaction (12, 13) has an introduction which is as elaborate as the one listing the Roman dates (IIIc): the prohibitions mentioned pertain to bloodletting, the planting of vineyards, the taming of animals and the undertaking of something new. This all-encompassing nefariousness is not encountered in any of the other formats or redactions in English manuscripts. After the introduction, this redaction continues with the formulaic list of dates, e.g. "Mense Ianuario die .i. 7 ante*quam* exeat die .vii." (in the month of January, the first day and before it ends the seventh day).[71] (12, 13) are identical. The two texts were copied in different foundations and a century apart, which makes it unlikely that they share a common exemplar.

The second redaction of the Latin stand-alone format with formulaic dates (31) contains the usual injunctions against bloodletting, medicinal potions and the commencement of something new. The formulas are phrased more concisely than those of (12, 13), which, in combination with a brief introduction, gives the impression that (31) represents a stripped redaction of that of (12, 13).

The most interesting redaction for Anglo-Saxonists is the Old English text on the twenty-four Egyptian Days. This redaction is attested three times (1-3). The Egyptian Days in these texts have already been discussed in the light of the variant set of dates for December in (1). (1-3) contain more information than any redaction or format of the twenty-four Egyptian Days known to me. The text opens with an introduction which refers to medical experiment:

> The doctors of old wrote in Latin books that there are always two days in each month on which it is very hurtful to drink any [medicinal] potion or to let blood, because there is a time on each of these days that if one opens

[70] Salmasius (1648: 816-18), Schmitz (1877: 307-08, 312-18), Wickersheimer (1966: 31 [XXII.6], 40 [XXVIII.6], 51-52 [XXXVIII.1], 53 [XL], 58-59 [XLVIII.6], 141 [XCII.3], 155-56 [CII.2,3], 158 [CVIII.1], 174-75 [CXIV.2]), Stuart (1979: 241-43).

[71] Text 8.3/13, l. 4.

> a vein on this time, it will cause death or protracted pain. A doctor knew this and bled his horse on such a time, and it lay dead immediately.[72]

This opening may have come into being in the translation of the text, because the reference to the doctor who bled his horse to test the validity of the theory is not found in Latin texts on the twenty-four Egyptian Days.[73] Mention is made of the Egyptian Hours (an tid is on ælcum þara daga), but they are not listed.[74] After the introduction follows a formulaic list of dates: "the first day in March, that is the month 'hlyda', and the fourth day before its end".[75] The list stands out in that it does not begin with the month of January, but with March. The reader is not left in the dark as to the reason for this change, for the list is followed by this paragraph:

> We put the month of March, which is called "hlyda", first in this account, because it [the month] forms the beginning after proper reckoning of the entire year, and almighty God created all creatures in this month.[76]

The reference to the vernacular name of March, the concern with time reckoning (rihtan getele) and the theological justification for the proper start of the year are strongly reminiscent of the work of Ælfric.[77] Ælfric's homily *Octabas et circumcisio Domini* attempts to counter all kinds of customs on the first of January with the help of doctrine and the computus by pointing out that these superstitions were for foolish people, and by observing that 1 January is not the first day of the year at all.[78]

After this Ælfrician justification for the choice of March as the first month, (1-3) continue with a rudimentary moonbook, which I discussed above.[79] The influence of Ælfric's *De temporibus anni* is felt in this moonbook as well. The moonbook is followed by yet another injunction against bloodletting, which ends with the following statement: "nis þis nan wiglung. ac wise menn hit afunden þurh þone halgan wisdom swa heom god ælmihtig gedihte" (this is no divination, but wise men discovered it through the holy wisdom as the almighty God revealed to

---

[72] Translation of text 8.3/1, ll. 1-5.

[73] Because of this reference to horse bleeding, Smith (1919-33: I.70) drew attention to this passage in his opus *The Early History of Veterinary Literature and its British Development.*

[74] The same applies to the 'Si tenebrae' redaction of the hexameter verses.

[75] Translation of text 8.3/1, l. 7.

[76] Translation of text 8.3/1, ll. 20-22.

[77] An excellent analysis of the influence of Ælfric on the Old English translation of the twenty-four Egyptian Days is provided by Henel (1934-35: 341-46).

[78] Clemoes (1997: 224-31).

[79] See pp. 351-52.

them).[80] These words echo phrases exclusively found in Ælfric's homilies *Octabas et circumcisio Domini* (nis þis nan wiglung ac is gecyndelic þing þurh gesceapenysse) and *De auguriis* (þis nis nan wiglung).[81] Similarly, the phrase with which the days are introduced in (3), "swa swa us seicgaþ bec" (as the books tell us), is found almost exclusively in Ælfric's writings.[82] In short, the translator of the twenty-four Egyptian Days was thoroughly familiar with the computistical and homiletic works of Ælfric, while Ælfric was at home in some prognostic genres, including the Egyptian Days.[83] The order of the formulaic list of dates, the explanation for starting with March, the rudimentary moonbook and the additional injunction against bloodletting are not encountered in Latin witnesses of the twenty-four Egyptian Days and must, therefore, have originated in the process of translation. Text (3) ends with a goose prohibition which is not included in (1, 2). This prohibition is presumably a condensed version of the three Egyptian Days, and is not encountered in this form in Latin texts on the twenty-four Egyptian Days.[84] In view of the many indications that the translator modified the source text and added a considerable amount of new material partly based on Ælfric's works, (1-3) represent one of the few instances where it can actually be said that the Anglo-Saxons did more with a prognostic text than plain translation.[85]

The Old English texts on the twenty-four Egyptian Days survive in three manuscripts: (1) Caligula A. xv (s. xi² (*c.* 1073), Christ Church, Canterbury); (2) Vitellius E. xviii (1062, New Minster, Winchester); and (3) Harley 3271 (s.xi¹ (1032?), New Minster, Winchester?). They form one redaction, but they deviate in certain ways. First, (3) contains a goose prohibition which (1, 2) lack. Second, (3) has a rubric (**DE DIEBVS MALIS**) which (1, 2) lack (but then many short texts in Harley 3271 had rubrics added). Third, the text of (3) was copied in the wrong order: the introduction and the list of dates follow the justification for March, the rudimentary moonbook, the second injunction and the goose prohibition. Fourth, the dates for December are from the variant set in (1) and

[80] Text 8.3/1, ll. 27-29.

[81] See pp. 97-101, 117-21.

[82] A proximity search in Healey and Venezky (2000) on "swa", "us" and "bec" revealed that the phrase is attested frequently in Ælfric's works, but hardly anywhere else except in 8.3/3 and the *Anglo-Saxon Chronicle* entry for 1009.

[83] See pp. 99-101.

[84] See pp. 338-40.

[85] Another exception is the Old English sunshine prognostic, see pp. 483-84.

from the basic series in (2, 3). Fifth, there are some differences in phrasing, notably the following:

> (1, 2) **N**u syndon hit þas dagas swa swa hit her onsegð.
> (3) **N**u synd hit þas dagas swa swa us seicgaþ bec:-[86]

and

> (1) **O**n maius monðe se þridda dæg is derigendlic. 7 se seofoða ær his ende.
> (2) **O**n on [*sic*] þam monðe þe we maius hatað. se þridda dæg is derigen(dlic) `7 se s(e)ofeða ær his utga(nge.)´
> (3) eft is on þan monþe þe we maios hatet se þridda dæg dergendlic: 7 se seoueþa ær his ende.[87]

and

> (1) nis þis nan wiglung. ac wise menn hit afunden þurh þone halgan wisdom swa heom god ælmihtig gedihte.
> (2) (Nis þis na)n wilung. ac wise menn hit afundon þurh þone halgan gast. `swa swa him dihte god:–´
> (3) Nis þis nan wigelung ac wise men hit afundan þuruh þæne halgan wisdom swa swa him gedihte godd.[88]

These verbal differences may be the result of omissions, variation in word choice, and auto-completion mistakes ("halgan gast" instead of the not so usual collocation "halgan wisdom"). It is highly improbable that (1-3) are independent translations of a Latin exemplar, especially in view of the aforementioned additions which reveal an Ælfrician influence that probably only came into being in the process of translation. Within the extensive corpus of texts on the twenty-four Egyptian Days in English and continental manuscripts, the translation exemplified by (1-3) occupies a unique place in being a literary creation in its own right rather than a straightforward translation.

---

[86] Texts 8.3/1, l. 6, and 8.3/3, l. 7, respectively.
[87] Texts 8.3/1, l. 10, 8.3/2, ll. 11-12, and 8.3/3, ll. 12-13, respectively
[88] Texts 8.3/1, ll. 27-29, 8.3/2, ll. 29-31, and 8.3/3, ll. 30-32, respectively

Edition[89]

8.3/1 London, British Library, Cotton Caligula A. xv, fols 130v/6-131r/4

Ða ealdan læces gesetton on ledonbocum *þæt* on ælcum monðe beoð æfre twegen dagas þa syndon swiðe d`e´rigendlice ænigne drenc to drincanne. oþþe blod to lætenne forþam þe an tid is on ælcum þara daga gif man ænige æddran geopenað on þara tide *þæt* hit bið lifleast. oððe langsum sar. þæs cunnede sum læce 7 let his horse blod on þære tide. 7 hit læg sona dead.

Nu syndon hit þas dagas swa swa hit her onsegð.

Se forma dæg on martio. þæt is on hlydan monðe. 7 se feorða dæg ær his ende.

On þam oðrum monðe þe we aprelis hatað se teoða dæg is derigendlic. 7 se ændlyfte ær his ende

On maius monðe se þridda dæg is derigendlic. 7 se seofoða ær his ende.

On iunius	monðe se	.x.	dæg. 7 ær his ende se .xv.
On Iulius	monðe se	.xiii.	dæg. 7 ær his ende se .x.
On agustus	monðe se	.i.	dæg. 7 ær his ende se .ii.
On septe*mber*	monðe se	.iii.	dæg. 7 ær his ende se .x.
On octob*er*	monðe se	.iii.	dæg. 7 ær his ende se .x.
On noue*mber*	monðe se	.v.	dæg. 7 ær his ende se .iii.
On Dece*mber*	monðe se	.vii.	dæg. 7 ær his ende se .x.
On Ianuari*us*	monðe se	.i.	dæg. 7 ær his ende se .vii.
On februari*us*	monðe se	.iiii.	dæg. 7 ær his ende se þridda.

We gesetton on foreweardan þissere endebyrdnesse þone monað martius þe menn hatað hlyda. forþa*m* he is annginn æfter rihtan getele ealles þæs geares. 7 se ælmihtiga god on þam monðe gesceop ealle gesceafta.

Nu eft be þam monan is mycclu*m* to warnienne *þæt* man on .iiii. nihta ealdne monan. oþþe on .v. nihta menn blod ne læte swa us bec seggað ærþa*m* þe se mona 7 seo sǽ beon anræde.

ac we gehyrdon seggon sumne wisne mann *þæt* nan mann ne leofode þe him blod lete on ealra halgena mæssedæg. oþþe gif he gewundod wære. nis þis nan wiglung. ac wise menn hit afunden þurh þone halgan wisdom swa heom god ælmihtig gedihte.

Text is continuous. Entries for June-February are in columns | **4** lifleast] *read* his ~ *(see 8.3/2,3)* | **5** his] h- < · | **10** seofoða] ~ < [feorða] | **16** ær] æ- < [h] | **22** god] -d < a | **26** wisne] w- < ·, *the curve points upward like that of a* 'wyn', *the ascender resembles that of a* 'þ' *cut short*; ~ ‖ ⟨*f.131r*⟩.

[89] Order of the texts: 1-3, 12, 13, 31, 14, 16, 24, 25, 22, 26, 20, 7, 18, 17, 21, 28, 30, 5, 10, 19, 23, 8, 27, 6, 9, 11, 15, 29, 32, 33, 4.

8.3/2 London, British Library, Cotton Vitellius E. xviii, fol. 15r/16-15v/6

Þa ealdan læcas gesettan on ledenbocum. þ*æt* on ælcum monðe beoð æf(re) twegen dagas. þe syndon swiðe derigendlice ænigum menn drenc to drincanne. oþþe blod to lætanne. forþam þe an tid is on ælcum þæra daga. gif man ænige æddran geopenað on þære tide. þ*æt* hit bið his lif(least) oððe langsum sar. þæs cunnade sum læce. 7 let his horse blod on þære tide. and hit læg sona dead:–

Nu syndon hit þas dagas. swa swa hit her onsegð.

þ*æt* is se forma dæg on martio on hlydan monðe. 7 se feorða dæg ærþam þe he on weg fa(reð)

On þam oðrum monðe þe we aprilis hatað. s(e) teoþa dæg is deri(gendlic) and se endlyfta dæg ær his utgange.

On on þam monðe þe we maius hatað. se þridda dæg is derigen(dlic) `7 se s(e)ofeða ær his utga(nge.)´

On iunius monðe se teoða. 7 ær his ende se fifteoða.

On iulius se þreotteoða. 7 ær his ende se teoða.

On agustus se forma. 7 ær his ende se oðer.

On september se þridda. 7 ær his ende se teoða.

7 **O**n oc(tober eac se þridda. 7 ær his ende se teoða.)

On nouember se fifta. 7 ær his ende se þridda.

On december se twelfta. 7 ær his ende se seofenteoða.

On ianuarius se forma. 7 ær his ende se seofeða.

On februarius se feorða. 7 ær his ende se þridda.

We gesetton on foreweardan on þyssere endebyrd(nesse þone) monað **M**artius. þe menn hatað hlyda for(þam he is angin æfter) rihtum getele ealles þæs geares. 7 **S**e ælmih(tiga god on þam) monðe gesceop ealle gesceafta.

(Nu eft be þam monan is mycclum to warnienne) þ*æt* man on feower nihta ealdne monan. oððe on fif nihta (menn blod) ne læte. swa swa us secgað bec. ærþa*m* þe se mona. 7 seo sæ be(on anræde).

(Ac w)e gehyrdon secgan sumne mann. þ*æt* nan mann ne leofode. (þe him) blod lete on ealra halgena mæssedæg. oððe gif he gewundod wære. (Nis þis na)n wilung. ac wise menn hit afundon þurh þone halgan gast. `swa swa him dihte god:–´

Text is continuous except the list of months (each month starts on a new line except for October). Margins damaged; text illegible and partly lost at the edges. Förster's edition of this text (1929) is deficient because of the fire damage and his working from photographs | **11 On** on] *read* On *(dittography)* | **11-12** `7... utga(nge.)´] *transposition indicated* | **17** 7... teoða.)] *Förster did not see that the entry for October followed that of September, which is why he thought it had been omitted by the scribe* | **19** se$_{1}$] s- < · | seofenteoða] *Förster read* seofe(ða), *which caused him considerable confusion (see pp. 353-54)* | **24** gesceafta.] ~ ‖ ⟨*f. 15v*⟩ | **28** sumne] *read* ~ wisne *(see 8.3/1,3)* | **30** gast] *read* wisdom *(see 8.3/1,3)* | **30-31** `swa... god:–´] *transposition indicated.*

8.3/3 London, British Library, Harley 3271, fols 90v/20-91r/24

DE DIEBVS MALIS.

Þa ealdan læcas gesettan on ledenbocun: þ*æt* on ælcu*m* monðe beoð æfre twegen dagas þe syndan swyðe derigendlice ænigne drenc on to ðicgenne: oððe blod ón to lætenne: forðan þe an tid is ón ælcum þæra daga gif man ænige æddran geopenað on þære tíde: þ*æt* hit bið his lifleast. oððe langsum sar; þæs cunnode sum læce. let his horse blod on þære tide. 7 hit læg sona dead.

Nu synd hit þas dagas swa swa us seicgaþ bec:-

se forma dæg on martio þæt is on hlydan monþe. 7 se feorþa dæg ærþam þe he fare aweg.

on þam oþran monþe þe we apriles hatat: se tyoþa dæg is dergendlic: 7 se endlyfta dæg ær his utgange;

eft is on þan monþe þe we maios hatet se þridda dæg dergendlic: 7 se seoueþa ær his ende.

On iunius se teoþa 7 ær his ende se fifteoþa.

On iulius se þreotteoða 7 ær his ende se teða.

On augustu*s*. se forma: 7 ær his ende se oðer.

On septemb*er* se ðridda. 7 ær his ende se teoða.

On octob*er*. eac se ðridda: 7 ær his ende se teoða.

On nouemb*er*. se fifta: 7 ær his ende se þridda.

On decemb*er*. se twelfta: 7 ær his ende se se`o´fanteoða.

On ianuarius. se forma: 7 ær his ende se seofoða.

On februarius se feorða: 7 ær his ende se ðridda:

We gesetton on foreweardan on þysre endebyrdnesse þone monaþ martiu*m* þe menn hatat hlyda forþan he is angin æfter rihtum getele ealles þæs geares 7 se ælmihtiga god ón þam monþe gescop ealle gesceafta;

Nu æft be þam monan is miclum to warnienne þæt mon on fyuwer nihtan monan oþþe on fif nihta men blod ne læte swa swa us secgað bec ærþan þe se mona 7 syu sæ beon anræde

eac we gehyrdan seggan sumne wisne man þ*æt* nan man ne lyfode þe him lete blod on ealra halgena mæssedæig oþþe gif he gewundad wære; Nis þis nan wigelung ac wise men hit afundan þuruh þæne halgan wisdom swa swa him gedihte godd.

gyt her to eacan is to warnienne þ*æt* man ne þicge goseflæsc on þane æftemestan dæi hlydan monþes ne on þæne æftemestan dæig december manþe goseflæsc byþ æfre unhalwende þam untruman swa swa ma oþra metta þe we ne magan her secggan.

Paragraphs three to six ⟨*90v/20-91r/4*⟩ *precede one and two* ⟨*91r/5-24*⟩ | **8** þæt] -t < i | **20** se`o´fanteoða] seafanteoða, -`o´- < a_1; a_1 *not erased or expunged* | **23** martiu*m*] martiū[m]; *read* martius | **26** æft] æft[·] | **33** eacan] ~ ‖ ⟨*f. 91r*⟩ | **34** manþe] *read* monþes.

8.3/12 London, British Library, Cotton Caligula A. xv, fols 129v/27-130r/12

Non interficias nec sanguis relaxetur. nec uinea plentet*ur*. nec messis incipiatur colligere. nec uinea ematur nec uendatur. Nec animalia domentur. Nec ulla quę ad profectum pertinere debeant incipiantur. (quia isti dies maledicti sunt a) domino.

Mense **I**anuario	**i**	Et antequa*m* exeat die **vii**
Mense **F**ebruario	**iiii**	& anteq*ua*m exeat die **iii**
Mense **M**artio	**i**	& anteq*ua*m exeat die **iiii**
Mense **A**prelis	**x**	& anteq*ua*m exeat die **xi**
Mense **M**aius	**iii**	& anteq*ua*m exeat die **vii**
Mense **I**unius	**x**	& anteq*ua*m exeat die **xv**
Mense **I**ulius	**xiii**	& anteq*ua*m exeat die **x**
Mense **A**gustus	**i**	& anteq*ua*m exeat die **ii**
Mense **S**eptember	**iii**	& anteq*ua*m exeat die **x**
Mense **O**ctober	**iii**	& anteq*ua*m exeat die **x**
Mense **N**ouember	**v**	& anteq*ua*m exeat die **iii**
Mense **D**december	**vii**	Et antequa*m* exeat die **x**

Introduction is continuous; the list of the months is in columns | **1** relaxetur] relaxe- < [rexlax] | plentet*ur*] *read* plantetur | **3** (quia... a)] ~ *erased, but text 8.3/13 shows that the erasure, though intended, is misguided* | **4** domino.] ~ ‖ ⟨*f. 130r*⟩ | **16 D**december] *read* December.

8.3/13 London, British Library, Cotton Tiberius C. vi, fol. 114r/8-18

Non int*er*ficias nec sanguis relaxet*ur*. nec uinea plantet*ur*. Nec messis incipiat*ur* collig*ere*. Nec uinea emat*ur*. nec uendat*ur*. nec a*nim*alia domen*tur*. nec ulla q*ue* ad p*ro*fectum p*er*tin*er*e debeant *in*cipia*ntur*. q*uia* isti dies maledicti s*un*t a d*om*ino.
Mense Ianuario die .i. 7 anteq*uam* exeat die .vii.
Mense Frebuario die .iiii. 7 anteq*uam* exeat die .iii.
M*ense* Marcio die .i. 7 anteq*uam* exeat die .iiii.
M*ense* Ap*r*il*is* die .x. 7 an*te*q*uam* exeat die .xi.
M*ense* Mai*us* die .iii. 7 an*te*q*uam* exeat. Die .vii.
M*ense* Iuni*us* die .x. 7 an*te*q*uam* exeat die .xv.
M*ense* Iuli*us* Die .xiii. 7 an*te*q*uam* exeat Die .x.
M*ense* Aug*ustus*. die .i. 7 an*te*q*uam* exeat die .ii.
M*ense* Sept*ember*. Die .iii. 7 an*te*q*uam* exeat Die .x.
M*ense* Octob*er* Die .iii. 7 an*te*q*uam* exeat Die .x.
M*ense* Noue*mber*. Die .v. 7 an*te*q*uam* exeat die .iii.
M*ense* Dece*mber* Die .vii. 7 an*te*q*uam* exeat Die .x.

5 Frebuario] *read* Februario | **7** .xi.] -i < v.

8.3/31 Oxford, St. John's College, MS 17, fol. 40vb/32-49

De dieb*us* ęgyptiacis q*ui* maledicti s*un*t in anno.

His dieb*us* n*on* debent ho*min*es se flebotomare. nec potione*m* accip*er*e. nec ullu*m* op*us* inchoare.

Ian*uarii* .i.º die. 7 in fine .vii.º

Feb*ruarii* .iiii.º die. 7 in fine .iii.º

Mart*ii* .i. die. 7 in fine .iiii.º

Ap*ri*l*is* .x. die. 7 in fine .xi.

Ma*ii* .iii. die. 7 in fine .vii.

Iun*ii* .x. die. 7 in fine .xv.

Iul*ii* .xiii. die. 7 in fine .x.

Aug*usti* .i. die. 7 in fine .ii.

Sept*em*b*ris* .iii. die. 7 in fine .x.

Oct*o*b*ris* .iii. die. 7 in fine .x.

Nou*em*b*ris* .v. die. 7 in fine .iii.

Dec*em*b*ris* .vii. die. 7 in fine .x.

Each entry starts on a new line. Entries for June-December in columns | **12** Sept*em*b*ris*] -b- < d.

8.3/14 London, British Library, Cotton Titus D. xxvi, fol. 5r/1-13

Incipiunt dies aegiptiaci qui in anno obseruandi sunt p*er* unu*m*que*m*que m*en*se*m* ii. duo non iteratur homo. non uinea plantatur. non m*es*sis trituretur. **N**on causa sequatur. non opus quod ad p*er*fectu*m* esse deb*et* facere. quia maledicti sunt .iiii. NŌN. Ian*uarii* .iii. NŌN apr*ilis*. ix. KŁ febr*uarii* .ix. KŁ. mai .vi. ID̄. FEBR*VARII* .ii. NŌN mai .vi. KŁ. mart*is* .xvi. KŁ. iun*ii* .v. NŌN mar*tis* .v. ID̄. iun*ii* .vi. KŁ apr*ilis* .xvi. KŁ iul*ii* NŌN iulii .xi. KŁ agusti .vii. ID̄ agustus. xiii. KŁ. Sept*embris* .iiii. NŌN. Sept*em*b*ris* .vii. KŁ. oct*o*b*ris* .v. NŌN. oct*o*b*ris*. vii KŁ noue*m*b*ris*.

2 ii. duo] *read* ii. *(dittography)* | **3** p*er*fectu*m*] *read* profectum | quia] *read* ~ hi dies a domino | **4,5** mai] *read* maii | **6** agustus] *read* agusti.

8.3/16 London, British Library, Cotton Titus D. xxvii, fol. 22r-22v/16

IANI PRIMA DIES. 7 SEPTIMA FINE TIMETVR.-

Periculosum est flebotomari in principio mensis ianuarii. hoc est kł ianuarii. & ante eius exitum die .vii.ª hoc e*st* .vii.ª kł febr*uarii*.

2 ianuarii$_1$] *read* ~ dies primus | **3** .vii.ª$_2$] *read* .viii.ª.

AST FEBRVI QVARTA EST PRECEDIT TERTIA FINEM.
principio mensis februarii die quarto. hoc est .ii. nonas febr*uarii*. & ante eius exitum dies tertius hoc e*st* .iiii.[a] kł martii.

MARTIS PRIMA NECAT CVIVS SIC CVSPIDE QVARTA EST.
In principio mensis martii die primo hoc e*st* kł martii. & ante eius exitum die quarto. hoc e*st* .v. kł. aprilis.

APRILIS DECIMA EST VNDENO A FINE MINATVR.
I principio mensis aprilis dies decimus. hoc e*st* .iiii.[a] idus aprilis. & ante eius exitum die undecimo: hoc e*st* .xii. kł. maii.

TERTIVS. EST. MAIO LVPVS EST ET SEPTIMVS ANGVIS.
A principio mensis mai die tertio. hoc e*st* .v. nonas mai. & ante eius exitum die septimo. hoc e*st* .viii. kł. iunii.

IVNIVS IN DECIMO QVINDENVM FINE SALVTAT.
A principio mensis iunii. die .x.[o] hoc e*st* .iiii. idus iunii. & ante eius exitum die .xv. hoc e*st* .xvi. kł. iulii.

TREDECIMVS IVLII DECIMA INNVIT ANTE KALENDAS.
A principio mensis iulii die tertio decimo. hoc e*st* .iii. idus iulii. & ante eius exitum die decimo. hoc e*st* .xi. kł. augusti.

AVGVSTI NEPA PRIMA FVGAT DE FINE SECVNDAM.
A principio mensis augusti die primo hoc e*st* kł augusti. & ante eius exitum die secundo. hoc e*st* `.iii.[a]´ kł septembris.

TERTIA SEPTEMBRIS VVLPIS FERIT A PEDE DENAM.
A principio mensis septembris die tertio. hoc e*st* .iii. nonas septembris. & ante ei*us* exitum die decimo. hoc e*st* xi kł octobris.

TERTIVS OCTOBRIS GLADIVS DECIMO ORDINE NECTIT.
A principio mensis octobris die .iii. hoc e*st* .v. nonas octobris. & ante eius exitum die decimo hoc e*st* xi kł nouembris.

QVINTA NOVEMBRIS ACVS VIX TERTIA MANSIT IN VRNA.
A principio mensis nouembris. die .v. hoc e*st* nonas nouembris. & ante eius exitu*m* die tertio. hoc e*st* .iiii. kł decembris.

5 principio] *read* A ~ *(see 8.3/24,25)* | **11 I**] *read* A *(see 8.3/24,25)* | **14** $mai_{1,2}$] *read* maii | **23** augusti.] ~ ‖ ⟨*f. 22v*⟩.

DAT DVODENA COHORS SEPTEM INDE DECEMQ*VE* DECEMBRI.

A principio mensis decembris die xii. hoc e*st* .ii. idus decembris. & ante eius exitum die .xvii. hoc e*st* xviii kł ianuarii.

Sup*er* omnes hos. sunt etiam isti obseruabiles. **A**b initio mensis augusti. dies primus lunę. insup*er* & de martio ac decembri nouissimi dies eiusde*m* feriæ. in quibus & esus cuiuslib*et* anseris p*ro*ibetur.

8.3/24 London, British Library, Harley 3271, fol. 120v/1-20

`IAN*VARIVS*´

`Ia*ni* prima dies & septima fine timetur´

In principio mensis Ianuarii. dies primus. `kł ian*uarii*´ & ante eius exitum dies septimus. `hoc *est* vii. kł febr*uarii*´

`Ast februi quarta *est* precedit t*er*tia fine*m*´

A principio mensis februarii. dies quartus. & ante eius exitum dies. t*er*tius `hoc *est* iiii kł `mi*n*ar´´

`Martiu*s*´

`martis prima negat cuius sic cuspide quarta *est*´

In principio mensis martii. dies .i. `kł mar*tii*´ & ante eius exitu*m* dies .iiii.$^{tus}$ `hoc *est* v. ƙ apr*ilis*´

`Aprelis decima *est* undeno a fine timetur´

A principio mensis aprelis dies .x.^{mus} & ante eius exitum dies .xi.^{mus} hoc *est* xii. kł mai*i*.

`Tertius *est* maio lupus est & septimus anguis´

A principio mensis mai*i* dies .iii. & ante eius exitum dies .vii.^{mus}

`Iunius in decimo quindenu*m* fine salutat´

A principio mensis iun*ii* dies .decimus. & ante eius exitu*m* dies .xv.^{mus}

This text has been revised extensively with interlinear additions and additions in the left and top margins: (1) January and March are mentioned in the left margin; (2) calendar dates for the Egyptian Days of January-March were added in the left margin; April has the calendar date for the second Egyptian Day in original position, and after that dates are lacking altogether (for the calendar dates, which I have not provided here when they are absent in the MS, see 8.3/16,25); (3) hexameter verses were added between the lines, preceded by the comment `hoc ipsum metrice´ *added in the top margin. This text is part of the first* β*-sequence in Harley 3271; the second copy is carried out with more care* | **3** `kł ian*uarii*´] *in top margin, to the left* | **4** `hoc *est* vii. kł febr*uarii*´] *two lines down, also in the left margin:* `[vii kł febr*uarii*]´ | vii.] *read* viii. | **7** `mi*n*ar´] `mīar´; *read* martii | **9** negat] *read* necat.

`Tredecimus iulii decima innuit ante kalendas´
A principio mensis iulii dies .xiiii.^{mus} & ante eius exitum dies .x.^{mus}

`Agusti nepa prima fugat de fine secunda´
In principio mensis augusti. dies .unus. & ante eius exitum dies .ii.^{us}

`Tertia septembris uulpis ferit a pede denam´
A principio mensis septembris dies .iii. & ante eius exitum dies decimus.

`Tertius octobris gladius decimo ordine nectit´
A principio mensis octobris dies .iii. & ante eius exitu*m* dies .decim*us*.

`Quinta nouembris acus uix tertia mansit in urna´
A principio mensis nouembris dies .v. & ante eius exitum dies .tertius.

`Dat duodena cohors septe*m* inde dece*m*que decembri´
A principio mensis decembr*is*. dies .xii. & ante eius exitum dies .xvii.

Sup*er* om*ne*s hos sunt *et*iam isti obseruabiles. Ab initio mensis augusti. dies primus lunę. insup*er* & de martio. ac decembri nouissimi eiusdem ferię in quibus & esus cuiuslib*et* anseris p*ro*hib*et*ur.

20 .xiiii.^{mus}] *read* .xiii.^{mus} | **31-32** dies primus lunę] ~ *glossed by* se forma monandæg | **32** nouissimi] *interlinear explanatory gloss: scilicet* dies.

8.3/25 London, British Library, Harley 3271, fol. 122r-122v/7

VERSVS AD DIES AEGYPTIACOS. INVENI`A´NDAS.

IANI PRIMA DIES ET SEPTIMA. FINE TIMETVR. **IANVAR*IVS*.**
In principio m*en*sis ianuarii dies prim*us*. hoc *est* kł ian*uarii*. & ante ei*us* exitu*m* dies septim*us*. hoc *est* viii. kł febr*uarii*.

FEBRVAR*IVS*.
AST FEBRVI QVARTA EST. PRECEDIT TERTIA FINE*M*.
A principio m*en*sis febr*uarii* dies quart*us*. hoc *est* ii. NŌN febr*uarii*. & ante ei*us* exitu*m* dies tertius. hoc *est* iiii. kł mar*tii*.

Entries for the Egyptian Days start on a new line; the goose prohibition is continuous. The rubricated names of the months are on the right-hand side of the page opposite the prose explanations of the hexameter verses. Henel (1934-35) did not print these names | **1** INVENI`A´NDAS] INVENI[E]NDAS, [E] < `A´.

MARTIVS.

MARTIS P*RI*MA NECAT CVIVS SIC CVSPIDE QVARTA EST.

In principio m*en*sis mar*tii*. dies prim*us*. hoc *est* kł mar*tii*. & ante eius exitu*m* dies quartus. hoc *est* v. kł apr*ili*s.

APRELIS DECIMA EST. VNDENO A FINE TIMETVR. **APRILIS.**

A principio m*en*sis apr*ilis*. dies decim*us*. hoc *est* iiii. id̄ apr*ilis*. & ante ei*us* exitu*m* dies undecim*us*. hoc *est* xii kł mai.

TERTIVS EST MAIO LVPVS EST ET SEPTIMVS ANGVIS. **MAIVS.**

principio m*en*sis maii dies tertius. hoc *est* v. NŌN. mai. & ante ei*us* exitu*m*. dies septimus. hoc *est* viii. kł iun*ii*.

IVNIVS IN DECIM*O*. QVINDENV*M* FINE SALVTAT. **IVNIVS.**

A principio m*en*sis iunii. dies .x.*mus* hoc *est* iiii. id̄. iun*ii*. & ante ei*us* exitu*m* dies quint*us* decim*us*. hoc *est* xvi. kł iulii.

TREDECIMVS IVLII DECIMA INNVIT \`ante´ KALENDAS. **IVLIVS.**

A principio m*en*sis iulii dies xiii.*mus* hoc *est* iii. idus iulii. & ante eius exitum dies .x.*mus* hoc *est* xi kł agusti.

AGVSTI NEPA PRIMA FVGAT DE FINE SECVNDA. **AGVSTVS.**

In principio m*en*sis agusti dies p*rimus* id *est* kł ag*usti*. & ante ei*us* exitu*m* dies secundus. hoc *est* \`iii. kł sept*embris*;´

SEPTEMB*ER*.

TERTIA SEPTEMBRIS VVLPIS FERIT A PEDE DENAM.

A principio m*en*sis sept*em*br*is*. dies tertius hoc *est* iii. NŌN septembr*is*. & ante eius exitum dies decimus id *est* xi. kł octobr*is*.

OCT*OBER*.

TERTIVS OCTOBRIS GLADIVS DECIMO ORDINE NECTIT:

A principio m*en*sis octobris. dies tertius hoc *est* v. NŌN. & ante eius exitu*m* dies decimus. hoc *est* xi. kł nouembr*is*.

NOVEMB*ER*.

QVINTA NOVEMBRIS ACVS VIX TERTIA MANSIT IN VRNA.

A principio m*en*sis nou*em*br*is* dies .v. hoc *est* NŌN nouembris. & ante exitu*m* dies .iii.*us* hoc *est* iiii. kł decembr*is*.

15 mai] *read* maii | **17** principio] read A ~ *(see 8.3/16,24)* | mai] *read* maii | **27** \`iii. kł sept*embris*;´] *transposition from line above indicated* | **29** A] ~ *on erasure* | **34** NŌN.] *read* ~ octobris | **38** exitu*m*] *read* eius ~.

DECEMB*ER*.

DAT DVODENA COHORS SEPTEM INDE DECEMQ*VE* DECEMBRI.

A principio m*en*sis dece*m*bri*s* dies .xii.^{mus} hoc *est* ii. id̄. decembri*s* & ante eius exitum dies .xvii.^{mus} hoc *est* xviii. kł ianuarii

Super om*ne*s hos: sunt etia*m* isti obseruabiles. **A** principio m*en*sis agusti dies primus lune insuper & de martio ac decembre dies nouissimi eiusdem ferię in q*ui*b*us* & esus cuiuslibet anseris p*ro*hibetur.

40 DECEMB*ER*.] ~ ‖ ⟨*f. 122v*⟩ | **44 A** principio] *read* ab initio *(see 8.3/16,24); probably an eye slip (see l. 42)* | **45** decembre] decembri *8.3/16,24.*

8.3/22 London, British Library, Egerton 3314, fol. 50r/3-50v/1

DE DIEB*VS* EG*YPTIACIS*.

Si tenebre ęgyptiis greco sermone uocantur;
Inde dies mortis tenebrosos iure uocamus;
Bis deni biniq*ue* dies scribuntur in annos;
In quib*us* una sol*et* mortalib*us* hora timeri;
Mensis quisq*ue* duos captiuos posid*et* horu*m*;
Ne simul hos uinctos homines ne peste trucident;
Iani p*ri*ma dies & septima fine timetur;
Ast f*e*br*ui* quarta e*st* p*re*cedit tertia fine*m*;
Martis p*ri*ma necat cui*us* e cuspide quarta e*st*;
April*is* decima est undena & fine timetur;
Tercius maio lupus est & septim*us* anguis;
Iunius undecim*us*o q*ui*ndenu*m* a fine salutat;
Tredecim*us* iulii. decimo innuit ante k*alendas*;
Augustus nepa p*ri*ma fugat de fine s*ecun*dam;
Tertia septe*m*bris uulpis ferit a pede denam;
Tertius octobris gladius decimum;
Quinta noue*m*bris acus uix t*er*tiam mansit in urna;
Dat duodena cohors se*m*pte*m* i*n* dece*m*q*ue* dece*m*bris;
His caueas ne quid p*ro*pr*i*o de sanguine demas;
Nullu*m* op*us* i*n*cipias nisi forte ad gaudia tendat;
Et caput & fine*m* m*en*sis i*n* corde teneto;
Nec i*n* medio ima ruas sed clara p*er* ęthera uiuas;

Each entry starts on a new line | **2** ęgyptiis] *read* ęgyptus | **4** annos] *read* anno | **7 N**e] *read* Nec | **10** e] *read* sic | **13** undecim*us*o] *with an* -us *abbreviation over* -m-; *read* in decimo | **15 A**ugustus] *read* Augusti | **17** decimum] *read* ~ ordine nectit | **18** t*er*tiam] *read* t*er*tia | **19** se*m*pte*m*] sēptē; *read* septem | i*n*] *read* inde *(*-de *probably forgotten because of* decemque *following)* | **22** teneto;] ~ ‖ ⟨*f. 50v*⟩ | **23 N**ec] *read* Ne.

8.3/26 London, British Library, Sloane 475, fols 216v/4-217r/6

Si ténębrę ęgýptus grecos sermóne uocántur.
In die dies mortis tenebrosus iure uocam*us*.
Bis deni biniq*ue* dies scribúnt*ur*. *in* annó.
In q*ui*b*us* una sol*et* mortahora timéri.
Mensis q*ui*sq*ue* duos captiuos posid*et* heru*m*.
Nec simul hos uinctos homines repeste trucidánt.
Iani p*ri*ma dies & septimá fine timetur.
Ast februi quarta est p*re*cedit t*er*tia fine*m*;
Mantis p*ri*ma necat cuius sic cuspide quarta est.
App*re*lis decima est unde & fine*m* miratur.
Tertio*us* est maio lup*us*. & septim*us* anguis;
Iunius in decimo quindęnu*m* a fine salutat*ur*.
Terdecim*us* iulii. decimo innuit ante calendas;
Angustí nepa príma fugat de fine secu*n*da*m*
Tercia septe*m*bris uulpis ferat a pede dena*m*.
Tercius hóctobris gládius decimu*m* ordine nectit.
Quinta nouembris acus uix tercia mansit in urna.
Dat duodena choors septe*m* inde dęce*m*q*ue* dece*m*ber.
His caueas ne quis p*ro*p*ri*o de sanguinę demas.
Nullu*m* opus incipias. nisi forte ad gaudia temdat.
Vt cáput & fine*m* m*en*sis. in corde teneto.

The last line is missing | **1** grecos] *read* greco | **2** In die] *read* Inde | tenebrosus] *read* tenebrosos | **4** mortahora, h- < ci; *read* mortalibus hora | **5** heru*m*] *read* horum | **6** repeste] *read* ne peste | **9** Mantis] *read* Martis | **10** unde & fine*m* miratur] *metrically,* miratur *is the correct reading in the unemended line, but read* undeno a fine minatur | **11** Tertio*us*] *read* Terti*us* | anguis] -n- < · | **12** salutat*ur*] *read* salutat | **14** Angustí] *read* Augusti | **15** ferat] *read* ferit | **16** ordine] ~ ‖ ⟨*f.* 217r⟩ | **20** temdat] *read* tendat.

8.3/20 London, British Library, Egerton 3314, fol. 18r/1-25

Histis mortiferam cognoscite uersib*us* horam.

die horam fine dies horam
Dat prima umdenam ianus. pede: septima sextam.
horam die fine dies horam
Februus octauam quarta pede: tertia denam.
die horam dies horam
Mar prima primam. finalis quarta secundam.
die hora die hora
In decimo prima est. undeno undenaq*ue* aprilis.

Each entry starts on a new line | **3** umdenam] *read* undenam | **7 M**ar] *read* Mars.

dies horam fine dies horam
Tertius in maia sextam. pede: septima denam.
die horam dies horam
In decimo sextam iunius. quindenaq*ue* quartam.
die horam fine dies horam
Tredecimo undenam iulius pede: denus eamdem.
die hora hora die
Augusti in prima est par. septima fine *secun*da.
dies horam dies fine horam
Tertia septembris parilem. decimus pede quartam.
dies horam dies fine horam
Tertius octobris quintam. decimus pede nonam.
horam die fine dies horam
Octauam quinta noni. pede: tertia quintam.
dies horam horam fine dies
Septima dat primam. sextam pede dena decembris

11 maia] *read* maio | **23** noni] *read* noui.

8.3/7 Cambridge, Trinity College, R. 15. 32, p. 37

KŁ IAN*VARII*. Iani prima dies. & septima fine tim*et*ur.
KŁ FEB*RVARII*. Ast februi quinta e*st* undenaque serui*et* umbris.
KŁ MAR*TII*. Martis prima necat cuius quasi cuspide quarta est.
KŁ APR*ILIS*. Aprilis decima est undena a fine minatur.
KŁ MAI*I*. Tertius est maio lupus est & septimus anguis.
KŁ IVN*II*. Iunius in decimo quindenum a fine salutat.
KŁ IVL*II*. Tredecimus iulii decimo innuit ante kalendas.
KŁ AG*VS*T*I*. Augusti nepa prima fugat de fine secundam.
KŁ SEPT*EMBRIS*. Tertia septembris uulpis ferit a pede denam.
KŁ OCT*OBRIS*. Tertius octobris gladius decimo ordine nectit.
KŁ NOV*EMBRIS*. Quinta nouembris uix tertia mansit in urna.
KŁ DEC*EMBRIS*. Dat duodena cohors septem inde decemq*ue* decembri.

Each entry starts on a new line | **11** uix] *read* acus ~ | **12** duodena] -u- < y.

8.3/18 London, British Library, Cotton Vitellius A. xviii, fols 3r-8v

⟨Jan⟩	Vicenam quintam iani primamque caueto.
	Rorat aquarius hanc. manet altera sub capricorno.
⟨1 Jan⟩	Dies eg
⟨25 Jan⟩	.Dies egiptiacus.
⟨Feb⟩	Quarta dies februi. uicenaque sexta timetur
	Rorat aquarius hanc. sub piscibus illa tenetur.
⟨4 Feb⟩	Dies Egiptiacus.
⟨26 Feb⟩	Dies Egiptiacus.
⟨Mar⟩	Prima necat martis. quartamque a fine timemus.
	Istius pisces aries ius optinet huius.
⟨1 Mar⟩	.Dies egiptiacus.
⟨28 Mar⟩	.Dies egiptiacus.
⟨Apr⟩	Denam & uicenam aprilis scito esse nociuam.
	Possidet hanc aries. taurus sibi uendicat illam.
⟨10 Apr⟩	.Dies egiptiacus.
⟨20 Apr⟩	.Dies egiptiacus.
⟨May⟩	Tercia de Maio nocet. & uicesima quinta.
	Sub tauro manet hec. & sub geminis latet illa.
⟨3 May⟩	.Dies.
⟨25 May⟩	.Dies eg
⟨June⟩	Dena necat iulii. quindena a fine minatur.
	Vtraque sub geminis occidit. & insidiatur.
⟨10 June⟩	.Dies egiptiacus.
⟨16 June⟩	.Dies egiptiacus.
⟨July⟩	Tredecima in iulio et uicena secunda (noc)ebit.
	Subditur hec cancro. subponitur illa leoni.
⟨13 July⟩	.Dies egiptiacus.
⟨22 July⟩	Dies egiptiacus.
⟨Aug⟩	(Augu)sti prima. simul & tricena cauenda est.
	hanc leo perstringit. sub signo uirginis illa est.
⟨1 Aug⟩	Dies
⟨30 Aug⟩	.Dies
⟨Sept⟩	Tercia septembris. nocet & uicesima prima.
	Virgo possidet hanc. illam retinet sibi libra.
⟨3 Sept⟩	Dies egiptiacus.
⟨21 Sept⟩	.Dies egiptiacus.
⟨Oct⟩	Octobris ternum fuge. uicenumque secundum.
	Sub libra manet hic. & scorpius optinet illum.

Egyptian Day entries are later additions to the calendar | **1** ⟨*f. 3r*⟩ | **3** *eg*] *read egiptiacus* | **5** ⟨*f. 3v*⟩ | **9** ⟨*f. 4r*⟩ | **13** ⟨*f. 4v*⟩ | **17** ⟨*f. 5r*⟩ | **20** *eg*] *read egiptiacus* | **21** ⟨*f. 5v*⟩ | *iulii*] *read iunii* | **25** ⟨*f. 6r*⟩ | **29** ⟨*f. 6v*⟩ | **33** ⟨*f. 7r*⟩ | **37** ⟨*f. 7v*⟩.

39 ⟨3 Oct⟩ .*D*ies *e*giptiacus.
⟨22 Oct⟩ .*D*ies *e*giptiacus.
⟨Nov⟩ *Q*u*inta nouembris obest. ternam de fine cauete.*
42 *Scorp*ius *hanc pungit. latet illa sub architenen*te.
⟨5 Nov⟩ .*D*ies *e*giptiacus.
⟨28 Nov⟩ .*D*ies *e*giptiacus.
45 ⟨Dec⟩ *Dat duodena necem. nocet & q*uin*dena dec*em*bris.*
*Vtraq*ue *letif*eru*m uulnus timet architenentis.*
⟨7 Dec⟩ *D*ies
48 ⟨12 Dec⟩ [*D*ies. *e*giptiacus.]
⟨15 Dec⟩ *D*ies *e*giptiacus.

41 ⟨*f. 8r*⟩ | **45** ⟨*f. 8v*⟩ | **48** [Dies. *e*giptiacus.]] ~ *erased, but still clearly legible and hence included in Wormald (1934). The three entries for December probably indicate confusion between the dates mentioned in the verses and the alternative set of dates sometimes listed in calendars (see pp. 354-56).*

8.3/17 London, British Library, Cotton Vitellius A. xii, fols 72v-77v

⟨Jan⟩ **I**ani p*ri*ma dies & septima fine minat*ur*.
⟨Feb⟩ **A**st februi quarta est p*re*cedit t*er*tia fine*m*.
3 ⟨26 Feb⟩ Dies egy*ptiacus*
⟨Mar⟩ **M**artis p*ri*ma necat. cui*us* sub cuspide q*ua*rta est
⟨Apr⟩ Ap*ri*lis decima e*st* undena `a´ fine timet*ur*
6 ⟨May⟩ Terci*us* in maio lup*us est* & septim*us* anguis.
⟨June⟩ Iuni*us* undecimo. Quindenu*m* a fine remordet
⟨July⟩ **T**redecim*us* iulii decimo innuit ante kalendas.
9 ⟨Aug⟩ **A**ugusti nepa p*ri*ma fugat de fine *se*cu*n*da.
⟨Sept⟩ **T**ertia septe*m*bris uulpes ferit a pede dena*m*
⟨Oct⟩ Terci*us* octob`r´iss gladi*us* decima*m* ordine nectit.
12 ⟨Nov⟩ **v** nouembris uix t*er*cia mansit in urna.

1 ⟨*f. 72v*⟩ | **2** ⟨*f. 73r*⟩ | **4** ⟨*f. 73v*⟩ | sub] *read* sic | **5** ⟨*f. 74r*⟩ | **6** ⟨*f. 74v*⟩ | **7** ⟨*f. 75r*⟩ | undecimo] *read* in decimo | **8** ⟨*f. 75v*⟩ | **9** ⟨*f. 76r*⟩ | **10** ⟨*f. 76v*⟩ | uulpes] *read* uulpis | **11** ⟨*f. 77r*⟩ | octob`r´iss] s_1 < r; *read* octobris | decima*m*] *read* decimo | **12** ⟨*f. 77v*⟩ | uix] *read* acus ~.

8.3/21 London, British Library, Egerton 3314, fols 18v-30r

⟨Jan⟩	**Iani p*rima* dies. & .vii.^{ma} a fine timetur.**
⟨Feb⟩	**Ast febr*ui* quarta e*st* p*re*cedit tertia finem.**
⟨Mar⟩	**Martis prim*a* necat. cui*us* sic cuspide quarta est:-**
⟨Apr⟩	**Aprilis .x.^{ma} est. undeno a fine timetur.**
⟨May⟩	**[Ter]tius a maio lupus est. & septimus anguis:-**
⟨June⟩	**Vndecimus iunius quindenu*m* a fine salutat.**
⟨July⟩	**Tredecim*us* iulii decimo innuit ante kalendas:-**
⟨Aug⟩	**Augusti nepa p*ri*ma fugat de fine s*ecun*da.**
⟨Sept⟩	**Tertius septe*m*bris uulpis ferit a pede denam.**
⟨Oct⟩	**TERTIVS OCTOBRIS GLADIVS DECEM IN ORDINE NECTIT:-**
⟨Nov⟩	**QVINTA NOVEMBRIS ACVS VIX T*ER*CIA MANSIT IN VRNA:-**
⟨Dec⟩	**Dat duodena choors septe*m* inde dece*m*q*ue* dece*m*br*is*.**

1 ⟨*f. 18v*⟩ | ⟨*f. 19v*⟩ | **3** ⟨*f. 20v*⟩ | **4** ⟨*f. 21v*⟩ | **5** ⟨*f. 22v*⟩ | **[Ter]tius**] **[Ter]** *erroneously erased to make room for the large KL initial customary in calendars* | **6** ⟨*f. 23v*⟩ | **Vndecimus**] *read* In decimo | **7** ⟨*f. 24v*⟩ | **8** ⟨*f. 25v*⟩ | **9** ⟨*f. 26v*⟩ | **10** ⟨*f. 27v*⟩ | **12** ⟨*f. 28v*⟩ | **14** ⟨*f. 29v*⟩.

8.3/28 Oxford, Bodleian Library, Douce 296, fols 1r-6v

⟨Jan⟩	**IANI PRIMA DIES ET SEPTIMA FÍNE TIMETVR.**
⟨Feb⟩	**AST FEBRVI .IIII. EST PRĘCEDIT TERTIA FINEM.**
⟨Mar⟩	**Martis prIMA NECAT CVI*VS* SIC CVSPIDE QVARTA EST.**
⟨Apr⟩	**Aprilis decima est undeno a fine minatur.**
⟨May⟩	**Tertius est maio lupus est & septimus anguis.**
⟨June⟩	**uni*us* in decimo quindenum a fine salutat.**
⟨10 June⟩	**Dies aegypti**
⟨July⟩	**Tredecimus iulii decimo innuit ante kalendas.**
⟨13 July⟩	**Dies mala.**
⟨Aug⟩	**Augusti nepa prima fugat de fine secundam.**
⟨Sept⟩	**Tertia septembr*is* uulpis ferit a pede denam.**
⟨Oct⟩	**Tertius octobris gladius decimo ordine nectit.**
⟨Nov⟩	**Quin nouembris acus uix tertia mansit in urna.**
⟨Dec⟩	**Dat duodena cohors .vi.^{tem} inde decemq*ue* December.**

1 ⟨*f. 1r*⟩ | **2** ⟨*f. 1v*⟩ | **3** ⟨*f. 2r*⟩ | **5** ⟨*f. 2v*⟩ | **6** ⟨*f. 3r*⟩ | **7** ⟨*f. 3v*⟩ | **uni*us***] *read* Iunius | **8 aegypti**] *read* aegyptiacus | **9** ⟨*f. 4r*⟩ | **11** ⟨*f. 4v*⟩ | **12** ⟨*f. 5r*⟩ | **13** ⟨*f. 5v*⟩ | **14** ⟨*f. 6r*⟩ | **Quin**] *read* Quinta | **15** ⟨*f. 6v*⟩ | **.vi.^{tem}**] *read* .vii.^{tem}.

8.3/30 Oxford, St. John's College, MS 17, fols 16r-21v

⟨Jan⟩ **IANI PRIMA DIES ET SEPTIMA FINE TIMETVR.**
⟨1 Jan⟩ **D*ies* mala.**
⟨25 Jan⟩ **D*ies* egyptiaca *id est* mala.**
⟨Feb⟩ **AST FEBRVI QVARTA EST SED SEPTIMA SERVIET VMBRIS.**
⟨Mar⟩ **MARTIS PRIMA NECAT CVIVS QVASI CVSPIDE QVARTA EST.**
⟨4 Mar⟩ **D*ies* mala.**
⟨Apr⟩ **APRILIS DECIMA EST VNDENE A FINE MINATVR.**
⟨May⟩ **TERCIVS \`IN´ MAIO LVPVS EST ET SEPTIM*VS* ANGVIS.**
⟨June⟩ **IVNIVS IN DECIMO QVINDENV*M* A FINE SALVTAT.**
⟨July⟩ **Tredecim*us* iulii decimo innuit ante kalendas.**
⟨Aug⟩ **AVGVSTI NEPA PRIMA FVGAT DE FINE SECVNDAM.**
⟨Sept⟩ **TERTIA SEPTEMBRIS VVLPIS FERIT A PEDE DENAM.**
⟨Oct⟩ **TERTIVS OCTOBRIS GLADIVS DECIMO ORDINE NECTIT.**
⟨Nov⟩ **QVINTA NOVE*M*BRIS ACVS VIX TERCIA MANSIT IN VRNA.**
⟨Dec⟩ **DAT DVODENA COHORS SEPTEM INDE DECEMQ*VE* DECEMBER.**

1 ⟨*f. 16r*⟩ | **4** ⟨*f. 16v*⟩ | **6** ⟨*f. 17r*⟩ | **9** ⟨*f. 17v*⟩ | **10** ⟨*f. 18r*⟩ | \`**IN**´] ~ *over* [**EST**] | **11** ⟨*f. 18v*⟩ | **12** ⟨*f. 19r*⟩ | **13** ⟨*f. 19v*⟩ | **14** ⟨*f. 20r*⟩ | **15** ⟨*f. 20v*⟩ | **17** ⟨*f. 21r*⟩ | **19** ⟨*f. 21v*⟩.

8.3/5 Cambridge, Trinity College, O. 7. 41, fols 1v-7r

⟨Jan⟩ Iani p*ri*ma dies: & septima fine timet*ur*.
⟨1 Jan⟩ dies egypt*iacus*
⟨25 Jan⟩ D*ies* egypt*iacus*
⟨Feb⟩ Ast februi quarta *est*: p*re*cedit t*er*cia fine*m*.
⟨4 Feb⟩ dies egypt*iacus*
⟨26 Feb⟩ D*ies* egypt*iacus*
⟨Mar⟩ Martis p*ri*ma necat cui*us* de cuspide q*ua*rta *est*.
⟨1 Mar⟩ D*ies* egypt*iacus*
⟨29 Mar⟩ D*ies* egipt*iacus*
⟨Apr⟩ Ap*ri*l*is* decimo e*st* undeno \`7´ fine minat*ur*.
⟨10 Apr⟩ D*ies* egypt*iacus*
⟨20 Apr⟩ D*ies* egypt*iacus*
⟨May⟩ Terci*us* *in* maio lup*us* e*st* & septim*us* anguis.
⟨3 May⟩ D*ies* egypt*iacus*
⟨25 May⟩ D*ies* egypt*iacus*
⟨June⟩ Iuni*us* *in* decimo q*u*indenu*m* a fine salutat.
⟨10 June⟩ D*ies* egypt*iacus*
⟨16 June⟩ D*ies* egypt*iacus*

1 ⟨*f. 1v*⟩ | **5** ⟨*f. 2r*⟩ | **9** ⟨*f. 2v*⟩ | **10** de] *read* sic.

12 *entry should have been on 28 March* | **13** ⟨*f. 3r*⟩ | **14** \`7´] ~ < [a], *but read* a | **17** ⟨*f. 3v*⟩ | **21** ⟨*f. 4r*⟩.

⟨July⟩ Tredecimus iulíí decimo innuit ante kalendas.
⟨13 July⟩ D*ies* egypt*iacus*
⟨22 July⟩ D*ies* egypt*iacus*
⟨Aug⟩ Augusti nepa p*ri*ma fugat de fine *secun*da.
⟨1 Aug⟩ D*ies* egypt*iacus*
⟨30 Aug⟩ D*ies* egipt*iacus*
⟨Sept⟩ Tercia septe*mbris* uulpes ferit a pede dena*m*.
⟨3 Sept⟩ D*ies* egypt*iacus*
⟨21 Sept⟩ D*ies* egypt*iacus*

25 ⟨*f. 4v*⟩ | **29** ⟨*f. 5r*⟩ | **29** fugat] *syntactical gloss over ~:* `*uel* it´ | **33** ⟨*f. 5v*⟩ | uulpes] *read* uulpis.

⟨Oct⟩ T*er*ci*us* octob*ris* puls*us* .x. *in*ordine nectit.
⟨3 Oct⟩ D*ies* egypt*iacus*
⟨22 Oct⟩ D*ies* egypt*iacus*
⟨Nov⟩ Quinta noue*mbris* ac*us* uix *ter*cia mansit in urna.
⟨5 Nov⟩ D*ies* egypt*iacus*
⟨28 Nov⟩ D*ies* egypt*iacus*
⟨Dec⟩ Dat duodena chohors septe*m* *in*de dece*m*q*ue* dece*m*b*ri*.
⟨7 Dec⟩ D*ies* egypt*iacus*
⟨22 Dec⟩ D*ies* egypt*iacus*

37 ⟨*f. 6r*⟩ | puls*us*] *read* gladius | **38** *in*ordine] *read* ordine | **41** ⟨*f. 6v*⟩ | **45** ⟨*f. 7r*⟩.

8.3/10 London, British Library, Arundel 60, fols 2r-7v

⟨Jan⟩ **IANI PRIMA DIES ET SEPTIMA FINE TIMETVR.**
⟨1 Jan⟩ **d*ies***
⟨25 Jan⟩ **d*ies***
⟨Feb⟩ **AST FEBRVI QVARTA EST PRECEDIT TERTIA FINEM.**
⟨4 Feb⟩ **d*ies***
⟨Mar⟩ **Martis p*ri*ma necat cuius sicuspide quarta est.**
⟨1 Mar⟩ **d*ies***
⟨28 Mar⟩ **d*ies***
⟨Apr⟩ **APRILIS DECIMO EST VNDENO a fine MINATVR.**
⟨10 Apr⟩ **d*ies***
⟨20 Apr⟩ **d*ies***

1 ⟨*f. 2r*⟩ | **6** ⟨*f. 2v*⟩ | **10** ⟨*f. 3r*⟩ | **11 sicuspide**] *read* sic cuspide | **15** ⟨*f. 3v*⟩.

⟨May⟩ **TERTIVS EST MAIO LVPVS EST ET SEPTIM*VS* ANGVIS.**
⟨3 May⟩ **d*ies***
⟨25 May⟩ **d*ies***
⟨June⟩ **IVNIVS IN DECIMO QVINDENV*M* A FINE SALVTAT.**
⟨10 June⟩ **d*ies***
⟨16 June⟩ **d*ies***
⟨July⟩ **TREDECIM*VS* IVLII DECIMA INNVIT ANTE K*A*L*EN*DAS.**
⟨13 July⟩ **d*ies***
⟨22 July⟩ **d*ies***
⟨Aug⟩ **AVGVSTI NEPA PRIMA. FVCAT DE FINE S*EC*V*N*DA.**
⟨1 Aug⟩ **d*ies***
⟨30 Aug⟩ **d*ies***
⟨Sept⟩ **TERTIA SEP*TEMBRIS* VVLPIS FERIT**

20 ⟨*f. 4r*⟩ | **25** ⟨*f. 4v*⟩ | **30** ⟨*f. 5r*⟩ | **35** ⟨*f. 5v*⟩ | **36 FVCAT**] *read* fugat | **38 d*ies***] *~ in left margin* | **40** ⟨*f. 6r*⟩.

A PEDE DENAM.
⟨3 Sept⟩ **d*ies***
⟨21 Sept⟩ **d*ies***
⟨Oct⟩ **TERTIVS *EST* OCTOBRIS GLADIVS .X. ORDINE NECTIT.**
⟨3 Oct⟩ **d*ies*.**
⟨Nov⟩ **QVINTA NOVEMBRIS ACVS VIX .III.**

45 ⟨*f. 6v*⟩ | **49** ⟨*f. 7r*⟩.

MANSIT I*N* VRNA.
⟨5 Nov⟩ **d*ies***
⟨28 Nov⟩ **d*ies***
⟨Dec⟩ **DAT DVODENA COHORS .VII. INDE DECE*MQVE* DECE*M*BRI.**
⟨12 Dec⟩ **d*ies***
⟨15 Dec⟩ **d*ies***

54 ⟨*f. 7v*⟩.

8.3/19 London, British Library, Cotton Vitellius E. xviii, fols 2r–7v

⟨Jan⟩ **Iani prima dies & septima fine timetur.**
⟨1 Jan⟩ **D*ies*.**
⟨Feb⟩ **Ast februi quarta est precedit tertia finem.**
⟨4 Feb⟩ **D*ies* mala.**
⟨Mar⟩ **Martis prima necat cui*us* sic cuspide quarta est.**
⟨28 Mar⟩ **D*ies* M*ala*.**
⟨Apr⟩ **Aprilis decima est undeno a fine mina(tur.)**
⟨10 Apr⟩ **D*ies* mala.**
⟨20 Apr⟩ **D*ies* mala.**
⟨May⟩ **Tertius maio lupus est et septimus ang(ui)s.**
⟨3 May⟩ **D*ies***
⟨25 May⟩ **Dies mala.**
⟨June⟩ **Iunius in decimo quindenu*m* a fine salutat.**
⟨10 June⟩ **D*ies* M*ala*.**
⟨16 June⟩ **D*ies* M*ala*.**
⟨July⟩ **Tredecim*us* iulii decimo innuit ante kalendas.**
⟨Aug⟩ **Augusti nepa prima fugat de fine s*ecun*dam.**
⟨1 Aug⟩ **D*ies* M*ala*.**
⟨30 Aug⟩ **D*ies* M*ala*.**
⟨Sept⟩ **(Tertia) septembris uulpis ferit a pede denam.**
⟨3 Sept⟩ **(Dies) mala.**
⟨Oct⟩ **(Tertius est octo)bris gladius decimo ordine nec(tit.)**
⟨3 Oct⟩ **D*ies* m(ala.)**
⟨24 Oct⟩ **D*ies* M*ala*.**
⟨Nov⟩ **Quinta nouembris acus uix t*er*tia mansi(t in urna.)**
⟨5 Nov⟩ **D*ies* M*ala***
⟨28 Nov⟩ **Dies M*ala*.**
⟨Dec⟩ **(Dat duode)na cohors .vii. inde dece*mque* dece*m*bri.**
⟨12 Dec⟩ **Dies m*ala*.**
⟨15 Dec⟩ **Dies m*ala*.**

1 ⟨*f. 2r*⟩ | **4** ⟨*f. 2v*⟩ | **7** ⟨*f. 3r*⟩ | **11** ⟨*f. 3v*⟩ | **15** ⟨*f. 4r*⟩ | **Tertius**] *read* ~ est | **20** ⟨*f. 4v*⟩ | **25** ⟨*f. 5r*⟩.

28 ⟨*f. 5v*⟩ | **33** ⟨*f. 6r*⟩ | **37** ⟨*f. 6v*⟩ | **40** *Wildhagen entered this Egyptian Day in his edition, though he later listed the date as missing (1921: 97)* | **41** *entry should have been on 22 October* | **42** ⟨*f. 7r*⟩ | **47** ⟨*f. 7v*⟩.

8.3/23 London, British Library, Harley 863, fols 1r-6v

⟨Jan⟩	**Iani p*ri*ma dies & septima fine time*tur*.**
⟨1 Jan⟩	**DIES MALA.**
⟨25 Jan⟩	D*ies*
⟨Feb⟩	**Ast februi .iiii. est precedit tercia fine*m*.**
⟨4 Feb⟩	D*ies*
⟨26 Feb⟩	D*ies*
⟨Mar⟩	**Martius prima necat cuius sic cuspide .iiii. e*st*.**
⟨1 Mar⟩	D*ies*
⟨28 Mar⟩	D*ies*
⟨Apr⟩	**Ap*ri*lis decimo e*st* undeno a fine minatur**
⟨10 Apr⟩	**.D*ies***
⟨19 Apr⟩	**D*ies***
⟨May⟩	**Tercius e*st* maio lupus est 7 septim*us* anguis.**
⟨3 May⟩	**D*ies*.**
⟨25 May⟩	**D*ies*.**
⟨June⟩	**Prima necat iunii q*uin*dena a fine mina*tur*.**
⟨10 June⟩	**.D*ies*.**
⟨16 June⟩	**.D*ies*.**
⟨13 July⟩	**.D*ies*.**
⟨22 July⟩	**D*ies***
⟨1 Aug⟩	**.D*ies*.**
⟨30 Aug⟩	**D*ies***
⟨3 Sept⟩	**.D*ies*.**
⟨21 Sept⟩	**.D*ies*.**
⟨3 Oct⟩	**.D*ies*.**
⟨22 Oct⟩	**.D*ies*.**
⟨5 Nov⟩	**.D*ies*.**
⟨28 Nov⟩	**.D*ies*.**
⟨7 Dec⟩	**.D*ies*.**
⟨22 Dec⟩	**D*ies***

1 ⟨*f. 1r*⟩ | **Iani**] ~ [··········] | **5** ⟨*f. 1v*⟩ | **9** ⟨*f. 2r*⟩ | **Martius**] *read* Martis | **14** ⟨*f. 2v*⟩ | **17** *entry should have been on 20 April* | **18** ⟨*f. 3r*⟩ | **23** ⟨*f. 3v*⟩ | **Prima**] *read* Dena | **28** ⟨*f. 4r*⟩ | **30** ⟨*f. 4v*⟩ | **.Dies.**] ~ *in left margin* | **31 Dies**] ~ *in left margin* | **32** ⟨*f. 5r*⟩ | **.Dies.**] ~ *in left margin* | **34** ⟨*f. 5v*⟩ | **36** ⟨*f. 6r*⟩ | **38** ⟨*f. 6v*⟩.

8.3/8 Cambridge, University Library, Kk. 5. 32, fols 50r-55v

⟨1 Jan⟩	D*ies*
⟨25 Jan⟩	D*ies*
⟨4 Feb⟩	D*ies*
⟨1 Mar⟩	D*ies*
⟨27 Mar⟩	D*ies*
⟨28 Mar⟩	D*ies*
⟨10 Apr⟩	D*ies*
⟨20 Apr⟩	D*ies*

1 ⟨*f. 50r*⟩ | **3** ⟨*f. 50v*⟩ | **4** ⟨*f. 51r*⟩ | **5** *this Egyptian Day is spurious* | **7** ⟨*f. 51v*⟩.

8.3/27 Oxford, Bodleian Library, Digby 63, fols 40r-45v

⟨2 Feb⟩	dies mala.
⟨3 Mar⟩	**d**ies egiptiagus.
⟨7 June⟩	**d***ies* mala.
⟨3 July⟩	**d**ies egipciagus.
⟨2 Sept⟩	**d**ies mala.
⟨3 Oct⟩	**d***ies* mala.
⟨13 Dec⟩	**d**ies mala.

1 ⟨*f. 40v*⟩ | **2** ⟨*f. 41r*⟩ | **3** ⟨*f. 42v*⟩ | **4** ⟨*f. 43r*⟩ | **5** ⟨*f. 44r*⟩ | **6** ⟨*f. 44v*⟩ | **7** ⟨*f. 45v*⟩.

8.3/6 Cambridge, Trinity College, R. 15. 32, pp. 15-26

⟨1 Jan⟩ *Dies mala*
⟨25 Jan⟩ *Dies mala*
3 ⟨4 Feb⟩ *Dies mala*
⟨26 Feb⟩ *Dies mala*
⟨1 Mar⟩ *Dies mala*
6 ⟨28 Mar⟩ *Dies mala*
⟨10 Apr⟩ *Dies mala*
⟨20 Apr⟩ *Dies mala*
9 ⟨3 May⟩ *Dies mala*
⟨25 May⟩ *Dies mala*
⟨10 June⟩ *Dies mala*
12 ⟨16 June⟩ *Dies mala*
⟨13 July⟩ *Dies mala*
⟨22 July⟩ *Dies mala*
15 ⟨1 Aug⟩ *Dies mala*
⟨30 Aug⟩ *Dies mala*
⟨3 Sept⟩ *Dies mala*
18 ⟨21 Sept⟩ *Dies mala*
⟨3 Oct⟩ *Dies mala*
⟨22 Oct⟩ *Dies mala*
21 ⟨5 Nov⟩ *Dies mala*
⟨28 Nov⟩ *Dies mala*
⟨12 Dec⟩ *Dies mala*
24 ⟨15 Dec⟩ *Dies mala*

Egyptian Day entries are later additions to the calendar | **1** ⟨*p. 15*⟩ | *mala*] -a < i | **3** ⟨*p. 16*⟩ | **5** ⟨*p. 17*⟩ | **7** ⟨*p. 18*⟩ | **9** ⟨*p. 19*⟩ | **11** ⟨*p. 20*⟩ | **13** ⟨*p. 21*⟩ | **15** ⟨*p. 22*⟩ | *Dies mala*] ~ *in lefthand corner* | **17** ⟨*p. 23*⟩ | **19** ⟨*p. 24*⟩ | **21** ⟨*p. 25*⟩ | **23**⟨*p. 26*⟩.

8.3/9 London, British Library, Additional 37517, fols 2r-3r

⟨1 Jan⟩ *Dies*
⟨25 Jan⟩ *Dies*
3 ⟨4 Feb⟩ *Dies*
⟨26 Feb⟩ *Dies*
⟨10 Mar⟩ *Dies*
6 ⟨21 Mar⟩ *Dies*
⟨3 Apr⟩ *Dies*
⟨24 Apr⟩ *Dies*
9 ⟨3 May⟩ *Dies*
⟨25 May⟩ *Dies*
⟨10 June⟩ *Dies*
12 ⟨26 June⟩ *Dies*
⟨13 July⟩ *Dies*
⟨22 July⟩ *Dies*

15 ⟨30 Aug⟩ *Dies*
⟨13 Sept⟩ *Dies*
⟨20 Sept⟩ *Dies*
18 ⟨3 Oct⟩ *Dies*
⟨22 Oct⟩ *Dies*
⟨5 Nov⟩ *Dies*
21 ⟨28 Nov⟩ *Dies*
⟨12 Dec⟩ *Dies*
⟨15 Dec⟩ *Dies*

1 ⟨*f. 2ra*⟩ | **5** ⟨*f. 2rb*⟩ | **9** ⟨*f. 2va*⟩ | **13** ⟨*f. 2vb*⟩ | **15** *Entry for 1 August may be lost because the stub which holds the leaf may have been pasted over it. Alternatively, the exemplar of the calendar may have featured an Egyptian Day entry in front of the date (which is not unusual for 1 August), in which case the scribe may have overlooked the entry* | **16** ⟨*f. 3ra*⟩ | **20** ⟨*f. 3rb*⟩.

8.3/11 London, British Library, Arundel 155, fols 2r-7v

⟨1 Jan⟩	***DIES ĘGYPTIACVS.***
⟨25 Jan⟩	***DIES ĘGYPTIACVS.***
⟨4 Feb⟩	***DIES ĘGYPTIACVS.***
⟨26 Feb⟩	***DIES ĘGYPTIACVS.***
⟨1 Mar⟩	***DIES ĘGYPTIACVS.***
⟨28 Mar⟩	***DIES ĘGYPTIACVS.***
⟨10 Apr⟩	***DIES ĘGYPTIACVS.***
⟨20 Apr⟩	***DIES ĘGYPTIACVS.***
⟨3 May⟩	***DIES ĘGYPTIACVS.***
⟨25 May⟩	***DIES ĘGYPTIACVS.***
⟨10 June⟩	***DIES ĘGYPTIACVS.***
⟨13 July⟩	***DIES ĘGYPTIACVS.***
⟨22 July⟩	***DIES ĘGYPTIACVS.***
⟨1 Aug⟩	***DIES ĘGYPTIACVS.***
⟨30 Aug⟩	***DIES ĘGYPTIACVS.***
⟨3 Sept⟩	***DIES ĘGYPTIACVS.***
⟨21 Sept⟩	***DIES ĘGYPTIACVS.***
⟨3 Oct⟩	***DIES ĘGYPTIACVS.***
⟨22 Oct⟩	***DIES ĘGYPTIACVS.***
⟨5 Nov⟩	***DIES ĘGYPTIACVS.***
⟨28 Nov⟩	***DIES ĘGYPTIACVS.***
⟨7 Dec⟩	***DIES ĘGYPTIACVS.***
⟨22 Dec⟩	***DIES ĘGYPTIACVS.***

Entries for the Egyptian Days are latter additions to the calendar | **1** *⟨f. 2r⟩* | **3** *⟨f. 2v⟩* | **5** *⟨f. 3r⟩* | **7** *⟨f. 3v⟩* | **9** *⟨f. 4r⟩* | **11** *⟨f. 4v⟩* | **12** *⟨f. 5r⟩* | **14** *⟨f. 5v⟩* | **16** *⟨f. 6r⟩* | **18** *⟨f. 6v⟩* | **20** *⟨f. 7r⟩* | **22** *⟨f. 7v⟩.*

8.3/15 London, British Library, Cotton Titus D. xxvii, fols 3r-8v

⟨1 Jan⟩	**Dies**
⟨25 Jan⟩	**Dies**
⟨4 Feb⟩	**Dies**
⟨26 Feb⟩	**Dies**
⟨1 Mar⟩	**Dies**
⟨28 Mar⟩	**Dies**
⟨10 Apr⟩	**Dies**
⟨20 Apr⟩	**Dies**
⟨3 May⟩	**Dies**
⟨25 May⟩	**Dies**
⟨10 June⟩	**Dies**
⟨16 June⟩	**Dies**
⟨13 July⟩	**Dies**
⟨22 July⟩	**Dies**
⟨1 Aug⟩	**Dies**
⟨30 Aug⟩	**Dies**
⟨3 Sept⟩	**Dies**
⟨21 Sept⟩	**Dies**
⟨3 Oct⟩	**Dies**
⟨22 Oct⟩	**Dies**
⟨5 Nov⟩	**Dies**
⟨28 Nov⟩	**Dies**
⟨12 Dec⟩	**Dies**
⟨15 Dec⟩	**Dies.**
⟨25 Dec⟩	**Dies**

1 *⟨f. 3r⟩* | **3** *⟨f. 3v⟩* | **5** *⟨f. 4r⟩* | **7** *⟨f. 4v⟩* | **9** *⟨f. 5r⟩* | **11** *⟨f. 5v⟩* | **13** *⟨f. 6r⟩* | **15** *⟨f. 6v⟩* | **17** *⟨f. 7r⟩* | **19** *⟨f. 7v⟩* | **21** *⟨f. 8r⟩* | **23** *⟨f. 8v⟩* | **25** *this day is spurious (see p. 358).*

8.3/29 Oxford, Bodleian Library, Hatton 113, fols iii recto-viii verso

⟨1 Jan⟩ **D**ies mala.
⟨25 Jan⟩ **D**ies mala.
3 ⟨4 Feb⟩ **D**ies mala.
⟨26 Feb⟩ **D**ies mala.
⟨1 Mar⟩ **D**ies mala.
6 ⟨28 Mar⟩ **D**ies mala.
⟨10 Apr⟩ **D**ies mala.
⟨20 Apr⟩ **D**ies mala.
9 ⟨3 May⟩ **D**ies mal*a*.
⟨25 May⟩ **D**ies mala.
⟨10 June⟩ **D**ies mala.
12 ⟨16 June⟩ **D**ies mala.
⟨13 July⟩ **D**ies mala.
⟨22 July⟩ **D**ies mala.
15 ⟨1 Aug⟩ **D**ies m*ala*.
⟨30 Aug⟩ **D**ies ęgiptiacus.
⟨3 Sept⟩ **D**ies ęgiptiacus.
18 ⟨21 Sept⟩ **D**ies ęgiptiacus.
⟨3 Oct⟩ **D**ies mala.
⟨23 Oct⟩ **D**ies egipt*iacus*.
21 ⟨5 Nov⟩ **D**ies ęgiptiacus.
⟨28 Nov⟩ **D**ies mala.
⟨12 Dec⟩ **D**ies mala.
24 ⟨15 Dec⟩ **D**ies egiptiacus.

1 ⟨*f. iii recto*⟩ | **3** ⟨*f. iii verso*⟩ | **5** ⟨*f. iv recto*⟩ | **7** ⟨*f. iv verso*⟩ | **9** ⟨*f. v recto*⟩ | **11** ⟨*f. v verso*⟩ | **13** ⟨*f. vi recto*⟩ | **15** ⟨*f. vi verso*⟩ | **17** ⟨*f. vii recto*⟩ | **19** ⟨*f. vii verso*⟩ | **20** *entry should have been on 22 October* | **21** ⟨*f. viii recto*⟩ | **23** ⟨*f. viii verso*⟩.

8.3/32 Rome, Vatican City, Bibliotheca Vaticana Apostolica, Reg. lat. 12, fols 7r-12v

⟨4 Feb⟩ **Dies mala.**
⟨26 Feb⟩ **Dies mala.**
3 ⟨1 Mar⟩ **Dies mala.**
⟨28 Mar⟩ **Dies mala.**
⟨10 Apr⟩ **Dies mala.**
6 ⟨20 Apr⟩ **Dies mala.**
⟨3 May⟩ **Dies mala.**
⟨25 May⟩ **Dies mala.**
9 ⟨10 June⟩ **Dies mala.**
⟨16 June⟩ **Dies mala.**
⟨13 July⟩ **Dies mala.**
12 ⟨1 Aug⟩ **Dies mala.**
⟨30 Aug⟩ **Dies mala.**
⟨21 Sept⟩ **Dies mala.**
15 ⟨3 Oct⟩ **Dies mala.**
⟨23 Oct⟩ **DIES mala.**
⟨5 Nov⟩ **Dies mala.**
18 ⟨28 Nov⟩ **Dies mala.**

1 ⟨*f. 7v*⟩ | **3** ⟨*f. 8r*⟩ | **5** ⟨*f. 8v*⟩ | **7** ⟨*f. 9r*⟩ | **9** ⟨*f. 9v*⟩ | **11** ⟨*f. 10r*⟩ | **12** ⟨*f. 10v*⟩ | **14** ⟨*f. 11r*⟩ | **15** ⟨*f. 11v*⟩ | **16** *entry should have been on 22 October* | **17** ⟨*f. 12r*⟩.

8.3/33 Salisbury, Cathedral Library, MS 150, fols 3r-8v

⟨2 Jan⟩ **DIES EGYP*TIACVS***
⟨25 Jan⟩ **DIES EGYP*TIACVS***
⟨6 Feb⟩ **Dies Egyptiacus.**
⟨4 Apr⟩ **DIES EGYPTIACVS.**
⟨11 Apr⟩ **Dies Egyptiacus.**
⟨4 May⟩ **DIES EG*YPTIACVS***
⟨25 May⟩ **D*IES* EGYP*TIACVS***
⟨20 June⟩ **DIES EGYPTIACVS.**
⟨6 July⟩ **DIES EGYPTIACVS.**
⟨13 July⟩ **DIES EGYPTIACVS.**
⟨4 Oct⟩ **DIES EGYPTIACVS.**
⟨24 Nov⟩ **DIES EGYPTIACVS.**
⟨12 Dec⟩ **DIES EGIPTIACVS.**

1 ⟨*f. 3r*⟩ | **3** ⟨*f. 3v*⟩ | **4** ⟨*f. 4v*⟩ | **6** ⟨*f. 5r*⟩ | **8** ⟨*f. 5v*⟩ | **9** ⟨*f. 6r*⟩ | **11** ⟨*f. 7v*⟩ | **12** ⟨*f. 8r*⟩ | **13** ⟨*f. 8v*⟩.

8.3/4 Cambridge, Corpus Christi College, MS 422, pp. 29-40

⟨25 Jan⟩ **DIES MA*LA*.**
⟨12 Mar⟩ **DIES.**
⟨23 Mar⟩ **DIES MALA.**
⟨3 Apr⟩ **DIES MALA.**
⟨21 Apr⟩ **DIES M*ALA*:**
⟨23 May⟩ **DIES MALA**
⟨7 June⟩ **DIES MALA.**
⟨14 July⟩ **DIES.**
⟨22 July⟩ **DIES MALA**
⟨30 Aug⟩ **DIES.**
⟨7 Sept⟩ **DIES MALA**
⟨24 Nov⟩ **DIES MALA**
⟨11 Dec⟩ **DIES MALA.**
⟨27 Dec⟩ **DIES MALA.**

1 ⟨*p. 29*⟩ | **2** ⟨*p. 31*⟩ | **4** ⟨*p. 32*⟩ | **6** ⟨*p. 33*⟩ | **7** ⟨*p. 34*⟩ | **8** ⟨*p. 35*⟩ | **10** ⟨*p. 36*⟩ | **11** ⟨*p. 37*⟩ | **12** ⟨*p. 39*⟩ | **13** ⟨*p. 40*⟩.

9 Lunaries

Alias

moonbook, selenodromium

Description

In classical and medieval times, the moon was one of the planets which was believed to exercise a far-reaching influence on the sublunar sphere, i.e. our planet earth.[1] This influence pertained to the natural world, time reckoning and prognostication. The moon was held to be important for the tides and the durability of timber (nature), for the calculation of Easter (computus), and for the future (prognostication). That the natural world and time reckoning were dependent upon the moon is, in Ælfric's words, "gecyndelic þing þurh gesceapenysse" (a natural thing through creation).[2] The effects of the moon upon the future, however, are representative of "wiglung" (divination). "Wiglung" is far from "gecyndelic" and constitutes, therefore, an unacceptable use of the days of the moon.[3]

Ælfric may have objected, but the moon was a convenient asset for prognostication in classical and medieval times. This is not so illogical if it is kept in mind that the moon was being studied for so many other things, notably for time reckoning and the Easter cycle. A focus on and general awareness of lunar time must have facilitated the transmission of lunar prognostics. Indeed, many lunaries are found in the computus in English manuscripts.[4]

Aspects of the moon are employed as a structural feature in a number of prognostic genres:[5]

	Apuleian Spheres	lunaries	month prognosis	moonbooks	moon colour	unlucky days
lunar aspect	all days of the moon	all days of the moon	day of new moon	regular series of days of the moon	colour	selected days of the moon
structural level	secondary	primary	secondary	primary	primary	primary
n	13	39	1	10	1	3

table 24: lunar aspects in prognostic genres

[1] Cf. Jastrow (1905-12: II.457-577), Henel (1934b), Förster (1944: 1-5), Gundel (1927: 136-46), Gundel and Gundel (1959: 41-54, 69-71, 77-80; 1966: 263-69), Taavitsainen (1988: 37-39), Means (1992: 376-85; 1993: 24-25).

[2] Ælfric, *Octabas et circumcisio Domini* (Clemoes 1997: 230/195-96).

[3] The issue of natural versus divinatory influence is discussed in full on pp. 115-20.

[4] See pp. 29-39.

[5] Moonbooks are not attested as stand-alone texts in English manuscripts. They are found in texts on the Dog Days and the twenty-four Egyptian Days.

That the moon is a popular asset to prognostication is seen by the sixty-seven attestations of prognostics with a lunar element. Of the six prognostic genres listed, five use days of the moon, against one which depends upon the colour of the moon. Only two genres employ all the days of the moon, while three use a selection in the form of a regular series (the six fives of moonbooks, for instance); a single day of the moon (the weekday on which new moon falls for the month prognosis); or an arbitrary selection (the two unlucky days per month fall on predetermined days of the moon). The structural level on which the lunar component is employed differs: as a primary means of structuring, the lunar aspect is essential because it helps shape and give meaning to a prognostic; as a secondary means, the lunar aspect supports the structure but does not define its shape or meaning. For instance, in the month prognosis, the future is predicted by the weekday on which the new moon occurs. The structure of the text is determined by the weekdays, and the day of new moon is a static piece of information which plays no further role. In contrast, lunaries are ordered by the days of the moon, which assign an outcome to bloodletting, dreams and the like. Therefore, the moon is used as the main organising principle of the text in lunaries.

More than half of the lunar prognostics are lunaries, a prognostic genre which is structured by the days of the moon. The word 'lunary' is not the only term used to designate the genre under discussion; some scholars employ the words 'lunarium' or 'moonbook'.[6] A good introduction to the semantic field of temporal lunar prognostics is provided by Taavitsainen.[7] She applied the word 'moonbook' throughout as a general term for prognostics using the moon's age. Taavitsainen distinguished three genres covered by the term 'moonbook': 'lunaries proper', 'zodiacal lunaries' and 'mansions of the moon',[8] the difference lying in the how time is defined. Of the three genres distinguished by Taavitsainen, lunaries are the only ones attested in English manuscripts. The Anglo-Saxons showed a deep interest in lunaries, which is illustrated by the existence of no less than eleven lunaries in Tiberius A. iii.

Lunaries proper (henceforth lunaries) are "perpetual prognostications according to the thirty days of the moon from one new moon to the

[6] Thorndike (1923-58: I.680, 682).

[7] Taavitsainen (1988).

[8] Taavitsainen (1988: 23, 45-48). Cf. Gundel and Gundel (1959: 77-80; 1966: 264-65), Svenberg (1963: 3-4).

next".[9] Lunaries make use of the synodic month, which lasts 29.5 days and which is the lunar cycle measured from new moon to new moon. The thirty entries of a lunary signify a rounded synodic month of thirty days which starts with new moon. The Latin lunaries transmitted in English manuscripts do not usually carry rubrics, but when they do, the titles use the word 'lunaris' to identify the text.[10]

Zodiacal lunaries are "tracts that count the joint influence of the twelve signs of the zodiac and the moon".[11] This genre consists of twelve entries which reflect the location of the moon with regard to the signs of the zodiac; it has not been attested in Anglo-Saxon manuscripts.[12] To my knowledge, the earliest English zodiacal lunaries are in the twelfth-century manuscript Egerton 821.

The mansions of the moon, finally, are structured by the "the moon's passage in the zodiac",[13] i.e. the sidereal month of 27.3 days, which is measured with reference to the moon's circuit of the stars as seen from the earth. Both the synodic month (from new moon to new moon) and sidereal month (the moon's circuit of the stars) were known in Anglo-Saxon times, as Ælfric's *De temporibus anni* illustrates:

> Truly the moon year has twenty-seven days and eight hours.... This is the moon year, but its month is more, which is when the moon travels new from the sun until it returns to the sun again, old and tired, and is displayed again through the sun [i.e. new moon]. In the moon month are counted twenty-nine days and twelve hours, this is the moon month, and its year is when it travels through all twelve star signs.[14]

This quotation elucidates that the synodic month was designated as the lunar month, and the sidereal month as the lunar year. It seems confusing that the moon year is shorter than the moon month, but the reason,

[9] Taavitsainen (1988: 23).

[10] For instance, texts 9.2.2/6,7, 9.2.4/7, 9.2.5/6, respectively. On the medieval vocabulary for lunaries, see Weißer (1982: 20-21), Taavitsainen (1988: 48-50).

[11] Taavitsainen (1988: 23).

[12] For more information on zodiacal lunaries, see Svenberg (1963), Taavitsainen (1988, 1994), Means (1993).

[13] Taavitsainen (1988: 47).

[14] "Soðlice þæs monan gear hæfð seofon 7 twentig daga 7 eahta tida.... Þis is þæs monan gear, ac his monað is mare, þæt is ðonne hê gecyrð niwe fram ðære sunnan oð þæt hê eft cume hire forne gean, eald 7 ateorod, 7 eft ðurh hî beo ontend. On ðam monðe sind getealde nigon 7 twentig daga, 7 twelf tida, þis is se mônlica monað, 7 his gear is þæt hê underyrne ealle ða twelf tunglan" (*De temporibus anni* IV.22, 29-30; Henel 1942: 32, 34). Cf. Bede's *De temporum ratione* XXXVI (Jones 1943: 249).

as Ælfric himself indicates, is that the moon year means the circuit through the constellations, and is as such comparable to the solar sidereal year. The prognostic genre known as the mansions of the moon is called thus because the sidereal month moves through twenty-eight constellations known as 'mansions'. Even though the Anglo-Saxons were familiar with the sidereal month through the computus, they did not turn this knowledge to prognostic use.[15]

The threefold division of lunar prognostics proposed by Taavitsainen is not the only one possible.[16] In the first critical edition of a number of collective lunaries, Svenberg distinguished between Greek lunar prognostics, which he called 'selenodromia', Latin 'lunaria' (for lunaries proper), and 'zodiakallunaria' (for zodiacal lunaries).[17] In his later work, Svenberg employed the terms 'lunaria' (for lunaries proper) and 'zodiologia' (for zodiacal lunaries and the mansions of the moon).[18] Thorndike designated temporal lunar prognostics as 'moonbooks', with a further specification into the genre of the 'lunarium', i.e. the lunary proper.[19] The first Middle English lunary to have been published was described by Craig with the Latin term 'lunationes', Anglicised as 'lunations'.[20] In his first article on the prognostics, Förster had no name for lunaries yet; he used the description "the influence of the moon on the fulfilment of dreams" for dream lunaries.[21] Later, Förster coined the German word 'Lunare' for the lunaries proper in his study of Tiberius A. iii, though he primarily identified the lunaries descriptively: "month calendar [Monatskalender], what is to be undertaken or refrained from on each day of the month", i.e. a collective lunary; "dreambook according to moon days [Mondtagen]", i.e. a dream lunary; "birth prognosis from the day of the month [Monatstage] of birth", i.e. a birth lunary, etc.[22] From the words 'Monatskalender', 'Mondtagen' and 'Monatstage', it would appear that Förster regarded lunaries as a calendric genre which followed

[15] For more information on the mansions of the moon, see Weinstock (1949), Yampolsky (1950), Taavitsainen (1988), Means (1993).

[16] Cf. Förster (1944: 5-6), Taavistainen (1988: 50-51).

[17] Svenberg (1936: 2-3, 140-52). Cf. Wistrand (1942: 19-20).

[18] Svenberg (1963: 3-4).

[19] Thorndike (1923-58: I.680).

[20] Craig (1916: xxxviii, xxxix).

[21] "die Einfluß des Mondes auf die Erfülling der Träume" (Förster 1903: 356).

[22] "Monatskalender, was an einem jeden Monatstage zu unternehmen oder zu lassen sei", "Traumbuch nach Mondtagen", "Nativitätsprognose aus dem Monatstage der Geburt" (Förster 1908c: 32-34).

the calendar months. This is not true, however, because elsewhere Förster employed the word 'Monatstage' for "the thirty days of the moon".[23] Förster used the word 'Lunare' for lunaries proper, but Gundel took the same word to mean lunar prognostics in general.[24] In his exhaustive study of collective lunaries, Förster has argued for adoption of the term 'Mondbücher' for all kinds of temporal lunar prognostics, and the term 'Lunare' for moon prognostics which make use of the thirty days of the moon of the synodic month.[25] Förster did not propose a further subdivision into the mansions of the moon and zodiacal lunaries (the latter are based on the twenty-eight days of the sidereal month and are therefore not 'Lunare' in Förster's eyes, it would seem). Braswell's definition of lunar prognostics with regard to Middle English texts does not distinguish between the three genres proposed by Taavitsainen: a lunary is "calculated either by the cycle the moon makes throughout its twenty-eight to thirty *mansions* or days, or by its zodiacal cycle through the twelve signs".[26] This grouping is also adhered to by Means.[27]

There seem to be as many genre divisions as there are scholars of the lunar prognostics. One genre that has been ignored by all, however, is what I have termed 'moonbook', viz. a text listing a regular series of days of the moon on which bloodletting proves fatal. Texts of this kind are sometimes integrated in texts on the Dog Days and on the twenty-four Egyptian Days.[28] These moonbooks are called 'lunationes' in some manuscripts,[29] a term employed by Craig to denote lunaries proper. Henel, who studied the moonbooks (my use of the term) called the text an "account of a series of unlucky moon ages", and simply "bloodletting instruction".[30]

To avoid the confusion that will necessarily arise over the widely different denotations of lunar prognostic genres, here are my definitions: (1) 'lunar prognostic' = any prognostic which makes use of aspects of the moon (see table 24), to be divided into a temporal and a non-temporal branch; (2) 'lunary' = prognostic which makes use of the thirty days of

[23] "die dreißig Mondphasen" (Förster 1912c: 16).

[24] Gundel (1927: 136).

[25] Förster (1944; 5-6).

[26] Braswell (1978: 189; 1984: 346).

[27] Means (1992: 378-82; 1993: 1, 25-50).

[28] See pp. 276-79, 351-52.

[29] E.g. in text 6/14, l. 7.

[30] "Aufzählung einer Reihe unglücklicher Mondalter", "Aderlaßvorschrift" (Henel 1934-35: 339, 346).

the lunar synodic month from new moon to new moon; (3) 'zodiacal lunary' = prognostic which makes use of the place of the moon in the twelve signs of the zodiac; (4) 'mansions of the moon' = prognostic which makes use of the passage of the twenty-eight days of the lunar sidereal month; (5) 'moonbook' = prognostic which presents a regular series of days from the synodic month on which certain actions prove fatal. In short, I adopt Taavitsainen's division with the exception of the term 'moonbook' which is the general term for the three temporal lunar prognostics distinguished in Taavitsainen's scheme, but is a specific kind of lunar prognostic in mine.

Lunaries can be subdivided into several genres which fall apart into two groups: collective lunaries, which contain predictions for a variety of occasions, and specific lunaries, which predict the outcome of one topic only. Specific lunaries deal with what actions should be undertaken, the character and course of life of a newborn child, appropriate times for bleeding, the predictive value of dreams, or the course of and possible recovery from illness.[31] Collective lunaries comprise all these topics plus two which are never encountered in isolation in English manuscripts: the return of a fugitive or runaway slave and the recovery of stolen or lost goods. Both Weißer and Taavitsainen observed that early lunaries are often specific ones, while in the later Middle Ages collective lunaries were favoured.[32] This is borne out by the Anglo-Saxon evidence: thirty-six specific lunaries against three collective ones. In contrast, the number of collective lunaries in Middle English exceeds that of specific lunaries.[33] Below, I discuss the lunary genres in some detail.

[31] Cf. Wistrand (1942: 11-12), Förster (1944: 6-7, 32-33), Weißer (1982: 15-20), Taavitsainen (1988: 98-101). Classical specific lunaries display a larger range of topics, mainly on health issues, cf. Gundel and Gundel (1959: 80).

[32] Weißer (1982: 423-24), Taavitsainen (1988: 84).

[33] Taavitsainen (1988: 62-63).

9.1 Lunary, Collective

Literature

Birch (1878: 506; 1892: 278); Camus (1891: 207-11); Jastrow (1905-12: II.457-577); Förster (1908c: 32-33; 1912c: 37-42; 1944); Budge (1913: II.560-65); Craig (1916: xxxviii-xlii); Thorndike (1923-58: I.680-82); Gundel (1927: 136-46); Svenberg (1936, 1939, 1963); Wistrand (1942); Gundel and Gundel (1959: 77-80; 1966: 263-69); Martin (1977: 15-16); Weißer (1982); Braswell (1984: 346-47); Hunt (1987: 170); Taavitsainen (1988); Kieckhefer (1989: 86); Hollis and Wright (1992: 264); Günzel (1993: 31-32); Means (1993); Epe (1995: 60-61, 63); Wallis (1995: 115-17); Liuzza (2001: 188); DiTommaso (2005: 259-79; 402-46; 2006: 119-26)

Attributions

medieval: Abraham, Adam, Aristotle, Armogynes, Augustine, Avicenna, Bezogar, Boethius, Daniel, David, Gregory, Haly, Hemagyons, Ioanton, Melampus, Merlin, Nechepso Nemroth Chaldeus, Noah, Petosiris, Ptolemy, Sergrondyth, Socrates, Solomon, Virgil

Branch of Superstition

observation of times: days of the moon

Texts

L/OE: 1. London, British Library, Cotton Tiberius A. iii, fols 32v-35v
L: 2. London, British Library, Cotton Titus D. xxvii, fols 27r-29v
3. London, British Library, Sloane 475, fols 211r-16v

Description

Collective lunaries having been studied exhaustively by Svenberg, Wistrand, Förster, Weißer and Taavitsainen; the reader is referred to the work of these scholars for additional information.[1] I limit myself to a brief overview of the genre.

The aim of a collective lunary is to predict the outcome of a number of issues depending upon the days of the moon. Latin collective lunaries typically deal with these aspects: agenda, birth, bloodletting, dreams, fugitives, illness and property.[2] The agenda component reveals what kinds of actions are appropriate for each days of the moon. The topics

[1] Svenberg (1936, 1939, 1963), Wistrand (1942), Förster (1944), Weißer (1982), Taavitsainen (1988). I am particularly indebted to Taavitsainen's clear presentation of the research on collective lunaries carried out in the past, which has served as a model for the description below.

[2] Cf. Wistrand (1942: 11-12), Förster (1944: 6-7, 32-33), Weißer (1982: 15-20), Taavitsainen (1988: 98-101).

addressed in the agenda part range from trade, the education of children, travelling, marriage, agricultural matters and moving house. Sometimes the agenda part is preceded by a statement asserting the overall quality of the day on a particular day of the moon, e.g. "it is useful to undertake all things".[3] The birth component reveals the character, walk of life and career opportunities of a newborn child.[4] These birth predictions can be quite elaborate, and often a distinction is made between boys and girls. Sometimes birthmarks are mentioned as well. The birth component in collective lunaries contains more information than specific birth lunaries, which address only one aspect, for instance whether the child will live or die, or its dominant character traits.[5] The detailed birth components in collective lunaries may have been developed at a later stage. The varying amount of detail presented in the birth component is one of the criteria used by Svenberg in his classification of the collective lunaries.[6] The bloodletting component is not always present in collective lunaries, but (1) includes such information.[7] Information on bloodletting is thought to be a later addition transferred from bloodletting lunaries to already existing collective lunaries.[8] The dream component of collective lunaries and dream lunaries does not predict the outcome of dreams on the basis of the subject, which is the domain of dreambooks,[9] but on the basis of the day of the moon on which the dream takes place. The prediction limits itself to whether or when a dream comes true, and what effect the dream will have. The illness component reveals the outcome of an illness depending upon the day of the moon on which the illness started.[10] The predictions range from death to life, with a whole range of discomforts or recovery scenarios in between.[11] There are two components present in collective lunaries which do not exist as specific lunaries in Latin: the possible return of fugitives or slaves, and the chance of recovering stolen or lost property.[12] The reason for the lack of specific lunaries

[3] "omnibus rebus agendis utilis est" (e.g. text 9.1/1, l. 3).

[4] An extensive discussion of the birth component is in Weißer (1982: 87-98).

[5] See pp. 426-28.

[6] Svenberg (1936: 17-18). See pp. 402-04.

[7] In Middle English collective lunaries, the bloodletting component may mention the body parts from which one should be bled, cf. Taavitsainen (1988: 101).

[8] Weißer (1982: 29-31).

[9] See pp. 290-96.

[10] For an exhaustive discussion of the illness component, see Weißer (1981: 98-134).

[11] This variation is reminiscent of that in some Apuleian Spheres (see p. 182).

[12] On the fate of the fugitive when he is caught in Middle English collective lunaries, see Taavitsainen (1988: 99).

dealing with these topics is unclear. It is striking that even in collective lunaries the entries for loss are not always present for each day of the moon.[13] This might be an indication that the fugitive and property components were considered of limited interest.

An intriguing chicken-and-egg question with regard to collective lunaries is whether they engendered specific lunaries, or whether specific lunaries were the building blocks of collective lunaries. Svenberg, who was the first to bring together a corpus of collective lunaries, could not decide which type begot the other, and neither could Förster.[14] Wistrand wrote an extensive critique of Svenberg's study, and proposed that collective lunaries were composed of specific ones, not the other way around.[15] Svenberg's failure to compare the different types of collective lunaries, Wistrand opined, was occasioned by the fact that Svenberg had regarded collective lunaries as coherent units rather than as compilations of specific lunaries. The usefulness of breaking collective lunaries into their component parts for reasons of comparison has been demonstrated by Wistrand.[16] Moreover, he illustrated that specific lunaries can be used to explain obscure passages in collective lunaries, while the reverse is not possible.[17] According to Weißer, this observation demonstrates the originality of specific lunaries as component parts of collective lunaries.[18] Weißer also noted the existence of sequences of specific lunaries in manuscripts. He claimed that such sequences had been made to furnish an overview of the same range of predictions as in collective lunaries, but with better readability.[19] I have identified one such series of lunaries, the α-sequence, which is attested seven times in English manuscripts.[20] The arrangement in columns, as in St. John's College 17, fol. 4r, and Lambeth Palace 427, fol. 3r, permits a clear overview of predictions both within one specific field, e.g. birth (arranged in columns), and on one specific day of the moon (arranged in rows). The fact that this kind of clarity is not afforded by collective lunaries supports Weißer's claim. Another argument in favour of the construction of collective lunaries from specific lunaries is the absence of certain types of specific

[13] See table 39.

[14] Svenberg (1936: 3, n. 2), Förster (1912c: 42).

[15] Wistrand (1942: 5-18).

[16] *Ibid.*

[17] Wistrand (1942: 9).

[18] Weißer (1982: 22).

[19] Weißer (1982: 22-23).

[20] See pp. 60-61.

lunaries in medieval manuscripts. If collective lunaries were decompiled to form specific lunaries, one would expect specific lunaries to occur that predict the return of a fugitive or runaway slave and the recovery of stolen or lost goods, but these are not found in Latin manuscripts while the other five areas of prediction are. If, on the other hand, specific lunaries were compiled into collective lunaries in early times, specific fugitive and property lunaries may have fallen out of fashion before the arrival of the lunary genre in Western Europe.

The case for the genesis of collective lunaries from specific lunaries has not gone unchallenged, however. Förster and Weißer pointed out that the oldest attested Latin collective and specific lunaries date from the ninth century, which leaves the matter of precedence unresolved.[21] The oldest attested (Egyptian) lunaries are collective rather than specific, but Greek lunaries (Svenberg's 'selenodromia') exist in both specific and collective forms.[22] Again, it is hard to draw conclusions about originality from the classical analogues of the Latin lunaries. Nevertheless, it is now generally assumed that "collective lunaries are compilations of specialized texts", in the words of Taavitsainen.[23]

Svenberg distinguished three types of Latin collective lunaries, which he claimed came into existence in different periods and derived from different sources. Svenberg's types I and II were thought to have been created in the pre-Christian era, while type III was supposed to represent a thirteenth-century translation of a Byzantine selenodromion.[24] This notion has been refuted by Wistrand, who denied the existence of direct links between Greek and Latin collective lunaries.[25] Nevertheless, the Latin collective lunaries are thought to have come into being in the third to ninth centuries, possibly from Byzantine sources.[26]

It is possible to group collective lunaries in various ways. The types outlined by Svenberg are as follows: I has no remarkable features; II is comparable to I but with more elaborate birth predictions; III is a loose-knit and variable group which shares references to biblical events.[27]

---

[21] Förster (1944: 8), Weißer (1982: 422).

[22] Svenberg (1936: 140-52), Wistrand (1942: 19-20), Förster (1944: 8-10), Gundel and Gundel (1959: 80; 1966: 266).

[23] Taavitsainen (1988: 84).

[24] Svenberg (1936: 142-52).

[25] Wistrand (1942: 19-20).

[26] Förster (1944: 34-36), Weißer (1982: 24-25, 75-76, 421-24), Taavitsainen (1988: 84).

[27] Svenberg (1936: 17-18).

Wistrand agreed that types I and II go back to two distinct redactions, but he thought that type III is a mixed bag of unrelated redactions.[28] Förster proposed a classification on the basis of the prefatory matter of the lunaries, i.e. the short introductions which sometimes precede the predictions for each day of the moon and which reveal: (1) the light of the moon; (2) the birth of pagan gods; or (3) events from the Bible (Svenberg's type III).[29] Most commonly, the introductions are absent (variant 4). In addition to the variation in introductions, Förster distinguished collective lunaries as follows: α, a short text; β, with elaborate birth predictions; and γ, a not particularly remarkable text.[30] Weißer adopted Wistrand's scheme of inspecting the composition and order of the elements for each day of the moon, and arrived at three groups, based on the order of the elements and the form of the birth predictions.[31] I have listed the order and presence of the components of the Anglo-Saxon collective lunaries elsewhere.[32] Taavitsainen discovered that the Middle English collective lunaries are not as easily categorised as older texts.[33] The earlier English collective lunaries, in contrast, fit neatly into the types and groups outlined in previous studies:

	Svenberg/Wistrand	Förster	Weißer
(1, 3)	type II	variant 4, group β	group 1
(2)	type I	variant 4, group α	group 3

table 25: classification of English collective lunaries

The Anglo-Saxon collective lunaries, then, belong to two distinct types no matter what scheme is used. (1, 3) belong to the same group, but they are not directly related, nor do they belong to one redaction.[34] This is apparent through extensive differences in phrasing and content and the presence certain components, particularly bloodletting predictions.[35] (1)

[28] Wistrand (1942: 17-18).

[29] Förster (1944: 10-32). These introductory topics are seen as separate themes comparable to the component parts of collective lunaries by Weißer (1982: 18). See also Taavitsainen (1988: 93, 101-07).

[30] Förster (1944: 36-41).

[31] Weißer (1982: 63-76).

[32] See table 39.

[33] Taavitsainen (1988: 130-32).

[34] Svenberg (1936) distinguished three redactions of type II lunaries in his text edition. Texts 9.1/1 and 9.1/3 represent two of these. Weißer (1982: 65-66) found that (3) is the more original form.

[35] See table 39.

represents a redaction to which the bloodletting instructions have been added at a later date, because early collective lunaries do not have a bloodletting component.[36]

There are not many collective lunaries in the vernacular from the eleventh century or earlier. Later collective lunaries in the vernacular have been attested in Old French, Middle English, Middle High German, Middle Dutch, Welsh, Scandinavian and Syriac.[37] The eleventh-century collective lunary (1) is special in that it is accompanied by a complete interlinear gloss in Old English. Förster opined that the Old English gloss existed in an older form, which he dated to possibly the first half of the eighth century on the basis of the presence of an antiquated inflectional ending '-i' in the Old English word "nontidi" (the hour of nones).[38] Förster already allowed for the possibility that "nontidi" is an error for "nontide", but there are more compelling reasons why an eighth-century date for the Old English gloss is highly unlikely. First, prognostics were extremely rare in Western Europe before the ninth century, and were probably unknown in England at the time.[39] It is, therefore, improbable that an Anglo-Saxon scribe had the opportunity to translate a complete collective lunary in the eighth century. It is even more improbable that this complete gloss was kept for over three centuries to be copied into an existing Latin collective lunary which turns out to be of exactly the same type and redaction.[40] Second, all Latin prognostics with Old English glosses were copied in the eleventh century.[41] Third, both the Old English gloss and the Latin text have the bloodletting instruc-

[36] Weißer (1982: 29-31).

[37] Middle English texts in Taavitsainen (1987, 1988), Means (1993); Middle High German in Weißer (1982); Old French in Camus (1891: 207-11); samples of collective lunaries in all the vernaculars mentioned in Förster (1944), except for the Syriac one, which is translated by Budge (1913: II.560-65). Further references in Beccaria (1956: 204 [51.5], 378 [133.29]), Wickerheimer (1966: 140-41 [XCII.2]).

[38] Förster (1944: 52-57).

[39] Most prognostic genres entered England in the second half of the tenth century at the earliest.

[40] There are only seven instances where the Old English gloss deviates from the Latin text, cf. Förster (1944: 54-55). On the other hand, it is significant that the gloss and Latin text do agree on a curious misreading in Latin. Text 9.1/1, l. 95 (and 9.1/3 and Erlangen 674, which both postdate 9.1/1), reads "puer natus granosus" instead of "puer natus gratiosus". The Old English gloss has "cild acenned corngesælig" (l. 94). The *hapax legomenon* "corngesælig" (rich in corn) is an attempt on the part of the translator to interpret the erroneous Latin "granosus". It is unlikely that the supposedly eighth-century Latin lunary used in the translation had the same peculiar misreading.

[41] See p. 83.

tions for each day of the moon, and these instructions are not attested in early collective lunaries. In any case, the earliest Latin collective lunary is from the ninth century, as Förster himself observed.[42] A gloss which antedates the earliest extant Latin lunary by about a century and which includes bloodletting instructions only found in later texts is remarkable to say the least. In conclusion, I think that the running gloss was either composed on the spot or that it was in the exemplar of (1).

Edition

9.1/1 London, British Library, Cotton Tiberius A. iii, fols 32v/16-35v/14

de obseruatione lune & q*ue* cauenda s*unt*

mona se forma on eallu*m* þingu*m* dondum nytlic ys cild acenned bið mære
Luna prima omnibus rebus agendis utilis est. puer natus erit illustris.
glæw wis gestæflæred on wætere gedyrfed gif he ætwint langlife he bið
astutus. sapiens. litteratus. in aqua periclitatus. si euaserit. longeuus erit.
mæden acenned ungewemmed clæne milde wlitig weru*m* gelicgende rihtlice
puella nata. intemerata casta. benigna. speciosa. uiris placens. ęque
toscedenne on æfteweardan ylde heo bið on bedde lange licgende. tacen heo hefð
discernens. in postera ętate erit. in lecto longe recumbens. signum. hab*et*
on muðe oððe on bruan se þe bið lange he handlað swa wæt swa
in ore. uel in supercilio. qui recumbit longe languescit. quicquid
hine swefnað on blisse hit bið gewyrfed forþi ne yfel selDAN god hit getacnað
somniauerit. in gaudium conuertetur. quia neq*ue* malu*m* raro bonum significat
7 blod lætan oððe wanian ealne dæg mona god ys.
& sanguinem minere tota die luna bona e*st*.

mona se oðer on eallu*m* þingu*m* to dondu*m* nytlic ys bicgan syllan scyp
Luna .ii. omnibus rebus agendis utilis est emere. uendere nauim
astigan. cild acenned wis milde geap gesælig mæden eallswa se þe
ascendere. puer natus. sapiens. benignus. astutus. felix. puella similiter. qui
lið raðe acofrað swefen næfð gefremincge nys na god mona
iac*et* cito conualescit. somnium non hab*et* effectum. non est bona luna
blod wanian
sanguinem minuere.

2 dondum] *read* to ~ | **4** glæw] -l- < a | gedyrfed] *read* bið ~ *(see l. 5)* | **5** periclitatus] *read* periclitatur | **6** gelicgende] *i.e.* gelicigende *(see l. 164)* | **8** toscedenne] *i.e.* toscedende | **10** bruan] *read* oferbruan | bið] *read* lið | handlað] *read* adlað | **18,19** ascendere.] ascen‖dere., *but* astigan.‖ ⟨*f. 33r*⟩.

[42] Förster (1944: 8).

mona se ðridda weorcu onginnan na gedafanaþ butan *þæt* bið geedcenned stifician
Luna .iii. opera incipere non congruit. nisi quod renascitur. stirpare.
nytenu tymian baras fyran wyrttun na saw þu forþi ydele wyrta
animalia domare. uerres castrare. ortum non seras quia uarię herbę
beoð accennede *þæt* bið forstolen raþe he bið fundon se þe gelið raðe he hamacgað
nascuntur. quod fura*tur* cito inuenitur. qui recumbit cito conualescit.
oððe lan fræcednysse he þolað cild acenned geþancfull grædig be þingum
aut longum periculum sustinebit. puer natus. animosus. cupid*us* de rebus
fremedum seldan he bið eald ungodan deaðe he swylt meden ealswa 7
alienis. raro erit senex. non bona mo`r´te morietur. puella similiter. &
geswincful feala wera gewilnað 7 heo ne bið eald swefen ydel ys
laboriosa. multos uiros cupit. & non erit uetula. Somnium uacuu*m* est.
nis na god mona blod lætan.
non est bona luna sanguinem minuere.

mona se feorþa wercu onginnan cildru on scole betæcen nytlice ys se þe flæhð raþe
Luna .iiii.[ta] opera incipere. pueros in scolam mittere utilis est. qui fugit cito
funden se þe gelyð rað he swylt oððe uneaþe he ætwnt se þe bið acennd
inuenitur. qui recumbit cito moritur. u*el* uix euadat qui nascitur
forligende gear twelfe gif he wint wælig he bið fræcednysse he hæf mæden
fornicator. annos duodecim. si euaserit diues erit. periculum hab*et*. puella
þæt selfe swefne swa wæder swa god swa yfel gefre*m*minge hit hæfð fra*m* tide
similiter. somnium siue bonum siue malum. effectum hab*et* ab hora.
þær syxtan oð nón god mona blod lætan
sexta. usq*ue* nonam. bona luna sanguinem min*uere*.

mona se fifta þu na selle offrunga forþi aðsware se þe flyhð raðe
Luna quinta non dabis sacramentum quia p*er*iurium. qui fu`g´it cito
he bið gecydd dead oððe gewriðan he bið gecyrred stale earfoðlice bið funden cild
nuntiatur mortuus. uel ligatus reuertitur. furtum difficile inuenitur. puer
acenned uneaðe ætwint æfter fif gear oft unnytt swylt mæden wyrst
natus uix euadit. post quinq*ue* annos sepe inutilis. moritur puella pessima
swelt forþi yfeldæda 7 wyrtgælstre se þe gelið he swelt swefnu
moritur. quia malefica & herbaria qui recumbit moritur. Somnia

25 stirpare] *i.e.* exstirpare | **27** uarię] *read* uanę *(the gloss correctly reads* ydele*)* | **28** he$_{1}$] *read* hit | hamacgað] *i.e.* amagað | **30** lan] *read* lange | **37** luna] -n- < e | **38** nytlice] *read* nytlic | **40** funden] *read* bið ~ *(Latin* inuenitur*)* | rað] *read* raðe | ætwnt] *read* ætwint | acennd] *read* acenned | **41** euadat] *read* euadet | **42** forligende] -r- < l | wint] *read* ætwint | hæf] *read* hæfð | **44** wæder] *read* wæðer | **46** þær] *read* þære | **48** offrunga] að *is a better gloss for* sacramentum *(see Förster 1944: 92-93, n. 1)* | aðsware] mansware *is a better gloss for* periurium *(see Förster 1944: 93-94, n. 2); read* ~ bið *(see l. 49)* | **49** periurium] *read* ~ est *(see Svenberg 1936)* | **52** wyrst] *read* ~ deaðe *(see l. 53)* | **53** pessima] *read* ~ morte *(see Svenberg 1936)* | **54** swefnu] *read* ~ uncuðu *(see l. 55)* | **55** Somnia] *read* ~ suspensa *(see Svenberg 1936).*

sint gefremmige habbað nis na god mona blod lætan
sunt. effectum habent. non est bona luna sanguinem minuere.

mona se sixta stalu bið funden se þe gelið lange 7 liðelice he adlað se þe
Luna sexta furtu*m* inuenitur. qui recumbit diu & leniter languescit. qui
bið acenned þriste mære swiðe aberd wif he gear nigontyne ætwint
nascitur audax. magnus. multum astutus. Si annos .x^{cem}viiii.^{uem} euaserit.
gesælig he bið tacn hefð on swiðram handu mæden acenned clæne weru*m*
fortunatus erit. Signum hab*et* in dextera manu. puella nata. casta. uiris
gecweme \`þancful´ *oððe* andfæncge on eallum godum swefne synt gewisse
accepta. grata in omnibus bonis. Somnia sunt certa
nelle þu awreon nys na god mona blod lætan.
noli reuelare. non est bona luna sanguinem minuere.

mona se syofoða blod lætan lac niman oððe temian hælan god ys
Luna .vii. sanguinem minuere medicare *ue*l domare. castrare bonum est.
flema bið gemet þyfð gestrangað cild acenned snoter gemendful
fugitiuus inuenitur. furtum conualescit. puer natus prudens memoriosus.
strang gelæred stefwis soðfæst lufwende tacn on andwlitan mæden
strenuus doctus. litteratus. uerax. amabilis. Signum in fronte. puella
felaspecol weru*m* *and*fæncge tanc onofer bruwe swiþran 7 on breoste wynstran
uerbosa. uiris accepta. Signum insuper cilio dextro. & in mamilla sinistra.
seoc mid lætedomu*m* bið geheled swæfnu gewisse synt oft late oð æfen god
eger medicamentis sanatur. Somnia certa sunt sepe tarda. usq*ue* sero. bona
mona blod lætan
luna sanguinem minere.

mona se ehtoða sædu on eorðan sendan beon awendan fra*m* stowe to stowe god
Luna .viii. semina in terram mittere apes mutare de loco ad locu*m* bonum
hit ys stalu na bið funden cild acenned uncuð strang swiðe he bið gedyrfed
est. furtum non inuenitur. puer natus ignotus. strenuus. multum. periclitatur
on wætere gewislice tacn hæfð on sidan swiðran. mæden tacn on oferbruwe
in aqua. presertim signum hab*et* in latere dextro. puello signum in supercilio

56 mona] -on- < ·· | **58** bið] *read* na ~ *(see l. 59)* | **59** inuenitur] *read* non ~ *(see Svenberg 1936)* | **60** aberd] *i.e.* abered | wif] *read* gif | **62** swiðram handu] *read* swiðran handa | **63** casta.] c- < ·;· ~ ‖ ⟨*f. 33v*⟩ | **64** \`þancful´] *over* andfæncge | **68** god] g- < o | **69** *uel* domare. castrare] *i.e.* pecora domare uel castrare | **70** gestrangað] *read* bið funden *(see l. 71)* | snoter] -n- < · | **71** conualescit] *read* inuenitur *(~ makes no sense in the lost or stolen property component)* | **72** tacn] -c- < i | **74** felaspecol] *not* felasprecol *(as in l. 192)* | tanc] *read* tacn | **74** onofer bruwe] *read* on oferbruwe*; ~ is senseless but in accordance with the Latin (see l. 75)* | **75** insuper cilio] *read* in supercilio | **76** lætedomu*m*] *read* læcedomum | oð] ~[ð] | **77, 79** bona luna sanguinem minere] *the collective lunaries of Svenberg's types I and II (see pp. 402-03) have a bloodletting component in the agenda part of day 7. Some redactions of type II have added bloodletting instructions for all days of the moon, which leads to a doubling of the bloodletting instruction for this day of the moon* | **80** stowe] -t- < · | **85** puello] *read* puella.

swiþran oft 7 his mære nytlice sceanfæst anu*m* were eðhylde heo ne bið
dextro. sepe & est magna utilis. uerecunda. uno uiro contenta non erit.
swefen raðe gewyrð gefyld gode betæc se þe gelið raðe swylt
somnium cito fi*et* completum. d*e*o commenda. qui recumbit. cito moritur.
ealne dæg god mona blod lætan.
tota die bona luna sanguinem minuere.

mona se nigoþa on eallu*m* nitingum to dondu*m* god ys wyrtun don se þe flyhð
Luna .ix. omnibus causis agendis bona est. ortum facere. qui fuit
raþe bið funden seoc raþe gewyrpð cild acenned corngesælig geap srang
cito inuenitur. eger cito conualescit puer natus granosus. astutus. strenuus.
smylte he bið geswenct oð gear seofone tacn on swiþran hand gyf he
serenus periclitatur usq*ue* ad annos septem. signum in dextera manu. Si
þritig geara leofoð wælig he bið mæden carful þancful nytwyrþe clæne tacn
xxx^{ta} annos uixerit. diues erit. puella studiosa grata. utilis. casta. signum
ealswa cwapa hæfð swæfnen raþe hit gewyrð bedigla ys na god mona blod
ut puer hab*et*. somnium cito fi*et*. cela non est bona luna sanguinem
lætan
minuere.

mona se teoða on eallu*m* þingu*m* to dondu*m* god on hus niwe infaran cildru
Luna .x.^{ma} omnibus rebus agendis bona. in domum nouam. intrare pueros
on scole betacen cild acenned gimeleas geswincful on forman ylde mæden
in scolam mittere. puer natus. neglegens. laboriosus. in prima *et*ate puella
milde wultewestre þurh ylde bed 7 bed heo deð se þe gelið raðe he styrfð
benigna lętifica per *et*atem melius ac melius agit. qui recumbit cito moritur
oððe genunge he ariseð swefnu ydele sint fram tide þære syxtan æfen god mona
aut cito surgit. Somnia uana sunt. ab hora .vi.^{ta} usq*ue* sero bona luna
blod lætan
sanguinem minuere.

mona se ændlefta wyldæda biddan treowu ceorran beon infaran nytlic ys
Luna .xi. beneficium petere. arbores abscidere. apes inuadere utilis e*st*.
cild acenned weallende abereð modful on langfære ylde bet he deð mæden
puer natus. feruidus. callidus. animosus. in postera ę*t*ate melius agit. puella

86 sceanfæst] *read* scamfæst | **92** nitingum] *read* intingum | **93** fuit] *read* fugit | **94** corngesælig] *read* gesælig; ~ *is a literal gloss of the Latin* granosus *(see l. 95)* | srang] *read* strang *(the same scribe drops the* 't' *more often, see 7/4)* | **95** granosus] *read* gratiosus *(on this erroneous reading, see p. 404, n. 40)* | **98** mæden] -d- < · | **100** cwapa] *read* cnapa | swæfnen] *read* swefen | bedigla ys na god] bedigla *over* cela, ys *over* est, na god *over* bona | **108** bed 7 bed] *i.e.* bet 7 bet | **109** lętifica] *read* lanifica *(the gloss reads* wultewestre*)* | **110** fram] f- < w | þære syxtan] *over* .vi.^{ta} usq*ue*; *read* ~ oð *(*usq*ue not glossed)* | **111** uana] ~ ‖ ⟨*f. 34r*⟩ | **114** ceorran] *read* ceorfan | **116** abereð] *read* abered | langfære] æftewyrden *is a better gloss for* postera *(see Förster 1944: 106-07, n. 8).*

tacn on anwlitan 7 on breoste hæbende wis heo bið clæne on ylde ungodu*m*
signum in fronte. & in mamilla habens. Sapiens erit. casta in ętate non bona
120 deaðe heo swylt seoc lang andlað oððe rædlice aris swefne betwuh feower
morte morietur. eger diu languescit uel celeriter surgit. Somnium inter .iiii.^{or}
dagas gewyrð beo þu ealswa. god mona nys blod lætan
123 dies fi*et* esto. Similiter bona luna non est saguinem minuere.

mona se twelfta on e`a´llum weorcum nytlic ys sawan wif lædan wæg
Luna .xii.^{ma} omnibus operibus utilis est seminare. uxorem ducere. iter
126 faran cild acenned god luflic tacn on handa swiþran hæfð oððe on
pergere. puer natus. bonus. amabilis. Signu*m* in manu dextera hab*et*. uel in
cneowe fræcenful mæden tacn on breoste hæfð wlitig ac na lang
129 genu periculosus. puella signum in mamilla hab*et*. speciosa. se non diuturnam
lif heo adrycð seoc oððe he lange lað oððe he swylt swefne ys gewis
uitam agit. eger uel diu languescit u*el* moritur. Somnium est. certum.
132 orsorh beo þu ealne dæg god ys mona blod lætan
securis esto tota die bona est luna sanguinem minuere.

mona se þreotteoþa fræcenful to angennene þinc ne þu mid freondu*m* na flit
135 **Luna** xiii. periculosa. ad incipiendas res. nec cum amicis c`o´ntendas.
se þe flehð raþe bið funden cild acenned þancfull tacn abuta eagan hæbbende
qui fugit. cito inuenitur. puer natus. animosus. Signum circa oculos habens.
138 þriste reaful ofermod hi*m* sylfum gelicigende na lange ne leofað mæden tacn
audax rapax. Superbus. sibi soli placens. non longe uiuit. puella signu*m*
on neccan hæfð oððe on þeo ofermodig þancfull þriste on lichaman mid
141 in ceruice hab*et* uel in femore superba animosa. temeraria in corpore cum
manegu*m* weru*m* raþe heo swilt seoc raðe ætwint oððe lange he hadlað swefn
multis uiris cito moritur. Eger cito euadit. uel diu languescit. Somnium
144 binnan dagu*m* nigon bið gefylled fra*m* tide þere syxtan god mona blod
infra dies .ix.^{uem} compl*et*ur. ab hora .vi.^{ta} usq*ue* sero bona l*una* sanguine*m*
lætan
147 minuere.

mona se feowerteoðe e`a´llu*m* god þingu*m* god þeawas bicgan wif
Luna .xiiii.^{ma} omnibus bonis rebus bona. mancipia emere. uxore*m*
150 lædan cildru on scole betæcan cild acen`n´ed ceapman tacn abutan eagan
ducere. pueros in scola*m* mittere. puer natus mercator signu*m* circa oculos.
oððe on þeo hæfð þriste modig hi*m* silfan licigende raðe swelt mæden
153 uel in femore hab*et*. audax. superbus sibi soli placens cito moritur. puella

120 andlað] *read* adlað | aris] *read* arist | **122** beo] *read* wær ~ *(see l. 123)* | **123** esto] *read* cautus ~ *(see Svenberg 1936)* | saguinem] *read* sanguinem | **126** luflic] -u- < f | on$_2$] on[·] | **127** in$_2$] -n < u | **128** na] ~ < [··] | **129** se] *read* sed | **130** lað] *read* adlað | **135** c`o´ntendas] `o´ < [e] | **136** abuta] *read* abutan | **141** animosa] -ni- < m | **144** þere syxtan] *over* .vi.^{ta} usq*ue; read* ~ oð æfen *(*usq*ue* sero *not glossed)* | **148** god$_1$] *read* godum.

tacn on neccan hæfð modig dyrstig manega weras gewilnigende
signum in uertice hab*et*. Superba temeraria. multos uiros desiderans. cito
swilt seoc gif raðe gewerpð. swefen on sceortu*m* timan gefre*m*minge
moritur. eger si non cito conualescit. Somnium breui tempore effectum
hæfð liflic ys mona blod lætan
hab*et*. uitalis est luna sanguinem minuere.

mone se fifteoða gewitnyssa syllan hit nis trum cild acenned fræcenful
Luna .xv^ma^ testimonium dare non est. firmum. puer natus. periculosus.
tacn on tuxle winstran hæfð cu*m*liðe fræcednisse hæfð of ysen
Signum in humero sinistro hab*et*. benign*us*. hospitalis. periculum hab*et* de ferro.
oððe on wætere mæden sca*m*fæst geswincful clæne wæru*m* gelicgende seoc gif
uel in aqua. puella uerecunda. laboriosa. casta. uiris placens. eger si
heo æfter þri*m* dagu*m* na arist he bið geswenct swefn na derað na ys
post triduum non resurgit. periclitatur. somnium non nocebit. non est
god mona blod lætan
bona luna sanguin*em* minuere.

mona se syxteoða nanu*m* þingu*m* nytlice stalu*m* se þe aweg gewit dead he bið gecyd
Luna xvi^ta^ nullus rebus utilis nisi furtis. qui recedit. mortuus nuntiatur.
cild acenned cu*m*liðe þancul staðolfæst ylde betere 7 betere tacn ansine
puer natus hospitalis. efficax. Stabilis. in ętate melior ac melior. Signum in facie
hæfð mæden tacn on sidan swiðran abered eallu*m* gelufad seoc her beforan
hab*et*. puella signum in latere dextro. astuta. omnibus amata. eger ut sup*ra*.
swefen æfter langu*m* timan bið gefylled 7 facn bið god ys mona blod
Somnium post multum tempus expletur. & dolus erit. bona est luna sanguinem
lætan.
minuere.

mona se seofonteoða nan ys geseligra onginnan sawan cildru on scolo
Luna septima decima. nulla est felicior incipere. serere. pueros. in scolam
betæcan cild acenned fræcenful freo`n´dheald abered wis gestæflæred þriste
mittere. puer natus. periculosos. amicabiles astutus. Sapiens litteratus. audax

154 gewilnigende] *over* desiderans cito*; read* ~ raðe *(*cito *not glossed)* | **156** gif] *read* ~ na *(*non *not glossed)* | raðe] *read* ~ swylt raðe *(see l. 157)* | **157** cito] *read* ~ moritur cito *(see Svenberg 1936)* | conualescit.] ~ ‖ ⟨*f. 34v*⟩ | **158** liflic] *read* nytlic *(see l. 159)* | **159** uitalis] *read* utilis *(~ makes no sense in the bloodletting component, see also Svenberg 1936)* | **160** mone] *read* mona | **162** tuxle] *read* eaxle | cu*m*liðe] *read* milde ~ *(*benign*us not glossed)* | ysen] *read* ysene | **164** gelicgende] *i.e.* gelicigende *(see l. 6)* | **166** heo] *read* he *(misreading probably because of the previous account of the birth of a girl, but the present prediction is an illness component)* | arist] -s- < l | **170** nytlice] *read* nytlic*; ~ over* utilis nisi*; read* nytlic buton *(*nisi *not glossed)* | **171** nullus] *read* nullis | **172** staðolfæst] -a- < ·*; read ~* on *(*in *not glossed)* | tacn] *read ~* on *(*in *not glossed)* | **174** her beforan] *over* ut sup*ra; read* swa ~ *(*ut *not glossed)* | **175** eger] -g- < · | **180** geseligra] -li- < u | scolo] *read* scole | **183** periculosos] *read* periculosus | amicabiles] *read* amicabilis.

soðfæst mæden word*um* gelæred on eallum þingum nytlic clæne wælig seoc lange
uerax. puella uerbis docta. in omnibus rebus utilis. casta. diues. eger diu
186 adlað swefne raðe gewyhð na ys god mona blod lætan
egrotabit. Somnium cito fi*et*. non est bona luna sanguinem minuere.

mona se ehteoða eallum to dodum nytlice gemacan on huse gelædan cild`r´u on
189 **Luna** xviii^{ua} omnibus agendis utilis. coniugem in dom*um* ducere. pueros in
hus oððe on scole cild acenned ofercumen tacn abutan cneow hefð
dom*um* u*e*l in scolam. puer natus. inuictus signum circa geniculum hab*et*.
192 ungedefe ofermod felasprecol mæd tacn oððe cild clæne geswincful
inquietus. superbus multiloquax. puella signum ut puer. casta. laboriosa.
gehealdend on eftran ylde betere seoc raþe arist swefen binnan dagu*m*
195 seruatrix. in posteriori ętate melior. eger cito surgit. Somnium inter dies
tyn beoð gefylled ealne dæg god mona blod lætan
.x.^{cem} completur tota die bona l*una* sanguine*m* minuere

198 mona se nigonteða ellum þingu*m* to dondu*m* nytlice cild acenned milde abered
Luna .xviiii^{na} omnibus rebus agendis utilis. puer natus. benignus. astutus.
swiðe wis wexende betere 7 betere tacn on oferbruwe mæden
201 multum sapiens. crescendo melior ac melior. Signum in supercilio. puella
ealswa swa cwapa on anu*m* were heðhylde heo ne bið seoc raðe gewyrpð þurh
similiter ut puer in uno. uiro contenta non erit. eger cito conualescit. p*er*
204 læcecræft swefne binnan fif dagu*m* geopenud bið fra*m* tide
medicinam. somniu*m*. inter .v.^{que} dies patefactus erit. ab hora .i.^{ma}
oðða nigoðan nys na god mona blod lætan
207 usq*ue* nonam. non est bona luna sanguinem minuere.

mona se twentigoþa eallu*m* þingu*m* ydelust ys cild acenned yrðlincg gep
Luna .xx.^{ma} omnibus rebus uanissima. est puer natus agricola. astutus.
210 mæden ealswa weras forhogað seoc lange adlað raðe na arisað swefen
puella similiter uiros spernit. eger diu languescit. cito non surgit. somnium
mæden ealswa weras forhogað seoc lange adlað raðe na arisað swefen
213 puella similiter uiros spernit. eger diu languescit. cito non surgit. somnium
na to gelefenne nys na god mona blod lætan
non credendum. non est bona luna sanguinem minuere.

186 gewyhð] *read* gewyrð | **188** dodum] *read* dondum | nytlice] *read* nytlic | **189** omnibus] *i.e.* omnibus rebus | **188,190** on hus oððe on scole] *read* on scole betæcan *(see ll. 189,191)* | **189,191** in dom*um* u*e*l in scolam] *read* in scolam mittere *(see Svenberg 1936)* | **190** ofercumen] *read* unofercumen *(Latin* inuictus*)* | **192** felasprecol] -p- < r | mæd] *read* mæden | oððe] *read* swa *(misreading of* aut *for* ut*)* | **196** mona] -o- < · | **198** ellum] *read* eallum | nytlice] *read* nytlic | **202** cwapa] *read* cnapa | **203** uno.] ~ ‖ ⟨*f. 35r*⟩ | **204** tide] *read* ~ þære forman *(*.i.^{ma} *not glossed)* | **205** patefactus] *read* patefactum | **206,207** oðða] *read* oð ða*;* ~ *over* usq*ue*.

mona se an7twentigoða untytlice to wyrcenne buton swurdwyrhtan 7 þu sylst
Luna .xx^{ma}i.^{ma} non utilis operandi. nisi gladiatoribus & si dederis
na underfehst eft stalu raðe bið funden cild acenned geswicful mildheort
non recipies iterum. futurum cito inuenitur. puer natus. laboriosus. misericors.
gestæflæred weldonde mæden tacn on neccan oððe on breoste swiþran
litteratus. bene agens puella signum in ceruice. uel in mamilla dextra.
geswincful clæne on eallum gelufod anum were eðhelde seoc earfoðlice ætwint
laboriosa. casta. in omnibus amata. uno uiro contenta. eger difficile euadit.
oððe raðe he swylt swefen ydele synt oð þa þriddan tide god ys mona
uel cito moritur. somnia uacua sunt. usq*ue* ad horam .iii.^{am} bona est luna
blod lætan
sanguinem minuere.

mona se twa7twentigoðe nytlice biicgan þeawas cild acenned læce mæden
Luna .xx.^{ma}ii.^{da} utilis emere mancipia. puer natus. medicus. puella
ealswa þearfena seoc raðe bið gestrangod nytlic ys mona blod lætan
similiter. paupercula. eger cito confortatur. utilis est luna sanguine*m* minuere.
swefnu gewisse beoð gif hi beoð gehealdene on gemynde.
Somnia certa erunt. si fuerint retenta in memoria.

mona se þri7twentigoða eallu*m* to dondu*m* nytlic. cild acenned folclic mæden
Luna .xx.^{ma}iii.^{a} omnibus agendis utilis. puer natus. popularis. puella.
þancful seoc lange he adlað oððe raðe swylt swefen na to gelyfenne na
animosa. eger diu languescit. uel cito moretur. somnium non credendum nec
on mode to healdenne oððа syxtan tide god mona blod lætan.
in animo retinendum. usq*ue* ad horam .vi. bona lu\`n´a sanguine*m* minuere.

mona se feower7twenti to ongynnenne þinc nytlic cild acenned winnende mæden
Luna .xx.^{ma}iiii.^{ta} ad incipiendas res utilis. puer natus. pugnans. puella
strang seoc raðe he swylt swefen naht ys on uhtan god mona blod
fortis. eger cito moritur Somnium nichil est. in matutino bona luna sanguinem
lætan
minuere.

mona se fif7twenti huntoþas began nytlic cild acenned grædig mæden grædig
Luna .xx^{ma}v.^{ta} uenationes exercere utilis. puer natus. cupidus. puella cupida.

216 untytlice] *read* unnytlic | þu] *over* si; *read* gif ~ *(*si *not glossed)* | sylst] *read* ~ feoh *(see l. 217)* | **217** operandi] -n- < · | dederis] *read* ~ pecuniam *(see Svenberg 1936)* | **218** geswicful] *read* geswincful *(dropping of* 'n' *by this scribe is attested more often, see 7/4)* | **219** futurum] *read* furtum | **224** swefen] s- < · | **228** nytlice] *read* nytlic | biicgan] *i.e.* bicgan *(on doubling of* 'i', *see 7/4)* | **230** ealswa] -l- < · | þearfena] *read* þearfend | **234** þri7twentigoða] þ- < t | **236** swefen] -e$_{1}$- < f | **237** moretur] *read* moritur | **238** oððа] *read* oð ða; ~ *over* usq*ue* | **240** feower7twenti] *i.e.* feower7twentigoða *(change from cardinal to ordinal number also in subsequent days)* | **242** raðe] r- < ·.

wulltewestre seoc binnan þri*m* dagu*m* cuð bið se dæg swefne binnan nigon
lanefica. eger infra triduum manifestus erit dies. Somnia intra dies
dagu*m* swutele beoð fra*m* þære syxtan tide oð nón god mona blod
.ix.^{uem} manifesta erunt ab hora .vi.^{ta} usq*ue* nonam bona luna sang*uinem*
latan
minuere.

mona se syx7twenti cild accenned gemindig mæden geradod seoc raðe he swylt
Luna .xx^{ma}vi.^{ta} puer natus mementuosus. puella citata. eger cito moritur.
swefen swa her beforan fra*m* undertid oð nón nys na god mona blod
Somnia ut supra. ab hora .iii.^{a} usq*ue* nonam non est bona luna sanguinem
lætan
minuere.

mona se seofon7twenti cild acenned stoter mæden wyrðful wis seoc leofað
Luna .xx.^{ma}vii.^{ma} puer natus. prudens. puella honesta. sapiens. eger uiu*et*.
swefenu habbað gefremmincge naht na deriað ealne dæg god mona
Somnia habent effectum. nichil nocebunt. tota die bona luna
blod latan.
sanguine*m* minuere.

mona se eahta7twenti cild accenned geswincful on eallu*m* geleafful mæden
Luna .xx.^{ma}viii.^{ma} puer natus. laboriosus. in omnibus credulus. puella
gehyrsum getriwe seoc raðe geeþrað swefnu swa her beforan fra*m* nontidi oð
obediens. fidelis. eger cito ual*et*. Somnia ut supra. ab hora. nona usq*ue*
æfen god mona blod lætan.
sero bona luna sanguinem minuere.

mona se nigon7twenti cild acenned geleafful 7 rice mæden wis 7 wælig
Luna .xx.^{ma}ix.^{na} puer natus credulus. & eminens. puella. Sapiens. & diues.
swefnu. god 7 gewiss ealswa god mona blod lætan
Somnium bonum & certum. Similiter bona luna sanguine minuere.

mona se þritti cild acenned gesæligust milde mæden gesælig geþwære seoc
Luna .xxx.^{ma} puer natus. felicissimus. benignus. puella. felix. mansueta. eger
swinð ac he leofað swefnu binnon þrim dagu*m* beoð onwrigene hwilan
laborat. sed uiu*et*. somnia. infra triduu*m* reuelabuntur. interdum

248 bið se dæg] *read* bið *(see l. 249)* | **249** erit dies] *read* erit *(this makes no sense in the illness component, see also Svenberg 1936)* | **251** sanguinem] sanḡ ‖ ⟨*f. 35v*⟩ | **255** momentuosus] *read* momentosus | **256** undertid] *i.e.* underntid | **260** stoter] *read* snoter | **267** .xx.^{ma}viii.^{ma}] *read* .xx.^{ma}viii.^{ua} | **268** nontidi] -o- < ; *read* nontide | **272** geleafful] *read* gelæred *(see l. 273)* | **273** credulus] *read* eruditus *(see Svenberg 1936)* | **275** sanguine] *read* sanguinem | **278** swinð] *read* swincð.

to warnienne nys na god mona blod lætan.
cauendum est. Non [est] bona luna sanguine*m* minuere.

endiað swefnu witigan.
Finiunt somnia Danielis prophetę.

280 nys na] *read* ys na ys *(see l. 281)* | **281** est. Non [est]] [est] *erroneously expunged, probably by the glossator, who could not make sense of the Latin and glossed* nys na *for* est. Non. *However,* est *belongs to the dream component, and* Non [est] *to the bloodletting component; the expunction is therefore unwarranted, and the Old English gloss should be emended from* nys na *to* ys na ys.

9.1/2 London, British Library, Cotton Titus D. xxvii, fols 27r/8-29v

ARGVMENTVM LVNARE AD REQVIRENDV*M* QVOMODO *VE*L QVALITER OBSERVETVR.

Luna .i. hec dies ad omnia agenda. utilis est. **I**n lecto qui inciderit diu languesc*et*. & longa infirmitate patietur. **E**t quidquid uideris in gaudium conuertetur. & si uideris te uinci. tu tamen uinces omnes inimicos tuos. **I**nfans si fuerit natus uitalis erit.

Luna .ii. similiter hęc dies ad omnia agere utilis e*st* emere. uendere. nauim ascendere. it*er* facere. sementem seminare. p*ro*pagines facere. ortum struere. terram p*ro*scindere. furtum factum cito inuenietur. Infirmus cito conualesc*et*. & si uideris somnium siue bonum siue malum non ponas in animo quia nullum effectum hab*et*. **I**nfans cito crescit. & non erit uitalis.

Luna .iii. de om*n*ibus quę agenda sunt abstinere oport*et*. nisi solum q*uod* uis ut non renascatur utile est extirpare. **I**n ortum nullum penitus opus exerceatur. quia uane nascunt*ur*. herbe. furtum factum cito inuenietur. **S**ompnu*m* si uideris nullu*m* effectum hab*et*. **I**n lectum qui inciderit non euad*et*. **I**nfans mediocriter cresc*et* & non erit uitalis.

Luna .iiii. omnia op*era*. incipere bonum e*st* molendi nos edificare. aqueductus aperire. qui fugerit cito inuenietur. **I**n lectum qui inciderit aut cito morietur. aut uix euad*et*. **S**ompnum si uideris effectum hab*et*. spera. & consule d*eum*. **I**nfans tractator regni erit.

Luna .v. sacramentum dare non e*st* bonum sed periculosum. **Q**ui fu`g´erit aut mortuus aut ligatus annuntiabitur. furtum factu*m* inuenietur. In lectum qui inciderit cito moriet*ur*. **S**omnia suspensa erunt. s*ecun*d*u*m quod uideris fi*et* tibi. caue consiliu*m* ne prodas. Infans iuuenis morietur.

9 Infirmus] -us < [· ·] | **10** non ponas in animo] *diacritic signs over* non *and* in animo *may indicate that the word order was to be changed into* non in animo ponas | **12** om*n*ibus] -us < [·]; ~ ‖ ⟨*f. 27v*⟩ | **17** molendi nos] *read* molendinos.

Luna .vi. utile e*st* uenatum p*er*gere. furtum non inuenietur. Infirmus diu languesc*et*. **S**omnum certum erit. sed caue ne dicas alteri. cautus esto. consilium detegere noli. fi*et* enim extra tuum decretum. Infans uitalis & felix erit.

Luna .vii. sanguinem minuere bonum e*st* & pectus purgare. **Q**ui fugerit cito inuenietur. **E**ger si medicatus fuerit. cito sanabitur. & somniu*m* ueru*m* erit. presens & futurum & post longa t*em*p*o*ra. Infans bonus erit. utilis & uitalis.

Luna .viii. sem*en* seminare. & apes mutare bonum est. **E**ger diu languesc*et*. & n*on* euad*et*. **S**ompnium tuum cito fi*et* *secundum* id q*uod* uideris. & si aduersa uideris ad oriente*m* te uerte. Infans in omnib*us* erit adquisitor & iuuenis decid*et*.

Luna .viiii. in om*n*ib*us* agentibus inchoare bonu*m* e*st* & somnium cito manifestabitur. Infra dies .xii. eger diu egrotabit & sanabitur. Infans bonus erit & uitalis.

Luna .x. omnib*us* rebus bonum e*st* inchoare. & sompniu*m* uanu*m* erit. tamen infra die*m* .iii. euenire sol*et*. **Q**ui in laborem inciderit. n*on* diu p*er*manebit. Infans multas regiones circuibit.

Luna .xi. bonum e*st* in uinea*m* ingredere. somnium sine p*er*iculo explebitur. infra triduum & non est falsum. Infans adquisitor erit in omnibus.

Luna .xii. in om*n*ib*us* reb*us* agentibus bonu*m* e*st* inchoare. & somnium firmu*m* erit. & cu*m* omni gaud`i´o fi*et*. *secundum* q*uod* uideris. & infra dies .ix. **E**ger diu languebit & surg*et*. Infans religiosus erit.

Luna .xiii. aliq*uo*d opus inchoare non e*st* bonum. **S**omniu*m* infra dies .ix. explebitur. *secundum* q*uod* uideris. tam*en* te ipsum cautum agas & sollicitu*m*. **E**ger longo t*em*p*o*re cubabit. **I**nfans emptor erit. & iracundus & non erit uitalis.

Luna .xiiii. omnia que agenda sunt bonu*m* e*st* inchoare. **S**omniu*m* infra dies .xii. conplebitur fi*et* iuxta q*uod* uidisti. cum om*n*i gaudio psalmis & orationib*us*

Luna .xv. non e*st* bonum inchoare ullum opus. **S**omniu*m*. bonu*m* & effectum hab*et*. Infans iuuenis moriet*ur*

Luna .xvi. p*ost* longum tempus fi*et* somniu*m*. est na*m*q*ue* utilis. **E**ger diu languebit & uix euad*et*. Infans uitalis erit & paup*er*.

Luna .xvii. **S**omniu*m* q*uod* uidisti fi*et* infra dies .xx. & in secreto cubili tui aliquid uidebis sine p*er*turbatione. Infirmus uix euad*et*. **I**nfans felix erit.

27 enim] ~ ‖ *⟨f. 28r⟩* | extra] -r- < ·; *read* extraneis | decretum] *read* secretum *(see Svenberg 1936)* | **35** Infra dies .xii.] ~ *may belong to the dream rather than the illness component (see Svenberg 1936)* | **37** diem] diē; *read* dies | **41** inchoare] -h- < o | **42** fi*et*.] ~ ‖ *⟨f. 28v⟩* | **48** cum... orationib*us*] *a transposition mark after ~ seems to indicate that ~ should follow the word* opus *in l. 49, which is also followed by a transposition mark; this cannot be correct because the present reading is supported by other collective lunaries (see Svenberg 1936).*

Luna .xviii. **E**uenire sol*et* somniu*m* infra dies .xxx. sed p*ro*pter hoc deprecare d*e*u*m* tuu*m*. ut in bonu*m* mittat. Infirm*us* multo t*em*pore iacebit. sed eaud*et*. Infans iuuenis morietur.

Luna .xviiii. **S**imilitudo somnii in secreto tuo uidebis infra dies .x. caue ne plus qua*m* duob*us* dicas. quia ualde auguriosu*m* e*st* **E**ger p*er* medicina*m* sanabitur. Infans in magno honore erit.

Luna .xx. **S**omniu*m* ne dicas ullo homini caute eni*m* agere debes. erit siquide*m* lic*et* a longe. Eger cito surg*et* sanus. Infans felix erit. & fortissim*us* bellator.

Luna xxi. quodcumq*ue* in sompnio uideris bonum e*st* lic*et* an aliquid sit p*er*uerse. Eger non diu languebit. Infans erit latro fortissimus.

Luna .xxii. uerum e*st* somniu*m* & certum. **E**ger cito sanabitur. Infans religiosus erit.

Luna .xxiii. dicere `somnu*m*´ socio debes. quia aliquando sol*et* accidere infra dies .viii. Eger p*ro*pe surg*et* sanus. Infans luxuriosus erit nimis.

Luna .xxiiii. **O**mne quod uideris de tua salute p*ro*mittit. **E**ger morietur. Infans girouagus erit.

Luna .xxv. precaue metus futuros. sol*et* eni*m* euenire infra dies xv. Eger sustinebit maximam iniuria*m*. Infans inopia*m* patietur.

Luna .xxvi. ad gaudium ueni*et* somnum tuum sed de inimicoru*m* insidiis sollicitu*m* te facito. Eger cito conualescit. Infans amabilis erit ualde.

Luna .xxvii. **S**ollicitus esto quia infra diem ipsum euenire sol*et*. aliquando in bonu*m* aliquando in malum. Eger uere diu languebit Infans mediocris erit. nec diues nec pauper.

Luna xxviii. Totum somnium q*uod* uidisti. ad letitiam ueni*et* tibi. Eger aliquid languebit. sed euad*et*. Infans neglegens erit & uagus.

Luna .xxviiii. hylaritate*m* & gaudium significat. **E**ger non morietur. Infans bonus erit & suauis.

Luna .xxx. Similitudinem aliquam infra dies .ix. dies uidebis aut totum somnium. Eger numquam sanus erit. Infans de fortuna tractabit. EXPLICIT:-

59 e*st*] ~ ‖ ⟨*f. 29r*⟩ | medicina*m*] -e- < i | **61** erit] *read* explebitur *(see Svenberg 1936)* | **63** an] *delete* ~ | **73-77** *the predictions of days 26 and 27 should be exchanged in accordance with readings in other collective lunaries (see Svenberg 1936)* | **76** uere] *read* uero | languebit] ~ ‖ ⟨*f. 29v*⟩ | **82** dies$_{2}$] *delete* ~.

9.1/3 London, British Library, Sloane 475, fols 211r-16v/4

æc dies utilis est omib*us* reb*us* agendis. Puer natus erit inlustris astutus sapiens literatus. & in aqua p*er*iclitabit & si euaserit posteriori etate melior ȩrit Puella nata litterata casta benigna speciosa uiris placens; In lecto qui inciderit diu languis cir & longa infirmitate patietur In sonis. quicquid. uideris in gaudiu*m* conuertetur nihil dubium. sis quia neq*ue* malu erit;

Luna .ii. Similiter utilis dies e*st* ererȩ uenderei nauem ascendere; It*er* p*er*gere hospitu*m* petere. ueste noua*m* induere. sessu*m* ponere sponsabas facere. sementes in terra*m* picere fodire fortis & instituere; furtum si fuerit insidiante domestico. cito inueniat*ur* Puer natus erit felix obtimus si seruus fuerit. lib*er* morietur; Puella nata erit benigna. uiris respuens. *et* unum uirum. conte*n*ta non erit. In lecto q*ui* inciderit. cito conualesc*et*. & sanabibt*ur*. Somniu*m* nullu*m*. efȩctu*m*.

Luna .iii. húnc die*m* q*ui*cq*ui*d potuerit te abstinere expedit: Etiam si uolueris in ciuitate*m* ingredere & emere non erit congruum. neq*ue* in agru*m*. op*er*ari nisi solum q*uo*d renascat*ur*; Vtile est stirpare. animalia donare nec in ortu*m* aliq*ui*t feras q*ui*a herbe uane nascunt*ur*; Furtum si fuerit factum cito i*n*uen`i´et*ur*; In lecto q*ui* ceciderit. aut cito co*n*uolescet. Aut longa*m* febre sustinebit; Puer natus erit animus & cupidus de reb*us* alienis. difficile q*ui* senex erit bona*m* morte*m*. non moriens; Puella nata erit. cupida de rȩbus aliȩnis laboriosa & multis uiris. cupida erit. & non p*er*ueni*et* ad senetue*m* habet.

Luna .iiii. Diem ha`n´c op*er*a incipere bonum est. puerum in scolis mittere. Aq*ue*ductu adducere. molendinum bonum est incip*ere* q*ui* fugerit. celerius inuenietur; In lecto qui ceciderit aut cito moriet*ur*. aut sim loco mutauerit uix euad*et*; Puer nat*us* erit. laboriosus & fornicabit*ur* usque i*n* annos .xii. si euaserit diues moriet*ur* & p*er*iculu*m*. habebit. p*er*mulltu*m*; Puella nata erit laboriosa. & cupida & morte mala morietur; So*m*niu*m* siue bonu*m*. siue malu*m*. nichil nocebit;

Text lacks day 14. The lunary opens a new quire. This edition is indebted to that of Svenberg (1936) and the corrections by Svenberg (1939, 1963) and Wistrand (1942) | **1** æc] *read* Luna .i. hæc | omib*us*] *read* omnibus | **2** posteriori] *read* in ~ | **3** languis cir] *read* languescit | **4** sonis] *the scribe frequently writes* son- *or* sonn- *for* somn- | **5** dubium] *read* dubius | neq*ue* malu] *read* neque bonum neque malum | **6** ererȩ uenderei] *read* emerȩ uendere | **7** hospitu*m*] *read* hospitium | sponsabas] *read* sponsalias | **8** picere] *read* proicere | fortis & instituere] *read* hortos instruere *(see Wistrand)* | si] *read* ~ factum | insidiante] *read* indicante | **8-9** domestico] *read* domestica | **9** inueniat*ur*] ~ ‖ ⟨*f. 211v*⟩ | **10** *et*] *read* sed | **11** sanabibt*ur*] *read* sanabit*ur* | efȩctu*m*] *read* ~ habet | **12** uolueris] -o- < u | **14** donare] *read* domare | **14-15** feras] *read* seras | **17** animus] -ni- < iri; *read* animosus | **18** erit.] ~ ‖ ⟨*f. 212r*⟩ | multis] -i- < a | **19** senetue*m*] *read* senetutem | habet] *read* somnium nullum effectum ~ | **21** Aq*ue*ductu] *read* Aqueductum | **22** sim] *read* si | mutauerit] *read* non ~ *(?, see Svenberg 1936, 1963)* | **23** fornicabit*ur* usque i*n* annos .xii.] *derived from* fornicator annos .xii. *(?, see Svenberg 1963).*

Luna .v. Sacram*en*tu*m* dare n*on* est bonu*m* si fuerit qui fgerit mortuus adnuntiabit*ur*; Legat*us* similit*er* furtum factu*m* difficile i*n*uenit*ur*. Puer nat*us* erit i*n*fans difficile q*ui* euad*et* post annos quinq*ue*. Si euaserit inutilis morietur; puella nata non erit uitalis. Et si d`iu´u`i´xerit pessima morteritura erit aut malefica aut erbaria. Et in lecto q*ui* cecimo inęt*ur*. & uniu*m*sa sonia susspensę*runt*;

l*una* .vi. Vęnarę apru*m* feras. Petras accip*er*e utile est. fouea*m* facere co*n*gruu*m* *est*. furtu*m* factu*m* n*on* i*n*uenietu*r*. Infirm*us* diuęs leuit*er* longuescet. fugitiuus i*n*uent*us* adnuntiabit*ur*; Puer nat*us* erit. audax & magn*us* & multu*m* astut*us*. In anno .xxx.iiii. si ęuaserit fortunat*us* erit. Puellana erit laboriosa in inima. ętatę & i*n* senectute si uiserit p*er*manebit. Et q*uod* uoluerit sacrificare expedi*et* cito; Et erit casta uiris accepta grata i*n* omib*us* bonis et q*uod*cu*m*q*ue* so*m*niu*m*. uideris certissimu*m* erit. Caut*us* esto ut*er*ę co*n*xilio túo & alio eu*m* ne p*ro*das.

Luna .vii. Húnc die*m* forcipęs ponęrę sanguine*m* minere om*nem* genus i*n*firmitatis medicare p*er*utiile *est*. Pec*us* domare siue castrare. co*n*gruu*m* *est* Qui fugeris inuenietu*r*. Furtu*m* factu*m* co*n*uolesc*et*. Puer nat*us* prudens erit temoriosus. stremorios dat*us* literatus uerax amicabilis; Puella nata erit uerbosa docta uiris accepta Eger medicam*en*tis sanabit*ur*. & sonnia certa erit.

LVVNA .viii. Húnc die*m* sementes facere siuę omne*m* genus sementis in terra p*ro*icere bonu*m* est. Siue apes mutare p*er*utilis est. Furu*m* factu*m*. n*on* i*n*uenietu*r*. Puer si nat*us* erít i*n*not*us* strenuu*us* multu*m* p*er*inclinabit*ur* in aq*ua*. Puella nata. erit laboriosa & p*ropter* uiros curiosa magna utiles uereco*n*da. casta s*et* uno uiro teco*n*tentia n*on* erit; Eger n*on* diu languebit sed cito morietu*r* & so*m*niu*m* cito fi*et* si d*eo* fuerit co*mmen*datu*m*.

Luna .viiii. Ille dies om*n*ib*us* gram*inibus* utile *est* Ortu*m* facere fontes inundare co*n*gruu*m* *est*. Qui fugerit cito i*n*uenietu*r*. Eger cito co*n*falescet. Puer natus granossus fi*et* & erit i*n* om*n*ib*us* reb*us* astut*us* & p*er*iclitabit usq*ue* i*n* annos .viii. & si uexerit annis .xxx. diues erit. Puella nata erit sapiens casta studiosa gra utilis casta. Sonniu*m* cito fi*et* & d*eum* illud. opor co*mmen*dare.

26 fgerit] *read* fugerit | **27** Legat*us*] *read* Ligatus | erit] *read* moritur *(see Svenberg 1963)* | **28** q*ui*] *delete* ~ | post] ~ ‖ ⟨*f. 212v*⟩ | **29** d`iu´u`i´xerit] *read* diu uixerit | morteritura] *read* moritura | **30** cecimo inęt*ur*] *read* ceciderit morietur | uniu*m*sa] *delete* ~ | susspensę*runt*] *read* susspensa ę*runt* | **31** Petras] *derivation from* accipitres *suggested in Svenberg (1963)* | **32** diuęs leuit*er*] *read* diu & leniter | **34** Puellana] *read* puella nata | in inima] *read* in ima *(dittography of* in *followed by* ima *(=*prima*))* | **35** uiserit] *read* uixerit diues | sacrificare] *read* lanificare | **36** omib*us*] *read* omnibus | **38** .vii.] ~ ‖ ⟨*f. 213r*⟩ | om*nem*] *read* omne | **39** p*er*utiile] *read* perutile | fugeris] *read* fugerit | **40-41** temoriosus. stremorios dat*us*] *read* memoriosus. strenuus doctus | **43** LVVNA] *read* Luna | **44** Furu*m*] *read* Furtum | **45** nat*us*] *read* ~ fuerit | i*n*not*us*] *i.e.* ignotus | strenuu*us*] *read* strenuus | p*er*inclinabit*ur*] *read* periclitabitur | **47** teco*n*tentia] *read* contenta | erit;] ~ ‖ ⟨*f. 213v*⟩ | **49** gram*inibus*] gram̄ *(see Svenberg 1936)* | inundare] *read* mundare *(see Svenberg 1939, 1963)* | **50-51** granossus] *this reading occurs in 9.1/1 as well (see also p. 404, n. 40)* | **52** casta] *delete* ~ *(this is a double, see ll. 52-53)* | gra] *read* grata | **53** opor] *read* oportet.

Łc DecyMA. Omib*us* agendis utile est. **M**ancipia emere uendere granaria *in*lu*us*trare pomaria inputrare edificáre i*n* domu*m* noua*m* introíre. Pueru*m* i*n* scola*m* tradęre. Puer nat*us* erit amicabilis. & i*n*uinctabilis sinistra. u*el* man*us* dext*ra* erit bon*us*. Ite*m* laboriosus in prima etatę p*er*iclitabit i*n* mare & euad*et*. Puella nata erit benigna & se*mper* ueniente etate melius in melius ag*et*. Eger a`u*m*´e cito moriet*ur* aut cito surg*et* & so*m*nia uana erit.

L*una* .xi. Vindemia i*n*gredere naue*m*. ascendere beneficiu*m* petere & dare filio adaptare arbores a*m*putare. sues suppotares aues inuasire; Puer natus erit amicabilis seruid*us* calid*us* animosus posteriori ętatę melius agit. Puella nata erit sapiens casta. ualitudinaria. in etatę n*on* bona moriet*ur*. In lecto q*ui* incidérit diu languescit. aut celeri*us* surg*et*. & so*m*nium i*n*fra dies .iii. fi*et* cónsumatu*m* caut*us* esto

L*una* .xii. Die hác om*n*ib*us* op*er*ib*us* agendis. bonu*m* est; Seminare urórem ducęre. sponsalia facęré it*er* p*er*gere Puer nat*us* erit bon*us*. & p*er*iculu*m* habębit. p*er*multu*m*. Puella nata erit speciosa s*et* non diurna uita exgut. In lecta q*ui* i*n*ciderit. aut languescet. aut cito moriet*ur*. & somniu*m* ęrit certu*m* sęcur*us* esto.

L*una* .xiii. P*er*iclitat*ur* neq*ue* co*n* amicis co*n*te*n*dere. neq*ue* feniciare exspedit q*uod*cu*m*q*ue* uolueri`s´. unde imarę. aut uua*m* p*re*mere suos supponere p*ro*pagines facere Qui fugerit cito inueniet*ur*; Puer nat*us* erit uiciosus. audax. rapax sup*er*b*us* sibili placens & i*n* magna etatę*m*. uiu; Puella nata erit sup*er*ba in animó & tęnęra in corpore multos uiros. habens. s*et* cito moritu*rr*a erit; In lecto q*ui* inciderit aut cito euad*et*. aut diu languesc*et*. & so*m*niu*m* it*er* diues .viiii. erit co*n*su*m*matu*m*. & certissimu*m* erit;

⟨Entry for day 14 missing⟩

L*una* .xv. Artificiu*m* cu*m*q*ue* fundare aut testam*en*tu*m* dare n*on* est firmu*m*. Puer natus erit p*er*iculos`u´s. astut*us*. hospitales. benign*us* & p*er*iculu*m* habebit de férro. aut de aqua. Puella nata erit uerecu*n*da laboriosa uiris placens. In lécto q*ui* ceciderit p*er*iclitabit*ur*. ac post triduu*m* surg*et*. & sonniu*m* nichil nocebit;

54 Łc] *read* Luna | Omib*us*] *read* Omnibus | emere] e- < o | **54-55** i*n*lu*us*trare] *read* inlustrare*(?, see Svenberg 1936)* | **55** inputrare] *i.e.* imputrare | edificáre] *read* uineas ~ *(see Svenberg 1936)* | **56** i*n*uinctabilis] *read* inuincibilis | sinistra] *read* signum ~ | man*us*] *read* manu | **58** a`u*m*´e] a[t]e, `ū´ < [t]; *read* aut | **60-61** adaptare] ~ [filio] *([filio] underlined to indicate deletion)* | **61** suppotares] *read* suppotare | aues] *read* apes | **62** seruid*us*] *read* feruidus | **63** casta.] ~ ‖ *⟨f. 214r⟩* | ualitudinaria] -d- < t | bona] *read* ~ morte | **64** .iii.] *read* .iiii. *(see Svenberg 1936)* | **65** urórem] *read* uxorem | **66** habębit] ~ *on erasure* | **67** diurna] *read* diuturna | exgut] *read* exigit | lecta] *read* lecto | **70** uolueri`s´] uolueri[t], [t] > `s´; *read* uoluerit | unde imarę] *read* uindemiare | **72** sibili] *read* sibi soli | uiu] *read* uiuet | **73** moritu*rr*a] *read* moritura | **74** it*er* diues] *read* infra dies | **77** cu*m*q*ue*] *read* quodcumque | **78** p*er*iculos`u´s] p*er*iculosis, -`u´- < i_2 *(not expunged or erased)* | hospitales] -sp- < st *(ligature)*; ~ ‖ *⟨f. 214v⟩*.

Luna .xvi. Nullis est utilis héc dies nisi fortis & gladiatorib*us* barba*m* aut capillos tondere est. Qui recessit mortuus adnuntiabit*ur*. Puer nat*us* erit hospitalis efficax. & conualesc*et* & stabilis erit & intate*m*. melior. Puela nata erit astuta om*ni*b*us* amata. & quicquid uoluerit lanificáre cito. co*n*ualesc*et*. Eger sustinebit sicut sup*er*ius dix*it*. & sonniu*m* p*ost* multu*m* te*mpus* fi*et* exspletu*m* & dolus erit.

Luna .xvii. Nulla feliciora terta*m* p*ro*scindęre stum*en*ta serere. Pueru*m* scole tradare medicam*en*tu*m* facere aras daræ. Puer natus erit p*er*iculosus amicabilis. astut*us* sapiens; Literatus. audax ueraxq*ue*. Puella nata erit uerbosa docta in om*n*ib*us* reb*us* utilis casta lanifica. facultate*m* optima*m* habens. In lecto q*ui* ceciderit diu egrotabit. & sonniu*m* cito fi*et* manifestu*m*.

Ł.VN .xviii. héc dies omib*us* age*n*dis utilis est sponsalias. facere puerum. scole tradere c*o*nguie*m* in bonu*m* ducere. Puęr natus erit inuictus. inq*ui*etus multiloquax sup*er*ib*us*. Puella nata erit laboriosa. Seruatrix. casta imposteriora etate melius egit. In lecto q*ui* inciderit. cito conualesc*et*. & sonniu*m*. infra dies .x fid expletu*m*.

Luna .xviiii. Héc dies om*n*ib*us* reb*us* utilis est. Hidrias facere. pecocara mutare uxore*m* accipere pueru*m* scole tradere. & q*ui*cquid. uolueris agere utilis est. Puer natus erit fidelis benign*us* astutus & inclitu*m* sapiens se*mper* ętatę sibi crescentę melior erit. Puella nata erit benígna astuta sapiens s*et* uno uiro c*on*temta erit; In lecto. q*ui* ceciderit cito c*o*nualesc*et* & medicaminib*us* curabit*ur*. & sonium infra dies .& patefactu*m* erit.

Luna .xx. Vanisimu*m* est híc dies om*n*ib*us* op*er*ib*us* agendis; Bonu*m* est uotis reddere t*er*ra*m* p*ro*scindere granaria inlustrare. pueru*m*. in solis tradere uęste*m* noua*m* induere; Puer nat*us* erit egricola*r*ris. benign*us* astut*us*. litterat*us*. Iudex in post teri ętatę erit. Puella nata erit lanefica astuta morib*us* bona uiros spernęas; & q*ui* in lecto ceciderit aut diu languesc*et* aut cito surg*et*. Q*ui* fugerit mortuus adnuntiabit*ur* aut ligat*us*; & sonniu*m* non est credendu*m*.

Luna .xxi. Híc dies hichil utilis est. op*er*andi. nisi gladitorib*us* mendacib*us* Pecunia*m* si dederis n*on* recipiæs. furtu*m* factu*m* cito inueniæt*ur* Puer nat*us* erit lactat*or*

81 fortis] *read* furtis | **82** est] *read* bonum ~ | **83** intate*m*] *read* in etatem | **84** cito] *read* ~ expediet | co*n*ualesc*et*. Eger sustinebit] *read* Eger sustinebit & conualescet *(see Svenberg 1963)* | **86** terta*m*] *read* terram | stum*en*ta] *read* frumenta *(see Svenberg 1963)* | **87** aras daræ] *read* aras dedicare *or* arma dare | **89** facultate*m*] *read* felicitatem | **91** Ł.VN] *read* Luna | omib*us*] *read* omnibus | sponsalias.] ~ ‖ ⟨*f. 215r*⟩ | **92** c*o*nguie*m* in bonu*m*] *read* coniugem in domum | **93** sup*er*ib*us*] *read* superbus | imposteriora] *read* in posteriora | **94** egit] *read* agit | fid] *read* fiet | **96** pecocara] peco | cara; *read* pecora | **97** utilis est.] -s e- < st *(ligature)* | **98** inclitu*m*] *read* multum | **99** s*et*] *i.e.* sed | c*on*temta] *read* contenta non | **101** &] *read* v | **103** solis] *read* scolis | **104** egricola*r*ris] egricolaris; *read* egricolaris | **105** post teri] *read* posteriori | spernęas;] *read* spernęns; ~ ‖ ⟨*f. 215v*⟩ | **107** ligat*us*] *read* ~ reducetur | **108** hichil] *read* nichil | gladitorib*us*] *read* gladiatoribus & | **109** lactat*or*] *read* tractator.

laboriosus miserat*us* litterat*us* dóctus bene agens. Puella nata erit laboriosa grata casta in om*n*ib*us* amata unu*m*. uiru*m* possidebit. In leto q*ui* ceciderit difficile euad*et*. Sonnia uana er*unt*.

L*una* .xxii. hęc díęs ne agendia locutionib*us* facere bonu*m* est care emere mancípia. Puer nat*us* erit mundic*us*. Puella nata similit*er*: Ego cito co*n*fortabit*ur*. Et sonnia cetera er*unt* si tamen fuerint retenta;

L*una* .xxiii. Om*n*ib*us* reb*us* agendis utile ęst. Puer natus. erit popularis. Puella nata erit animosa. Eger n*on* diu longuesc*et* q*ui*a aut cito conualesc*et* aut cito morietu*r*. So*m*niu*m* n*on* est crede*n*tiu*m* nec in animo tenendu*m*.

L*una* xxiiii; Om*n*ib*us* reb*us* incipiendis utile est. Puer nat*us* erit pugnans. Puella nata erit fotas. Eger cito morięt*ur*. Et so*m*nia nichil erit.

L*una* .xx.v. Om*n*ib*us* ueracionib*us* exercere utilis est Puer natus erit cupid*us*. Puella nata erit cupida. & lanifica. Eger infra triduu*m*. erit manifestus. Et so*m*niu*m* p*er* omines p*er*ęgrinos inuingu*n*tur; Et q*ui*cq*ui*d uideris. inter dies .viiii erit manifestu*m*.

L*una* .xxvi. Puer natus erit momentosus. Eger cito cit. moriet*ur*. & sonniu*m* ita fi*et*. sicut sup*er*ius dix*it*.

L*una* .xx.vii. Puer natus erit prudens. Puella nata erit honesta sapiens. Et q*ui* in lecto ceciderit ad uita*m* surg*et*. & so*m*niu*m* effectu*m*. habebit & scias eu*m* actu*m* esse futúru*m*.

L*una* .xx`v´iii. Puer nat*us* erit laboriosus & in om*n*ib*us* credend*us*. Puella nata ęrit obediens & fidelis. & qui in lęcito ceciderit cito co*n*fortabit*ur*. & so*m*niu*m* sic*ut* supperius dix*it*.

L*una* .xxviiii. Puer natus. erit erudit*us*. & emigens. puella nata erit sapiens diues. & so*m*niu*m*. bonu*m* erit. & certu*m* futuru*m* tam*en*.

L*una* .xxx. Puer nat*us* erit fidelissim*us* & benign*us*; Puella nata ęrit felix. bęnígna q*ui*eta mansueta Et q*ui* in lécto cęcidęrit p*er*ueni*et*. q*ua*si mortuus s*et* ad uita*m* uertet*ur*; Et so*m*niu*m* infra triduu*m*. reuelabit*ur*; Int*er*du*m* tam*en* cautę agendu*m* est.

110 miserat*us*] *read* misericors | **111** leto] *read* lecto | **113** ne agendia] *read* mercandia | **114** mundic*us*] *read* mendicus | Ego] *read* Eger | **115** cetera] *read* certa | retenta] -t_1- < c; *read* ~ in memoria | **118** crede*n*tiu*m*] *read* credendum | **120** fotas.] *read* fortis; ~ ‖ ⟨*f. 216r*⟩ | **121** .xx.v.] v < i | ueracionib*us*] *read* uenacionibus | **122-23** so*m*niu*m* p*er* omines p*er*ęgrinos inuingu*n*tur] *read* somnia omines peregrinos iniunguntur *(see Svenberg 1963)* | **125** cito cit] *read* cito *(dittography?)* | **130** credend*us*] credulus *9.1./1* | **131** lęcito] *read* lecto | **133** emigens] *read* eminens | **135** fidelissim*us*] felicissmus *9.1/1* | **136** mansueta] mansue‖ta ⟨*f. 216v*⟩ | s*et*] *i.e.* sed | **137** uertet*ur*] *read* conuertetur.

9.2.1 Lunary, Specific, Agenda

Literature

Jastrow (1905-12: II.457-577); Förster (1908c: 35; 1912c: 37-45; 1944); Budge (1913: II.556-59); Thorndike (1923-58: I.680-82); Svenberg (1936); Wistrand (1942); Weißer (1982); Taavitsainen (1988); Kieckhefer (1989: 86); Hollis and Wright (1992: 264); Wallis (1995: 115-17); Epe (1995: 61); Liuzza (2001: 188); DiTommaso (2005: 259-79; 402-46; 2006: 119-26)

Branch of Superstition

observation of times: days of the moon

Texts

OE: 1. London, British Library, Cotton Tiberius A. iii, fols 39v-40r
2. Oxford, Bodleian Library, Hatton 115, fols 152v-53v

Description

The genre boundaries of agenda lunaries are not always recognised. Förster claimed that a Latin version of (1) was included in the same manuscript on folio 65r (viz. 9.2.3/3).[1] The text he referred to, however, is a bloodletting, not an agenda lunary. The confusion was presumably caused by the fact that bloodletting lunaries do not usually state their purpose except in their rubrics, and 9.2.3/3 lacks a rubric. In a later article, Förster devoted a section to 'Tagwähllunare' (agenda lunaries) in which he mixed up agenda lunaries with collective lunaries.[2] Likewise, Hollis and Wright as well as Liuzza described the two Old English agenda lunaries as if they are incomplete collective lunaries,[3] which is surprising in view of the amount of research carried out on this topic since Förster's studies on the lunaries. Although agenda lunaries are used as building blocks for collective lunaries, the two genres should not be confused: collective lunaries predict a whole range of events,[4] whereas agenda lunaries limit themselves to specific actions to be undertaken or refrained from.

The purpose of an agenda lunary is to give advice on undertakings which are particularly good or bad on days of the moon. The predictions have a highly practical value and pertain to agriculture, hunting and fishing, travel, relationships and diplomatic affairs, trade and household activities, e.g. the sensible advice for the sixth days of the moon: "put

[1] Förster (1908c: 35). Cf. Thorndike (1923-58: I.680, n. 1).

[2] Förster (1912c: 37-45).

[3] Hollis and Wright (1992: 264), Liuzza (2001: 188).

[4] See pp. 399-401.

[fresh] hay in your bed; then you will have none of the customary pain in it, but you will be glad thereof".[5] In contrast to collective lunaries, in which the agenda component is sometimes preceded by a prediction of the overall quality of the day, agenda lunaries do not report whether a day is good or bad in general.[6]

To my knowledge, Old English (1, 2) are two of the very few medieval agenda lunaries in existence.[7] Agenda lunaries, zodiacal agenda lunaries, and agenda mansions of the moon have been attested in Middle English.[8] Weißer reported three agenda lunaries, but at least one of these (possibly all three of them), in St. John's College 17, is a bloodletting lunary.[9]

No source or Latin redaction has been identified which could have provided the original from which (1, 2) were translated. Both texts are incomplete: (1) has three entries and (2) has seventeen. The texts resemble each other closely in phrasing and content, but since (1) breaks off so early, and (2) contains more information for days two and three, (2) cannot be a copy of (1). Reversely, (1) cannot have been copied from (2), since the former antedates the latter by more than a century. (1) is so short that a comparison of the vocabulary has little significance. Both texts probably were copied in Christ Church, Canterbury. Since the two manuscripts of (1, 2) share more vernacular prognostics in identical redactions, it is likely that one exemplar was available for both (1) and (2).

---

[5] Translation of text 9.2.1/2, ll. 15-16.

[6] A specific lunary of this kind is in the *Syriac Book of Medicines* (Budge 1913: II.556-57).

[7] The Old French agenda lunary which Förster (1944: 159) claimed was published by Camus (1891: 207-11 [not 207-41]) is in fact a collective lunary.

[8] Means (1993).

[9] Weißer (1982: 57-58). Although I have not seen the other two manuscripts in question, I am fairly certain that Weißer's references pertain to bloodletting lunaries, for two reasons. First, the same confusion has arisen more often as explained earlier (Förster 1908c: 35), and as Weißer himself realised (1982: 30). Second, one of the two supposed agenda lunaries is followed by a birth lunary in the manuscript. If this is so, it is more likely that the lunaries are part of the α-sequence (see pp. 60-61), i.e. bloodletting + birth and not agenda + birth.

Edition

9.2.1/1 London, British Library, Cotton Tiberius A. iii, fols 39v/24-40r/4

On anre nihte ealdne monan. far þu to cinge. bide þæs þu wille he þe þæt gifð. gang in to him on þa þriddan tide þæs dæges. oððe þænne þu wene þ*æt* sæ sy full.

On twa nihtne monan far to. 7 bige land þ*æt* þine yldran ahton. þonne miht þu hit alysan.

On .iii. nihtne monan. far þonne on þin land. 7 þu his wel gewealtst. 7 sec þine frynd. 7 hi þe beoð bliþe.

1 wille] ~ ‖ ⟨*f. 40r*⟩.

9.2.1/2 Oxford, Bodleian Library, Hatton 115, fols 152v/4-153v/16

ON annihte monan fær to cyninge. 7 bidde þes þu wille. ge þ*æt* g*e*feð gang in to him on þa þridda tid þes deges. oðð þon*ne* þu wyte þ*æt* sǽ si ful.

On .ii. nihte monan gang. þ*en*no 7 byge land þæt þine yldran ær ahton. þon*ne* meht þu hit alésan. 7 on .ii. nihte mona he byð god to fǽranne on oðer land. 7 wyf to onfonne to riht life.

On .iii. nihtte monan far þon*ne* on þin land. 7 þu hys þonne wel gewaldest. 7 sec þine freonde 7 he beoð blyðe. 7 .iii. nihta mona byð god an to fixanne.

On .iiii. nyhta monan sibba þa cidenda men. 7 þu hie gesibbast. 7 on þone dæg sec þine fiend 7 þu hie gemetest. 7 hi ge beoð gewaldne. Se .iiii. nihta mona se byð god þæm érgendan hys sul ut to done. 7 þem grindere his cweorn. 7 þem cipemen hys cipinge to anginnane.

On .v. nihte monan gang to þinu*m* þeahtere 7 he þon*ne* þe in eallu*m* þingu*m* wel geþengeð. 7 sec on þone dæg þine frend. 7 se þeo stelað on þone dæg. ne geáhsað hit manna.

On .vi. nihtne monan dó þon*ne* hig on þin beð. ðonne hafast þu þæron nenige wunelic sar. ac þu þer byst gefeonde he is eac god circan on to timbrane. 7 eac scipes timber on to anginnanne.

On .vii. nihtne monan bidde þine laford he þe seleð. 7 gyf þu wille fedan cynigas bearn. oððe æðeles monnes geleod hine in þin hus 7 in þines hiredes 7 fed hine þon*ne* byð þe þ*æt* god. Se .vii. nihta mona is god on to fixiane 7 æðeles monnes wergild an to manianne.

Text is incomplete and ends with day 17 | **1** ge] *read* he þe | **2** oðð] *read* oððe | **3** þ*en*no] þn̄o; *read* þonne | **7** he] *read* hie | **12** þon*ne*] þ[i]on*ne* | **13** þeo] *read* þe | dæg.] ~ ‖ ⟨*f. 153r*⟩ | **15** beð] *read* bed | **19** geleod] *read* geled.

Se .viii. nihta monan geuntrumað ne léofað he lange. ac he ys gód on oðer land to feranne. 7 wyf to brigane.

On .ix nihtte monan. fer to cyniges bene gang in to him æt fulre séo. þon*ne* byst þu gesundful wyð hine.

On .x. nihtne monan bidde swa hwas swa þu wylle. hyt þe byoð gere. Se .x. nihta mona he ys god to standanne mid æðelu*m* monnu*m*. 7 to sprecanne hymb heora weorc. 7 éac byscop an to césane. 7 éaldormen. 7 cynigas.

On .xi. nihta eald mona fǽr on swa hwelce héalfe middangeardes swa þu wylle. ne sceð þe nænig wiht ne man dior. 7 he byð god an to cwellanne micle fixas on sæ.

On .xii. nihte monan byð god tó féranne ofer sæ. 7 on hird to ferenne. 7 æac to gewyfianne.

On xiii.[a] nihte mone æld fær in niwe hus. 7 nim eal mid þeo þrio fata ful ǽles 7 meolce. 7 hyt byð æac god ceap to mílciane.

On .xiiii. nihte monan is god ælc telg*e* to anginnanne ærest. 7 on niwne hired to fǽrenne. 7 preost to halgiene. 7 nunnan halig ref to anfone.

On xv. nihte. monan. hys god to fixianne. 7 huntu*m* heortas to secanne. 7 wildeswin.

On .xvi. nihte monan far offer sǽ. 7 site on þes scipes fórðstefna. ðon*ne* geseces þu þ*æt* land swa þeo leof`e´st beoð. 7 freond findest begeondan þæm sǽ. 7 he is god hordern ón to scæwiene. 7 minster to gereranne. 7 to sættenne.

On .xvii. nihte mone gyf þu wylle hus timbran. ber þ*æt* timber:-

23 brigane] *i.e.* bringane | **24** byst] [·]byst | **29** eald mona] *the first word of this collocation can be both inflected (i.e.* ealdne monan*) and uninflected, as in this case. The uninflected form is most commonly found in computistical tables of the duration of moonshine, e.g. Cockayne (1864-66: III. 222-24), and rules for finding movable feasts, e.g. Henel (1934a: 42-43), cf. Healey and Venezky (2000: proximity search of* eald *and* mona*); see also 9.2.2/2 and 9.2.4/2* | **30** dior] *read* ne ~ | cwellanne] ~ ‖ ⟨*f. 153v*⟩ | **34** eal] *read* eac | **35** ceap] *read* sceap | **40** far] -r < n | offer] *read* ofer.

9.2.2 LUNARY, SPECIFIC, BIRTH

Literature

Birch (1878: 478-79; 1892: 256); Jastrow (1905-12: II.457-577); Förster (1908c: 34, 36, 39-40; 1912c: 16-30; 1944); Thorndike (1923-58: I.680-82); Svenberg (1936); Wistrand (1942); Gundel and Gundel (1966: 69-70); Weißer (1982); Taavitsainen (1988); Kieckhefer (1989: 86); Hollis and Wright (1992: 264); Günzel (1993: 31-33); Epe (1995: 61-62); Wallis (1995: 115-17); Liuzza (2001: 187); DiTommaso (2005: 259-79; 402-46; 2006: 119-26)

Attribution

medieval: Daniel

Branch of Superstition

observation of times: days of the moon

Texts

OE: 1. Cambridge, Corpus Christi College, MS 391, p. 716
2. London, British Library, Cotton Caligula A. xv, fol. 132r
3. London, British Library, Cotton Tiberius A. iii, fol. 41rv
4. Oxford, Bodleian Library, Hatton 115, fol. 148v

L/OE: 5. London, British Library, Cotton Tiberius A. iii, fol. 36v

L: 6. London, British Library, Cotton Tiberius A. iii, fol. 65rv
7. London, British Library, Cotton Titus D. xxvi, fols 7v-8r
8. Oxford, St John's College, MS 17, fol. 4rb

Description

An exhaustive discussion of birth lunaries and their relationship to the birth component of collective lunaries is provided by Weißer.[1] Birth lunaries foretell the future of a newborn child in very broad lines. The entries are concise and pertain to dominant character traits ("religiosus", "bellator") or vitality ("uitalis", "iuuenis tolletur"). The detail of the birth component in collective lunaries is not matched by birth lunaries. In the former, the character and walk of life are described elaborately for both boys and girls, often accompanied by a description of birthmarks. A comparison between the two birth predictions illustrates the difference:

> (9.1/1) The first [day of the] moon.... a boy born will be illustrious, clever, wise, learned, endangered in water, but if he escapes, he will be long in life. A girl born will be pure, chaste, mild, beautiful, pleasing to men, of right

[1] Weißer (1982: 87-98).

discrimination, in later life she will lie in bed long; she has a birthmark on her mouth or eyebrow.[2]

and

(9.2.2/5) Who is born on the first [day of the] moon will be lively.[3]

The birth component of the collective lunary differentiates between boys and girls and presents the character in considerably more detail than does the birth lunary.[4] Some days of the moon in collective lunaries also mention the future profession of newborn children.[5] No Latin birth lunary has been identified that contains as much information as the birth component of collective lunaries. It is therefore assumed that the birth component was expanded only after its inclusion in collective lunaries.[6] For some reason, an analogous expansion did not take place in birth lunaries, which is why these texts remained brief.

Some Latin birth lunaries carry a rubric which reveals the authority behind the text (6, 7): "**Incipit Lunaris s*ancti* danielis de natiuitate `infa*ntium*´**" (6). The same attribution to Daniel forms the explicit of the collective lunary in Tiberius A. iii: "Finiunt somnia Danielis prophetę".[7] This collective lunary immediately follows an alphabetical dreambook. It may be that the two texts were copied as a unit, in which case the explicit might simply be a mistaken or misplaced reference to the dreambook (also known as the *Somniale Danielis*) rather than belonging to the collective lunary, which deals with more than just dreams. Only birth and collective lunaries are attributed to authorities in the Middle Ages.

Birth lunaries have been transmitted in Latin and the vernacular, including Old and Modern English.[8] The earliest witnesses date from the ninth century (e.g. the text in Harley 3017). Medieval birth lunaries in vernaculars other than Old English must exist, but they have not been

[2] Translation of text 9.1/1, ll. 3-11.

[3] Translation of text 9.2.2/5, ll. 2.

[4] The amount of information presented in the birth component can be used to distinguish several types of collective lunaries, cf. Svenberg (1936: 17-18), Wistrand (1942: 7-11). See pp. 402-03.

[5] A complete list of professions is in Weißer (1982: 89-97).

[6] Weißer (1982: 88-89).

[7] Text 9.1/1, l. 283.

[8] Latin texts are listed in Förster (1912c: 16), Svenberg (1936: 5), Beccaria (1956: 200 [50.8]), Weißer (1982: 57-58). Editions of Latin texts in Förster (1912c: 18-21), Wistrand (1942: 8-9), Modern English in Förster (1912c: 26-30).

published or listed, to my knowledge. In Anglo-Saxon manuscripts, birth lunaries occur in a limited number of contexts, to wit in computi (2, 8) and prognostic sections (1, 3-7). Within these contexts, birth lunaries are predominantly encountered in the α-sequence (1, 4, 6-8).[9]

Förster maintained that the Latin birth lunaries he identified (which includes 5-7), go back to one redaction. Indeed, texts (5-7) agree entirely in phrasing, content and order of the entries. (8) employs different phrasing in two places: "**Lun*a* xix** Honorabilis erit" versus "Luna .xix. In honore erit" (on the nineteenth day [of the moon] he will be honourable), and "**Lun*a* xxvii** Amabilis erit" versus "Luna xxvii. amicos [*sic*] erit" (on the twenty-seventh day [of the moon], he will be amiable/friendly).[10] Nevertheless, the overall similarity of (8) to (5-7) is close enough to conclude that the English Latin birth lunaries form one redaction.[11] The Old English lunaries are not as closely related among themselves as the Latin ones. Förster distinguished two redactions which went back to two different Latin source redactions.[12] The first redaction, the Old English gloss to (5), is based upon the Latin text of (5). The second Old English redaction (1-4) descended from an unidentified Latin source. Within the second redaction, texts (2, 3) are identical. The manuscripts containing these hail from Christ Church, Canterbury; Tiberius A. iii is dated to about fifteen years before the Norman Conquest, Caligula A. xv to about ten years after. In view of the close similarities between (2, 3), and the common origin and date of the manuscripts, the texts must have shared a common exemplar.[13] Text (1) and the incomplete lunary (4) are probably two separate translations not derived from or related to the translation of (2, 3). Förster thought that the Latin source texts used for the translations belong to one redaction.[14]

[9] On this sequence, see pp. 60-61.

[10] Texts 9.2.2/8, ll. 19, 27, and 9.2.2/7, ll. 20, 28, respectively.

[11] The continental birth lunary printed by Wistrand (1942: 8-9) does not correspond as closely to texts 9.2.2/5,6,7 as does 9.2.2/8.

[12] Förster (1912c: 17-18).

[13] This also applies to the dream lunaries (9.2.4/2,3).

[14] Förster (1912c: 17-18).

Edition

9.2.2/1 Cambridge, Corpus Christi College, MS 391, p. 716

Onre .i. nihte ealdne monan þ*æt* cild þ*æt* swa bið acenned þ*æt* bið liflic.
On .ii. n*ihte* aldne monan þ*æt* bið seoc 7 sicle.
On .iii nihte aldne monan se leofað lange.
On .iiii. þ*æt* bið on wurðunge geond feola ðeode
On .v. nihte aldne monan þ*æt* geong sweltað
On .vi. nihte þ*æt* bið lang lifes gesælig.
On .vii. nihte ealdne monan se leofeð lange on wurðunge
On .viii. nihte þ*æt* iung sweltað.
On .ix. nihte aldne se bið frecenlice acenned.
On .x. se bið þrowere.
On .xi. nihte aldne monan se bið landes ofergænge.
On .xii. nihte aldne monan se bið on allum þingum wurðful.
On xiii. nihte. se bið æwfest 7 rihtwis.
On .xiiii. n*ihte* in allum þingum he bið welgetyd.
On xv. se geong sweltað.
n xvi se bið in allum þingum nytwyrðe.
O.n xvii. nihte se bið sona gewiten.
On xviii. nihte se bið earm 7 geswingful on his life
On xix. on weorðunge
On xx. þ*æt* bið sona gefaren
n xxi þ*æt* bið on godre weorðunge.
On xxii. unheore feohtling.
On xxiii. se bið þeof 7 sceaðe.
On x`x´iiii. se bið geswingful on his life.
On xxv. se bið halsum in his lif.
n xxvi. þ*æt* bið weorces gælsa
On xx.vii. se bið on frecnum þingum acenned.
On xxviii ne bið se naðer ne welig ne arm.
On xxix. se bið forsæwen.
On xxx. se bið freondliðe

1 Onre .i.] *read* On .i. *but more probably* On anre *(see 9.2.2/2, 9.2.4/2,3)* | **4** wurðunge] -r- < n. | **6** gesælig] *read* 7 ~ | **7** nihte] ni- < m | **8** iung] iung[e] | **9** aldne] *read* ~ monan | **12** nihte] ni- < m | **16** n] *read* On | allum] -m *partly illegible through hole* | nytwyrðe] nytw[·]yrðe | **17 O**.n xvii.] *read* On .xvii. | **18 O**n] -n < x | **21** n] *read* On | **23** þeof 7 sceaðe] *read* þeofsceaðe *(see 9.2.2/2,3; on this compound, see Förster 1912c: 24-25, n. 6); the simplex reading ~ is supported by at least one Latin birth lunary (see 9.2.2/8)* | **24** x`x´iiii.] x[v]iiii, -`x´- < [v] | **25** halsum] *i.e.* gehealdsum | **26** n] *read* On.

9.2.2/2 London, British Library, Cotton Caligula A. xv, fol. 132r/9-35

Gif mann bið akenned on anre nihte ealne monan. se bið lang lifes 7 welig.
Gyf he bið on tweigra nihta akenned. se bið a seoc 7 unhal.
Gif he bið on þreora nihta. se leofað lange.
Gif he bið on .iiii. nihta akenned se bið a in wordu*m*.
Gif he bið on .v. nihta adl on geogoðe gewiteð.
Gif he bið on .vi. nihta adlig. se bið. lang lifes 7 gesælig.
Gif he bið on .vii. nihta se bið a weorð 7 lyfað lange.
Gif he bið on .viii. nihta eald se swelteð sona.
Gif he bið on .ix. nihta se bið frecenlice akenned.
Gif he bið on .x. nihta se bið þrowere.
Gif he bið on .xi. nihta se bið landes ofergenga.
Gif he bið on .xii. nihta eald se bið on eallum þingum wurðfull.
Gif he bið on .xiii. oþþe on .xiiii. nihta se bið æwfæst 7 rihtwis.
Gif he bið on .xv. nihta se bið sona gefaren.
Gif he bið on .xvi. nihta se bið on eallum þingum nytwurðe.
Gif he bið on .xvii. nihta se bið sona gewitan.
Gif hif he on .xviii. nihta oððe. on .xix. se bið gesælig.
Gif he bið on .xx. nihta se bið sona gefaren.
Gif he bið on .xxi. nihta so bið on godre weorþunge.
Gif he bið on .xxii. nihta se bið unearh fihtling.
Gif he bið on .xxiii. nihta se bið þeofsceaða.
Gif he bið on .xxiiii. nihta se bið geswincfull on his life.
Gif he bið on .xxv. nihta se bið gehealtsum his lifes.
Gif he bið on .xxvi. nihta se bið weoreces gælsa.
Gif he bið on .xxvii. nihta se bið to frecnum þingum akenned.
Gif he bið on .xxviii. nihta se ne bið naðor ne earm ne welig.
Gif he bið on .xxix. oþþe on .xxx. nihta eald monan akenned. se bið gód 7 frendliðe.

Mitchell's claim (1995: 18) that he did not regularise the spelling of the Old English texts he cited is void in view of his editions of this text and 3.1.1/1 | **1** ealne] *read* ealdne | **4** wordu*m*] *read* ~ leas *(see 9.2.2/3)* | **5** adl] *read* eald *(a similar misreading in 9.2.2/3, but this is a birth lunary, not an illness lunary)* | **6** adlig] *read* eald *(a similar misreading in 9.2.2/3)* | **13** æwfæst] -f- *has closed curve, but horizontal stroke indicates an* 'f' | **17 G**if hif he] *read* Gif he bið | **19** so] *read* se | **24** weoreces] *i.e.* weorces | **26** ne$_2$] [e]ne | **27** eald monan] *see 9.2.1/2.*

9.2.2/3 London, British Library, Cotton Tiberius A. iii, fol. 41r/12-41v/8

Gif man biþ acenned on ane nihtne ealdne monan. se lang lifes. 7 welig bið.
Gif he bið on tweigra nihta acenned. se bið a seoc. 7 unhal.
Gif he biþ on þreora nihta. se lyfað lange.
Gif he bið on iiii.^{or} nihta accenned. se bið a in wordum leas.
Gif he biþ .v. nihta adl him on geoguþ gewiteþ.
Gif he bið .vi. nihta. adli se bið. lang lifes 7 gesælig.
Gif he bið .vii. nihta. se bið a weorð. 7 lifeþ lange.
Gif he biþ .viii. nihta eald se swelteð sona.
Gif he bið .ix. nihta se byð frecenlice accenned.
Gif he biþ .x. nihta se biþ þrowere.
Gif he byþ .xi. nihta se bið landes ofergenga.
Gif he byþ .xii. nihta eald. se biþ on eallum þingu*m* wurðfull.
Gif he bið .xiii. oððe .xiiii. nihta se bið æwfæst 7 rihtwis.
Gif he bið .xv. nihta se bið sona gefaren.
Gif he byð .xvi. nihta. se byþ on eallum þingum nytwyrþe.
Gif he bið .xvii. nihta. se bið sona gewiten.
Gif he bið .xviii. oððe .xviiii. nihta. se bið gesælig.
Gif he bið .xx. nihta. se byþ sona gefaren.
Gif he bið .xxi. nihta se bið on goddre weorþunge.
Gif he bið .xxii. nihta. se biþ unerh fihtling.
Gif he bið .xxiii. nihta. se byð þeafsceaþa.
Gif he byþ .xxiiii. nihta. se bið geswincfull on his life.
Gif he byð .xxv. nihta. se biþ gehealtsum. his lifes.
Gif he biþ xxvi. nihta. se byð weorces gælsa.
Gif he bið .xxvii. nihta se bið to frecnum þingum acenned.
Gif he biþ .xxviii. nihta. se ne biþ naþor ne earm ne welig.
Gif he bið .xxix. nihta. oððe .xxx. se bið god. 7 freondliþe.

1 ane nihtne] *read* anre nihte *(see 9.2.2/2, 9.2.4/2,3)* | **5** adl him] *read* eald *(a similar misreading in 9.2.2/2, but this is a birth lunary, not an illness lunary)* | **6** adli] *read* eald *(a similar misreading in 9.2.2/2)* | **7** lifeþ] -þ < s | **15** .xvi.] -v- < [x] | **18** nihta.] ~ ‖ ⟨*f. 41v*⟩.

9.2.2/4 Oxford, Bodleian Library, Hatton 115, fol. 148v/1-18

SE ðe bið acenned on annihtne mona. se bið lange. lifes. 7 weleði.
Se þe bid on .ii. nihta ealdne monan. se bið seoc.
Gif he bið acenned on .iii. nihtne monan. se leofaþ lange 7 hydig.

Text ends with day 14 | **2** bid] *read* bið.

Gif he biþ feower nihta eald: he bið rice.
Se on .v. nihtne bið geboren. gung `he´ gewitað.
Se þe bið acenned on .vi. nihtne. se biþ lange lifes. 7 geselig.
Se þe bið acenned on vii. nihta ealdne mona. se leofaþ lange on wurþunge.
Gif se mona bið eahta nihta ealð. se gewiteþ sona.
Gif he bið acenned on nigan nihtne ealdne monan. se biþ fræcendlice acenned.
Se ðe bið acenned on .x. nihtne ealne monan. se bið ðrowere.
Gif man biþ acenned on xi. nihta ealdne monan. se bið landes ofergenga.
Se biþ acenned on xii. nihta ealne monan. se biþ lifes. 7 on eallum his þingum weorþ mannum mid gode.
Gif man bið acenned on xiii. nihta ealdne monan. se bið rices waldend. 7 godcunde.
Gif man biþ acenned on xiiii. nihta ealne mone. se bið ælces godes wyrþe.

5 Se] *read* ~ þe | **8** ealð] *read* eald | **9** nihtne] *read* nihta *(contamination of* nigan nihtne ealde monan *and* nigan nihta ealdne monan*)* | **10** nihtne ealne] *read* nihta ealdne | **12** Se] *read* ~ þe | ealne] *read* ealdne | **16** ealne] *read* ealdne.

9.2.2/5 London, British Library, Cotton Tiberius A. iii, fol. 36v/8-22

se þe acenned bið liflic he bið
Luna .i. qui natus fuerit. uitalis erit.
medeme he bið
Luna secunda: mediocris erit.
untrum he bið
Luna tertia: infirmus erit.
trahtnere cyninga he bið
Luna .iiii.^{ta} tractatur regnum erit.
geog he bið genumen
Luna .v.^{ta} iuuenis tolletur.
liflic he bið
Luna sexta: uitalis erit.
liflic 7 notwurðe he bið
Luna vii.^{ma} uitalis & utilis erit.
geog he afealleð
Luna .viii.^{ua} iuuenis decid*et*.
ealra strinend he bið
Luna .ix.^{na} omnium adquisitor erit.
he abuten færð fela rica
Luna .x. circuibit multa regiones.

Text lacks entry for day 17 | **8** tractatur] *read* tractator | regnum] *read* regum | **9,15** geog] *i.e.* geong *(on loss of* 'n', *see ll. 25,29, and 7/4, l. 66)* | **20** multa] -l- < i; *read* multas.

ealra strinend he bið
Luna .xi.^{ma} omnium adquisitor erit.
æwfæst he bið
Luna .xii: reliosus erit.
wiðerweard letted he bið
Luna .xiii.^{ma} aduersus impeditor erit.
ealra trahtnere he bið
Luna x^{ma}iiii:^{ta} omnium tractator erit.
geog swylt
Luna .x^{ma}v.^{ta} iuuenis morietur.
liflic 7 þearfa he bið
Luna .x^{ma}vi.^{ta} uitalis & pauper erit.
na lange he ne leofað
⟨Entry for day 17 missing⟩
Luna .xviii. non diu uiu*et*.
on wyrðscipe he bið
Luna xix. in honore erit.
feohtere he bið
Luna .xx: bellator erit.
sceaþa þancful he bið
Luna xxi. latro ingeniosus erit.
geswincful he bið
Luna .xxii. laboriosus erit.
widcuð he bið
Luna .xxiii. uulgarus erit.
genihtsu*m* he bið
Luna xxiiii. copios erit.
fræcnyssa feala he þolað
Luna xxv. pericula multa patietur.
na welig na wædla bið
Luna xxvi. nec diues nec pauper erit.
freond he bið
Luna xxvii: amicus erit.
gimeleas he bið
Luna xxviii: neglegens erit.
god 7 forsceawere he bið
Luna .xxviiii: bonus & prouisor erit.
ceapa feala he asmeað
Luna xxx: negotia multa tractabit.

24 reliosus] *read* religiosus | **25** letted] *i.e.* lettend *(see l. 9)* | **29** geog] *i.e.* geong *(see l. 9)* | swylt] *read* he ~ | **47** copios] *read* copiosus | **50** bið] *read* he ~ | **53** amicus] amicosus *9.2.2/6,* amabilis *9.2.2/8.*

9.2.2/6 London, British Library, Cotton Tiberius A. iii, fol. 65r/22-65v/6

Incipit Lunaris s*ancti* danielis de natiuitate `infa*ntium*´.

Luna .i. q*ui* natus fuerit. uitales erit.
Luna .ii. mediocris erit.
Luna .iii. infirmus erit.
Luna .iiii. tractator regum erit.
Luna .v. iuuenis tolletur.
Luna .vi. uitalis erit.
Luna .vii. uitalis & inutilis erit.
Luna .viii. iuuenis decid*et*.
Luna .ix. omniu*m* adquisitor erit.
Luna .x. circuibat multas regiones.
Luna .xi. omniu*m* adq*ui*sitor erit.
Luna .xii. religiosus erit.
Luna .xiii. aduersus impeditor erit.
Luna .xiiii. tractator erit.
Luna .xv. iuuenis morietur.
Luna .xvi. uitalis & pauper erit.
Luna .xvii. infelix erit.
Luna .xviii. non diu uiu*et*.
Luna .ixx. in honore erit.
Luna .xx. bellator erit.
Luna .xxi. latro ingeniosus erit.
Luna .xxii. laboriosus erit.
Luna .xxiii. uulgaris erit.
Luna .xxiiii. copiosus erit.
Luna .xxv. p*er*cula multa patietur.
Luna .xxvi. nec diues. nec pauper erit.
Luna xxvii. amicosus erit.
Luna xxviii. neglegens erit.
Luna xxi.x. bonus & prouisor erit.
Luna .xxx. negotia multa tractabat.

1 **`infa*ntium*´**] **infa** *added under the line close to the right margin* | **2** uitales] *read* uitalis | **8** inutilis] *read* utilis *(see 9.2.2/5,7,8)* | **11** circuibat] *read* circuibit | **14** .xiii.] -ii- < v | **15** tractator] *read* omnium ~ *(see 9.2.2/5,7,8)* | **16** morietur.] ~ ‖ ⟨*f.* 65*v*⟩ | **20** .ixx.] *read* .xix. *(but see 9.2.3/3)* | **26** p*er*cula] *read* pericula | **31** tractabat] *read* tractabit.

9.2.2/7 London, British Library, Cotton Titus D. xxvi, fols 7v/2-8r/13

incipit lunares S*ancti* danielis de natiuitate.

Luna .i. qui natus fuerit uitalis erit.
Luna .ii. mediocris erit.
Luna .iii. infirmus erit.
Luna .iiii. Tractator regum erit.
Luna .v. Iuuenis toll*etur*.
Luna .vi. Vitalis erit.
Luna .vii. Vitalis & utilis erit.
Luna .viii. Iuuenis decid*et*.
Luna .ix. om*n*iu*m* adquisitor erit.
Luna .x. circuibit multas regiones.
Luna .xi. Om*n*ium adquisitor erit.
Luna .xii. Religiosus erit.
Luna xiii. Aduersus impeditor erit.
Luna .xiiii. Om*n*ium tractator erit.
Luna .xv. Iuuenis morietur.
Luna .xvi. Vitalis & paup*er* erit.
Luna xvii. Infelix erit.
Luna xviii. non diu uiu*et*.
Luna .xix. In honore erit.
Luna .xx. Bellator erit.
Luna .xxi. Latro ingeniosus erit.
Luna .xxii. Laboriosus erit.
Luna xxiii. Vulgarus erit.
Luna .xxiiii. Copiosus erit.
Luna .xxv. p*er*icula multa patię*tur*.
Luna .xxvi. Nec diues nec paup*er* erit.
Luna .xxvii. Amicos erit.
Luna .xxviii. Neglegens erit.
Luna .xxviiii. Bonus & proui erit.
Luna .xxx. Negotia multa tractabat.

1 lunares] *read* lunaris | **17** pauper] ~ ‖ ⟨*f. 8r*⟩ | **28** Amicos] *read* Amicus *(see 9.2.2/5)* *or* Amicosus *(see 9.2.2/6)* | **30** proui] proui[os]; *read* prouisor | **31** tractabat] *read* tractabit.

9.2.2/8 Oxford, St. John's College, MS 17, fol. 4rb/1-30

Luna i *Qui* nat*us* fuerit uitalis erit;
Luna ii Mediocris erit.
Luna **iii** Infirm*us* erit.
Luna **iiii** Tractator regni erit.
Luna **v** Iuuenis tollet*ur*.
Luna **vi** Vitalis erit.
Luna **vii** Vitalis & utilis.
Luna **viii** Iuuenis decidet.
Luna **ix** O*mn*i*um* adq*ui*sitor erit.
Luna **x** Circu*m*ibit multas regio*n*es;
Luna **xi** O*mn*i*um* adq*ui*sitor erit.
Luna **xii** Religios*us* erit.
Luna **xiii** Adu*er*sus i*m*peditor erit.
Luna **xiiii** O*mn*i*um* t*ra*ctator erit.
Luna **xv** Iuuenis moriet*ur*.
Luna **xvi** Vital*is* & paup*er* erit.
Luna **xvii** Infelix erit.
Luna **xvii`i´** Non diu uiu*et*;
Luna **xix** Honorabilis erit.
Luna **xx** Bellator erit.
Luna **xxi** Latro & ingenios*us* erit.
Luna **xxii** Laboriosus erit.
Luna **xxiii** Wlgaris erit.
Luna **xxiiii** Copiosus erit.
Luna **xxv** P*er*icula multa patiet*ur*.
Luna **xxvi** Nec diues nec paup*er* erit.
Luna **xxvii** Amabilis erit.
Luna **xxvii`i´** Negligens erit.
Luna **xxix** Bon*us* & p*ro*uisor erit.
Luna **xxx** Negotia multa t*ra*ctabit;

Text is in columns | **4** regni] regum *9.2.2/6,7* | **10** Circu*m*ibit] Circūibit; *read* Circuibit | **21** Latro & ingenios*us*] latro ingeniosus *9.2.2/5,6,7; the Old English translations commonly read* þeofsceaða *(9.2.2/2,3), which indicates that the Latin may have been regarded as a compound (but see 9.2.2/1).*

9.2.3 LUNARY, SPECIFIC, BLOODLETTING

Literature

Migne (1861-1904: I.959-62); Birch (1878: 477, 496; 1892: 255, 269); Jastrow (1905-12: II.457-577); Förster (1908c: 39; 1912c: 36-37; 1944); Thorndike (1923-58: I.680-82); Henel (1934-35: 333-35); Svenberg (1936); Jones (1939: 88-89); Wistrand (1942); Weißer (1982); Braswell (1984: 347); Taavitsainen (1988); Kieckhefer (1989: 86); Hollis and Wright (1992: 269); Cameron (1993: 27); Günzel (1993: 31-33); Epe (1995: 62); Wallis (1995: 115-17); Liuzza (2001: 187); DiTommaso (2005: 259-79; 402-46; 2006: 119-26)

Attribution

post-medieval: Bede

Branch of Superstition

observation of times: days of the moon

Texts

L/OE: 1. Cambridge, Corpus Christi College, MS 422, p. 27
L: 2. London, British Library, Arundel 60, fol. 1r
3. London, British Library, Cotton Tiberius A. iii, fol. 65r
4. London, British Library, Cotton Titus D. xxvi, fol. 6rv
5. London, British Library, Cotton Titus D. xxvii, fol. 2r
*6. London, British Library, Cotton Vitellius E. xviii, fol. 1*r*[1]
7. London, British Library, Harley 3271, fol. 102v
8. London, Lambeth Palace Library, MS 427, fol. 3r
9. Oxford, Bodleian Library, Bodley 579, fol. 56r
10. Oxford, St. John's College, MS 17, fol. 4ra[2]

Description

With no fewer than ten English bloodletting lunaries, nine of which have survived, the genre has been poorly researched in the past.[3] As I pointed out before, Förster and Weißer confused agenda and bloodletting lunaries because the latter often do not state explicitly that they pertain to bleeding.[4] The difference between the two genres is obvious all the same: agenda lunaries mention specific actions to be undertaken or refrained from, and bloodletting lunaries merely mention good and bad times, e.g.

[1] This text has not survived. Indications for its existence are discussed below.

[2] Text 9.2.3/10 consists of an original text (10a) which have undergone extensive revision at a later date (10b).

[3] The most extensive studies of the genre are by Förster (1912c: 36-37) and Henel (1934-35: 333-35).

[4] See pp. 422-23.

"**L**una **i. T**ota die bona est", and "**L**una **ii. N**on est bona" (2). Fortunately, there are two indications which substantiate that texts containing such brief statements are indeed bloodletting lunaries. First, some texts have a rubric that explains their purpose: "**AD SANGVINEM MINVENDVM**" (2), "**De flebotomatione *uel* de minuendo sanguine**" (4), or "**DE SANGVINE MINVERE**" (7). Second, the bloodletting component of collective lunaries, which was added to the text at a later date,[5] explicitly states its intent as an aid in regulating bloodletting, for instance "the moon is all day good for bloodletting".[6]

Bloodletting lunaries are simple devices which, by their nature, do not allow any freedom of interpretation. The predictions reveal good and bad days of the moon for bloodletting, with occasionally a specification of a part of the day on which bleeding is particularly good. On the fourth day of the moon, for instance, "bleeding is good in the early morning".[7] Förster saw similarities with Babylonian astrology, which also took into account the hour of day.[8] Weißer drew a comparison with the Egyptian practice of dividing the day into three parts.[9] Indeed, in the Egyptian lists of lucky and unlucky days (not the Egyptian Days as the Anglo-Saxons knew them!),[10] the days are divided into three parts, each of which could be lucky or unlucky.[11] It is tempting to see evidence of the antiquity of the bloodletting lunaries in the link with Egyptian customs, but no such link can be substantiated. The late inclusion of a bloodletting component into Latin collective lunaries, its absence in Greek selenodromia, and the earliest attestation of bloodletting lunaries in the ninth century may be indicative of a medieval rather than classical or pre-Christian genesis of the genre. Weißer mentioned Babylonian and Assyrian bloodletting injunctions, but whether these are lunaries or not is not specified.[12]

Bede's writings are sometimes regarded as signs of the existence of bloodletting prognostics, including lunaries, in the late eighth century. The pseudo-Bedan treatise *De minutione sanguinis, siue de phlebotomia*,[13] is seen by some as a sign for the bloodletting prognostics to be older than

[5] See p. 400.
[6] Translation of text 9.1/1, l. 15.
[7] Translation of text 9.2.3/2, l. 6.
[8] Förster (1944: 91, n. 18).
[9] Weißer (1982: 30-31).
[10] See p. 333.
[11] Cf. Dawson (1926).
[12] Weißer (1982: 31).
[13] Migne (1861-1904: I.959-62).

the first attested texts.[14] Thanks to Jones's efforts, *De minutione* can no longer be construed in this way. An error which persists to this day is an interpretation of the description of St. John of Beverley healing a nun who had been bled at the wrong time, in Bede's *Ecclesiastical History*, as evidence of bloodletting lunaries in Bede's time.[15] The relevant passage from the *Ecclesiastical History* is discussed in more detail elsewhere.[16] All in all, there is no concrete evidence that bloodletting lunaries existed in the early Middle Ages.

In English manuscripts, bloodletting lunaries are attested in a limited number of contexts. The most common place is the computus (1, 2, 5, *6*, 8-10), followed by prognostic sections (3, 4) and the use of a bloodletting lunary as guest material (7).[17] Although bloodletting lunaries are undeniably medical in intent, their absence from medical sections in Anglo-Saxon manuscripts is conspicuous. The insertion of bloodletting lunaries into a computus or prognostic section is not haphazard. In both contexts, the bloodletting lunary is placed in the α-sequence, a fixed unit of four lunaries and a birth prognostic (3, 4, 8, 10).[18] Additionally, bloodletting lunaries may precede the calendar in the computus (1, 2, 5, *6*). The ties between the manuscripts containing (1, 2, 5) have been pointed out by Henel,[19] who also made a case for the existence of a now-lost bloodletting lunary preceding the calendar of Vitellius E. xviii (i.e. *6*).[20] The apparently random positioning of the earliest bloodletting lunary (9) in the computus of Bodley 579 and the guest text (7) in the miscellany Harley 3271, is in contrast with the careful placement in the other Anglo-Saxon manuscripts, where the lunary is embedded in an α-sequence or a lunary/calendar unit. This deliberate placement would suggest that the value of bloodletting lunaries as tabular items in computistical or lunar sequences came to be recognised.

In 1912, Förster wrote that he did not know of any bloodletting lunaries in the vernacular.[21] In the same year, James published the only bloodletting lunary in Old English (the gloss to 1) in his *Descriptive Catalogue of the*

[14] See pp. 278-79.

[15] E.g. Cameron (1993: 27), Liuzza (2001: 202).

[16] See pp. 115-17.

[17] On these contexts, see chapter two.

[18] See pp. 60-61.

[19] Henel (1934a; 1934-35: 335).

[20] Henel (1934a: 26, n. 78). The lost bloodletting lunary in Vitellius E. xviii is not discussed in Pulsiano's analysis of the computus of this manuscript (1998b).

[21] Förster (1912c: 36).

Manuscripts in the Library of Corpus Christi College Cambridge.[22] Since then, a Provencal and an Old French bloodletting lunary have come to light.[23] For some reason, vernacularisation of the bloodletting lunaries remained a marginal phenomenon. Continental Latin bloodletting lunaries have been attested, mostly from the eleventh century or later.[24]

I distinguish four redactions for the Anglo-Saxon Latin bloodletting lunaries, which coincide to a large extent with the contextual situation outlined above. The earliest text, (9), offers a straightforward binary system of entries ("bona est" or "mala est") without specification into parts of the day. The other redactions offer occasional advice on particularly beneficial hours. The second redaction is composed of the bloodletting lunaries in the lunary/calendar sequence in the computus (1, 2, 5, presumably *6*), plus the guest prognostic in Harley 3271 (7). Apart from some minor alterations in the arrangement of the entries (e.g. "bona est" where other texts read "non est bona"), there is enough agreement between the texts to regard them as one redaction. Within redaction two, (2, 5) deviate from (1, 7) on two occasions. For days twenty-five and twenty-eight, (1, 7) read "non est bona", but (2, 5) read "malum est"; for day twenty (1, 7) read "non est bona", but (2 (and possibly) 5) read "bona est". Therefore, I see these two groups as variant versions of redaction two. The feminine declension "bona" is used throughout in the second redaction, while the third redaction exhibits a preference for neuter "bonum". The third redaction is formed by the bloodletting lunaries belonging to the α-sequence (3, 4, 8, 10a). These differ in various places from the texts of the second redaction. The advice on days ten, twelve and twenty-nine is in direct opposition. Furthermore, the advice does not coincide entirely for some days, e.g. "ab hora .iii. & .vi. bona est" (redaction two) versus "tota die bonum est" (redaction three), and "ab hora .v. bona est" versus "ab hora .viii. bonum est". Redaction three consists of two versions which differ from each other in three places, viz. (3) and (4, 8, 10a). The fourth redaction, finally, is the revision of (10), viz. (10b), by the expunction and substitution of about half the entries. The changes are so extensive that the text is no longer similar to any of the other three redactions.

[22] James (1912: II.316).

[23] Förster (1944: 8, n. 2).

[24] References in Förster (1912c: 36), Svenberg (1936: 5), Beccaria (1956: 121 [8.10], 213 [55.23], 379 [133.33]), Weißer (1982: 57).

The English bloodletting lunaries hail from only three places and were copied in a relatively short period. Redaction one is from Canterbury and otherwise unattested. Both versions of redaction two are from New Minster, Winchester. The first version of redaction three is from Christ Church, Canterbury, while the second version is from New Minster, Winchester and Thorney Abbey. Redaction four is from Thorney Abbey. The earliest redaction is one, dating from the 980s. Redaction two was copied in the period 1023-73. Version one of the third redaction dates from about 1050, while the earliest witness of version two is from the first half of the eleventh century and the next from the first quarter of the twelfth. Redaction four is from the early twelfth century. For a genre with such a short textual history, the diversity is remarkable. Moreover, it is unprecedented that changes between and within text redactions can be tied to specific locations so clearly.

Edition[25]

9.2.3/1 Cambridge, Corpus Christi College 422, p. 27

	gimenett
Luna i	**B**ona est. her hit is (god tima.)
Luna ii	**N**on est bona. nis hi(t her god tima.)
Luna iii	**A**b hora t*er*tia bona est. fr(am ðære .iii. tide.)
Luna iiii	**I**n matutina bona e*st*. on (ærne mergen.)
Luna v	**N**on est bona. nis hit her god ti(ma.)
Luna vi	**N**on est bona. nis hit hér gód tíma.
Luna vii	**O**m*n*i die bona est. ealne dæg hit is gód.
Luna viii	**D**e nona usq*ue* ad nocte*m* bona e*st*. fra*m* none.
Luna viiii	**N**on est bona. nis hit her gód tíma.
Luna x	**N**on est bona. nis hit her gód tíma.
Luna xi	**N**on est bona. nis hit her god tima.
Luna xii	**N**on est bona. nis her gód tíma.
Luna xiii	**A** quinta ora bona e*st*. fra*m* ðære .v. tídæ.
Luna xiiii	**B**ona est. her hit is gód tíma.
Luna xv	**N**on est bona. nis hit her gód tíma.
Luna xvi	**I**nutilis est. nis hit her nytwirðlic.
Luna xvii	**B**ona est. her hit is gód tíma.

The top right-hand corner of the page as been torn out, so the endings of the first six lines are lost | **13** nis] *read* ~ hit.

[25] Order of the texts: 1, 7, 2, 5, 3, 4, 8-10 (NB text *6* is now lost).

Luna xviii	**N**on est bona. nis hit her god tima.
Luna xix	**M**elior est. her hit is betere.
Luna xx	**N**on est bona. nis hit her gód tíma.
Luna xxi	**I**n matutina bona e*st*. on ærne mergen.
Luna xxii	**A**b ora .iii.[ia] ad .vi.[tam] bona. fra*m* underne oð middæg
Luna xxiii	**A**b ora quinta bona e*st*. fra*m* ðære .v. tide.
Luna xxiiii	**B**ona est. her hit is gód tíma.
Luna xxv	**N**on est bona. nis hit her gód tíma.
Luna xxvi	**B**ona est. her hit is god tíma.
Luna xxvii	**T**ota die bona est. ealne dæg hit is gód.
Luna xxviii	**N**on est bona. nis hit her gód tíma.
Luna xxviiii	**B**ona est. her hit is gód tima.
Luna xxx	**N**on est bona. nis hit her god tima.

23 bona] *read* ~ est | **27** **B**ona est] *other texts read* non est bona/-um.

9.2.3/7 London, British Library, Harley 3271, fol. 102v/1-16

DE SANGVINE MINVERE:–

LVNA **i.**	**T**ota die bona est.
LVNA **ii.**	**N**on est bona.
LVNA **iii.**	**A**b hora .iii. bona est.
LVNA **iiii.**	**I**n matutina bona est.
LVNA **v.**	**N**on est bona.
LVNA **vi.**	**N**on est bona.
LVNA **vii.**	**O**m*n*i die bona est.
LVNA **viii.**	**D**e nona usq*ue* ad noctem bona est.
LVNA **ix.**	**N**on est bona.
LVNA **x.**	**N**on est bona.
LVNA **xi**	**N**on est bona.
LVNA **xii.**	**N**on est bona.
LVNA **xiii.**	**A**b hora quinta bona est.
LVNA **xiiii**	**B**ona est.
LVNA **xv.**	**N**on est bona.
LVNA **xvi**	**I**nutilis est.
LVNA **xvii.**	**B**ona est.
LVNA **xviii**	**N**on est bona.
LVNA **xix.**	**M**elior est.
LVNA **xx.**	**N**on est bona.
LVNA **xxi.**	**I**n matutina bona est.
LVNA **xxii.**	**A**b hora .iii. & .vi. bona est.
LVNA **xxiii.**	Ab hora .v. bona est.
LVNA **xxiiii.**	Bona est.
LVNA **xxv.**	Non est bona.
LVNA **xxvi.**	Non est bona.
LVNA **xxvii.**	Om*n*i die bona est
LVNA **xxviii.**	Non est bona
LVNA **xxix**	Bona est.
LVNA **xxx.**	Non est bona.

Text is in columns.

9.2.3/2 London, British Library, Arundel 60, fol. 1r

AD SANGVINEM MINVENDVM.

Luna i	**T**ota die bona est.
Luna ii	**N**on est bona.
Luna iii	**A**b hora .iii. bona est.
Luna iiii	**I**n matutina bona est.
Luna v	**N**on est bona.
Luna vi	**N**on est bona.
Luna vii	**O**m*ni* die bona est.
Luna viii	**D**e nona usq*ue* ad noc-te*m* bona est.
Luna viiii	**N**on est bona.
Luna x	**N**on est bona.
Luna xi	**N**on est bona.
Luna xii	**N**on est bona.
Luna xiii	**A**b hora .v. bona est.
Luna xiiii	**B**ona est.
Luna xv	**N**on est bona.
Luna xvi	**I**nutilis est.
Luna xvii	**B**ona est.
Luna xviii	**N**on est bona.
Luna xix	**M**elior est.
Luna xx	**B**ona est.
Luna xxi	**I**n matutina bona est.
Luna xxii	**A**b hora .iii. & vi. bona est.
Luna xxiii	**A**b hora .v. bona est.
Luna xxiiii	**B**ona est.
Luna xxv	**M**alum est.
Luna xxvi	**N**on est bona.
Luna xxvii	**T**ota die bona est.
Luna xxviii	**M**alum est.
Luna xxix	**B**ona est.
Luna xxx	**N**on est bona.

Text is in columns. Text is framed in four coloured rectangles; columns are demarcated by double vertical lines.

9.2.3/5 London, British Library, Cotton Titus D. xxvii, fol. 2r

Ad sanguinem minuendam.

Luna i	Tota die bona est.
Luna ii	**N**on est bona.
Luna iii	**A**d hora .iii. bona est.
Luna iiii	In matutina bona est.
Luna v	**N**on est bona.
Luna vi	**N**on est bona.
Luna vii	Omni die bona est.
Luna viii	**D**e nona usque ad noctem bona est.
Luna viiii	**B**ona est.
Luna x	Non est bona.
Luna xi	**N**on est bona.
Luna xii	**N**on est bona.
Luna xiii	Ad hora .v.^{ta} bona
Luna xiiii	**B**ona est.
Luna xv	**N**on est bona.
Luna xvi	Inutilis est.
Luna xvii	**B**ona est.
Luna xviii	**N**on est bona.
Luna xviiii	Melior est.
Luna xx	**N**on est.
Luna xxi	**I**n matutina bona est.
Luna xxii	Ad hora .iii. & .vi. bona est.
Luna xxiii	**A**d hora .v. bona est.
Luna xxiiii	**B**ona est.
Luna xxv	Malum est.
Luna xxvi	**N**on est bona.
Luna xxvii	**T**ota die bona est.
Luna xxviii	**B**ona est.
Luna xxviiii	Malum est.
Luna xxx	**N**on est bona.

Text is in columns. Left margin faded | **1 minuendam**] *read* minuendum | **11 Bona est**] *other texts read* non est bona/-um | **15** bona] *read* ~ est | **22 Non est**] *read* Bona est *(see 9.2.3/2, the version closest to 9.2.3/5) or* Non est bona *(see 9.2.3/1,7)* | **31,32** *the predictions for days 28 and 29 should be swapped (see 9.2.3/2).*

9.2.3/3 London, British Library, Cotton Tiberius A. iii, fol. 65r/1-11

Luna .i. tota die bonum est.
Luna .ii.[a] non est bonum.
Luna .tertia. bona est.
Luna iiii. in matutina bonum est.
Luna .v. non est bonum.
Luna .vi. non est bonu*m*.
Luna septima. tota die bonum est.
Luna .viii. de nona usq*ue* ad sero bonu*m* est.
Luna .ix. non est bonum.
Luna .x. bonum est.
Luna .xi. non est bonu.
Luna .xii. bonum est.
Luna .xiii. bonum est usq*ue* ad hora nona.
Luna .xiiii. bonu*m* est.
Luna .xv. non est bonum.
Luna .xvi. inutilis est.
Luna .xvii. tota die bonu*m* est.
Luna .xviii. non est bonu*m*.
Luna ixx. melior est.
Luna .xx. tota die bonu*m* est.
Luna .xxi. in matutina b*onum*.
Luna .xxii. tota die bonu*m* est.
Luna .xx.iii. ab hora viii. b*onum* est.
Luna .xx.iiii. bonum est.
Luna .xx.v. non est bonu*m*.
Luna .xx.vi. melior est.
Luna .xxvii. tota die bonu*m* e*st*.
Luna .xxviii. Similiter.
Luna .xxix. n*on* e*st* b*onum*. nec .xxx.

12 bonu] *read* bonum | **21** ixx.] *read* xix. *(but see 9.2.2/6)* | **23** b*onum*] *read* ~ est | **28** melior est] *other texts read* non est bona/-um | **30** Similiter] *other texts read* non est bona/-um.

9.2.3/4 London, British Library, Cotton Titus D. xxvi, fol. 6r/2-6v/9

De flebotomatione *ue*l de minuendo sanguine

Luna prima. Tota die bonum est.
Luna .ii. non est bonu*m*.
Luna .iii bona *est*
Luna .iiii. in matutina bona est.
Luna .v. non est bonu*m*.
Luna .vi. n*on* est bonu*m*.
Luna .vii. Tota die bonu*m* est.
Luna .viii. de n*ona* usq*ue* ad sero bonu*m* est.
Luna .ix [non] est bonu*m*.
Luna .x.
Luna .xi. non est bonu*m*.
Luna .xii. bonu*m* est.
Luna .xiii. bona est usq*ue* ad hora nonna.
Luna .xiiii. bonu*m est*
Luna .xv. non est bonu*m*.
Luna xvi Inutilis est.
Luna .xvii. Tota dię bonum est.
Luna .xviii. n*on* est bonu*m*.
Luna xix. melior est.
Luna xx. Tota die bonu*m* est.
Luna .xxi. In matutina bona est.
Luna .xxii. Tota die bonum est.
Luna .xxiii. Ab hora .viii. bonum est.
Luna .xxiiii. bonum est.
Luna .xxv. Non est bonu*m*.
Luna .xxvi. non est bonu*m*.
Luna .xxvii. Tota die bonum est.
Luna .xxviii. non est bonu*m*.
Luna .xxix. non est bonu*m*.
una .xxx. Similiter.

12 [non]] ~ *erroneously erased (see 9.2.3/8,10)* | **13** .x.] *read* ~ bonum est | **17** nonna] *read* nona | **24** xx.] ~ ‖ ⟨*f. 6v*⟩ | **34** una] *read* Luna.

9.2.3/8 London, Lambeth Palace Library, MS 427, fol. 3ra

Luna i	Tota die bonu*m est*
Luna ii	Non *est* bonu*m*.
Luna iii	Bonu*m est*
Luna iiii	In matutina bonu*m est*
Luna v	N*on* es bonu*m*m.
Luna vi	Non *est* b*onum*
Luna vii	Tota die b*onum est*
Luna viii	De nona usq*ue* ad sero bonu*m est*
Luna ix	Non est bon*um*.
Luna x	Bonu*m est*
Luna xi	N*on est* bonu*m*.
Luna xii	Bonu*m est*
Luna xiii	Bonu*m est* usq*ue* ad hora*m* nona*m*
Luna xiiii	Bonu*m est*
Luna xv	Non *est* b*onum*.
Luna xvi	Inutilis *est*
Luna xvii	Tota die b*onum est*
Luna xviii	Non *est* b*onum*.
Luna xix	Melior *est*
Luna xx	Tota die b*onum est*
Luna xxi	In matutino b*onum*
Luna xxii	Tota die b*onum*
Luna xxiii	Ab hora .viii. b*onum est*
Luna xxiiii	Bonu*m est*
Luna xxv	Non est b*onum*.
Luna xxvi	Non est b*onum*.
Luna xxvii	Tota die b*onum*
Luna xxviii	N*on* e*st* b*onum*
Luna xxix	Non *est* b*onum*
Luna xxx	Similiter

Text is in columns. This text, together with 9.2.4/8, is framed in two double-lined rectangles | **5** es] *read* est | bonumm] bonūm; *read* bonum | **23** matutino] *read* matutina | b*onum*] *read* ~ est | **24,29** b*onum*] *read* ~ est.

9.2.3/9 Oxford, Bodleian Library, Bodley 579, fol. 56r/6-20

LVNA PRIMA BONA EST

Luna secunda	bona est
Luna tertia	bona est
Luna quarta	bona est
Luna quinta	mala est
Luna sexta	mala est
Luna septima	bona est
Luna octaua	mala est
Luna nona	bona est
Luna decima	bona est
Luna .xi.	bona est
Luna .xii.	mala est
Luna .xiii.	bona est
Luna .xiiii.	bona est
Luna .xv.	mala est
Luna .xvi.	bona est
Luna .xvii.	bona est
Luna .xviii.	mala est
Luna .xviiii.	bona est
Luna .xx.	bona est
Luna .xxi.	mala est
Luna .xxii.	bona est
Luna .xxiii.	bona est
Luna .xxiiii.	bona est
Luna .xxv.	mala est
Luna .xxvi.	mala est
Luna .xxvii.	bona est
Luna .xxviii.	mala est
Luna .xxix.	mala est
Luna .xxx.	mala est

Text is in two columns: days 1-15, 16-30.

9.2.3/10 Oxford, St. John's College, MS 17, fol. 4ra/1-30

Luna **.i.**	**T**ota die bona *est.*
Luna **ii**	[**N**on *est* bona.] `Bona *est.*´
Luna **iii**	[**B**ona *est.*] `Non *est* bona.´
Luna **iiii**	[**I**n matutina bona *est.*] `Ab hora .vi. usq*ue* ad .ix. bona *est.*´
Luna **v**	**N**on *est* bona.
Luna **vi**	**N**on *est* bona.
Luna **vii**	**T**ota die bona *est.*
Luna **viii.**	**D**e nona usq*ue* ad uesp*erum* bona *est;*
Luna **ix**	[**N**on *est* bona.] `Vital*is est.*´
Luna **x.**	**B**ona *est.* `A .vi. usq*ue* sera*m* bona *est.*´
Luna **xi.**	[**N**on *est* bona.] `Similit*er.*´
Luna **xii**	**B**ona *est.*
Luna **xiii**	**B**ona *est* usq*ue* ad hora*m* nona*m;*
Luna **xiiii.**	**B**ona *est.* `A .vi. hora usq*ue* ad sera*m.*´
Luna **xv**	[**N**on *est* bona.] `Vitalis *est.*´
Luna **xvi**	**I**nutilis *est.*
Luna **xvii**	**B**ona *est.*
Luna **xviii**	**N**on *est* bona.
Luna **xix**	[**M**elior.] `Non *est* bona.´
Luna **xx**	**T**ota die bona *est.*
Luna **xxi**	**I**n matutina bona *est.* `usq*ue* ad .iii.´
Luna **xxii**	**T**ota die bona *est.*
Luna **xxiii**	[**A**b hora .viii. bona *est.*] `Vsq*ue* .vi. b*ona.*´
Luna **xxiiii**	**B**ona *est.* `matutina hora.´
Luna **xxv**	**N**on *est* bona.
Luna **xxvi**	**N**on *est* bona.
Luna **xxvii**	**T**ota die bona *est.*
Luna **xxviii.**	[**N**on *est* bona.] `Ab .vi. usq*ue* sera*m* b*ona.*´
Luna **xxix.**	[**N**on *est* bona.] `Similit*er.*´
Luna **xxx**	[**S**imiliter;] `Non *est* bona.´

Text is in columns. This text has been extensively revised in a hand contemporary with that of the original redaction. The original and the variant are so dissimilar that they constitute two discrete redactions of which the original is paralleled in 9.2.3/4,8. The variant has no English analogue to my knowledge. In most cases the original readings have been expunged. Original readings that have been superseded but not expunged remained in use for the sense of the prediction (e.g. day 14), except in day 10, where the original reading should have been expunged. I have put original readings which have been supplanted and expunged in square brackets and the revisions in apostrophes, so the reader can verify the extent of the revisions | **4** `usq*ue*... *est.*´] *added under the line for lack of space, transposition indicated* | **8** bona *est;*] -na *est; written above the line for lack of space, transposition indicated* | **9** `Vital*is*´] *read* utilis *(~ would be more appropriate in a birth lunary than in a bloodletting lunary)* | **13** nona*m;*] -na*m; above the line for lack of space, transposition indicated* | **15** `Vitalis´] *read* utilis *(see l. 9)* | **23,28** `b*ona*´] *read* ~ est.

9.2.4 Lunary, Specific, Dreams

Literature

Birch (1878: 479; 1892: 257); Förster (1903: 356; 1908c: 33, 35; 1925-26; 1944); Jastrow (1905-12: II.457-577); Thorndike (1923-58: I.680-82); Mercati (1932); Svenberg (1936; 1939); Wistrand (1942); Schmitt (1966: 195); Martin (1977: 16-17, 25); Harmening (1979: 107); Fischer (1982a: 7, 165, n. 13); Weißer (1982); Taavitsainen (1988); Kieckhefer (1989: 86); Hollis and Wright (1992: 265); Günzel (1993: 31-33); Epe (1995: 62-63); Wallis (1995: 115-17); Liuzza (2001: 188): Haag (2003: 46-47); DiTommaso (2005: 259-79; 402-46; 2006: 119-26)

Branch of Superstition

observation of times: days of the moon

Texts

OE:	1. Cambridge, Corpus Christi College, MS 391, pp. 720-21
	2. London, British Library, Cotton Caligula A. xv, fols 131v-32r
	3. London, British Library, Cotton Tiberius A. iii, fols 37v-38r
	4. Oxford, Bodleian Library, Hatton 115, fol. 148r
L/OE:	5. London, British Library, Cotton Tiberius A. iii, fols 35v-36r
L:	6. Cambridge, Corpus Christi College, MS 391, pp. 718-20
	7. London, British Library, Cotton Titus D. xxvi, fol. 9rv
	8. London, Lambeth Palace Library, MS 427, fol. 3r
	9. Oxford, St John's College, MS 17, fol. 4rc

Description

An exhaustive study of the genre of dream lunaries was carried out by Förster.[1] Dream lunaries are unlike alphabetical dreambooks in that they do not interpret dream *topoi*. Instead, dream lunaries reveal whether a dream comes to pass in real life, and sometimes also within how many days fulfilment will take place.

Dream lunaries have been attested in Latin and the vernacular, including Old English, Welsh and Italian.[2] Förster claimed that the Latin dream lunaries descended from Byzantine texts, but the earliest witnesses of Greek dream lunaries are in fourteenth- and fifteenth-century manuscripts.[3] The earliest Latin dream lunaries date from the tenth centu-

[1] Förster (1925-26). I am greatly indebted to Förster's lucid presentation.

[2] Latin texts are listed by Förster (1925-26: 62-63), Beccaria (1956: 201 [50.14], 228 [91.13]), Weißer (1982: 57-58), vernacular texts by Förster (1925-26: 65, 92-93; 1944: 7-8, n. 1).

[3] Förster (1925-26: 62). See also Mercati (1932).

ry, but the fact that several redactions exist among the early texts would point to an older genesis.[4]

Text (6) differs from the other insular dream lunaries in that it includes a Psalm verse at the end of each entry, for instance "**L**una .i. quicquid uideris in gaudium. conuertitur **B**eatus uir qui non abiit [Ps 1:1]".[5] Two of the Latin dream lunaries found by Förster also include Psalm verses, but these do not coincide in all instances.[6] The inclusion of non-prognostic material in lunaries is not unusual. Weißer discerned the following categories of additional information: zodiacal elements, biblical events, Psalm verses, the light of the moon, the birthdays of gods and the duration of rain.[7] Of these, Psalm verses and biblical events seem to have been intended as a sign of clerical authority or approval of the lunaries. Several lunary genres include Psalm verses, notably collective lunaries.[8] Svenberg connected the Psalm verses in collective lunaries with Bible sortilege, specifically with regard to dream predictions.[9] It seems likely that the Psalm verses in collective lunaries were taken from dream lunaries, because these are the first to include such material.

Förster distinguished two groups of Latin dream lunaries which have little in common.[10] One of these includes (5-7) and presumably (8, 9), which were not known to Förster, but which are identical to (7). These Latin texts are treated by Förster as if they belong to one redaction, but this is not true, as a comparison of the order and contents of the entries makes clear. Rather, these Latin dream lunaries can be divided into three redactions, to wit (5), (6) and (7-9). Within the latter group, (8, 9) are closely related to each other, while they lack certain phrases present in (7). The Old English texts are grouped into three redactions by Förster: (1-3), (4) and (5). The last one is the Old English gloss to the Latin text of (5). The other two redactions cannot be traced to any Latin source text, so there must have been at least two more Latin redactions in addition to those identified by Förster. Within the first Old English redaction, (2, 3) are identical and represent a version that differs from (1).

---

[4] Förster (1925-26: 64-65).

[5] Text 9.2.4/6, l. 1.

[6] Förster (1925-26: 67-74, notes). On the order of the Psalm verses in lunaries, see Svenberg (1939: 76), Förster (1944: 30), Weißer (1982: 446-47).

[7] Weißer (1982: 18). Cf. Taavitsainen (1988: 101-07).

[8] Förster (1944: 30), Weißer (1982: 31), Taavitsainen (1988: 104-05).

[9] Svenberg (1939: 76-77). On psalter sortilege, see pp.176-78.

[10] Förster (1925-26: 62-64).

Edition

9.2.4/1 Cambridge, Corpus Christi College 391, pp. 720/4-721/11

Þonne se mone bið anre nihte eald swa hwæt swa þu gesihst þ*æt*e kymð to gesean.

On twam nihtum 7 on .iii. ne bið on þam swefne ne gód ne yfel.

On .iiii. 7 on .v. þ*æt* bið god wite þu þ*æt* on þinre heortan.

On .vi. nihte monan þ*æt* ðe þonne ðynce þ*æt* þu geseo sy þ*æt* fæst on þinum breostum heald þe georne þ*æt* ðu þone geþanc ne forleose

On vii nihte monan swa hwæt swa þe þonne on eage gebyreð æfter langre tide cymð seo geendung.

On .viii. 7 on .ix. nihte sona þe ætewð swa hwæt swa þe geswefnað gif þu unrotnesse geseo wend þin heafud eas(t bi)de god are.

On x nihte þin swefen agæð. butan frecednesse.

On xi nihte þ*æt* swefen kymð to geafean.

On twelf nihte 7 on .xiii. binnan .iii. nihtum þu gesihst þ*æt* ðe on swefne æteowde.

On .xiiii. nihte nafað þ*æt* nane fre*m*minge ne godes ne yfeles.

On xv. nihte monan scorte fulfremmednesse hafað þ*æt* swefen:

On .xvi. nihte monan æfter langre tide þ*æt* swefen agæð.

On xvii. 7 in .xviii. 7 on xix þ*æt* swefen bið god (7 o)n manegum dagum geendað.

On xx. 7 on xxi nihte ceapunge 7 hwearfunge 7 getacnað.

On xxii. 7 xxiii. seo meting bið geteres ful 7 geflites 7 costunge ne bið þ*æt* god swefen.

On xxiii. nihte þ*æt* getacnað gefean 7 hælo

On xxv. 7 xxvi. towardlice fyrhtu 7 brogan þ*æt* getacnað 7 on ix. dagum oððe on .x. þ*æt*e bið æteowed ac wend east bide god are.

On xxvii. 7 þe bið 7 on xxvii. 7 on xxix. þ*æt* swefen tacnað ealne gefean 7 eghwylcere agnesse 7 uneðnesse smyltnesse 7 glædnesse gehatað.

On xxx. nihte aldne monan efter twegra daga fyrste þ*æt* swefen agæð butan srecednesse.

1-2 gesean] *read* gefean *(see ll. 27-28)* | **6** georne] [·]georne | **17** langre] lang[e]re | **18** in] i- < o; *read* on | **19** ceapunge] -p- < n | hwearfunge] ~ ‖ ⟨*p. 721*⟩ | 7$_3$] *read* þæt | **20** geflites] -f- < 7 | **22** xxiii.] *read* xxiiii. | **24** wend] *read* ~ þin heafud *(see 9.2.4/2,3)* | **25** þe bið 7] *delete* ~ | xxvii.$_2$] *read* xxviii. | **26** agnesse] *i.e.* angnesse | **27-28** srecednesse] *read* frecednesse *(see ll. 1-2)*.

9.2.4/2 London, British Library, Cotton Caligula A. xv, fols 131v/16-132r/8

On anre nihta eald monan swa hwæt swa þe mæteð þ*æt* cymð to gefean.

On tweigra nihta eald monan. 7 on þreora næfþ*æt* swefen nænige fremednesse gódes ne yfeles.

On feower nihta. 7 on fifa. þ*æt* bið gód swefen wite þu þ*æt* georne on þinre heortan.

On .vi. nihta þ*æt* þe þonne þ*æt* þu geseo. þ*æt* beo fæst on þinum breostu*m*. wite þ*æt* þin þanc ne losige.

On .vii. nihta swa hwæt swa þe on eage byreð. æfter tide cymð seo endung.

On .viii. nihta. 7 on .ix. sona þ*æt* ypeð. swa hwæt swa þe geswefnað. gif þu unrotnysse gesawe. wend þin heafod east bide þe god are.

On .x. nihta þin swefen agæð butan frecednysse.

On .xi. þ*æt* swefen agǽð mid gefean.

On .xii. nihta. 7 on .xiii. binnan þrim nihton þu gesihst þ*æt* þe ær on swefne ætywde.

On .xiiii. nihta. næfð þ*æt* nænige fremednysse gódes ne yfeles.

On .xv. nihta sceortwyrplic þ*æt* bið.

On .xvi. nihta æfter langre tide hit agæð.

On .xvii. 7 on .xviii. 7 on .xix. nihta þ*æt* swefen bið god. 7 on manegum dagum geendað.

On .xx. 7 on .xxi. nihta þ*æt* tacnað ceapunge 7 hwearsunge.

On .xxii. 7 xxiii. nihta seo mætingc bið gecornes. 7 geflitnes. 7 eall costunge full. ne bið þ*æt* na gód swefen.

On .xxiiii. nihta. þ*æt* tacnað gesynto 7 hælo.

On .xxv. 7 on .xxvi. nihta þ*æt* tacnað toweardlice firhto 7 brogan. 7 on .ix. dagum oþþe. on .x. þ*æt* bið geypped. ac wend þin heafod east bide þe are.

On xxvii. 7 on .xxviii. nihta þ*æt* tacnað ealdne gefean. 7 ealle angnysse. 7 uneaðnysse. smyltnysse 7 glædnesse gehatað.

On .xxix. nihta eallswa þ*æt* ærre.

On xxx. nihta ær twegra nihta fyrste þ*æt* swefen agæð butan frecnum þingum.

1,2 eald monan] *the first word of this collocation can be both inflected (i.e.* ealdne monan, *cf. 9.2.4/3) and uninflected, as in this case (see 9.2.1/2)* | **6** þonne] read ~ þince *(see 9.2.4/1,3)* | **8** tide] *read* langre ~ *in accordance with 9.2.4/1 (but see 9.2.4/3)* | **9** ypeð] yweð *or* ypeð *(it is hard to distinguish between* 'wyn' *and* 'p' *in this instance)* | **12** .xi.] *read* ~ nihta | **20** hwearsunge] *read* hwearfunge | **21** gecornes] geteres ful *9.2.4/1 (but see also 9.2.4/3); on this reading, see Förster (1925-26: 84, n.1)* | geflitnes] *read* geflites *in accordance with 9.2.4/1 (but see 9.2.4/3)* | **23** gesynto] ge‖synto ⟨*f. 132r*⟩ | **25** are] *read* god ~ *in accordance with 9.2.4/1 (but see 9.2.4/3)* | **26** þ*æt*] *read* ~ swefen | ealdne] *read* ealne | ealle] *read* eall *(but see 9.2.4/3)* | **29** $nihta_2$] daga *9.2.4/1 (but see 9.2.4/3).*

9.2.4/3 London, British Library, Cotton Tiberius A. iii, fols 37v/5-38r/2

On anre nihte ealdne monan swa hwæt swa þe mæteð þ*æt* cymð to gefean.

On tweigra nihte monan. 7 on þreora. næfþ þ*æt* swefen nænige fremednesse godes ne yfeles.

On feower nihtne. 7 on fifa. þ*æt* byþ god swefen. wite þu þ*æt* georne on þinre heortan.

On syx nihta. þ*æt* þe þonne þince þ*æt* þu geseo. þ*æt* beo fæst on þinum breostum. wite þ*æt* þin geþanc ne leose.

On .vii. nihta swa hwæt swa þe on eage byreþ æfter tide cymð seo endung.

On .viii. nihte. 7 on .ix. sona þ*æt* ypeð swa hwæt swa þe geswefnaþ. gif þu unrotnesse gesawe. wend þin heafod east. bide þe god are.

On .x. nihta. þin swefen agæþ. butan frecnesse.

On xi. nihta þ*æt* swefen agæþ mid gefean.

On .xii. 7 on xiii. nihta. binnan þrim nihton þu gesyhst þ*æt* þe ær on swefne ætywede.

On xiiii. nihta. næfð þ*æt* nænige fremednesse. godes ne yfeles.

On .xv. nihta sceortwyrplic þ*æt* byþ.

On .xvi. nihta æfter langre tide hit agæð.

On .xvii. 7 on .xviii. 7 on .xix. nihta. þ*æt* swefen byþ god. 7 on manegum dagum geendað.

On xx. nihta. 7 on .xxi. þ*æt* tacnaþ. ceapunga. 7 hwearfunga.

On xxii. 7 on xxiii. nihta seo mæting byþ gecornes. 7 geflitnes. 7 eall costnunge full. ne biþ þæt na god swefen.

On .xx.iiii. nihta. þ*æt* tacnaþ

toweardlice firhto. 7 brogan. 7 on nigon dagum oððe on .x. þ*æt* byþ geypped. ac wend þin heafod east bide þe are.

On .xxvii. 7 on xxviii. nihta. þ*æt* swefen tacnaþ ealne gean. 7 ealle angsumnesse. 7 uneaðnesse smyltnesse. 7 glædnysse gehateþ.

On .xxix. nihta eallswa þ*æt* ærre.

On .xxx. nihta. ær tweigra nihta fyrste þ*æt* swefen agæð butan frecnum þingum.

Entries for days 24 and 25-26, originally one entry, have been split up on the basis of 9.2.4/1,2 | **8** tide] *read* langre ~ *in accordance with 9.2.4/1 (but see 9.2.4/2)* | **9** ypeð] yweð *or* ypeð *(it is hard to distinguish between* 'wyn' *and* 'p' *in this instance)* | **11** frecnesse] *i.e.* frecednesse | **21** gecornes] geteres ful *9.2.4/1 (but see also 9.2.4/2); on this reading, see Förster (1925-26: 84, n.1)* | geflitnes] *read* geflites *in accordance with 9.2.4/1 (but see 9.2.4/2)* | **23** tacnaþ] *read* ~ gesynto 7 hælo | **24** toweardlice] *read* On .xxv. 7 on .xxvi. nihta þæt tacnaþ ~ | **25** are] *read* god ~ *in accordance with 9.2.4/1 (but see 9.2.4/2)* | **26** gean] *read* gefean | ealle] *read* eall *(but see 9.2.4/2)* | **27** gehateþ] ~ ‖ ⟨*f. 38r*⟩ | **29** nihta$_2$] daga *9.2.4/1 (but see 9.2.4/2).*

9.2.4/4 Oxford, Bodleian Library, Hatton 115, fol. 148r

ÐÆre æresten nyhte þonne niwe mone byð ecymen. þ*æt* mon þonne in sweofne gesihþ. þ*æt* cymeð to gefean.
Þære æfteran niht. 7 þore ðriddan nyht: ne byoð þ*æt* naðer ne god ne yfel.
Ðære feorðan nyht. 7 þeora fiftan: wene heo godre gefremednesse.
Þære syxtan niht þ*æt* þu gesyx. swa hyt byoð. 7 þeo wyð eorfoþu geoscilt.
Þere seofoðan nyht. þ*æt* þu gesixt. swa hyt byð. 7 æst*er* mycelre tyde agæð.
Þære .viii. niht. 7 þere nigoþan. raþe þu gesihst. swefn þ*æt* bið able oðþe trega
Þere nigoðan niht þ*æt* þeo gemeteð. þ*æt* bioð butan festnesse.
⟨Entry for day 11 missing⟩
Þeore .xii. niht. 7 þeore .xiii. niht. ine þrim dagu*m* þu gesihst þin swefn
Þeore .xiiii. nithi. ne hafað þat nane gefrémédnesse.
Þeore .xv. niht: hit hafað litle gefremædnesse.
Þeore xvi. niht: æst*er* mycelre tide agæð þin sweofn.
Ðere xvii. niht. 7 xviii. 7 nigontene. in .iii. 7 c.um. daga bið goð swefn.
Ðonne se mona bið xx. niht. 7 .i. 7 xx. niht. þ*æt* bið scir oðþe ceap in þem swefne toweard.
Þonne heo byð .ii. 7 xx. niht eald. þ*æt* þu gesihst hit lengeð to gode gefean.
Þonne heo bið .iii. 7 xx. nihta eald. þ*æt* bid cid 7 geflit.
Ðonne heo bið .iiii. 7 xx. nihta eald. 7 v. 7 xx. 7 vi. 7 xx. nihta eald. þ*æt* bið weorðlic ege on nigon dagu*m*. oðþe on .x. þin swefn agæð.
Þonne heo bið .vii. 7 xx. 7 viii. 7 xx. nihta eald: ealne gefean þ*æt* bicneð.
Þonne heo bið .ix. 7 xx. 7 fulle .xxx. nthta eald. þ*æt* bið æfre buton fræcnesse;

Text lacks entry for day 11 | **4** þeora] þeora | **5** niht] -h- < t | gesyx] *read* gesyxt | **6** æst*er*] *read* æft*er* *(see l. 13)* | **7** niht] ni[t]ht | able] *read* adle | **8** nigoðan] *read* teoðan | festnesse] -s$_1$- < t | **11** nithi] *read* niht | **13** æst*er*] *read* æft*er* *(see l. 6)* | **14** goð] *read* god | **18** bid] *read* bið | **22** nthta] *read* nihta.

9.2.4/5 London, British Library, Cotton Tiberius A. iii, fols 35v/15-36r/13

swa wæt swa þu gesihst on blisse bið 7 gif þu gesihst þe
Luna prima quicquid uideris in gaudium erit. & si uideris te
beon ofercumene ofercymst ealle feond þine geunnendum gode.
uinci tu tamen uinces omnes inimicos tuos annuente deo.
gif þu gesihst swefnu nane gefremminge hefð na on mode þu asete
Luna .ii.[da] si uideris somnium. nullum effectum hab*et*. nec in animo ponas
oððe god oððe yfel
siue bonum siue malum.

3 ofercumene] ~ *over* tu tamen*; read* ~ þu ðeahhwæþere *(*tu tamen *not glossed).*

ealswilc swilce se oðer
Luna .iii.^{a} qualis & secunda.
gode gefremminge hæfð naht ne derað
Luna .iiii.^{ta} bonum effectum hab*et*. nichil noc*et*.
eallswa se feorþa
una .v.^{ta} sicut & quarta.
æfter þa*m* þe þu gesihst swa þe gewyrð digle geþeaht
Luna .vi.^{ta} *secundum* quod uideris ita tibi fi*et*. Secretum consilium
utlendisc nelle þu areccan
extraneis noli proferre.
swa hwæt swa þu gesihst æfter langum timan hit gewyrð
Luna .vii^{a} quicquid uideris. post multum tempus fi*et*.
gewisse sint ealle
Luna .viii.^{a} certa sunt omnia.
binnan twan dagu*m* gelipð
Luna .viiii.^{a} inter duos dies euenit.
swa hwæt swa þe swefnast nane gefremmige yfele hæfð
Luna .x.^{a} quicquid somniaueris. nullum effectum malum hab*et*.
lease sint ealle
Luna .xi.^{a} falsa sunt omnia.
gewisse sint ealle
Luna .xii.^{a} certa sunt omnia.
eallswilc
Luna .xiii.^{a} qualis .xii^{a}
gefremminge hæfð scortes timan
Luna .xiiii.^{a} effectum hab*et* breuis temporis.
eallswilc
Luna .xv.^{a} qualis .xiiii.^{a}
æfter langum timan hit gewyrð
Luna .xvi.^{a} post multum tempus fi*et*.
æfter dagu*m* endlufon hið gelipð
Luna .xvii.^{a} post dies .xi.^{cim} eueni*et*.
binnon twentigu*m* dagu*m* hit getimað
Luna .xviii.^{a} inter .xx.^{ti} dies conting*et*.
binnon dagu*m* feower hit gelimpð
Luna .xix. inter dies .iiii.^{or} eueni*et*.
ne þu sege swefen þin binnon dagu*m* seofoðan ac begim
Luna .xx. ne tu dixeris somnium tuum intra dies .vii.^{tem} sed obserua
gewiss
certitudinem.

14 una] *read* Luna | **17** utlendisc] -c < t; *read* utlendiscum | **23** twan] *read* twam | gelipð] *read* gelimpð *(see l. 39)* | **25** swa$_2$] -w- < · | þe] *read* þu | gefremmige] *i.e.* gefremminge *(on loss of* 'n', *see 7/4, l. 66)* | **26** hab*et*.] ~ ‖ ⟨*f. 36r*⟩ | **39** hið] *read* hit | gelipð] *read* gelimpð *(see l. 23)* | **45** seofoðan] *read* seofon.

gewiss
certitudinem.
eallswa uigessima
Luna .xx^{ma}i.^{ma} sicut & .xx.^{ma}
swa hwæt swa þu gesihst gewiss his to blisse becuman
Luna .xx^{ma}ii.^{da} quicquid uideris certum est ad gaudium p*er*tinere.
sacful geflit binnon dagu*m* þrim gelimpð
Luna .xxiii.^{a} rixalis contentio inter dies .iii. eueni*et*.
swa hwæt swa þu gesihst be hele þine hit bið
Luna .xxiiii^{a}. quicquid uideris de salute tua erit.
æge towyrd binnon dagu*m* ehta
Luna. .xx^{ma}v.^{ta} m*et*us futurus inter dies .viii.
binnon dagu*m* twentigu*m* hit gel*i*mpð
Luna .xxvi. inter dies uiginti eueni*et*.
eallswa
Luna .xx^{ma}vii.^{ma} sicut & xxvi.
ealle blisse tacn 7 ealle angsu*m*nysse bliþe
Luna .xx.^{ma}viii.^{ua} & xxix. omne gaudium significat. & omnem angustium hilaris
aflemð
aufert.
binnon þri*m* dagu*m* gewyrð swefen þin butan frecendnysse
Luna .xxx.^{ma} infra triduum fi*et*. Somnium tuum sine periculo

Am*en*.

65 tacn] *read* tacnað | **66** angustium] *read* angustiam.

9.2.4/6 Cambridge, Corpus Christi College, MS 391, pp. 718/23-720/3

Luna .i. quicquid uideris in gaudium. conuertitur **B**eatus uir qui non abiit.
Luna .ii. luna .iii. effectum habent nec in animo ponas. **A**dstiterunt reges terrę. **T**u autem d*omi*ne suscep*tor*.
Luna iiii. & v. effectum habent sed nichil nocent **E**t scitote q*uonia*m. **N**eq*ue* habitabit
Luna vi. quicquid uideris certissimum cautus és consilio tuo utere **L**aboraui in gemitu*m*.

On the use of Psalm verses in lunaries, see pp. 448. Note the order of the verses | **1 L**una... uideris] *the remainder (about half) of the line is left blank in the manuscript (for a rubric?)* | **B**eatus uir qui non abiit] *Ps 1:1 (all references are to the Gallican Psalter)* | **2** effectum] *read* nullum ~ *(see 9.2.4/5)* | **A**dstiterunt reges terrę] *Ps 2:2* | **3 T**u autem d*omi*ne suscep*tor*] *Ps 3:4* | **4 L**una] ~ ‖ ⟨*p. 719*⟩ | **E**t scitote q*uonia*m] *Ps 4:4* | **4-5 N**eq*ue* habitabit] *Ps 5:6* | **6-7 L**aboraui in gemitu*m*] *read* Laboraui in gemitu, *Ps 6:7*.

Luna vii. certissimum. **E**xurgat d*eus*. **D***eus* m*eus* inpoluta.
una viii. & ix. **C**ito fient que uideris. **V**olucres celi **E**t factus est refugium
Luna .x. effectum h*abet* sed nichil noc*et*. ana locuti sunt.
Luna xi intra dies .vii. fi*et* somnum tuum. **Q**uamdiu ponam consilio.
Luna xii quicquid uideris certissimum e*sse* scias caue. **Q**uorum os maledic*tione*
Luna .xiii. intra dies .ix. fi*et* **Q**ui ingreditur.
Luna .xiiii. & .xv. effectum h*abent* & in breui tempore fi*et*. **B**enedicam qui michi. **P**robasti cor m*eum*
Luna xvi. post tempus fi*et* dolus erit. **S**aturati sunt filii.
Luna xvii. qui(cqui)d uideris fi*et* **E**t apparuerunt
Luna xviii. & xix. Intra dies .x. fi*et* **M**itta tibi **P**ones eos ut clibanu*m*.
Luna xx. & xxi. ne cogites quid uideris. **S**perauit in d*omino* alua me ex ore leonis.
Luna .xxii. certissimu*m* est quod uideris **C**onfundantur omnes iniqua.
Luna xxiii. & xxiiii anissimum est. **Q**uis est homo **I**udica me d*omi*ne q*uoniam* ego in innocentia mea.
Luna xxv & xxvi. **I**ntra dies .ix erit. **T**ibi dixit cor meum. **S***ecun*d*u*m opera manuum.
Luna .xxvii. & xxviii effectum h*abent* non noc*ent*. m ira indignatio **E**sto michi in d*eum*
.xxix. effectum h*abet* non nocet. **S**up*er* inimicos meos
Luna xxx. **I**n triduum fi*et* somnum caue iligite d*omi*nu*m* om*nes* s*ancti* ei*us*

8 Exurgat d*eus*.] *Ps 67:2; possibly an erroneous reference for* Exsurge domine *Ps 7:7, which would fit the sequence of Psalm verses better* | **D***eus* m*eus* inpoluta] *Ps 17:31; this verse is redundant because one has already been quoted for this day of the moon* | **9** una] *read* Luna | fient] *read* fiet | **V**olucres celi] *Ps 8:9* | **E**t factus est refugium] *read* Et factus est dominus refugium, *Ps 9:10* | **10** ana locuti sunt] *read* Vana locuti sunt, *Ps 11:3* | **11 Q**uamdiu ponam consilio] *Ps 12:2* | **12** xii] [i]xii | **Q**uorum os maledic*tione*] *Ps 13:3* | **13 Q**ui ingreditur] *Ps 14:2* | **14 B**enedicam qui michi] *read* Benedicam domino qui michi, *Ps 15:7* | **15 P**robasti cor m*eum*] *Ps 16:3* | **16 S**aturati sunt filii] *read* Saturati sunt filiis, *Ps 16:14* | **17 E**t apparuerunt] *Ps 17:16* | **18 M**itta tibi] *read* Mittat tibi, *Ps 19:3* | **P**ones eos ut clibanu*m*] *Ps 20:10* | **19 S**perauit in d*omino*] *Ps 21:9* | **19** alua me ex ore leonis] *read* Salua me ex ore leonis, *Ps 21:22* | **20 C**onfundantur omnes iniqua] *Ps 24:4* | **21** anissimum] *read* Vanissimum | **Q**uis est homo] *Ps 24:12* | **21-22 I**udica me d*omi*ne q*uoniam* ego in innocentia mea] *Ps 25:1* | **23 T**ibi dixit cor meum] *Ps 26:8* | **23-24 S***ecun*d*u*m opera manuum] *Ps 27:4* | **25** m ira indignatio] *read* Quoniam ira in indignatione, *Ps 29:6* | **25-26 E**sto michi in d*eum*] *Ps 30:3.* | michi] ~ ‖ ⟨*p. 720*⟩ | **27** .xxix.] *read* Luna ~ | **S**up*er* inimicos meos] *read* Super omnes inimicos meos, *Ps 30:12* | **28** triduum] -r- < i | iligite d*omi*nu*m* om*nes* s*ancti* ei*us*] *read* Diligite dominum omnes sancti eius, *Ps 30:24*.

9.2.4/7 London, British Library, Cotton Titus D. xxvi, fol. 9r/6-9v/13

Incipit lunaris de somnis

Luna .i. quicquid uideri ad gaudiu*m* p*er*tin*et*.
Luna .ii. & .iii. affectus erit.
Luna .iiii. bonus & affectus erit.
Luna .v. & vi. s*ecun*d*u*m quod uideris fi*et*.
Luna .vii. quicquid uideris post multum tempus fi*et*.
Luna .viii. & .ix. cito uidebis.
Luna .x. q*ui*cquid uideris nullu*m* malum est.
Luna xi. somnus tuus sine p*er*icolo.
Luna xii. cum om*n*i gaudio fi*et* somnus tuus.
Luna .xiii. infra dies .vii. fi*et* somnus tuus.
Luna .xv. Nullu*m* bonu*m* effectum abes.
Luna .xvi. p*ost* multum temp*us* fi*et* somnus tuus.
Luna xvii Similiter.
Luna .xviii. & xix. infra dies .xx. fi*et* somnus tuus.
Luna xxi. & xxii. ad gaudium p*er*tin*et*.
Luna xxiii. rixam habebit & contentiones. sine ulla detractione.
Luna xxiiii aliqua*m* salute*m* p*ro*mittit.
Luna xxv. & xxvi. infra dies .x. fi*et* somnus tuus.
Luna xxvii. & xxviii. & xxix. ad gaudium pertin*et*.
Luna .xxx. infra duum fi*et* Somnus sine periculo.

2 uideri] *read* uideris | **9** p*er*icolo] *read* ~ fiet | **11** .xiii.] *read* ~ & .xiiii. *(see 9.2.4/8,9)* | fi*et*] ~ ‖ ⟨*f. 9v*⟩ | **12** abes] *read* abet, *i.e.* habet | **15** xix.] *read* ~ & .xx. *(see 9.2.4/8,9)* | **21** duum] *read* triduum *(see 9.2.4/8,9)*.

9.2.4/8 London, Lambeth Palace Library, MS 427, fol. 3rb

i Q*ui*cq*ui*d uid*er*is ad gaudiu*m* p*er*tin*et*
ii Affect*us* erit
iii Simili*ter*.
iiii Bon*us* 7 affect*us* erit
v S*ecund*um q*uo*d uid*er*i fiet.
vi Simili*ter*
vii Q*ui*cq*ui*d uid*er*is p*ost* multu*m* te*m*p*us* fiet.
viii Cito uideb*is*
ix Simili*ter*
x Q*ui*cq*ui*d uid*er*is nullu*m* malu*m* erit
xi So*mnus* tuu*us* sine p*er*ic*u*lo fiet
xii Cu*m* om*n*i gaudio fiet so*mnus*.
xiii Infra dies .vii. fiet so*mnus*
xiiii Simili*ter*
xv Nullu*m* bonu*m* effectu*m* hab*et*.
xvi P*ost* multu*m* tep*us* fiet
xvii Simili*ter*
xviii Infra dies xx. fiet
xix Simili*ter*
xx Simili*ter*
xxi Ad gaudiu*m* p*er*tinet.
xxii Simili*ter*
xxiii Rixa*m* habebit 7 co*n*tentiones
xxiiii Ad salute*m* p*er*tinet
xxv In eode*m* die uidebit*ur*
xxvi Infra .x. dies fiet
xxvii Ad gaudiu*m* p*er*tinet
xxviii Simili*ter*
xxix Simili*ter*
xxx Infra t*r*iduu*m* sin*e* p*er*c*u*lo fiet

Text is in columns. This text, together with 9.2.3/8, is framed in two double-lined rectangles. The Luna *column is absent in 9.2.4/8 since it is supplied in 9.2.3/8, which occupies the columns to the left of 9.2.4/8* | **5** uid*er*i] *read* uideris | **11** tuu*us*] *read* tuus | **16** tep*us*] *read* tempus | **30** p*er*c*u*lo] *read* p*er*ic*u*lo.

9.2.4/9 Oxford, St. John's College, MS 17, fol. 4rc/17-46

Lun*a* i	*Q*uic*q*u*i*d uid*e*ris ad gaudiu*m* p*e*rtin*et*;
Lun*a* ii	Affect*us* erit.
Lun*a* iii	Similit*er*.
Lun*a* iiii	Bon*us* & affect*us* erit.
Lun*a* v	S*ecundum* q*uod* uid*e*ris fiet.
Lun*a* vi	Similit*er*.
Lun*a* vii	*Q*uic*q*u*i*d uid*e*ris p*ost* multu*m* te*mpus* fiet.
Lun*a* viii	Cito uideb*is*.
Lun*a* ix	Similit*er*.
Lun*a* x	*Q*uic*q*u*i*d uid*e*ris nullu*m* malu*m* erit.
Lun*a* xi	So*mnus* tuus sine p*e*ric*u*lo fiet.
Lun*a* xii	Cu*m* o*mn*i gaudio fiet so*mnus*. `*Ea die aliq*uid *in*de *uideb*is. *7 die t*er*cia* *explebit*ur.´
Lun*a* xiii	Infra dies .vii. fiet so*mnus*.
Lun*a* xiiii	Similit*er*. `*Eode*m *die fiet.*´
Lun*a* xv	Nullu*m* bonu*m* effectu*m* h*abe*t.
Lun*a* xvi	P*ost* multu*m* te*mpus* fiet so*mnus*.
Lun*a* xvii	Similit*er*.
Lun*a* xviii	Infra dies .xx. fiet so*mnus*.
Lun*a* xix	Similit*er*.
Lun*a* xx	Similit*er*.
Lun*a* xxi	Ad gaudium p*e*rtin*et*.
Lun*a* xxii	Similit*er*.
Lun*a* xxiii	Rixa*m* habebit & co*n*tentiones.
Lun*a* xxiii`i´	Ad salute*m* p*e*rtinet.
Lun*a* xxv	In eode*m* die uidebit*ur*.
Lun*a* xxvi	Infra .x. dies fiet.
Lun*a* xxvii	Ad gaudiu*m* p*e*rtin*et*. `*Ode*m *die uideb*is.´
Lun*a* xxviii	Similit*er*.
Lun*a* xxix	Similit*er*.
Lun*a* xxx	Infra t*r*iduu*m* fiet sine p*e*ric*u*lo;

Text is in columns. Additions have been made to entries 12, 14 and 27, judging by the handwriting and the thickness of the pen used these additions were not made in one stint, nor were they the work of the scribe of the original text. The original entries have not been expunged, so it is unclear whether the additions were intended to supplant the original entries | **12-13** `t*ercia explebit*ur.´] *on line below for lack of space, transposition indicated* | **17** so*mnus*] s- < ·.

9.2.5 Lunary, Specific, Illness

Literature

Birch (1878: 479; 1892: 257); Förster (1903: 355; 1908c: 34, 35, 40; 1912c: 30-36; 1944); Jastrow (1905-12: II.457-577); Budge (1913: II. 536-38); Thorndike (1923-58: I.680-82); Svenberg (1936); Wistrand (1942); Weißer (1976; 1981; 1982); Braswell (1984: 347); Taavitsainen (1988); Kieckhefer (1989: 86); Hollis and Wright (1992: 265-66); Günzel (1993: 31-33); Epe (1995: 62); Wallis (1995: 115-17); Liuzza (2001: 187-88); DiTommaso (2005: 259-79; 402-46; 2006: 119-26)

Branch of Superstition

observation of times: days of the moon

Texts

OE: 1. Cambridge, Corpus Christi College, MS 391, pp. 717-18
2. London, British Library, Cotton Tiberius A. iii, fol. 40r

L/OE: 3. London, British Library, Cotton Caligula A. xv, fols 125vb-26r
4. London, British Library, Cotton Tiberius A. iii, fols 36v-37r

L: 5. London, British Library, Cotton Tiberius A. iii, fol. 65v
6. London, British Library, Cotton Titus D. xxvi, fols 8r-9r
7. Oxford, St John's College, MS 17, fol. 4rbc

Description

Illness lunaries have been studied exhaustively by Weißer.[1] These lunaries predict the outcome of an illness by the day of the moon on which the illness started. In its most basic form, an illness lunary reveals whether a sick person will live or die. Basic predictions may be elaborated upon to create complex ones, e.g. by adding information on the duration, severity or symptoms of the illness, or advice on medical consultation.[2]

The earliest attested illness lunaries date from the ninth century (e.g. in Harley 3017), but in view of the variation between the texts Weißer suspects an earlier genesis for the first translations into Latin from Greek.[3] The number of attested Latin and Greek illness lunaries is quite high in comparison with that of other specific lunaries.[4] Remarkably, the

---

[1] Weißer (1976, 1981, 1982).

[2] Weißer (1982: 99-108).

[3] Weißer (1982: 422).

[4] References and editions in Svenberg (1936: 5), Förster (1944: 6-7, n. 5), Beccaria (1956: 149 [26.9], 165 [34.23], 200-01 [50.9,11,12], 218 [57.5], 345 [117.7], 365 [129. 11]), Wickersheimer (1966: 53-54 [XLII], 57 [XLVIII.3], 74 [LXIII.9], 110 [LXXVI. 28]), Weißer (1982: 44-56).

illness lunary is the only specific lunary genre to have been translated into the vernacular so frequently.[5]

Weißer distinguished six groups of illness lunaries on the basis of the order and complexity of the predictions.[6] Texts (3-7) belong to an early group with little complexity.[7] Texts (1, 2) have not been categorised by Weißer, but in view of their early date and the general agreement in spirit with the predictions of (3-7), they must belong to the same group. Förster was aware of two redactions of Latin illness lunaries, one of which is represented by (3-6).[8] Text (7), which deviates in some entries from (3-6), can be regarded as a variant version of the same redaction. The Old English texts are divided into three redactions by Förster: (1), (2) and (3, 4).[9] Texts (3, 4) are identical in content, the only difference being that the Old English gloss in (4) is interlinear and on the same line as the Latin text in (3).

Edition

9.2.5/1 Cambridge, Corpus Christi College, MS 391, pp. 717-18/1

Se ðe onre nihte monan weorðeð untrum se bið on ðære able swiðe geswenced.
n .ii. nihta monan hraðe æfter sare he ariseð.
Gif on iii. he winneð 7 eft in þære untrumnesse se mon swelteð.
Gif on .iiii. he winneð 7 eft ariseð.
Gif on .v. ne gedegeð þe þa adle.
Gif on vi he winneð 7 ariseð.
On vii nihte aldne monnan he sceal feala findan butan him mihtig god milde wurþe færlice hine deað fram life alædeð
Gif he bið an viii ne leofeð he na lange.
Gif on ix. he bið lange seoc.
if on x. on his heortan unhælo cymð 7 he bið frӕcnoð
Gif on xi on langum sare he sargað 7 he gelomlice his hælo hafoð. eft

1 onre] *read* on anre *(see 9.2.2/1)* | able] -b- < l; *read* adle | **2** n] *read* On | **5** gedegeð] gede[·]geð | **7** monnan] *read* monan | **7-8** butan him mihtig god milde wurþe] *appeals to God's mercy are sporadically included in illness lunaries (see Weißer 1982: 106)* | **9** an] *read* on | **11** if] *read* Gif | frӕcnoð] *read* frӕcnod.

[5] Weißer (1982: 424-30).
[6] Weißer (1982: 114-24).
[7] Weißer (1982: 118-19).
[8] Förster (1912c: 31).
[9] Förster (1912c: 31-36).

Gif on xii he winneð 7 eft ariseð
On xiii lytel sticce he ligeð seoc
On (xii)ii he winneð 7 ariseð
Gif on .xv. fræclice bið his þing.
if on xvi. on þære stowe he ariseð
Gif on xvii he swinceð 7 eft ariseð.
On .xviii. he winneð 7 eft ariseð.
On .xix. he winneð 7 ariseð.
n xx. he ariseð.
On xxi. he bið lange seoc
On xxii rædlice he hal ariseð.
On .xxiii. he ariseð
n xxiiii he bið langa lama 7 swelteð
On xxv. he hraþe ariseð
Gif on xxvi. 7 on xxvii frecne bið þæs mannes þing þ*æt* ifel uneaðe beflið
On xx.viii. 7 on xxix. he of þam sare sone ariseð
Gif xxx he bið lange seoc þæhweðere ariseð.
Đis is eallum gemæne iungum 7 ealdum finit÷÷

17 if] *read* Gif | **21,25** n] *read* On | **25** langa] *read* lange | **29** ariseð.] ~ ‖ ⟨*p. 718*⟩ | **30** Đis... finit÷÷] ~ *not in Förster (1912c), supplied from the manuscript by Ker (1957).*

9.2.5/2 London, British Library, Cotton Tiberius A. iii, fol. 40r/5-21

On anre nihte ealdne monan se þe hine adl gestandeð. se bið frecenlice gestanden.
Gif hine on ii. nihta ealdne monan adl gestandeþ. sona he ariseþ.
Gif hine. on .iii. nihte gestandeð. se liþ fæste. 7 smylt.
Gif hine on iiii. nihta gestandeþ. se biþ geswenced. 7 þeah arist.
Gif se mona biþ .v. nihta eald. þone man mæg gelacnian.
Gif he bið vi. nihta ea. 7 hine adl gestandeð. se biþ lifes.
Gif he bið vii. nihta eald se swinceað lange.
Gif he biþ eahta nihta eald. 7 hine adl gestande. se bið hraþe sweltende.
Gif he bið .ix. nihta eald. se swinceað lange. 7 þeahhwæðere ariseþ. 7 ealswa .x. 7 xi.
Gif he bið .xii. nihta. sona `he´ ariseþ.
⟨Entry for day 13 missing⟩

Text lacks entry for day 13. Marginal note at beginning, in a later hand: hic est i*n*firmor*um* | **4** smylt] *read* swylt | **7** ea] *read* eald.

Gif he bið .xiiii. nihta eald. *uel* .xv. *uel* .xvi. *uel* xvii. *uel* .xviii. *uel* .xix. þ*æt* bið swiþe frecenlic on þam nihtum.

Gif he bið xx. nihta eald. se liþ lange 7 arist.

Gif he bið xxi. oððe .xxii. oððe xxiii. se liþ lange 7 swinceað. 7 arist.

Gif he bið .xxiiii. nihta se ligð fæste.

Gif he biþ on xxv. nihta. frecenlice se bið gestanden.

Gif he biþ gestanden þonne se mona byþ xxvi. oððe .xxvii. oððe xxviii. oððe xx`i´x nihta eald. se ariseþ.

Gif he biþ on xxx. nihta ealdne monan. gestanden. uneaðe he gewyrpð 7 þeah ariseþ.

9.2.5/3 London, British Library, Cotton Caligula A. xv, fols 125vb-126r

Lun*a* i.	qui inciderit difficile euad*et*.	Se þe afealð ea`r´foð`lice´ he ætwint.
Lun*a* ii.	cito consurg*et*.	Raðe he arisþ.
Lun*a* iii.	Non euad*et*.	He ne ætwint.
Lun*a* iiii.	Labor*et* & sarg*et*.	He swincð 7 arisð.
Lun*a* v.	Tricabit & surg*et*.	He sipað 7 arisð.
Lun*a* vi.	Non euad*et*.	He ne ætwint.
Lun*a* vii.	Medicina sanabitur.	mid læcedome he bið g*e*hæled.
Lun*a* viii.	Diu langu*et* & surg*et*.	Lange he adlað 7 arisð.
Lun*a* ix.	Langu*et*.	He adlað.
Lun*a* x.	Diu egrotat.	Lange he siclað.
Lun*a* xi.	P*er*iculo p*er*iclitat.	On frecednesse he dyrfð.
Lun*a* xii.	Surg*et*.	He arisþ.
Lun*a* xiii.	Aliquot tempus egrotat.	Sumne timan he sicclað.
Lun*a* xiiii.	Laborat & surg*et*.	He swincð 7 arisþ.
Lun*a* xv.	Periclitat.	He dyrfð.
Lun*a* xvi.	Locu*m* mitabit & surg*et*.	Stowe he awent 7 arisð.
Lun*a* xvii.	Tricabit & surg*et*.	He sipað 7 urisþ.
Lun*a* xviii.	Laborabit & surg*et*.	He swincð 7 arisð.
Lun*a* xix.	Similiter.	Eallswa.
Lun*a* xx.	Similiter.	Eallswa.
Lun*a* xxi.	Rem adiuuabit.	Ðingc he fultumað.
Lun*a* xxii.	Langu*et* & surg*et*.	He adlað 7 arisþ.

Text is in columns, the days of the moon on fol. 125vb, the predictions in Latin and Old English on fol. 126r. The Old English gloss is on the same line as the Latin | **5** Labor*et*] Labor&; *read* Laborat | sarg*et*] *read* surget | **11** he] h- < n | **12** P*er*iculo] P*er*i- *in lighter ink* | **17** mitabit] *read* mutabit | **18** urisþ] *read* arisþ | **19** **Lun***a*... arisð.] ~ *not in Cockayne (1864-66).*

Lun*a* xxiii.	Similiter.	Eallswa.
Lun*a* xxiiii.	Diu langu*et.*	Lange he adlað.
Lun*a* xxv.	Langu*et* & morietur.	adlað 7 he swelt.
Lun*a* xxvi.	Langu*et.*	He adlað.
Lun*a* xxvii.	Tricabit & surg*et.*	He sipað 7 arisþ.
Lun*a* xxviii.	Eger multum iacebit & morie*tur.*	Seoc swiðe he lið 7 swylt.
Lun*a* xxix.	Eger euad*et.*	Seoc ætwint.
Lun*a* xxx.	Eger laborabit & surg*et.*	Seoc he swincð 7 arisð.

26 adlað] *read* He ~ | **31** ætwint] *read* he ~.

9.2.5/4 London, British Library, Cotton Tiberius A. iii, fols 36v/23-37r/11

se þe afeallað earfoðlice
Luna .i. qui inciderit. difficile
he ætwint
euad*et.*
raþe he arist
Luna .ii.[a] cito consurg*et.*
he na ætwint
Luna .iii.[a] non euad*et.*
he swincð 7 arist
Luna .iiii. labor*et* & surg*et.*
he sipað 7 arist
Luna .v. tricabit & surg*et.*
he na ætwint
Luna .vi. non euad*et.*
mid læcedome he bið gehelend
Luna .vii. medicina sanabitur.
lange he adlað 7 arist
Luna .viii. diu langu*et* & surg*et.*
he adlað
Luna .ix. langu*et.*
lange he siclað
Luna .x. diu egrot*et.*
on fræcnysse he dyrfð
Luna xi: periculo periclitat.

10 labor*et*] labor&; *read* laborat | **12** tricabit] ~ ‖ ⟨*f. 37r*⟩ | **15** gehelend] *read* geheled | **22** egrot*et*] egrot&; *read* egrotat.

he arist
Luna xii. surg*et.*
sumne timan he siclað
Luna xiii: aliquod tempus egrotat
he swincð 7 arist
Luna .xiiii. laborat & surg*et.*
he dyrfð
Luna xv. periclitat.
stowe awent 7 he arist
Luna xvi: locum mutabit & surg*et.*
he sipað 7 arist
Luna .xvii: tricabit & surg*et.*
he swincð 7 arist
Luna xviii. laborabit & surg*et.*
ealswa
Luna .xix: Similiter.
ealswa
Luna xx: similiter.
þinc he fultumað
Luna xxi. rem adiuuabit.
he adlað 7 arist
Luna .xxii: langu*et* & surg*et.*
ealswa
Luna xxiii: Similiter.
lange he adlað
Luna xxiiii. diu langu*et.*
he adlað 7 he swelt
Luna .xxv. langu*et* & morietur.

38 laborabit] -a_2- < &.

he adlað
Luna xxvi. langu*et*.
he sipað 7 arirst
Luna xxvii: Tricabit & surg*et*.
seoc swiðe he lið 7
Luna xxviii: eger multum iacebit &
swelt
morietur.
seoc ætwint
Luna xxix. Aeger euad*et*.
seoc swincð 7 rist
una xxx. eger laborabit & surg*et*.

55 arirst] *read* arist | **61** ætwint] *read* he ~ | **63** swincð] *read* he ~ | rist] *read* arist | **64** una] *read* Luna.

9.2.5/5 London, British Library, Cotton Tiberius A. iii, fol. 65v/7-9

Luna .i. qui inciderit difficile euad*et*.
Luna .ii. cito consurg*et*.
Luna .iii. n*on* euad*et*.
Luna .iiii. labor*et* & surgit.
Luna .v. tricabit & surg*et*.
Luna .vi. non euad*et*.
Luna .vii. medicina sanabitur.

4 labor*et*] labor&; *read* laborat | surgit] *read* surget.

9.2.5/6 London, British Library, Cotton Titus D. xxvi, fols 8r/14-9r/5

Incipit lunares de aegris.

Luna .i. qui inciderit difficile euad*et*.
Luna .ii. Cito consurg*et*
una .iii. euad*et*.
Luna .iiii. labor*et* & surg*et*.
Luna .v. Tricabit & surg*et*.
Luna .vi. Non euad*et*.
Luna .vii. Medicina sanabitur
Luna viii. Diu langu*et* & surg*et*.
Luna .ix. Langu*et*.
Luna .x. Diu egrotat.
una .xi. periclina p*er*iclitat.
Luna .xii. Surg*et*.
Luna .xiii. Aliq*uo*t te*mpus* aegrotat
Luna .xiiii. Laborat & surg*et*.
Luna xv. p*er*iclitabitur.
Luna .xvi. Locum mutabit & surg*et*.
Luna .xvii. Tricabit & surg*et*.
Luna .xviii. Laborabit & surg*et*.
Luna .xix. Similiter.
Luna .xx. Similiter.
Luna .xxi. Readiuuabit.
Luna .xxii. Langu*et* & surg*et*.
Luna .xxiii. Similiter.
Luna .xxiiii. Diu laugu*et*.
Luna .xxv. Laugu*et* & morietur.
Luna .xxvi. Laugu*et*.
Luna .xxvii. Tricabit & surg*et*.
Luna xxviii. Aeger multu*m* iacebat &
moriętur.
Luna xxix. Aeger euad*et*.
Luna .xxx. Aeger laborabit & surg*et*.

1 lunares] *read* lunaris | **4** una] *read* Luna | euad*et*] *read* non ~ *(see 9.2.5/4)* | **5** .iiii.] ~ ‖ *⟨f. 8v⟩* | labor*et*] labor&; *read* laborat | **12** una] *read* Luna | periclina] *read* periculo *(see 9.2.5/4)*.

22 Readiuuabit] *read* Rem adiuuabit *(see 9.2.5/4)* | **25** laugu*et*] *read* languet | **26** Laugu*et*] *read* Languet | morietur] mo‖rietur *⟨f. 9r⟩* | **27** Laugu*et*] *read* Languet | **29** iacebat] *read* iacebit.

9.2.5/7 Oxford, St. John's College, MS 17, fol. 4rb/31-4rc/16

Luna **i**	Q*ui* cecid*er*it difficile euad*et*;
Luna **ii**	Cito *con*surget.
Luna **iii**	Non euadet.
Luna **iiii**	Laborabit & surget.
Luna **v**	Similiter.
Luna **vi**	Non euadet.
Luna **vii**	Medicina saluabit*ur*.
Luna **viii**	Diu languet & surg*et*.
Luna **ix**	Languet.
Luna **x**	Diu egrotabit.
Luna **xi**	Similit*er*.
Luna **xii**	Surget.
Luna **xiii**	Aliq*uo*d te*mpus* eg*ro*tabit.
Luna **xiiii**	Laborabit & surg*et*;
Luna **xv**	P*er*iclitabit*ur*.
Luna **xvi**	Surget.
Luna **xvii**	Tricabit & surg*et*.
Luna **xviii**	Laborabit & surg*et*.
Lun*a* **xix**	Similit*er*.
Lun*a* **xx**	Similit*er*.
Lun*a* **xxi**	Bene adiuuabit*ur*.
Lun*a* **xxii**	Languet & surg*et*.
Lun*a* **xxiii**	Similit*er*.
Lun*a* **xxiiii**	Diu languet.
Lun*a* **xxv**	Languet & moriet*ur*.
Lun*a* **xxvi**	Diu languet.
Lun*a* **xxvii**	Tricabit & surg*et*.
Lun*a* **xxviii**	Diu languet & moriet*ur*.
Lun*a* **xxix**	Euadet eger.
Lun*a* **xxx**	Eger laborabit & surg*et*;

Text is in columns | **14** surg*et*;] ~ ‖ ⟨*f. 4rc*⟩.

10 Month Prognosis

Literature

Jastrow (1905-12: II.457-577); Förster (1908c: 36); Thorndike (1923-58: I.679); Hollis and Wright (1992: 264); Epe (1995: 60); Liuzza (2001: 184)

Branch of Superstition

observation of times: weekdays

Text

OE: 1. London, British Library, Cotton Tiberius A. iii, fol. 40v

Description

The month prognosis predicts important events for each month, depending upon the weekday on which the new moon appears. The weekday structure is a familiar device also found in birth prognostics, brontologies and the year prognosis. Text (1) is uniquely attested. No known analogues in Latin or the vernacular have been identified for (1), but a Latin source must be presupposed as the entries can be rendered into a Latin formula word by word: "Đonne se mona bið acenned on sunnandæig. *þæt* tacnað..." could be a translation of "Si prima luna fuerit die dominico significat...".[1]

The predictions of (1) pertain to human affairs, such as peace, warfare, death and health. The first entry, for Sunday, stands out in its inclusion of meteorological and agricultural information: "it means three things in that month: rain, wind, mildness, and it means a lack of cattle, and the health of people".[2] Hollis and Wright saw correspondences between the month prognosis and the wind and sunshine prognostics,[3] but such similarities are illusory for two reasons. First, the weekday structure is unlike the twelve days of Christmas enumerated in the wind and sunshine prognostics. Second, the sunshine prognostic focusses on agriculture and produce, the wind prognostic on death, and the month prognosis on death and health. A comparison between the month prognosis and the wind and sunshine prognostics is, therefore, inept. Rather, the month prognosis is remarkably similar to the weekday brontology or the year prognosis (but then without the meteorological and agricultural content). All three genres show a preoccupation with death and health. It is tempting to presume a link between the three genres, but evidence is lacking. The unique attestation of (1) is not particularly helpful either. I

[1] Text 10/1, l. 1.

[2] Translation of text 10/1, ll. 1-3.

[3] Hollis and Wright (1992: 264).

am inclined to think that (1) could be a reworking of a year prognosis with (incomplete) omission of meteorological data, but I have not yet found a year prognosis which is close in content to (1).

Edition

10/1 London, British Library, Cotton Tiberius A. iii, fol. 40v/6-17

Đonne se mona bið acenned on sunnandæig. þ*æt* tacnað .iii. þing on þam monþe. þ*æt* is ren. 7 wind. 7 smyltnys. 7 hit tacnað. nytena wædla. 7 manna gesynto 7 hælo.

Gif he bið o monandæig acenned. þonne tacnað þ*æt* þam þe akennede beoð sare. 7 geongra manna heafod ece on þam monþe.

Gif he biþ on tiwesdæig akenned. þ*æt* tacnað eallum mannum gefean. 7 geongum geomrunge.

Gif he bið on wodnesdæig akænned. þ*æt* tacnað þ*æt* gesybsume weras wuniað betwyh holdum freondum.

Gif he on þunresdæig bið acenned þ*æt*. tacnað cynega hælo þurh læcecræfte.

Gif he bið on frigedæig akenned. þ*æt* bið god huntoð on þam monþe.

Gif he bið on sæternesdæig akenned. þonne tacnað þ*æt* gewinn. 7 blodgytas. 7 se þe hit mid suðanwinde onginne þonne hæfð he sige.

4 o] *read* on | **11** frigedæig] -ig < d.

11 Moon Colour

Literature

Birch (1878: 477); Bezold and Boll (1911: 25-37); Günzel (1993: 77-78)

Attribution

medieval: Pythagoras

Authors

Pliny, Bede

Branch of Superstition

observation of signs: colour of the moon

Text

L: 1. London, British Library, Cotton Titus D. xxvi, fols 5r-6r

Description

This text is not a prognostic in the ordinary sense. It is probably for this reason that Günzel discussed its contents under "miscellaneous texts" rather than under "prognostics" in her study and edition of Titus D. xxvi, xxvii.[1] Günzel's analysis is admirably concise and acute; the following account is much indebted to hers.

Günzel recognised a three-part structure in this text, consisting of: (1a) an account of distances between the earth, moon, sun and stars; (1b) weather predictions based upon the colour of the moon; and (1c) an account of the colours and visibility of the rainbow. The first and last items are not prognosticatory, but the second is. Part (1a), attributed to Pythagoras in the text, is taken from Byrhtferth's Glosses upon Bede's *De natura rerum* and *De temporum ratione*.[2] Part (1c), on the rainbow, is taken from Bede's *De natura rerum*.[3]

Part (1b) makes forecasts on the basis of the colours of the moon. The text belongs to a large group of lunar prognostics.[4] Text (1b) differs from the other lunar prognostics in one important respect: it is a non-temporal text. This is a remarkable feature because lunar (and solar) observations, whether they be superstitious or not, are mostly concerned with the passage of time. In comparison with other prognostics, there are two distinctions. First, the author of (1b) is known, viz. Bede, who introduced the

[1] Günzel (1993: 77-78).

[2] Günzel (1993: 28, 77) has based her views on the Byrhtferth Glosses upon an antiquated perspective by Jones (1938; 1939: 21-38). For more on Byrhtferth's authorship and the nature of the Glosses, see Gorman (1996).

[3] Günzel (1993: 78).

[4] See pp. 393-98.

topic of the colour of the moon in his *De natura rerum*.[5] There is only one other prognostic of which the author is known, i.e. the development of the foetus, derived from Vindicianus' *Gynaecia*.[6] Second, (1b) is excerpted from a larger work, while most other prognostics have probably always existed as independent texts. I know of two more exceptions: the text on the development of the foetus, which began as a chapter of the *Gynaecia*, and the texts on the Dog Days, which started out as parts of medical tracts on the humours or bloodletting.[7] Despite its atypical position within the prognostic corpus, (1b) displays the fundamental characteristic of a prognostic in that it predicts the future. The predictions are limited to the weather, particularly rain and storm. The origin of predictions using the colour of the moon are unknown, but dreambooks sometimes make mention of coloured moons, and Assyrian clay tables reporting a combination of shape and colour predictions have been found.[8]

Text (1) as a whole seems to be a brief compilation of meteorological notes. The motive for its compilation is obscure, but this is not the only curious piece of information in the first two quires of Titus D. xxvi, which consists mainly of prognostics.[9] Also included in Latin are treatises on the six ages of the world, and on the length of Christ and the wood of the cross. These two texts are immediately followed by four prognostics, text (1), and another eight prognostics. The combination of prognostics and notes is not exclusive to Titus D. xxvi: it is also encountered in the companion volume Titus D. xxvii, and in Caligula A. xv + Egerton 3314, Tiberius A. iii, Harley 3271 and Royal 2. B. v.[10] It would seem that what Warner and Gilson described as "chronological and other commonplaces" (prognostics and encyclopedic notes) were pieces of information of equal value.[11] In conclusion, I regard text (1) as representative of the contents of the first two quires of Titus D. xxvi as a whole.

---

[5] Günzel (1993: 78).

[6] See pp. 226-28.

[7] See pp. 153-57.

[8] Bezold and Boll (1911: 25-37). Jastrow (1905-12: II.457-577) printed several prognostic texts dealing with the moon, its shapes, eclipses, conjunctions with planets, stars and the sun, but none of these resemble text 11/1. An Assyrian prognostic on the colour of the sun has been attested, cf. Jastrow (1905-12: II. 607-08).

[9] See pp. 57-59.

[10] On the encyclopedic notes in Anglo-Saxon manuscripts, see Dekker (2007).

[11] Warner and Gilson (1921: I.41), with regard to the texts in question in Royal 2. B. v.

Edition

11/1 London, British Library, Cotton Titus D. xxvi, fols 5r/14-6r/1

PVithagoras u*ero* uir animi sagax scribit a terra ad luna*m* cxxvi milia stadioru*m* esse collegit a solem aute*m* ab ea duplu*m*. inde ad xii. signa triplicatu*m*.

Ex indiciis sicut fertur. **S**i luna .iiii. rubeat quasi auru*m* uento ostendit. **S**i pura sit serenitate*m*. **S**i in su*m*mo corniculo maculis ingrescit pluuia*m* indicat. **A**t sol se orto suo maculosus sub nube lat*et* pluuia*m*lem diem pręsagit. **S**i rubeat sincer*um*. si palleat te*m*pestuosum celum si mane rub*et* tempestuosu*m* significat diem. **S**i uesp*ere* rubicundu*m* aparuerit serenum crastinu*m* portendit diem.

Artus qui & hiris dicit*ur* quadricolor ex aduerso sole nubibusque formator. **N**am de celo igneum de aquis purpureum de aere iacinctiu*m* de terra gramineum trahit colore*m* & non cernitur nisi impleni luno.

1 **PV**ithagoras] *read* Pithagoras (*'*P' *is a light mark for the illuminator to make a rubricated* 'P'; *by accident* 'P' *was rubricated as* '**V**') | uir] *half a line is still available after* ~ *(for a rubric?)* | **2** a] *read* ad | inde] ~ ‖ ⟨*f. 5v*⟩ | **4** ingrescit] *read* nigrescit | **5** se] *read* si | pluuia*m*lem] pluuiālem; *read* pluuialem | **8** **A**rtus] *read* Arcus | formator] *read* formatur | **10** colore*m*] ~ ‖ ⟨*f. 6r*⟩ | impleni luno] *read* in plenilunio.

12 Regimen

Literature

Renzi (1852-59); Migne (1861-1904: I.759-86); Sudhoff (1908; 1909a-1909c); Thorndike (1923-58: I.676); Jones (1939: 73); Keil (1960); Reiche (1973); Stuart (1979); Taavitsainen (1988: 57-58); Mooney (1994); Adamson (1995); Wallis (1995: 112-15); Liuzza (2001: 224)

Attributions

medieval: Bede, Hippocrates

Branch of Superstition

observation of times: seasons, months

Text

L: 1. London, British Library, Harley 3271, fols 122v-23v

Description

A regimen is an aid in maintaining health that recommends appropriate types of food and drink or medical procedure in accordance with the time of year or the temperaments. A good introduction to this genre is Reiche's.[1] Many specimens have been edited in de Renzi's monumental but untrustworthy five-volume *Collectio Salernitana*.[2]

Regimens were known in classical times. The earliest Latin instances date from the ninth century, in which they already existed in relatively large numbers. Beccaria's catalogue of 145 medical manuscripts from the ninth to eleventh centuries contains over fifty references to regimens, some manuscripts containing no fewer than four texts.[3] In view of the many attestations in continental manuscripts, it is remarkable that the English pre-Conquest manuscripts have so far yielded but one text.[4]

---

[1] Reiche (1973). For a bibliography on regimens, see Wallis (1995: 133-34, n. 19).

[2] Renzi (1852-59).

[3] Beccaria (1956: 111 [5.8,11], 120 [8.6], 129 [11.2,3], 134 [15.2,4,5,7], 137 [16.21, 22], 140 [19.2], 143 [23], 148 [26.1], 165 [34.20], 171 [35.30], 178 [40.6], 179-80 [41. 2,9], 182 [43.7], 194-96 [48.7,13], 200 [50.4], 203 [51.3], 206 [52.7], 212 [55.21], 216 [56.13], 225 [62.1,6], 234 [68.5,6], 245 [73.17], 256-57 [78.12,15,19], 266-67 [83.5, 6,8], 287 [91.11], 295-96 [94.17], 308 [100.6,7], 315 [103.6], 318-19 [105.2], 321 [106.5], 365-66 [129.8,14], 378-80 [133.28,38], 382 [134.6], 384-85 [135.2,10]). Beccaria also included references to regimens in the manuscripts CUL Gg. 5. 35, Sloane 475 and 2839. More references are in Wickersheimer (1966: 13 [I], 24-25 [XI.2,3], 29 [XVIII.2], 39-41 [XXVIII.2,4,5,7,8], 47-48 [XXIX.21,22], 59 [XLVIII.7,8], 61 [XLIX.3], 67 [LX], 72 [LXIII.1], 108 [LXXVI.23], 119 [LXXVII.30], 131 [LXXXV. 8], 137-39 [LXXXVIII.2,8], 151 [XCIX.7], 157 [CIV.3]).

[4] The possible reasons underlying the rarity of this genre in English manuscripts are discussed on pp. 31-33, 44-45.

Regimens can be ordered by day, week, month or season. The monthly structure is the most commonly attested in medieval manuscripts, hence the designations 'Monatsregeln' and 'Monatsdiätetiken' in German.[5] Wallis has argued that the oldest (classical) regimens were seasonal, and that this structure changed when regimens came to be included in computi in the Middle Ages.[6] While it is true that regimens are frequently encountered in computi, I am not convinced that this inclusion caused the change in structure, especially because many monthly regimens are found in a medical rather than computistical context, also in early manuscripts. Moreover, the existence of a number of redactions among the earliest Latin monthly regimens would suggest that the monthly structure must have existed even before the inclusion of monthly regimens inclusion in computi. Whether monthly regimens came into being through the computus or not, the structure of choice for regimens in medieval manuscripts was the monthly one.

Monthly regimens show considerable variation, although the contents of the texts resemble each other very much. In general, regimens give advice on diet (beneficial herbs and drinks), hygiene (bathing) and health (bloodletting, medication). Some regimens include additional information on the humours or the twenty-four Egyptian Days.[7] The variation exhibited by regimens lies mainly in the amount and order of information. The texts can be quite lengthy, as (1) is, or very brief. As to the order in the texts, the monthly regimen may start with January or March.[8]

Regimens have been attributed to Hippocrates (e.g. 1) and Bede. For a change, the ascription to Bede is not the work of Renaissance scholars, as the title of the regimen in Sloane 475, fols 4v-6r illustrates: "**OBSERVATIO MENSIV*M*. S*E*C*VN*D*V*M BEDA*M***". Nevertheless, the inclusion of a regimen among Bede's works in Migne can be dismissed as a spurious attribution.[9]

Wallis wrote that Reiche had identified "fifty different types of monthly medical calendar", but this is not right.[10] Reiche mentioned that Bec-

---

[5] Cf. Reiche (1973: 116).

[6] Wallis (1995: 113-14). See also pp. 31-33.

[7] Cf. Wallis (1995: 114). Examples of Egyptian Days in regimens are in Reiche (1973: 117-18), Stuart (1979: 241-43), Sloane 475, fols 4v-6r.

[8] On March as the beginning of the year in texts on the twenty-four Egyptian Days, see p. 367.

[9] Migne (1861-1904: I.759-86), cf. Jones (1939: 73).

[10] Wallis (1995: 133, n. 19).

caria had identified over fifty texts, not types.[11] Beccaria distinguished twelve different types of regimens, and a few that are unclassifiable.[12] Reiche published eight redactions of continental monthly regimens, Stuart four.[13] The taxonomy of the genre has been poorly researched, as Reiche already noted,[14] despite the many text witnesses. In Beccaria's classification, (1) belongs to the 'Medicina Ypogratis' type on account of its title.[15] Text (1) does not resemble closely any of the texts printed by either Reiche or Stuart. In response to a letter by Jones, Sigerist observed that regimens "are all very similar but never quite identical", which are wise words that anyone who has ever tried to compare two regimens will be able to confirm.[16] Much research still needs to be done on this genre.

Edition

12/1 London, British Library, Harley 3271, fols 122v/29-123v/25

MEDICINA YPOGRATIS. QVID VSITARE DEBEATVR. PER SINGVLOS MENSES.

DE IANVARIO.

Mense ian*uario* non minuare sanguine*m*. potione*m* *con*tra effocatione*m* tantu*m* bibe. & electuariu*m* accipe. gingiber & reoponticu*m* usitare debes.

MENSE FEBRVARIO.

Mense FEB*RVARIO* de pollice uena*m* incide q*ui*a tunc febricitat terra. & om*n*ia que in ea sunt; & oximelle confici *con*ficienda accipere debes ad colera deducenda & flegma. melancoli*cum* q*uo*d pleris`q*ue*´ inueni`a´t*ur* habundare expellit p*er* uentre*m*. causa in capite circu*m*soluit & q*uo*d ex humore nascunt*ur* & ipsa n*on* p*er*mittit generare. apiu*m*. & agrimonia*m*. usitare debes.

Each entry starts on a new line | **1** YPOGRATIS] *i.e.* Hippocrates | **3** IANVARIO.] ~ ‖ ⟨*f. 123r*⟩ | **8** confici *con*ficienda] *delete* confici *(dittography)* | **9** melancoli*cum*] -a- < o | pleris`q*ue*´] -eris- *on erasure* | **11** usitare] u[s]sitare *(see ll. 13,28).*

[11] Reiche (1973: 113).
[12] Beccaria (1956: 443-44).
[13] Reiche (1973: 117-41), Stuart (1979: 241-43).
[14] Reiche (1973: 114).
[15] Beccaria (1956: 443).
[16] Cited in Jones (1939: 73).

MENSE MARTIO.

Mense mart*io* bonu*m* est balneum usitare sanguine*m*. minuære. potione*m* ad soluendum n*on* bibere. quia frigores generat. agram*en* usit*a*. & radices confectas. & sicera. & potu*m* dulcerata*m* & lubastica usitare debes.

MENSE APRILI.

Mense ap*r*i*li* de ulla radice n*on* manducare. q*ui*a tunc scabies & p`ru´rigines emittunt. bonu*m* est sanguine*m* minuære. potione*m* bibere. carnes recentes manducare. sanguine*m* inte*r*cutania*m* minuære. calidu*m* usitare. & betonica*m*. & pipenella*m*. `dolore*m* stomachi purgare. unguentu*m* calasticu*m* usitare.´

MENS*E* MAIO.

Mense mai*o* calidu*m* bibe. calidu*m* usita. caput purga. uena*m* epatica*m* incide. potione*m* ad soluendu*m*. bibe. cataplasma. in capite pone quia oculos turbulentos sana`t´ agram*en*. manducare. & absint`h´iu*m*. & semen maratri. usitare. aqua*m* ieiunus non bibe: de ullo capud. aut pede n*on* manducare. q*ui*a tunc de aere in rós uenena mala descendunt. & alia de t*er*ra surgunt.

MENSE IVNIO.

Mense iun*io* aqua*m* ieiuniis bibe. p*ro*pt*er* colera soluenda. saluia*m* usitare. ceruisa*m* non bibes. lactucas manduca acetu*m* bibe.

MENSE IVLIO.

Mense iul*io* uinu*m* modicu*m* bibe quia cerebro humores tunc p*ro*duc*et*. sanguine*m* n*on* minuære. potione*m* ad soluendu*m* non bibere. saluia*m*. & rudan. apiu*m*. & flores uuę usitare.

MENSE AVGVSTO.

Mense agus*to* caulos. n*on* manducare. quia uenefici sunt. p*ro*pt*er* uermes q*ui* illos comedunt. maluas. n*on* manducare: quia amara sunt tunc & colera. nigra nutriunt. agram*en* manducare. puleio. usitare.

13 usitare] u[s]sitare *(see l. 11)* | **15** dulcerata*m*] *read* dulceratum | **16** APRILI] -R- < L | **17** scabies] -c- < e | **20** `dolore*m*... usitare.´] *this phrase is added over* & betonica*m* & pipenella*m*, *but the exact insertion point is not indicated* | **23** cataplasma] ~ *glossed by Old English* cliþa. *This gloss is not incorporated in the* Old English Corpus Online *(Healey and Venezky 2000: search on* cataplasma *and* cliþa) | **25** pede] *read* pedes *or* pedem | **28** soluenda.] ~ ‖ ⟨*f. 123v*⟩ | usitare] u[s]sitare *(see l. 11)* | **31** humores] -e- < o | tunc] -c < d | **33** usitare] u- *on erasure* | **36** amara] -a *on erasure.*

MENSE. SEPTEMBRI.

Mense sept*embri* om*n*ia que \`uis´ accipias. quia tunt om*nes* escę. p*ro* fructu*m* *con*fecta sunt. lac caprinu*m* & anunculinum ieiunus bibe. p*ro*pt*er* sanguine*m* adducendu*m*. & coaucol\`u*m*´ ad te*m*perandu*m*. & pulmones curandos. casto & grano mastico usitare.

M*ENSE* OCT*OBRI.*

Mense octo*bri* racemos & musto usitare. quia corp*us* sanant. & solutione*m* faciunt & garoflo. usitare.

Mense nou*embri* non balneare. quia de calore balnei. humores mouent*ur*. q*uia* tunc sanguis coagulat*us*. \`e*st*´ bonu*m* est studiu*m* habere. quia tunc omn*es* humores sunt purgati. cinna\`mo´mum. usitare.

Mense dec*embri* bonu*m* *est* studiu*m* habere. uena*m* epatica*m* incidere. potione*m* ad soluendu*m*. bibere. spíco. usitare.

39 que] -e *on erasure* | tunt] *read* tunc | fructu*m*] *read* fructu | **40** anunculinum] -u$_1$- < n; annuclinum, anul nuclinum *(Reiche 1973: 128, 132)* | **41** coaucol\`u*m*´] coaucol[a], -\`u*m*´- < [a]; *read* coagulum*(?)* | casto] cast[·]o | **44** octo*bri*] o- < · | musto] -u- < ii | **45** garoflo.] -flo. *on erasure* | **46** nou*embri* non] -ou*embri* non *on erasure* | **46-47** mouent*ur*. q*uia* tunc sanguis] ~ *on erasure* | **48** purgati] -i < e | **49** epatica*m*] -a$_2$- < ⁖.

13 *SORTES SANCTORUM*

Literature

Pithou (1687: 370-73); Brand (1849-55: III.336-38); Hercher (1863); Chabaneau (1880a; 1880b); Rocquain (1880); Hartel (1886: 234-36); Winnefeld (1887); Harris (1888; 1901); Bolte (1901-06: IV.284-341); Dobschütz (1912: 54); Heinevetter (1912); Brandin (1914); Thorndike (1923-58: I.630, II.606); Förster (1936); Ducange *et al.* (1937-38: VII. 532-34, s.v. 2 *sors*); Dold (1948); Svenberg (1963: 6); Browne (1976); Harmening (1979: 191-204); Braekman (1981); Browne and Stewart (1983-2001); Kieckhefer (1989: 88); Stewart (1995); Liuzza (2001: 189-90); Klingshirn (2002)

Alias

Sortes Apostolorum

Branch of Superstition

divination: astragalomancy, cubomancy

Text

L: 1. Oxford, St. John's College, MS 17, fols 157vb-58va

Description

Like the only other divinatory text from Anglo-Saxon sources, the alphabet prognostic, (1) consists of a bare list of responses, ordered alphabetically in the former, and by a sequence of numbers in the latter. The entries of (1) are composed of a sequence of three numbers followed by an interpretation of the future. The sequence begins with c.c.c., and ends with i.i.i., while the range of the individual numbers is i-v and c. 'c' is to be interpreted as a "cursive ligature" of Roman v and i, probably not a modified form of Greek ς, i.e. 6, which complements the Roman numbers i-v.[1] The sequence can thus be resolved into a range from 1 to 6. (1) has fifty-six entries in all, one of which is lacking. The number of entries coincides with the number of possibilities in which a set of three numbers, each ranging from 1 to 6, can be resolved, if the result is sorted in descending or ascending order.[2]

[1] Klingshirn (2002: 95).

[2] The total number of possible combinations of three numbers thrown with three dice is 6*6*6 = 216. If the result of the throw is not sorted, any one of six permutations (the factorial for a combination of three numbers is six) of three numbers is a valid outcome. However, in 13/1 the result is sorted, so a throw of 316, for instance, must be resolved into 631 before it can be looked up in the text. The number of valid, sorted results for a throw with three dice is thus fifty-six: six for casting three identical numbers (xxx, in bold), thirty for casting two identical numbers and one dissimilar number (yyx

The working principle of (1) is not made explicit in the prognostic itself, but analogous texts usually have introductions.[3] This prognostic is to be operated with six-sided dice, either with one throw of three dice or three throws of one die.[4] Braekman published four Middle English redactions of the *Sortes Sanctorum*, and in the facsimiles of two of these three rectangles bearing the sides of dice are entered next to the interpretations.[5] This adds weight to the supposition that (1) is a form of astragalomancy (divination by means of knuckle bones or dice), specifically cubomancy (divination by means of six-sided dice).[6] The outcome of the throw is sorted in descending order, and the result is to be looked up in the text. The predictions given in the text "are cautiously optimistic, counseling the virtues of steadiness in adversity, wariness of one's neighbors, and above all trust in God".[7]

---

or yxx, in italics), and twenty for casting three dissimilar numbers (zyx, in roman type):

666			*331*	321	*311*	**555**			*221*	*211*	**444**			**111**
665	*655*			*332*	*322*	*554*	*544*			**222**	*443*	*433*		
664	654	*644*			**333**	*553*	543	*533*			*442*	432	*422*	
663	653	643	*633*			*552*	542	532	*522*		*441*	431	421	*411*
662	652	642	632	*622*		*551*	541	531	521	*511*				
661	651	641	631	621	*611*									

The total number of permutations for the fifty-six entries above is 336. The discrepancy between 336 possibilities and the number of combinations thrown with three dice, 216, can be explained as follows. First, all permutations for three identical numbers are possible ($x^ax^bx^c$, $x^ax^cx^b$, $x^bx^ax^c$, $x^bx^cx^a$, $x^cx^ax^b$ and $x^cx^bx^a$), but this is not taken into account. Second, only three out of six permutations for two identical numbers with one dissimilar number are distinguished (x^ax^by or x^bx^ay, yx^ax^b or yx^bx^a, x^ayx^b or x^byx^a). Third, all permutations for three dissimilar numbers are distinguished (xyz, xzy, yxz, yzx, zxy, and zyx). So five out of six permutations are not recognised for xxx, and three out of six for xxy, yxx and xyx (so (5*6) + (3*30) = 120 possibilities). If the 120 possibilities not distinguished in the total of unsorted combinations are added to those which are distinguished, the total is: 120 + 216 = 336. I should like to thank Anke Prinsen for her invaluable help in this matter.

[3] Klingshirn (2002: 94-96).

[4] Harris (1901: 48) argued that the number of possible results of one throw with three dice is fifty-six, and of three throws with one die 216. The difference between these results, however, depends upon whether the result is sorted or not.

[5] Braekman (1981: 23-46).

[6] Heinevetter (1912: 39). For drawings of knuckle bones and dice, see Heinevetter (1912: 30, 37, 45, 48-49).

[7] Klingshirn (2002: 95).

Several stone inscriptions of divination by means of dice demonstrate that astragalomancy was known in Greece.[8] In the inscriptions quoted in *Pauly* and Harris, the dice used are four-sided knucklebones (numbered 1, 3, 4 and 6), and the die is to be thrown five or seven times to obtain the right interpretation.[9] Braekman mentioned a Greek inscription which reports a four-sided die to be thrown three times.[10] Moreover, the Greeks also used six-sided dice thrown three times.[11] The emergence of codified Greek astragalomancy is placed in the second century AD.[12] Sanskrit, Arabic, Persian and Turkish witnesses of astragalomancy have been found as well.[13]

Another branch of divination connected to the *sors* under discussion is that in which specific questions are asked, and in which the answers are arranged in lists. An example of this type are the Greek *Sortes Astrampsychi*, ascribed to the Egyptian Astrampsychos and dated to the sixth or seventh century.[14] The questioner chooses a question from a numbered list, memorises the number of the question (x), and adds a randomly chosen number between 1 and 10 (n). In a separate table, the sum $x + n$ is cross-referenced with one of the decads. The questioner retrieves the relevant decad, of which the nth line contains the answer. Intentional complications, such as the table that refers the questioner to a decad based on the outcome of $x + n$, and favourable or unfavourable times to consult the *sors*, were added to heighten the oracular nature.[15] A text related to the *Sortes Astrampsychi* is the sixth- or seventh-century Latin *Sortes Sangallenses*, which constitutes the original text of the palimpsest manuscript St.

[8] Chabaneau (1880a: 160-61; 1880b: 264-65), Wissowa *et al.* (1894-1978: 1st series II.1793, s.v. *astragalomanteia*; 1st series II.1795, s.v. ἀστράγαλος; 1st series XIII.2.1458-62, s.v. *losung*; Suppl. IV.51-53, s.v. *astragalomanteia*), Harris (1901: 46-47), Heinevetter (1912), Braekman (1981: 6).

[9] Chabaneau (1880b: 265), Wissowa *et al.* (1894-1978: 1st series II.1793, s.v. *astragalomanteia*; Suppl. IV.51-52, s.v. *astragalomanteia*), Harris (1901: 47), Klingshorn 92002: 96-97). Harris (1901: 113-16) printed one of these stone inscription under the title *Sortes Alearum*. Heinevetter (1912: 4-26, 29) published several of these texts. Chabaneau (1880b: 266-68) translated one of the stone inscriptions.

[10] Braekman (1981: 6).

[11] Wissowa *et al.* (1894-1978: Suppl. IV.54-55, s.v. *astragalomanteia*).

[12] Wissowa *et al.* (1894-1978: Suppl. IV.51, s.v. *astragalomanteia*), Harris (1901: 162).

[13] Bolte (1901-06: IV.284-93), Braekman (1981: 7).

[14] Harris (1901: 49-56), Bolte (1901-06: IV.280-82), Braekman (1981: 6), Dold (1948: 9), Browne (1976), Stewart (1995).

[15] Harris (1901: 49-56). Edition of the *Sortes Astrampsychi* can be found in Hercher (1863), Harris (1901: 128-60), and, more reliably, in Browne and Stewart (1983-2001).

Gallen 908.[16] Here, the decads have been expanded to dodecads. Dold has argued that the answers of the dodecads correspond to a throw with one or two dice.[17] So instead of choosing a number between 1 and 10, as in the *Sortes Astrampsychi*, the questioner throws dice to find the answer to his query. This would effectively link the *Sortes Sangallenses* with astragalomancy.

The instances mentioned above testify to the long history of astragalomancy. The *Sortes Sanctorum*, or *Sortes Apostolorum* as they were also known,[18] are yet another branch of divination by means of dice. As Klingshirn has shown in his thorough study of the *Sortes Sanctorum*, this type of divination was strongly condemned in the *Decretum Gelasianum*, in the canons of various church councils from the fifth century onwards, and in penitentials.[19] Nevertheless, the first text witnesses date from the ninth century.[20] In addition to (1), a number of analogues have been found: in Latin in Egerton 821 and Ludwig XII. 5 (both of English origin), several continental versions in Latin from the ninth century onwards, and vernacular witnesses in Provençal, French and Middle English.[21] A comparison between the Latin *sortes* and (1) makes clear that a number of different redactions exist, but that they are similar in subject matter. The most notable difference between (1) and other Latin texts is the absence in (1) of the introduction.[22]

[16] Harris (1901: 56-59), Bolte (1901-06: IV.282), Dold (1948: 7-9), Braekman (1981: 6-7). Winnefeld (1887: 13-44), Harris (1901: 161-79) and Dold (1948: 20-115) have published the *Sortes Sangallenses*.

[17] Dold (1948: 10).

[18] On the complicated history of the name *Sortes Apostolorum* for the *Sortes Sanctorum*, see Klingshirn (2002: 98-104).

[19] Klingshirn (2002: 84-90, 104-14).

[20] Klingshirn (2002: 93)

[21] Hartel (1886: 234-36), Braekman (1981: 7-8, 17). Winnefeld (1887: 54-60) and Harris (1901: 180-84) edited one of the Latin *sortes*; another was published by Pithou (1687: 370-73), Rocquain (1880: 465-74), Chabaneau (1880a: 172-78), Harris (1901: 117-27) and Brandin (1914: 483-94). The Provençal *sors*, immured in a wall in the thirteenth or fourteenth century), discovered and first printed in 1866 (cf. Chabaneau 1880a: 157-58), was edited by Rocquain (1880: 465-74), Chabaneau (1880a: 167-72) and Harris (1901: 117-27). The Provençal *sors* makes use of coloured threads in the margins to choose from, rather than a throw of dice, but the text is comparable to that of its astragalomantic counterparts (Rocquain 1880: 461). Brandin (1914: 483-94) printed a French *Sortes Sanctorum*. Four of the Middle English *sortes* were edited by Braekman (1981: 21-46). Manuscripts are listed in Thorndike (1923-58: II.606, n. 4), Förster (1936: 241 n. 15), Thorndike and Kibre (1963: 1101, 1687), and Klingshirn (2002: 129).

[22] On the introduction, see Klingshirn (2002: 94-95).

Edition

13/1 Oxford, St. John's College, MS 17, fols 157vb/9-158va/8

.c.c.c. Animum tuum si dubitantem sentis crede primo modum deo adiuuante impetrabis quę uis;

.c.c.v. De quo consulis crede constanter. quia perueniet ad te quod speras;

.c.c.iiii. De quo cupis deum roga. & ipse adiuuabit te ut peruenias ad id quod desideras;

.c.c.iii. Quod postulas securus esto. & ueniet tibi cum gaudio magno. sed pone in deum cor tuum confidenter;

.c.c.ii. Elemosinam pauperibus tribue. & habe spem bonam in deum.

.c.c.i. De luce ad tenebras ire cupis. ubi nulla tibi consolatio est. uita tua carere desideras. sed cito cessa. & non age hoc quod cupis;

.c.v.v. Est uia incerta quam ire cupis. sed deus per suam misericordiam sanum te ducet.

.c.v.iiii. Magnum est quod rogas. & si uis ut fiat quod cogitas. quod non est in tua potestate sed in dei.

.c.v.iii. Non dubites quicquam de quo consulis. deum roga. bonum est tibi & illum timere;

.c.v.ii. Tu dubitas utrum fieri possit. & tamen te incredulo ad tuas manus ueniet;

.c.v.i. Cum magno labore peruenies ad quod desideras. roga deum humiliter. ipse te adiuuet. ideoque securus esto;

.c.iiii.iiii. Noli audire iniquam doctrinam. sed recede ab hoc consilio. & uide ne postmodum te pęniteat.

.c.iiii.iii. Sicut nauis in mari iactatur a fluctibus & dubitat an perueniat ad portum. sic tu dubitas in animo. & deo auxiliante peruenies ad quod desideras;

.c.iiii.ii. Si uicinus tuus ad te uenerit & blandis sermonibus uult te seducere. non credas ei. quia pęnitebit te dum non poteris emendare;

.c.iiii.i. Vide primum quod non est animus tuus stabilis. & praua sunt intra pectus tuum. emenda illa. & tunc tibi ueniet desiderium tuum quod tibi uertetur in gaudium;

.c.iii.iii. Quod cogitas non potest fieri. aliud cogita. & magnum lucrum habebis

.c.iii.ii. Petitio tua accepta erit. si in deum permanserit firma;

.c.iii.i. Via tibi difficilis est. tamen patiens esto. & deum roga. & inuenies desiderium tuum.

.c.ii.ii. De quo consulis si fides tua est firma. consequeris magnam gloriam a deo.

.c.ii.i. Dicis quod times. & inimici tui cadent. & adhuc multum tibi melius erit.

.c.i.i. Noli timere sed diligentius auge bonum sic poteris impetrare quod petis.

Text is continuous except for a break of two lines between entries .iii.ii.i. and .ii.ii.i. *This break exists because* .iii.i.i. *accidentally precedes* .iii.ii.i. *in the manuscript, which may have confused the scribe to such an extent that he omitted entry* .ii.ii.ii. *altogether* | **28** &] ~ ‖ ⟨*f. 158ra*⟩.

.v.v.v. Bonu*m est* q*uo*d petis. & ideo inuenies cito.

.v.v.iiii. In d*eum* co*n*fide & eu*m* in adiutoriu*m* quęre. & uinces inimicos tuos. si*cut* in uoluntate habes.

.v.v.iii. Sic*ut* seme*n* in t*er*ra serit*ur* & fruct*us* dilatat ut iteru*m* in t*em*p*or*e suo maiore*m* fructu*m* afferat. sic & illud q*uo*d petis te latet. ut gaudiu*m* t*ibi* mai*us* fiet cu*m* ueniet.

.v.v.ii. In uia ire cupis ubi nulla tua uia *est* & multi serpentes ante te s*un*t q*ui* t*ibi* cupiunt noc*ere*. *sed* recede ab hoc co*n*silio. & cogita ut n*on* p*er*das anima*m* tua*m*;

.v.v.i. Expecta patient*er*. q*uia* q*uo*d cupis cito ueniet in man*us* tuas cu*m* gaudio.

.v.iiii.iiii. Sic*ut* plu*m*bu*m* magno auro coop*er*it*ur*. sic q*uo*d cupis interi*us* malu*m* exteri*us* pulchre tegit*ur*. p*ro*pt*er* hoc n*on* desid*er*es q*uo*d n*on* potest fieri.

.v.iiii.iii. Spe*m* tua*m* ad d*eum* dirige. & ipse te adiuuet ut adu*er*sariu*m* uincas;

.v.iiii.ii. Si aliud cogitas & aliud ad te uenerit. d*eum* n*on* sp*er*nas. ideo caute age ne forte p*er*eas;

.v.iiii.i. Non ingrediaris ad istud te*mpus*. *sed* sustine q*uia* difficile accipies.

.v.iii.iii. Quę in manib*us* tuis. *sed* & a*ni*malia t*ibi* futura cici*us* uenient.

.v.iii.ii. Inimicu*m* q*ui* te uult noc*ere* fuge. noli tardare. *sed* lib*er*a te ne in morte*m* inc*ur*ras. q*uia* p*er* d*e*i adiutoriu*m* potes euad*ere*;

.v.iii.i. Noli e*ss*e desp*er*ans *sed* crede. q*uo*d ueniet t*ibi* desid*er*iu*m* bonu*m* cu*m* gaudio.

.v.ii.ii. Difficile p*er*uenit hoc & tam*en*. si d*eum* humilit*er* rogaueris i*m*petrabis.

.v.ii.i. Parata s*un*t quę petis. noli sollicit*us* e*ss*e. Secur*us* esto. q*uia* i*m*petrabi*s* quę cupis.

.v.i.i. Hac hora recede a me q*uia* n*on* possu*m* t*ibi* m*odo* ueru*m* dic*ere*. Veni alio die. & dica*m* q*uo*d uis uid*ere* & nichil uereare.

.iiii.iiii.iiii. Sustine modicu*m* \`te*mpus*´. & postea ueniet t*ibi* uoluntas tua.

.iiii.iiii.iii. Non habes q*uo*d petis. & nichil a*m*pli*us* quęras. q*uia* n*on* potest esse;

.iiii.iiii.ii. Noli timere. d*eus* te adiuuet. secur*us* esto;

.iiii.iiii.i. Impet*ra*s q*uo*d cupis. inimicosq*ue* tuos uinces.

.iiii.iii.iii. Q*ui*d co*ntra* me laboras in hęc co*n*sulendo ambula. q*uia* malu*m est* q*uo*d petis.

.iiii.iii.ii. Nauis t*ibi* ad portu*m* parata *est*. ideo lęt*us* esto. q*uia* t*ibi* d*eu*s in adiutoriu*m est*;

.iiii.iii.i. D*eum* n*on* times. multu*m* p*ro*mittis. & se*m*p*er* negligis. ora d*eum* ut sit t*ibi* propiti*us*. q*uia* ualde irat*us est*. & postea *quod* placabil*is est* roga eu*m*. & quę cupis cito co*n*seq*ue*ris.

.iiii.ii.ii. D*eus* adiuuet te. & uoluntate*m* tua*m* co*n*seq*ue*ris *quod* desid*er*as;

.iiii.ii.i. Tibi in a*nimo est* ut hoc possit fieri cu*m* i*m*pedim*en*to. & tam*en* null*us* t*ibi* potest i*m*pedire.

.iiii.i.i. Exalto a*nim*o. & sup*er*ba m*en*te cupis. & tam*en* inutile *est* q*uo*d desid*er*as;

53 in] *c. 13 letters missing before* ~ | **61** possu*m*] pos‖sum ⟨*f. 158rb*⟩ | **63** \`te*mpus*´] ~ *over* [petis], [petis] *underlined for deletion.*

.iii.iii.iii. Non tu gl*or*ieris in isto s*e*c*u*lo. s*ed* roga d*eu*m. ut t*ibi* det maiore*m* gl*o*-*ri*am;

.iii.iii.ii. Dulce habes. & amaru*m* cupis. & n*on* *im*pet*ras* q*uo*d cupis.

.iii.iii.i. Vide ne sp*er*es in diuitíís. Roga d*eu*m. & felicior eris.

.iii.ii.ii. Vnde sollicit*us* es. sustine longu*m* te*mpus*. & p*er*uenies ad hoc q*uo*d cupis.

.iii.i.i. Ia*m* t*ibi* ap*er*t*us* *est* ingress*us*. & ianua patet. si ex toto corde uadis. sed sustine meli*us* te*mpus*.

.iii.ii.i. In hac hora n*on* ingrediaris. q*uia* n*on* ueniet q*uo*d cupis.

.ii.ii.i. Pecunia*m* tua*m* ad lucru*m* mitt*er*e cupis. uide ut ad gaudiu*m* t*ibi* ueniet. q*uia* nimis p*er*iculosu*m* *est* q*uo*d cupis;

.ii.i.i. Tibi licitu*m* *est*. p*er*ge q*uo* cupis. cu*m* bonis actib*us* *im*petrabis;

.i.i.i. Non habes q*uo*d petis n*isi* uolueris cu*m* bonis actib*us* mereri. tam*en* pone in d*eu*m cor tuu*m* & inuenies quę cupis; FINIT;

ISTI PSALMI CANTANT*VR*; PS*ALMVS* Exaudi d*om*ine iusticia*m* mea*m*. **PS*ALMVS*** Ad te d*omine* leuaui an*imam*. **PS*ALMVS*** D*eu*s misereat*ur*. **PS*ALMVS*** Deus in adiutor*ium*. **PS*ALMVS*** In te d*omine* sp*er*aui **PS*ALMVS*** Inclina d*omine*. **PS*ALMVS*** Benedicite. **L**etania. **P**at*er* n*oste*r. **C**redo in d*eum*. **coll*ecta*.** **L**ib*er*a nos d*om*ine de potestate tenebraru*m*. & de manu mortis ęt*er*nę eripe nos. ut uoluntas tua sit in *om*nib*us* ap*er*ta absq*ue* ambiguitate p*er* hoc signu*m* sortis te nobis poscentib*us*. p*er* d*eum*.

84-86 *entry* .iii.i.i. *precedes* .iii.ii.i. *in the manuscript. The latter entry is followed by a two-line break after which the text resumes with entry* .ii.ii.i., *thereby skipping* .ii.ii.ii | **92** iusticia*m*] iu‖sticia*m* ⟨*f. 158va*⟩ | Exaudi... mea*m*] *Ps 16:1* | **93** Ad... an*imam*] *Ps 24:1* | D*eu*s misereat*ur*] *Ps 66:2* | **94** D*eus* in adiutor*ium*] *Ps 69:2* | In... sp*er*aui] *Ps 30:2* | **94-95** Inclina d*omine*] *Ps 85:1* | **95** Benedicite] *Ps 65:8*.

14 Sunshine Prognostic

Literature

Hellmann (1896b: 65-67); Förster (1903: 350; 1906: 369, n. 1; 1912a: 64-71); Jastrow (1905-12: II.577-612); Gundel and Gundel (1966: 269-70); Harmening (1979: 120); Hollis and Wright (1992: 263-64); Epe (1995: 58); Soldt (1995); Liuzza (2001: 184)

Alias

solare

Branches of Superstition

observation of signs: sunshine; observation of times: twelve days of Christmas

Texts

OE: 1. Cambridge, Corpus Christi College, MS 391, p. 713
2. Oxford, Bodleian Library, Hatton 115, fols 149v-50r

Description

Sunshine prognostics predict the future on the basis of sunshine on the twelve days of Christmas. The predictions focus on agriculture, husbandry, produce and the presence of metallic resources, for instance "many fruits will be on the trees", "the sea and all the rivers will be filled with fish", and "quicksilver will be easy to obtain".[1] The twelve-day structure is shared with the wind prognostic, but is not encountered in any other prognostic, to my knowledge. There are only three prognostic genres that make use of Christian feast days, to wit the wind and sunshine prognostics and some redactions of the year prognosis. A good study of the sunshine prognostic is Förster's.[2]

Texts (1, 2) are the earliest attested sunshine prognostics. Förster identified several witnesses in Latin, Middle High German and Swedish.[3] Early printed editions of the so-called 'Bauernpraktik' (the German name for the year prognosis) often include sunshine and wind prognostics, e.g. the facsimile published by Hellmann.[4] A Latin text presumably underlies (1, 2), but no such text has been found which antedates the translation into Old English. Texts (1, 2) differ in phrasing in some places.[5] Since (1) is incomplete, the later text (2) cannot be a copy. More-

[1] Translation of text 14/2, ll. 8, 13, 11, respectively.
[2] Förster (1912a: 64-71).
[3] Förster (1903: 350; 1912a: 66-71).
[4] Hellmann (1896b: Aii verso-Aiii recto).
[5] See Förster (1912a: 64).

over, (2) is most likely produced in Canterbury, while (1) is in a Worcester manuscript.

There are three noteworthy aspects of (1, 2). First, there is an emphasis on the discovery of metals, not encountered in any other prognostic: gold is mentioned twice, quicksilver once. The Latin text printed by Förster lists silver twice and gold once.[6] Second, (1, 2) refer specifically to the finding of metal "on ængelcynne" (among the English). This topicality is not found in any of the sunshine prognostics, nor in any of the other prognostics for that matter. Third, the Old English texts refer to the *Wonders of the East*: "the camels will carry off much gold from the ants which must guard the gold hoard".[7] This learned allusion is unique to the Old English sunshine prognostics. The references to the English and the *Wonders of the East* give the impression that an Anglo-Saxon compiler customised or rewrote (1, 2), which is unusual because most translations into the vernacular keep close to the Latin source text.

Edition

14/1 Cambridge, Corpus Christi College, MS 391, p. 713/1-19

kiningum 7 ricum mannum bið mycel syb þy geare.

Gif ðy iiii. dæge sunne scineð. þon*ne* oðbeoreð olfendas mycel gold þam æmetum þe þonne goldhord heoldan sculon.

Gif ðy .v dæge sunne scineð mycle blostma 7 blæda mid mannum frecednes 7 manna hus frecenessa þrowiað.

Gy vi dæge gif sunne scineð mycel meolc bið þy geare mid mannum.

Gif þy vii dæge sunne scineð beorhte drihten asent mycle wæstmas on treowum on þam geare

Gif þy viii dæge sunne scineð beorhte þonne bið cwicseolfer on angelkynne yðgeate

Gif on ix dæge sunne scineð god sendeð mycele fugeloð on þam geare

Gif ðy .x. dæge sunne scineð beorhte sǽ. 7 ealle ea beoð mid fixum afylde.

Gif þy xi dæge sunne scineð þonne bið mycel costung deaðes mid mannum.

Gif þy .xii. dæge sunne scineð men beoð wace on mislicum brocum 7 bið mycel sib;

3 sculon] -c- < t | **4** ðy] *ascender not crossed, but the length of the ascender is intended for* 'ð' *rather than a round* 'd', *which has a short ascender in this hand* | **6 G**y] *read* Ðy *(the scribe probably combined* Gif *and* Ðy; gif *occurs later in the same line to correct the mistake)* | **9** angelkynne] -k- < h | **13** mycel] m- *partly illegible through hole.*

[6] Förster (1912a: 66-67).

[7] Translation of text 14/2, ll. 6-7. See also p. 98.

14/2 Oxford, Bodleian Library, Hatton 115, fols 149v/24-150r/17

Þy forma dæg drihtnes gebyrde. gyf sunne scyneð. mycel gefea byoð mid mannum. 7 *ge*nihtsum.

Gyf þy æfteran dæg sunne scyneþ. þon*ne* byð on ængelcynne gold eaðbegeate.

Gyf þy þryddan dæg sunne scyneð. betweoh earmum mannu*m* mycel gefeoht byoð. 7 betweoh cynigum. 7 rycu*m* mannu*m* micel sib.

Gyf þy .iiii. dæge sunne scyneð. þon*ne* þa olfenda mycel gold oðberað þan ætmettu*m* þa þone goldhord healden scolden.

Gyf þy .v. deg*e* sunne scyneð. mycel blostman bleoda beoð þy gere.

Gyf .vi dæg*e* sunne scyneð driht sendeð mycele meolc.

Gyf .vii. dæg*e* sunne scineð. mycele westmas on treowu*m* beoð.

Gyf þy .viii. dæg*e* sunne scyneð. ðon*ne* byð cwicseolfor eaðgeate.

Gyf þi .ix. dæg*e* sunne scyneð. þonne god sendeð micelne fulluht on geare.

Gyf þi .x. dæg*e* sunne scyneð. þonne byð sé 7 ealle ǽa mid fixum ontined.

Gyf þi .xi dæg*e* sunne scyneð. micel costung byð deaðes mid mannu*m*.

Gyf þi .xii. dæg*e* sunne scyneð. men beoð wace. 7 byð micel sib on eorðan:-

3 ængelcynne] ~ ‖ ⟨*f. 150r*⟩ | **8** blostman] *read* ~ 7 | **9** Gyf] *read* ~ þy | driht] *read* drihten | **10** Gyf] *read* ~ þy.

15 Unlucky Days

Literature

Braswell (1984: 347); Förster (1903: 352; 1929: 261-65); Taavitsainen (1998: 54-55); Hollis and Wright (1992: 268); Epe (1995: 59); Hirsh (1997); Liuzza (2001: 186)

Branch of Superstition

observation of times: days of the moon

Texts

OE: 1. London, British Library, Cotton Caligula A. xv, fol. 130r
2. London, British Library, Cotton Vitellius E. xviii, fol. 9r

L: 3. Oxford, St. John's College, MS 17, fol. 40vb

Description

The unlucky days are yet another branch of the extensive body of texts which report unfavourable days.[1] The better-known counterpart to the unlucky days are the Egyptian Days, texts of which are attested in large numbers in medieval times. There are two unlucky days per month on which anything started will never be finished.[2] The texts consist of little more than a brief introduction and a list of days. These days are not to be confused with the twenty-four Egyptian Days, which fall on fixed dates. Unlucky days are ordered by days of the moon rather than dates.

Förster identified a number of texts on the unlucky days in Latin and the vernacular.[3] In the twelfth century, an Anglo-Norman text on the unlucky days was added to Tiberius C. vi, fol. 114r, along with a Latin text on the twenty-four Egyptian Days.[4] Förster claimed that the unlucky days go back to a Greek source. Texts (1, 2) are translations from a Latin text, but Förster confessed that he had not yet located a Latin text which may be representative of the source for the translation.[5] Text (3), not known to Förster, resembles (1, 2) to such an extent that it may be representative of the Latin source text. The manuscript of (3), however, postdates those of (1, 2) by about half a century, but then the examplar of St. John's College 17 probably already existed in the eleventh century.[6]

[1] See p. 330.

[2] For a list of days, see table 38.

[3] Förster (1903: 352; 1929: 264-65).

[4] See p. 85.

[5] Förster (1929: 264).

[6] See p. 85.

Edition

15/1 London, British Library, Cotton Caligula A. xv, fol. 130r/13-27

Syndon twegen dagas on æghwylcum monðe swa hwæt swa on þam dagum ongynð ne wurð hit næfre geendod.

On **I**anuarias	þonne se mona bið .iii. nihta eald 7 .iiii.		
On **F**ebruarius	þon*ne* he bið	v	nihta eald 7 vii.
On **M**artius	þon*ne* he bið	vi	nihta eald 7 vii.
On **A**prelis	þon*ne* he bið	v	nihta eald 7 viii.
On **M**aius	þon*ne* he bið	viii	nihta eald 7 ix.
On **I**unius	þon*ne* he bið	v	nihta eald 7 xvii.
On **I**ulius	þon*ne* he bið	iii	nihta eald 7 xiii.
On **A**gustus	þon*ne* he bið	viii	nihta eald 7 xiii.
On **S**eptember	þon*ne* he bið	v	nihta eald 7 ix.
On **O**ctober	þon*ne* he bið	v	nihta eald 7 xv.
On **N**ouember	þon*ne* he bið	vii	nihta eald 7 ix.
On **D**ecember	þon*ne* he bið	iii	nihta eald 7 xii.

And swa hit bið gyme se þe wylle.

Entries for February-December are in columns | **1** swa$_2$] *read* ~ man *(see 15/2)* | **3 I**anuarias] *read* Ianuarius | **8** xvii.] *read* xxvii. *(see 15/2,3)* | **13** ix.] ~ < [x] | **14** xii.] *read* xiii. *(see 15/2,3)* | **15** bið gyme se þe] ~ < [gyme se þe wylle.].

15/2 London, British Library, Cotton Vitellius E. xviii, fol. 9r/17-26

DE DIEBVS MALIS CVIVSQVE MENSIS:

(T)weigen dagas syndon on æghwilcu*m* monðe. þ*æt* swa hwæt swa man on þam
dagum onginneð. **N**e wurð hit næfre geendod. þæt is þonne
On ianuariu(s) þon*ne* se mona bið þreora nihta eald. **7** feowra.
7 On februarius. þonn he bið .fifa. **7** seofena eald.
7 On martius. þe syxta. **7** se seofeða.
7 On aprilis. se fifta. **7** se eahteþa.
7 **O**n maius. se eahteþa. **7** se nygeþa.
On iunius. se .v. **7** se .xxvii.
On iulius. se .iii. **7** se .xiii.
On agustus. se .viii. **7** se .xiii.
On september. se .v. **7** se .ix.

Margins damaged, but text is legible | **4** ianuariu(s)] -ua- *displaced through hole* | **5** þonn] *read* þonne | **6** þe] *read* se.

On october. se .v. **7** se .xv.
On nouember. se .vii. **7** se .ix.
On december. se þridda. **7** se þreotteoða
(b)utan ælcan tweon swa hit bið gewislice. gyme se þe wille:~

15/3 Oxford, St. John's College, MS 17, fol. 40vb/18-31

S*unt* in unoq*uo*q*ue* m*en*se duo dies. q*uo*d cu*m* in eis incipit*ur*. n*on* finit*ur* u*n*q*uam*.
In m*en*se ian*ua*rio: luna .iii.[a] & .iiii.[a]
In feb*ruario*: luna .v. & .vii.
In mart*io*. luna .vi. & .vii.
In apr*ili*. luna .v. & .viii.
In maio. lun*a* .vii`i´. & .ix.
In iun*io*. lun*a* .v. & .xxvii.
In iul*io*. lun*a* .iii. & .xiii.
In aug*usto*. l*una* .viii. 7 .xiii.
In sept*embri*. l*una* .v. 7 .ix.
In oct*o*b*ri*. l*una* .v. 7 .xv.
In nou*embri*. l*una* .vii. 7 .ix.
In dec*embri*. l*una* .iii. 7 .xiii.

Each entry starts on a new line, except that of January | **1** duo] duo[·].

16 Wind Prognostic

Literature

Hellmann (1896b: 65-67); Förster (1903: 350; 1912a: 55-64); Jastrow (1905-12: II.705-48); Harmening (1979: 120); Hollis and Wright (1992: 263-64); Epe (1995: 57-58); Liuzza (2001: 184)

Branches of Superstition

observation of signs: wind; observation of times: twelve days of Christmas

Text

OE: 1. Oxford, Bodleian Library, Hatton 115, fol. 149v

Description

The wind prognostic predicts the future on the basis of the wind on the twelve days of Christmas. The predictions focus on death and disaster, for instance "ordained men will die", and "there will be peril at sea and ships will perish".[1] The predictions are without exception negative in tone, which seems to indicate that wind and storms were regarded unfavourably. Wind is rarely used to predict the future in medieval prognostication.[2] The twelve-day structure of the wind prognostic is shared with the sunshine prognostic, but is not encountered in any other prognostic, to my knowledge. A good study of this genre is Förster's.[3]

Text (1) is the earliest attested wind prognostic. Förster identified several instances in Latin, Middle High German and Swedish.[4] Early printed editions of the so-called 'Bauernpraktik' (the German name for the year prognosis) often include sunshine and wind prognostics, e.g. the facsimile published by Hellmann.[5] A Latin text presumably underlies (1), but no such text has been found to antedate the Old English translation.

---

[1] Translation of text 16/1, ll. 2, 5.

[2] Förster edited a modern directional wind prognostic, a genre I have not found in medieval manuscripts, but which has a long history according to Förster (1912a: 64). The directional wind prognostic is based on the direction from which the wind blows on New Year's Eve.

[3] Förster (1912a: 55-64).

[4] Förster (1903: 350; 1912a: 54-63).

[5] Hellmann (1896b: Aiii recto).

Edition

16/1 Oxford, Bodleian Library, Hatton 115, fol. 149v/8-23

HER segh ymb drihtnes gebyrd. ymb þa .xii. niht hs tide.
Gyf se wind byoð on þa forma niht. gehadode weras sweltað.
Þære æfteran niht. 7 þere þriddan niht bið winð: þon*ne* wespnas forweorðað.
Þeore feorðan niht gif wind byð: lef byð lytel.
Ðære .v. niht gif wind byð: þon*ne* byð frecne on seo. 7 scipu forweorðað.
Ðere vi. niht gif wind byð. ðonn*e* adla byoð þy geare. on eorðan mislica.
Ðere vii. niht gyf win byoð: fir byð swyðe ryfe þy geare.
Ðere viii. niht gyf win byod. þon*ne* ældemen sweltað.
Ðere ix. niht gyf win byð. scep sweltað.
Ðære .x. niht gyf win byð: treow byoð fornerwede.
Ðære xi. niht gyf wind byoð. æale nyetenu forweorðað.
Þon*ne* xii. niht gyf winð byð: þon*ne* byoð micel gefeoht on eorðan:-

1 segh] *read* segþ | hs] *read* his | **3** bið] *read* gif ~ | winð] *read* wind | wespnas] *read* westmas | **4** niht] -h- < t | lef] *i.e.* hlaf | **6** ðonn*e*] ðonn̄ | **7,8,9,10** win] *read* wind | **8** byod] *read* byoð | ældemen] *i.e* ælde men *(Cockayne's suggestion* ealdormen *is unlikely because these prognostics refer to the death of old people more often)* | **10** treow] [··] ~ | **12** winð] *read* wind.

17 Year Prognosis

Literature

Hampson (1841: I.133-34); Migne (1861-1904: I.951); Birch (1878: 480, 505; 1892: 257-58, 277); Meyer (1881: 84-85); Camus (1891: 206-07, 211); Hellmann (1896b); Förster (1903: 347-50; 1908b: 296-301; 1908c: 33, 36; 1912b: 291-95; 1920: 52); Craig (1916: xxxii-xxxvii); Svenberg (1936: 6-7); Jones (1939: 87); Gundel and Gundel (1959: 72-75); Martin (1977: 21, 24); Harmening (1979: 120-45); Matter (1982); Braswell (1984: 347); Hunt (1987: 180, n. 126); Taavitsainen (1988: 52); Hollis and Wright (1992: 263); Günzel (1993: 33-34); Epe (1995: 56-57); Liuzza (2001: 183-84)

Alias

'Bauernpraktik', *Revelatio Esdrae*

Attributions

medieval: Esdras/Ezra, Ezekiel; post-medieval: Bede

Branch of Superstition

observation of times: weekdays, 1 January or Christmas Day

Texts

OE: 1. London, British Library, Cotton Tiberius A. iii, fols 41v-42r
2. London, British Library, Cotton Vespasian D. xiv, fol. 75v
3. Oxford, Bodleian Library, Hatton 115, fol. 149rv

L/OE: 4. London, British Library, Cotton Tiberius A. iii, fol. 36rv

L: 5. London, British Library, Cotton Titus D. xxvi, fols 10v-11v
6. London, British Library, Cotton Titus D. xxvii, fol. 25rv
7. London, British Library, Sloane 475, fol. 217rv
8. Oxford, St. John's College, MS 17, fol. 159rb

Description

It is traditionally observed that of all meteorological prognostic genres, the year prognosis was most widely distributed in the Middle Ages.[1] Year prognoses in Latin and the vernacular have been attested in many volumes from the late eighth century to the present day. Good studies of the genre are those of Hellmann, Craig and Matter.[2]

A year prognosis predicts the weather to come, harvest and agricultural conditions, and human affairs: "if the kalends of January falls on

[1] Hellmann (1896b: 7), Förster (1903: 347; 1912b: 291), Craig (1916: xxxii).

[2] Printed editions have been studied by Hellmann (1896b), manuscript versions by Craig (1916: xxxii-xxxvii). Matter (1982) discussed the origins of the genre and the transmission into Latin and English. Matter's article is copiously annotated.

Sunday, it will be a good winter and a windy spring, a dry summer and this year will be a very good year; sheep will grow, and there will be much honey, and there will be abundance and peace on earth".[3] Typically, a prognosis of the weather is given for each of the seasons, after which follows a description of the size of crops and produce (pertaining to harvest, vineyards, livestock, honey). The prediction ends with observations on the human condition, e.g. the death of old people or the establishment of peace. This final prediction is usually quite brief, though in later texts in particular, human affairs take up a large part of the predictions.[4]

The texts are ordered by the weekday on which 1 January (1, 4-6, 8) or Christmas (3, 7) falls. Sometimes it is not clear to which day a text pertains. Text (2), for instance, refers to the "first day of the year", leaving the time of New Year up to the reader.[5] Generally, the older texts use 1 January, while later ones employ either 1 January or Christmas.[6] Craig even found a manuscript in which the two arrangements were written side by side.[7] The oldest attested Latin year prognosis, in Leiden, Vossianus Lat. Q. 69, fol. 37vab (s. viii^{ex}), is based on the kalends of January.[8] Text (7), from around 1100, is the first Latin text to use Christmas Day; (3), from around 1150, is the earliest vernacular year prognosis to do so.[9] It is perhaps significant that the manuscript containing (3) also includes wind and sunshine prognostics, which are both arranged by the twelve days of Christmas. Matter placed the origin of the Christmas Day variant in England.[10] Hellmann dated the genesis of Christmas-based year prognoses after the year 1000.[11]

Craig observed that "it seems impossible to make any distinction between the two series" of kalends and Christmas Day year prognoses.[12] Indeed, a comparison of the contents of the entries for (1), which is kal-

[3] Translation of text 17/1, ll. 19-21.

[4] This is already apparent in text 17/8. Cf. Craig (1916: xxxiv).

[5] Translation of text 17/2, l. 1. The beginning of the year and 1 January do not necessarily coincide, cf. Harrison (1973), Harmening (1979: 121-45).

[6] Hellmann (1896b: 61-62).

[7] Craig (1916: xxxiii).

[8] Bremmer and Dekker (2006: 91, 100 [157.2.7e]). The text will be published by Bremmer.

[9] Matter (1982: 383) thought that the year prognosis in Digby 86 was the earliest Christmas Day variant in the vernacular, but this manuscript postdates Hatton 115.

[10] Matter (1982: 383).

[11] Hellmann (1896b: 62).

[12] Craig (1916: xxxiii).

ends-based, and (3), which is Christmas-based, reveals that the translator of (3) probably merely substituted "**KL** ianuarius" with "middeswintres messedeg":

> (1) If the kalends of January falls on Sunday, it will be a good winter and a windy spring, a dry summer and this year will be a very good year; sheep will grow, and there will be much honey, and there will be abundance and peace on earth.[13]

and

> (3) If Christmas Day falls on Sunday, it will be a good winter and a windy spring, a dry summer and the vineyards will be good; sheep will grow, and there will be honey in abundance, and all will be peace and abundance on earth.[14]

Although (1, 3) are not likely to be derived from a common Latin source, they do contain the same kind and roughly the same amount of information, the only substantial difference being the arrangement of 1 January versus Christmas Day. The step from kalends to Christmas entailed no more than a substitution in the structural part of the text: the predictions themselves did not change, as Craig noted.[15]

It is generally assumed that the year prognosis derived from a Greek text presented as the work of the prophet Ezra.[16] In medieval times, the year prognosis is attributed to Ezra (alias Esdras) or Ezekiel. The ascription to Bede is post-medieval and entirely spurious.[17] Hellmann was inclined to accept an early date for the emergence of a Latin year prognosis, but he did not therefore also believe in the authenticity of the ascription to Bede.[18] The emergence in Latin took place in a remarkably early period in the Middle Ages for prognostics: the oldest Latin texts date from the end of the eighth century.[19] To my knowledge, the only other prognostics in Latin known in this period are the Apuleian Sphere, the twenty-four Egyptian Days and the *Sortes Sanctorum*. The year prognosis

[13] Translation of text 17/1, ll. 19-21.

[14] Translation of text 17/3, ll. 1-3.

[15] Craig (1916: xxxiii).

[16] Hellmann (1896b: 62-63), Förster (1903: 247), Craig (1916: xxxiii), Matter (1982: 376-78).

[17] Migne (1861-1904: I.951). On the spurious nature of the Bedan attribution, see Jones (1939: 87).

[18] Hellmann (1896b: 59-60).

[19] Leiden, Vossianus Lat. Q. 69, fol. 37vab (s. viii^{ex}), and München, clm 14456, fol. 75v (before 824).

proved incredibly popular throughout the Middle Ages and up to the present. Craig identified a great number of manuscripts containing year prognoses, while Hellmann found fifty-nine printed editions from 1508 onwards.[20] In addition to year prognoses in Latin, texts have been attested in English, French, German, Danish, Norwegian, Icelandic, Swedish, Finnish, Frisian, Dutch, Italian, Spanish and Czech.[21]

Sigerist's observation that regimens "are all very similar but never quite identical",[22] would seem to apply to year prognoses as well. Texts of both genres have been transmitted in such large numbers that an attempt to devise a taxonomy of redactions and variants is exceedingly difficult. The Old English texts (1-4) show enough differences in phrasing and content to presume that they cannot derive from a common exemplar in Old English. The predictions follow a fixed pattern of weather prediction, produce and a limited account of human affairs. It is likely that the texts derive from different versions of one Latin redaction.[23] In the case of (4), the immediate source is the Latin text that served as the basis for the Old English glosses. The Latin texts vary greatly in content. Texts (4-6) would seem to form three versions of one redaction; (7) and (8) are witnesses of two more redactions. (8) differs from (1-7) in that the seasonal focus is largely lost in the former. The genre requires intensive study and preferably a comparison of the several hundreds of texts that must have survived in medieval manuscripts.

Edition

17/1 London, British Library, Cotton Tiberius A. iii, fols 41v/8-42r/5

KŁ ianuarius gif he byþ on monandæg. þonne biþ grimm 7 gemenged winter. 7 god lencten. 7 windig sumor. 7 hreohfull gear biþ. 7 adlseoce menn beoð on þam geare.

KŁ ianuarius. gif he bið on tiwesdæg. þonne byð dreorig winter. 7 grimm. 7 windig lencten. 7 renig sumor. 7 mænig wif swylt. 7 scipu frecedlice geyrnað. 7 cynincgas. 7 ealdormenn sweltað.

Entries 2-5 start on a new line, the rest is continuous | **1** monandæg] *it is unusual for a year prognosis to start with Monday (they commonly start with Sunday)* | **5** frecedlice] f- < r.

[20] Craig (1916: xxxii-xxxvii), Hellmann (1896b: 8-25), Matter (1982: 380-81, 387-92). See Förster (1903: 348-49; 1908b: 298-301; 1912b: 292-95), Harmening (1979: 134).

[21] Camus (1891: 206-07, 211), Hellmann (1896b: 36-54), Förster (1903: 348; 1908b: 298-301), Craig (1916: xxxiv-xxxvii).

[22] Cited in Jones (1939: 73).

[23] Cf. Förster (1908b: 298).

KŁ ianuarius gif he biþ on wodnesdæg. þonne bið heard winter. 7 yfel lencten. 7 god sumor. 7 eorþan. wæstmas. swiþe geswencte. 7 hunig ne genihtsumað. 7 gunge menn sweltað.

KŁ ianuarius gif he bið on þunresdæg. þonne biþ god winter. 7 windig. lencten 7 god sumor. 7 genihtsumnes on eorþan. wæstmum. 7 sib biþ ofer eorðan. 7 swaþeah sceap. 7 cild sweltað.

KŁ ianuarius gif he biþ on frigedæg. þonne bið missenlic winter. 7 god lencten. 7 god sumor. 7 micel genihtsumnes 7 sceapa eagan tedriað on þam geare.

KŁ ianuarius gif he biþ on sæternesdæg. þonne biþ snawig. winter 7 blawende lencten 7 renig sumor 7 eorþan wæstmas geswencte beoþ. 7 sceap. forwirðaþ. 7 ealde menn sweltaþ. 7 oðre menn adlseoce bioð. 7 mænigra eagan tedru bioð. 7 fyr ricsaþ on þam geare gærgerimes.

K ianuarius gif he biþ on sunnandæg þonne bið god winter 7 windig lencten. 7 dryge sumor. 7 swyþe god gear biþ þy geare. 7 sceap weaxað. 7 micel hunig biþ. 7 genihtsumnes. 7 sib byð on eorþan.

17 oðre] ~ ‖ ⟨*f. 42r*⟩.

17/2 London, British Library, Cotton Vespasian D. xiv, fol. 75v/3-21

Đonne forme gearesdæig byð sunendæig: hit byð god winter. 7 windig lænctetid. dryge sumer. god hærfest. 7 scep tyððrigeð. 7 hit byð grið. 7 wæstme manigfeald.

Đonne hit byð monendæig: hit byð scurfah winter. 7 god læncten. 7 windig sumer. 7 storemig. 7 geswyncfull hærfest.

Þonne hit byð tywesdæig: hit byð wæt winter. 7 windig læinten. 7 wæt sumer. 7 wifmæn swelteð 7 scipes forfareð. 7 cynges swelteð.

Þonne hit byð wodnesdæig: hit byð heard winter. 7 yfel læinten. god sumer. 7 geswyncfull hærfest. 7 hunig byð gæsne.

Đonne hit byð þuresdæg hit byð god winter. 7 windig læinten. god sumer 7 god hærfest.

Þonne hit byð fridæg hit byð hwerefinde winter. 7 god lænten. 7 god sumer. 7 god hærfest.

Đonne hit byð sæterdæig hit byð scurfah winter. 7 windig læinten. 7 ealle wæstmes yfeles gewænde. scep cwelleð 7 ealde mænn.

A marginal note in a post-medieval hand (Talbot's?) reads: (pro)gnostico*n* Anni. *In the bottom margin, a post-medieval hand (Nowell's?) added*: Wynter, Læncten. sumer hærfest hoc s*unt* no*m*i*n*a Anglor*um* 4[or] anni te*m*por*um*. *The same hand has underlined several words in the text, including the names of the seasons.*

17/3 Oxford, Bodleian Library, Hatton 115, fol. 149r/12-149v/7

Gif middeswintres messedeg b`i´ð on sunnandeg. þon*ne* bið god winter. 7 lengten windi. 7 drige sumer. 7 wingeardas gode. 7 sceap beoð weaxende. 7 hunii beoð genihtsu*m*. 7 eal sib bið genyhtsu*m*mo.

Gif he bið on monandeg se middeswintres messedæg. þon*ne* bið gemenged winter. 7 god lengten. 7 windig sumer. 7 ystig. 7 beoð gode wingeardas. 7 swiþ feorme mannu*m*.

Gif he bið on tiwesdeg. þon*ne* bið yfag winter. 7 windig lengten. 7 renig sumer. 7 moni wif sweltað. 7 scip beoð frecnode. 7 ciningas forweorðað.

Gif seo midwinter bið on wodnesdæg. þon*ne* bið heard winter. 7 grim. 7 yfel lengten. 7 god sumer. 7 wingeardas beoð geswincfulle. 7 hunig byð lesse.

Gif heo byoð on þunresdæg. þon*ne* byoð god winter. 7 windig lengten. 7 god sumor. 7 ælc god byð genihtsum in þem selfan geare.

Gyf se midwinter byð on frigendæg*e*. þon*ne* byð onwendædlic winter. 7 byð goð leingten. 7 goð sumer. 7 byð genihtsumes micel.

Gif se midwint*er* byð on seternesdeag. þon*ne* byð winter gedrefedlic. 7 windig lengten. 7 westmas swincað. 7 scep cwellað. 7 ealde men gewitað. 7 þa clenan beoð leahtrode;-

2 hunii] *read* huni | **3** genyhtsu*m*mo] genyhtsūmo; *read* genyhtsumo | **7** yfag] *read* ysig | **9** heard] -a- < · | **11-12** sumor.] ~ ‖ ⟨*f. 149v*⟩ | **13,14** goð] *read* god.

17/4 London, British Library, Cotton Tiberius A. iii, fol. 36r/14-36v/7

gif bið on dæg drihtenlicu*m* winter god bið 7 wynsum 7 wearm
Si fuerit kł ianuarius die dominico. hiems bona erit & suauis. ac calida.
windhladen 7 drige wingeard god sweap weaxað hunig genihtsumað
uer uentuosus. & sicca estas uindemia bona. oues crescent mel habundabit
ealde swealteð 7 sib gewyrð
senes morientur. & pax fi*et*.
gif bið on dæg monan winter gemeacged lænten god sumor windhladen
Si fuerit kł ianuarius die lunę. hiems mixta. uer bonus. estas uentuosa
7 cyældbære wingeard god strengð manna beon sweltað
& tempestuosa. uindemia bona. ualitudo hominum. apes morientur.
gif bið dæg martes winter æþelust lænten windhladen 7 renlic
Si fuerit kł ianuarius die martis hiems nobilissima. uer uentuosus & pluuialis

3 windhladen] ~ *over* uer uentuosus; *read* lænten ~ (uer *not glossed)* | wingeard] ~ *over* estas uindemia; *read* sumor ~ (estas *not glossed)* | sweap] *read* sceap | **7** gemeacged] *read* gemencged | **9** cyældbære] *read* cwældbære | **12** martis] -a- < o.

sumor god wif sweltað scypu beoð gedyrfed on widsæ wingeard
estas bona. mulieres morientur. naues perclitantur in pelago. uindemia
wingeard geswincful
uindemia laboriosa.
gif bið dæg wodnes winter heard 7 stið lænten yfel 7 sumor
Si fuerit kł ianuarius die mercuririi hiems dura & aspera. uer malus. & estas
god wingerd god hwæte god geonge sweltað hunig na bið
bona uindemna bona. frumentum bonum. iuuenes moriuntur. mel non erit.
cypmen swingað
mercatores laborabunt.
gif bið dæg þures winter god bið lenten windig sumor god 7
Si fuerit kł ianuarius die iouis hiems. bona erit. uer uentuosus. estas bona &
genihtsu*m*nys bið cyniigas 7 rædwitan forwyrþan sib gewyrð
habundantia erit.reges & principes peribunt. pax fi*et*.
gif bið dæg friggan winter stedfæst 7 swaw bið lænten god 7 sumor
Si fuerit kł ianuarius die ueneris hiems stabilis & nix erit. uer bonus & estas.
sar eagena wingerd god sfap 7 beon forwyrðaþ bileofa leof gewyrð
dolor oculoru*m*.u`i´ndemia bona. oues & apes peribunt. annona cara fi*et*;
gif bið dæg sæternes winter genipful snaw bið bigleofa leof bið
Si fuerit kł ianuarius die saturni. hiems caliginosa. nix erit annona cara erit.
wæstm genihtsumað e`a´lle adliað 7 ealde sweltað wingeard
fructus habundabit. homines egrotabunt & ueterani moriuntur. uindemia
god.
bona.

14 perclitantur] *read* periclitantur | **18** mercuririi] *read* mercurii | **20** uindemna] *read* uindemia | **24** hiems.] ~ ‖ ⟨*f. 36v*⟩ | **25** cyniigas] *i.e.* cynigas *(on doubling of* 'i', *see 7/4)* | **27** swaw] *read* snaw | **29** sfap] *read* scap | **31** genipful] -l < þ.

17/5 London, British Library, Cotton Titus D. xxvi, fols 10v/10-11v/6

incipiunt signa de temporib*us*.

Si die .i. f*eria* fueri`n´t kł ian*uarii* hiemps bona & uentosa erit. aestas sicca. & uindemia bona erit. boues crescent & mel abundanter erit. senes morientur. & abundantia & pax erit.

Si .ii. f*eria* fuerint kł ian*uarii*. hiemps mixta uer iocundu*m* aestas sicca & uentosa fi*et*. & tempestas erit & uindemia non bona & ualitudo homium erit & apes morientur.

2 uentosa] *read* uer uentosum *(spring is forgotten repeatedly and the customary storms have been attributed to winter, see ll. 8,12; see also 17/6,7)* | **5** iocundu*m*] iocund[a]*m*, -u_2- < [a] | uentosa] ~ ‖ ⟨*f. 11r*⟩ | **6** erit$_1$] er[un]t, -i- < [u] | homium] *read* hominum.

Si .iii. f*eria* fuerint kł ian*uarii*. hiemps pluuiosa erit & uentosa aestas sicca uindemia laborabit. mulieres morientur & reges peribunt.

Si .iiii. f*eria* fuerint kł ian*uarii*. hiemps dura & asp*era* erit. uer malu*m* & uentosum erit aestas bona & uindemia bona. frum*en*tu*m* bonu*m* & iuuenes morientur.

Si .v. f*eria* fuerint. kł ian*uarii*. hiemps bona & uentosa erit ęstas bona & uindemia bona. & abundantia erit & in illo anno principes siue reges p*er*ibunt.

Si .vi f*eria* fuerint. kł ian*uarii*. hiemps mutabilis erit. uér bonum aestas sicca & bona. & oculoru*m* dolor & uindemia bona erit. & oues peribunt.

Si .vii. f*eria* fuerint. kł ian*uarii*. hiemps turbolenta uér uentosum & fructus laboriosus erit oues peribunt & senes morient*ur*.

8,12 uentosa] *read* uer uentosum *(see l. 1)* | **15** erit.] ~ ‖ ⟨*f. 11v*⟩.

17/6 London, British Library, Cotton Titus D. xxvii, fol. 25r/8-25v/3

KŁ. IAN*VARII*. Si fuerit in prima feria. hiems bona erit. & uent*us* uentosus. & aestas sicca. & uindemia bona. & oues multiplicabuntur. & mel habundabit. & habundantia pacis.

KŁ. IAN*VARII*. Si fuerit in .ii. f*eria*. hiems mixta erit. & uernus bon*us*. & aestas uentosa. & uindemia bona. & ualitudo hominum.

KŁ. IAN*VARII*. Si fuerit in .iii. f*eria*. hiems ymbriosus & uentosus. & aestas pluuialis & te*m*pestas. & mulieres plurime moriunt*ur*. & naues periclitabuntur. & reges peribunt.

KŁ. IAN*VARII*. Si fuerit in .iiii. f*eria*. hiems dura & aspera. & uernus malus. & aestas bona. & uindemia laboriosa. & mel non erit.

KŁ. IAN*VARII*. Si fuerit in .v. f*eria*. hiems bona. & uernus uentosus. & aestas bona erit.

KŁ. IAN*VARII*. Si fuerit in .vi. f*eria*. hiems mutabilis. & uernus bonus. & aestas bona. & copiosa magna.

KŁ D*ECEMBRIS*. Si fuerit. in vii. f*eria*. hiems turbinosus. & uernus uentosus. & laboriosus & oues peribunt. & ueteres moriuntur. & case cremabuntur.

Each entry starts on a new line | **1** uent*us*] *read* uernus | **6** uentosus] *read* uernus ~ *(spring is forgotten repeatedly and the customary storms have been attributed to winter; see also 17/5,7)* | **14** magna.] ~ ‖ ⟨*f. 25v*⟩ | **15 D*ECEMBRIS*]** *read* Ianuarii.

17/7 London, British Library, Sloane 475, fol. 217r/7-217v/12

Natalis d*omi*ni p*ri*ma dies si acciderit dominica scitote hiemem benígnu*m* & uentososa*m* quadragessima*m*. estate*m*. arida*m*. uinea*n*s opulentas. oues. fetus. p*ro*ducentes. mel. sufficere. te*m*pestiues homines mori. & pace*m* in t*er*ris.
Si dies lune fuerit. scitote hiem men turbulente*m* quadragessima*m* optima*m*. estatę*m* uentosa*m*; mel paru*m* homines infirmos uineas non fructuosas.
Si uero mártis scitote esse*m* pluuiale*m* hiemę*m*. quadragessima*m* uentosa*m* estate*m* optima*m* feminas mori. reges périré clases p*er*iclitare.
Si dies mercurii. fuęrit scitóte hiemem. duru*m* & gelidu*m* quadragessima*m* pessima*m* uineas frúctíferas iuuenes mori mércatorés dispereunt.
Si dies iouis fugerit scitotę̇ hiemem esse bonu*m* quadragessima*m* uéntosa*m* estatę optima*m* omiu*m*q*ue* bónoru*m*. sufficientia*m*. homines. annosós mori reges pacatos & pace*m* in hominib*us*.
Si dies ueneris fuerit scitote hiémę́m. c*on*trariu*m* quadragessima*m* optima*m* estate*m* bona*m* agustu*m* opuléntu*m*. oculos. infirmos. oues. & apes mori;
Si dies fuerit sabbáti scitote. hiemem. graue*m* quadragessimam. uentosa*m* fructu*m* defici;

1 hiemem] hiem em̄ se ·; *i.e.* hiemem *with clumsy expunction of* se | **1-2** uentososa*m*] *read* uentosa*m (spring is forgotten repeatedly and the customary storms have been attributed to winter; see also 17/5,6)* | **2** uinea*n*s] uineā s; *read* uineas | **3** te*m*pestiues] *read* tempestiue | **4** hiem men] *read* hiemem | **6** esse*m*] essē; *read* esse | **7** clases] *i.e.* classes | **8** gelidu*m*] ~ ‖ ⟨*f. 217v*⟩ | **10** fugerit] -u- < li; *read* fuerit | estatę] *read* estatem | **11** omiu*m*q*ue*] *read* omniumque | **13** ueneris] u- < [s] | **15** quadragessimam] -r- < a.

17/8 Oxford, St. John's College, MS 17, fol. 159rb/5-38

Si p*ri*ma feria kł ian*uarii* fuerit. frugifer ann*us* erit. extremi ho*min*u*m* morient*ur*. frum*en*tu*m* & uinu*m* abundabit. apes p*ro*ficient. oues morient*ur*. naues p*er*iclitabuntur. gentes mouebunt*ur*. fremit*us* bello*rum* erit. pugna nulla. pax breuis: in m*en*se sept*em*bri g*ra*uis mortalitas & siluę p*ro*ficient;
Si *secun*da feria kł ian*uarii* fuerit. armo*rum* sonit*us*. mutatio genti*um* diu*er*saru*m*. scandala ubiq*ue*. nauigia p*ro*sp*er*a. messes da*m*natę. q*ua*drupedia plurima morient*ur*;
Si t*er*cia feria kł ian*uarii* fuerit. frugifer ann*us* erit. p*ro*sp*er*a negotia. te*m*pestates in aug*usto* & sept*em*bri. bella minime. & lites cessant;
Si q*ua*rta feria kł ian*uarii* fuerit. fames p*er* loca. uindemia par`c´a. messes fallent. piscatio multa. hib*ernus* fortis. ęstas pluuialis;

Each entry starts on a new line. Marginal note in a sixteenth(?)-century hand reads: Dictus in ········· prognostica Temporu*m* | **4** mortalitas] -s < · | **10** par`c´a] par[u]a, -`c´- < [u].

Si q*ui*nta feria kł ian*uarii* fuerit hiems ualida. & pestifera: g*ra*ndo plurima. p*ri*ncipes morient*ur*. clades q*ua*drupedu*m*. sang*ui*s plurim*us* effundet*ur*. in oriente abundantia multa. in meridie fames. in occidente monstrabit*ur* & aufert*ur*;

Si sexta feria fuerit. t*err*ę motus & p*ro*digia multa. monstruosa a*nim*alia nascent*ur*. noua signa appareb*unt*. feminę morient*ur*. plurimi fruct*us* da*m*nabunt*ur*. sterilitas messiu*m*. piscatio plurima. nauigia tuta;

Si septima feria kł ian*uarii* fuerit hib*er*nus bon*us*. uern*us* uari*us*. siccitas in ęstate. in autu*m*no aq*ua*tio multa. uindemia bona. glandis plurima. oues & porci morient*ur*. mel multu*m*. medietas ho*m*inu*m* diu*er*sis infirmitatib*us* p*er*iclitabit*ur*. in oriente fames. in mari belu ę & pisces morient*ur* plurimi. coruscationes & tonitrua in augusto m*en*se erunt;

15 fuerit] *read* kł ianuarii ~.

APPENDIX ONE

HANDLIST OF PROGNOSTICS IN ENGLISH MANUSCRIPTS OF THE NINTH TO TWELFTH CENTURIES

This appendix presents information on the English manuscripts containing the prognostic text corpus, and a detailed set of data for each individual prognostic in these manuscripts. The handlist includes all Old English and glossed prognostics, many Latin ones, and some prognostics now (partly) lost.

The lack of a thorough, descriptive catalogue by subject for Latin texts in English manuscripts makes the contribution of Latin prognostics to this list more haphazard than I would have wished.[1] The number of Latin prognostics would probably be more than doubled were a close inspection of all extant English manuscripts of the ninth to twelfth centuries carried out. Nevertheless, the texts which I have collected have proved useful as material to compare the vernacular texts against, though in some cases the Old English texts are among the earliest witnesses of a prognostic genre that we have. Many references to Latin prognostics can be found in the articles of Förster and Henel, and Ker's *Catalogue of Manuscripts Containing Anglo-Saxon*.[2] I located some Latin prognostics in catalogues of manuscripts while researching other matters, e.g. the texts on the three Egyptian Days and the three miraculous birthdays in CCCC 422, p. 49; texts I would probably not have found if it were not for James's *Catalogue of Manuscripts in the Library of Corpus Christi College Cambridge*.[3] Prognostics are sometimes not introduced as such in descriptions of the contents of manuscripts, which makes their discovery a matter of chance, as with the texts on the twenty-four Egyptian Days and the unlucky days in Tiberius C. vi, fol. 114r, recently introduced as "two notes".[4]

Each manuscript is introduced with the help of information provided in descriptions of manuscripts in catalogues. The number of reference

[1] Mooney (1998: 123) observed that "the principal difficulty in editing astrological and prognostic texts is finding them".

[2] Förster (1903, 1906, 1908a-c, 1910, 1911, 1912a-c, 1916, 1920, 1921, 1925, 1925-26, 1929, 1936, 1944), Henel (1934-35), Ker (1957).

[3] James (1912).

[4] Pulsiano (1994b: 41 [233.2]).

works I have consulted is not exhaustive. As is often the case with catalogues of manuscripts, the more one consults them, the wider the range in dates and places of origin for a given manuscript. My choices in these matters are not definitive, but merely provide me with a working basis. I have relied most of all on the work of Ker, Pulsiano and Doane, Gameson and Gneuss.[5] My main aim in the concise manuscript descriptions has been to discover where and when the prognostics were copied, and in which manuscript contexts they were incorporated. I refer the reader to the catalogues listed for each manuscript, should more information be desired.

The prognostics have not been numbered in order of appearance: each text has been assigned a unique number which codes for the prognostic genre and the specific text witness. Thus, the dream lunary in Tiberius A. iii, fols 35v/36r is referenced as 9.2.4/5 (lunary [9], specific type [2], dreams [4], taking fifth place in the list of dream lunaries).[6]

Entries in square brackets are excluded from the main text corpus and pertain to texts added at a later date in a language other than Latin or Old English, to non-insular prognostics attested in manuscripts which may also contain English prognostics, or to continental manuscripts which were transferred to England before the thirteenth century. These may be composite manuscripts (e.g. Sloane 475), or manuscripts brought to, and expanded in England (e.g. Digby 63). The ninth-century manuscript Harley 3017, which Liuzza advanced as a computus that may have been in England in Anglo-Saxon times is here excluded since there is no support for Liuzza's supposition.[7]

It has proved impossible for me continuously to integrate newly-found prognostics because this would entail continual revision throughout the book. Therefore, I have established a closed corpus of 174 prognostics. Prognostics found at a later date are described in the supplement.[8] Unfortunately, this has led to the exclusion of several manuscripts containing interesting collections of prognostics.

[5] Ker (1957), Pulsiano and Doane (1994-), Gameson (1999), Gneuss (2001).

[6] The lists of witnesses per genre are provided in the introductions in the text edition.

[7] On the alleged English provenance, see Derolez (1954: 212-17), Liuzza (2001: 223-24). For a critical note, see Gneuss (2003: 300). A comparison between English prognostics and those in Harley 3017 by me is forthcoming.

[8] On pp. 545-48.

CORPUS

Cambridge, Corpus Christi College, MS 9
AKA the *London-Cambridge Legendary*, the *Cotton-Corpus Legendary*
CCCC 9, pp. 61-458, was once part of a legendary with Nero E. i, vol. i and ii.[9]
DATE: overall: s. xi^{2}; additions s. xi^{ex}, xii^{in} (pp. 17-60); calendar: s. xi^{2}
ORIGIN: Worcester
CONTENTS: calendar, computus; saints' lives; legendary
LITERATURE: James (1912: I.21-30); Budny (1997: I.609-22 [41]); Ker (1957: 41 [29]); Gneuss (1981: 8 [36]; 2001: 30 [36]); Gameson (1999: 60 [54])

CCCC 9, pp. 3-14 *6/5*
TYPE: Dog Days
LANGUAGE: L
INCIPIT: **Dies caniculares.**
EDITION: Wormald (1934: 226-37 [18])

Cambridge, Corpus Christi College, MS 391
AKA **Portiforium Oswaldi*; *Portiforium Sancti Wulfstani*
CCCC 391 may have been made for, or owned by Wulfstan II, bishop of Worcester (1062-95).
DATE: overall: s. xi$^{3/4}$, 1064-69; additions s. xi^{2}-xiii; prognostics: 1064-69[10]
ORIGIN: Worcester
CONTENTS: computus; Gallican psalter; hymns, canticles; collectar; exorcisms, blessings, ordeals, prayers; offices; prognostics
LITERATURE: Wanley (1705: II.110 [K. 10]); James (1912: II.241-48); Turner (1916: lviii [13]); Förster (1925-26: 77-79); McLachlan (1929); Wormald (1952: 61-62 [11]); Ker (1957: 113-15 [67]); Hughes (1958-60: II.v-xi); Kauffmann (1975: 54 [3]); Gneuss (1981: 11 [104]; 2001: 37 [104]); Robinson (1988: I.57 [157]); Franzen (1991: 69-70); Hollis & Wright (1992: 259); Corrêa (1995: 57-58); Pulsiano (1995: 69-70 [38]); Budny (1997: I.629-43 [43]); Gameson (1999: 64 [86]); Liuzza (2001: 213-14 [W])

CCCC 391, pp. 712†-713/1-19[11] *14/1*
TYPE: sunshine prognostic (lacks entries for days 1 to beginning of 3)
LANGUAGE: OE
INCIPIT: kiningum 7 ricum mannum bið mycel syb þy geare.
EDITION: Förster (1906: 369 [incomplete], n. 1; 1912a: 65-66)[12]
LITERATURE: Wanley (1705: II.110 [II.1]); James (1912: II.246 [7]); Förster (1925-26: 78 [4]); Ker (1957: 114 [67.d. i]); Healey & Venezky (1980: 158 [Prog 1.1 (Först), B23.3.1.1]); Quinn & Quinn (1990: 133 [F401]); Hollis & Wright (1992: 257); Voigts & Kurtz (2000: 4.00); Liuzza (2001: 213 [W1])

CCCC 391, pp. 713/20-714/5 *5.1.3/1*
TYPE: brontology, temporal, weekday
LANGUAGE: OE
INCIPIT: **O**n anweardne gear gif hit þunreð ærest on sunnandæg
EDITION: Förster (1908a: 46); Liuzza (2004: 18)
TRANSLATION: Liuzza (2004: 19, n. 62)
LITERATURE: Wanley (1705: II.110 [II.2]); James (1912: II.246 [7]); Förster (1925-26: 78 [5]); Ker (1957: 114 [67.d. ii]); Healey & Venezky (1980: 158 [Prog 1.2 (Först), B23.3.1.2]); Quinn & Quinn (1990: 133 [F401]); Hollis & Wright (1992: 257); Voigts & Kurtz (2000: 118. 00); Liuzza (2001: 213-14 [W2])

---

[9] On the makeup of the original manuscript, see Ker (1957: 41), Gneuss (2001: 30, 65).

[10] In s. xiii^{1}, the Tremulous hand copied a fragment of the three Egyptian Days on p. 721/12-15.

[11] On this foliation, see pp. 52-53.

[12] Förster (1912a: 65-66) used 14/2 (Hatton 115) to add the missing lines.

CCCC 391, p. 714/5-10 *5.1.1.1/1*
TYPE: brontology, temporal, canonical hours (night office)
LANGUAGE: OE
INCIPIT: **G**if þunor cumeð on forantniht
EDITION: Förster (1908a: 47); Liuzza (2004: 18-19)[13]
TRANSLATION: Liuzza (2004: 19, n. 62)
LITERATURE: James (1912: II.246 [7]); Förster (1925-26: 78 [6]); Ker (1957: 114 [67.d.ii]); Healey & Venezky (1980: 158 [Prog 1.2 (Först), B23.3.1.2]); Quinn & Quinn (1990: 133 [F401]); Hollis & Wright (1992: 257); Voigts & Kurtz (2000: 118.00); Liuzza (2001: 213-14 [W2])

CCCC 391, p. 714/10-19 *5.2/1*
TYPE: brontology, non-temporal, compass directions
LANGUAGE: OE
INCIPIT: **G**if þunorrade bið hlynende of eastdæle
EDITION: Förster (1908a: 47-48); Liuzza (2004: 19)[14]
TRANSLATION: Liuzza (2004: 19, n. 62)
LITERATURE: James (1912: II.246 [7]); Förster (1925-26: 78 [7]); Ker (1957: 114 [67.d.ii]); Healey & Venezky (1980: 158 [Prog 1.2 (Först), B23.3.1.2]); Quinn & Quinn (1990: 133 [F401]); Hollis & Wright (1992: 257); Voigts & Kurtz (2000: 118.00); Liuzza (2001: 213-14 [W2])

CCCC 391, pp. 714/19-715/3 *5.1.1.2/1*
TYPE: brontology, temporal, canonical hours (day office)
LANGUAGE: OE
INCIPIT: **G**if ðunor æt þære þriddan tide dæges
EDITION: Förster (1908a: 48); Liuzza (2004: 18-19)
TRANSLATION: Liuzza (2004: 19, n. 62)
LITERATURE: James (1912: II.246 [7]); Förster (1925-26: 78 [8]); Ker (1957: 114 [67.d.ii]); Healey & Venezky (1980: 158 [Prog 1.2 (Först), B23.3.1.2]); Quinn & Quinn (1990: 133 [F401]); Hollis & Wright (1992: 257); Voigts & Kurtz (2000: 118.00); Liuzza (2001: 213-14 [W2])

CCCC 391, p. 715/4-26 *3.1.3/1*
TYPE: birth, temporal, weekday
LANGUAGE: OE
INCIPIT: **G**if mon bið acennen on sunnandæg oððe on nihte
EDITION: Förster (1912b: 297-300)
LITERATURE: Wanley (1705: II.110 [II.3]); James (1912: II.246 [7]); Förster (1925-26: 78 [9]); Ker (1957: 114 [67.d.iii]); Healey & Venezky (1980: 158 [Prog 1.3 (Först), B23.3.1.3]); Quinn & Quinn (1990: 133 [F401]); Hollis & Wright (1992: 257); Voigts & Kurtz (2000: 53.00); Liuzza (2001: 214 [W3])

CCCC 391, p. 716 *9.2.2/1*
TYPE: lunary, specific, birth
LANGUAGE: OE
INCIPIT: **O**nre .i. nihte ealdne monan *þæt* cild *þæt* swa bið acenned
EDITION: Förster (1912c: 21-26 [W])
LITERATURE: Wanley (1705: II.110 [II.4]); James (1912: II.246 [7]); Craig (1916: xl); Förster (1925-26: 78 [10]); Ker (1957: 114 [67.d.iv]); Healey & Venezky (1980: 158 [Prog 1.4 (Först), B23.3.1.4]); Quinn & Quinn (1990: 133 [F401]); Hollis & Wright (1992: 257); Voigts & Kurtz (2000: 132.00); Liuzza (2001: 214 [W4])

CCCC 391, pp. 717-18/1 *9.2.5/1*
TYPE: lunary, specific, illness
LANGUAGE: OE
INCIPIT: **S**e ðe onre nihte monan weorðeð untrum
EDITION: Förster (1912c: 34-36 [W]); Ker (1957: 114 [67.d.v])[15]

[13] Adapted Liuzza (2004: 19).
[14] *Ibid.*
[15] Ker printed the last line, which was lacking in Förster.

LITERATURE: James (1912: II.246 [7]); Craig (1916: xxxix); Förster (1925-26: 78 [11]); Weißer (1982: 45 [*Ca$_1$E]); Healey & Venezky (1980: 158 [Prog 1.5 (Först), B23.3.1.5]); Quinn & Quinn (1990: 133 [F401]); Hollis & Wright (1992: 257); Voigts & Kurtz (2000: 142.00); Liuzza (2001: 214 [W5])

CCCC 391, p. 718/2-8 *3.1.2/1*
TYPE: birth, temporal, 3 miraculous days
LANGUAGE: OE
INCIPIT: ry dagas synd on .xii. monðum mid iii nihtum
EDITION: Förster (1929: 260 [W])
COLLATION: Henel (1934-35: 346-47 [W])[16]
LITERATURE: James (1912: II.246 [7]); Förster (1925-26: 78 [12]); Ker (1957: 114 [67.d.vi]); Healey & Venezky (1980: 95 [Days 1.1 (Först), B23.2.1.1]); Quinn & Quinn (1990: 132 [F201]); Hollis & Wright (1992: 258); Voigts & Kurtz (2000: 173.00); Liuzza (2001: 214 [W6])

CCCC 391, p. 718/9-22 *8.1/1*
TYPE: Egyptian Days, three
LANGUAGE: OE
INCIPIT: **Ð**ry dagas synd on xii monðum þa synd swiðe unhalwende
EDITION: Förster (1929: 273-74 [W]); Franzen (1991: 69 [incomplete])[17]
LITERATURE: James (1912: II.246 [7]); Förster (1925-26: 78 [13]); Ker (1957: 114 [67.d.vii]); Healey & Venezky (1980: 95 [Days 1.2 (Först), B23.2.1.2]); Quinn & Quinn (1990: 132 [F201]); Hollis & Wright (1992: 258); Voigts & Kurtz (2000: 174.00); Liuzza (2001: 214 [W7])

CCCC 391, pp. 718/23-720/3 *9.2.4/6*
TYPE: lunary, specific, dreams (psalm verses follow each day)
LANGUAGE: L
INCIPIT: **L**una .i. quicquid uideris
COLLATION: Förster (1925-26: 67-74)[18]
LITERATURE: Wanley (1705: II.110 [II.5]); James (1912: II.246 [7]); Förster (1925-26: 78 [14]); Ker (1957: 114 [67.d. viii]); Liuzza (2001: 214 [W8])

CCCC 391, pp. 720/4-721/11 *9.2.4/1*
TYPE: lunary, specific, dreams
LANGUAGE: OE
INCIPIT: **Þ**onne se mone bið anre nihte eald swa hwæt swa þu gesihst
EDITION: Förster (1925-26: 79-86 [W])
LITERATURE: Wanley (1705: II.110 [II.6]); James (1912: II.246 [7]); Förster (1925-26: 79 [15]); Ker (1957: 114 [67. d.viii]); Healey & Venezky (1980: 158 [Prog 1.6 (Först), B23.3.1.6]); Hollis & Wright (1992: 257); Budny (1997: I.644 [57]);[19] Voigts & Kurtz (2000: 192.00); Liuzza (2001: 214 [W8])

[CCCC 391, p. 721/12-15[20]
TYPE: Egyptian Days, three days (lacks ending)
LANGUAGE: imitative OE (Tremulous Worcester hand)
EDITION: James (1912: II.246 [7]); Förster (1925-26: 77 [W]); Franzen (1991: 69)
LITERATURE: Ker (1957: 114 [67.e]); Healey & Venezky (1980: 95 [Days 1.3 (Först), B23.2.1.3]); Quinn & Quinn (1990: 132 [F201]); Hollis & Wright (1992: 258); Voigts & Kurtz (2000: 195. 00)]

[16] As variants to 3.1.2/3 (Vitellius E. xviii).

[17] In Franzen used to elucidate the version by the Tremulous Worcester hand (CCCC 391, p. 721).

[18] As variants to 9.2.4/5 (Tiberius A. iii).

[19] Budny described the last letter of "recednesse", the final word of 9.2.4/1.

[20] The only prognostic copied by the Tremulous hand is customarily included in the Old English text corpus, e.g. Ker (1957: 114), Healey and Venezky (2000). I have not included this text in the prognostic corpus because it dates from the thirteenth century.

Cambridge, Corpus Christi College, MS 422, Part B

AKA the *Red Book of Darley*

Parts A (pp. 1-26, s. x^{med} [*Solomon and Saturn*]) and B have been bound together probably since the twelfth century. The contents of part B shows similarities with that of Tiberius C. vi, the calendar with those in Arundel 60 and Vitellius E. xviii.

DATE: overall: *c.* 1061; additions s. xii; prognostics: *c.* 1061 (p. 27), s. xii (p. 49); calendar: *c.* 1061

ORIGIN: overall: New Minster, Winchester, for use at Sherborne; perhaps in Sherborne by s. xi^2; prognostics: New Minster, Winchester (p. 27), Sherborne (p. 49); calendar: New Minster, Winchester

CONTENTS: prognostics, calendar, computus; masses; benedictions, prayers; form of excommunication; hymns; prayer; ordeals; exorcism; offices, litanies, chant, benediction, lections

LITERATURE: Wanley (1705: II.149 [S. 16]); Warren (1883: 271-75); James (1912: II.315-22); Wormald (1952: 62-63 [14]); Ker (1957: 119-21 [70]); Hohler (1972); Temple (1976: 121 [104]); Gneuss (1981: 11 [111]; 2001: 38 [111]); Robinson (1988: 59 [165]); Hollis & Wright (1992: 260); Pfaff (1995a: 21-24); Corrêa (1995: 56-57); Budny (1997: I. 645-66 [44]); Liuzza (2001: 214-15 [D]); Graham *et al.* (2003: 81-97 [60, ASMMF 11.8]); Gittos (2005: 66-70)

CCCC 422, p. 27 *9.2.3/1*

TYPE: lunary, specific, bloodletting (top right corner torn out, endings of first five entries lost)

LANGUAGE: L/OE (linear gloss)

INCIPIT: gimenett [title] **L**una i **B**ona est. / her hit is (god tima.)

FACSIMILE: Graham *et al.* (2003: 11.8.1)

EDITION: Henel (1934-35: 334-35)

LITERATURE: James (1912: II.316 [II]); Ker (1957: 119 [70.B.a]); Healey & Venezky (1980: 95 [Days 2 (Henel), B23.2.2]); Quinn & Quinn (1990: 132 [F202]); Hollis & Wright (1992: 258); Voigts & Kurtz (2000: 84.00); Liuzza (2001: 214-15 [D1]); Graham *et al.* (2003: 89 [60])

CCCC 422, pp. 29-40 *8.3/4*

TYPE: Egyptian Days, twenty-four days

LANGUAGE: L

INCIPIT: **DIES MA*LA*.**

FACSIMILE: Budny (1997: II, pl. 604 [of pp. 28-29]); Graham *et al.* (2003: 11.8.2)

EDITION: Wormald (1934:184-95 [14])

CCCC 422, pp. 29-40 *6/4*

TYPE: Dog Days

LANGUAGE: L/OE

INCIPIT: **DIES CANICVLARES.** / hare dagas

FACSIMILE: Graham *et al.* (2003: 11.8.2)

EDITION: Wormald (1934:184-95 [14]); Meritt (1945: 56)

LITERATURE: Ker (1957: 119 [70.B.c]); Healey & Venezky (1980: 155 [OccGl 88 (Meritt), C88]); Quinn & Quinn (1990: 176 [H320]); Voigts & Kurtz (2000: 148.00)

CCCC 422, p. 49/4-8 *8.1/5*

TYPE: Egyptian Days, three days

LANGUAGE: L

INCIPIT: Isti sunt. tres dies anni. p*re* aliis obiseruandi

FACSIMILE: Graham *et al.* (2003: 11.8.2)

EDITION: James (1912: II.319 [II])

LITERATURE: Liuzza (2001: 214 [D2]); Graham *et al.* (2003: 90 [60.11])[21]

CCCC 422, p. 49/8-12 *3.1.2/4*

TYPE: birth, temporal, 3 miraculous days

LANGUAGE: L

INCIPIT: In anno sunt. tres dies & tres noctes.

FACSIMILE: Graham *et al.* (2003: 11.8.2)

---

[21] Graham *et al.* were unaware that this text and the next are two separate texts and quoted the incipit of the first and the explicit of the second.

EDITION: James (1912: II.319-20 [II])
LITERATURE: Ker (1957: 114 [67.d.vi], 174 [139.A.i]); Graham *et al.* (2003: 90 [60.11])[22]

Cambridge, Trinity College, O. 7. 41 (1369)
DATE: overall: after 1112, additions s. xiii, xiv; prognostic and calendar: after 1112[23]
ORIGIN: Colchester
CONTENTS: prognostic, calendar, computus with chronicle notes; mathematical notes; *De concordia evangelistarum*; Marianus Scotus's *Chronica*; the orders of the church; Hebrew alphabet, notes; arithmetic
LITERATURE: James (1900-04: III.379-82 [1369]); Gneuss (1981: 15 [198]); Robinson (1988: I.104 [383]);[24] Gameson (1999: 74 [170])

CTC O. 7. 41, fol. 1r 2/2
TYPE: Apuleian Sphere
LANGUAGE: L
INCIPIT: Racio spere pytagorice qua*m* apulei*us* descripsit.
LITERATURE: James (1900-04: III.379 [1369.1]); Thorndike (1923-58: I.692); Thorndike & Kibre (1963: 1315); Gameson (1999: 74 [170])

CTC O. 7. 41, fols 1v-7r 8.3/5
TYPE: Egyptian Days, twenty-four days
LANGUAGE: L
INCIPIT: Iani p*ri*ma dies: & septima fine timet*ur*. [verse] dies egypt*iacus* [entry]
LITERATURE: James (1900-04: III.379 [1369.2]);[25] Thorndike (1923-58: I.686, 695)

CTC O. 7. 41, fols 1v-7r 6/6
TYPE: Dog Days
LANGUAGE: L
INCIPIT: Dies caniculares.

Cambridge, Trinity College, R. 15. 32 (945)
The main scribe of the calendar and computus, Ælsinus, is one of the main scribes of Titus D. xxvi, xxvii
DATE: overall: s. xi^{in} (pp. 1-12, 37-218), 1035-36 (pp. 13-36); additions to the calendar s. xi^{1}, additions s. xi^{ex} (note on p. 36), more additions to the calendar s. xi^{ex}; calendar: 1035-36; Dog Days original to the calendar; Egyptian Days added s. xi^{ex}; prognostic: s. xi^{in} [26]
ORIGIN: overall: New Minster, Winchester, transferred to and expanded in St. Augustine's, Canterbury, s. xi^{ex}; calendar: New Minster, Winchester; additions St. Augustine's, Canterbury; prognostic: New Minster, Winchester
CONTENTS: astronomical notes; computus; arithmetic
LITERATURE: James (1900-04: II.363-66 [945]); Van de Vyver (1935: 140-41, 147); Wormald (1952: 64 [19]); Ker (1957: 135 [90]); Gneuss (1981: 15 [186]; 2001: 45 [186]); Robinson (1988: I.99 [357]); Liuzza (2001: 215 [Tr]); Wright & Hollis (2004: 31-39 [84, ASMMF 12.5])

CTC R. 15. 32, pp. 15-26 8.3/6
TYPE: Egyptian Days, twenty-four days

---

[22] *Ibid.*

[23] Robinson dated the manuscript to after 1112 with the help of the lunar tables. The singleton folding sheet, fol. 23, on which James and Gneuss based their estimate, has computistical tables dating to 1086.

[24] Robinson erroneously referred to shelf-mark 1360 instead of 1369.

[25] James (1900-04: III.379) wrote: "the usual verses Iani prima dies dies et septima fine timetur are given.... The Dies egyptiaci are also marked". This is one of the few references to Egyptian Days in English calendars I have encountered.

[26] James noted that 8.3/7 is in a larger hand, which might suggest that the text served as guest material. Gneuss, however, did not note anything of the kind.

LANGUAGE: L
INCIPIT: *Dies mala*
FACSIMILE: Robinson (1988: II, pl. 18 [of p. 15]); Wright & Hollis (2004: 12.5.1)
EDITION: Wormald (1934: 128-39 [10])
LITERATURE: Wright & Hollis (2004: 34-35 [84.6.e])

CTC R. 15. 32, pp. 15-26 *6/7*
TYPE: Dog Days
LANGUAGE: L
INCIPIT: **Dies caniculares incipiuntur.**
FACSIMILE: Wright & Hollis (2004: 12.5.1)
EDITION: Wormald (1934: 128-39 [10])

CTC R. 15. 32, p. 37/1-12 *8.3/7*
TYPE: Egyptian Days, twenty-four days
LANGUAGE: L
INCIPIT: KŁ IAN*VARII*. Iani prima dies. & septima fine tim*et*ur.
FACSIMILE: Wright & Hollis (2004: fiche 12.5.1)
LITERATURE: James (1900-04: II.363); Thorndike (1923-58: I.695); Thorndike & Kibre (1963: 651, 805); Gneuss (2001: 45 [186]); Liuzza (2001: 215 [Tr1]); Wright & Hollis (2004: 35 [84.6.n])

Cambridge, University Library, Kk. 5. 32, fols 49-60
DATE: overall: 1021-22 (fols 49-60); addition s. xi^{ex}; calendar: 1021-22
ORIGIN: St. Augustine's, Canterbury, transferred to Glastonbury (*c.* 1100)[27]
CONTENTS: computus, calendar; excerpts from Byrhtferth's *Enchiridion*
LITERATURE: Hardwick et al. (1856-67: III.701-02 [2074]); Ker (1957: 39 [26]); Gneuss (1981: 7 [26]; 2001: 29 [26]); Robinson (1988: I.37 [69]); Baker & Lapidge (1995: cxxi-cxxii [K])

CUL Kk. 5. 32, fols 50r-55v *8.3/8*
TYPE: Egyptian Days, twenty-four days
LANGUAGE: L
INCIPIT: D*ies*
FACSIMILE: Robinson (1988: II, pl. 16 [of fol. 51v])
EDITION: Wormald (1934: 72-83 [6])

CUL Kk. 5. 32, fols 50r-55v *6/8*
TYPE: Dog Days
LANGUAGE: L
INCIPIT: **Dies caniculares.** *hic incipiunt*
EDITION: Wormald (1934: 72-83 [6])

London, British Library, Additional 37517
AKA the Bosworth Psalter
DATE: overall: s. x, xi;[28] calendar: s. x/xi
ORIGIN: Canterbury (St. Augustine's?)[29]
CONTENTS: calendar; glossed Roman psalter; glossed canticles; litany; hymnal; monastic canticles; prayers
LITERATURE: Thompson et al. (1903-12: VII, pl. 163-64); Gasquet & Bishop (1908: 3-6, 34-39, 126-30); Gilson (1912: 65-67); Ker (1957: 161-62 [129]); Korhammer (1973); Temple (1976: 48-49 [22]); Watson (1979: I.79 [381]); Gneuss (1981: 20 [291]; 2001: 59 [291]); Pulsiano (1994b: 1-12 [166, ASMMF 2.1]); Orchard (1995; 2002: I.158-84)

Add. 37517, fols 2r-3r *8.3/9*
TYPE: Egyptian Days, twenty-four days
LANGUAGE: L
INCIPIT: D*ies*
FACSIMILE: Gasquet & Bishop (1908: pl. iv [of fol. 2r]); Watson (1979: II, pl. 23 [detail of fol. 2v]); Pulsiano (1994b: 2.1.1)
EDITION: Wormald (1934: 58-69 [5])

[27] Ker, Gneuss and Robinson opted for a Glastonbury origin.

[28] See Gneuss (2001: 59) for a survey of the dates of the contents.

[29] It has not yet been settled whether the manuscript is from Christ Church or St. Augustine's. Gneuss tentatively opted for Christ Church. Ker and Temple have argued for a St. Augustine's origin. N. Orchard's analysis places the calendar at least in St. Augustine's.

Add. 37517, fols 2r-3r 6/9
TYPE: Dog Days
LANGUAGE: L
INCIPIT: **DIES CANICVLARES INCIPIVNT.**
FACSIMILE: Pulsiano (1994b: 2.1.1)
EDITION: Wormald (1934: 58-69 [5])

London, British Library, Arundel 60
AKA the Arundel Psalter
DATE: overall: s. xi^2, 1073? (fols 1-132, 143-148), 1099 (fol. 149); additions s. xi^{ex} (fols 46v-52r); fols 133-142 added s. xii^2; prognostic and calendar: 1073?
ORIGIN: New Minster, Winchester
CONTENTS: prognostic, calendar, computus; glossed Gallican psalter; glossed canticles; litany; prayers; six ages of the world; list of bishops of Winchester
LITERATURE: Wanley (1705: II.291-92); Forshall (1834-40: I.13); Oess (1910: 1-25); Wormald (1952: 66 [25]); Ker (1957: 166-67 [134]); Kauffmann (1975: 53-54 [1]); Temple (1976: 120 [103]); Watson (1979: I.88 [436]); Gneuss (1981: 21 [304]; 2001: 60 [304]); Pulsiano (1994b: 13-18 [174, ASMMF 2.2]; 1995: 63 [7]); Gameson (1999: 95 [356]); Liuzza (2001: 215 [A])

Arundel 60, fol. 1r 9.2.3/2
TYPE: lunary, specific, bloodletting
LANGUAGE: L
INCIPIT: **AD SANGVINEM MINVENDVM.** [title] **Luna i Tota** die bona est.
FACSIMILE: Pulsiano (1994b: 2.2.1)
COLLATION: Henel (1934-35: 334-35)[30]
LITERATURE: Forshall (1834-40: I.13 [60.1]); Pulsiano (1994b: 14 [174.1]); Gneuss (2001: 60 [304]); Liuzza (2001: 215 [A1])

Arundel 60, fols 2r-7v 8.3/10
TYPE: Egyptian Days, twenty-four days
LANGUAGE: L
INCIPIT: **IANI PRIMA DIES ET SEPTIMA FINE TIMETVR.** [verse] ***dies*** [entry]
FACSIMILE: Pulsiano (1994b: 2.2.1)
EDITION: Wormald (1934: 142-53 [11])
LITERATURE: Liuzza (2001: 215 [A2])[31]

Arundel 60, fols 2r-7v 6/10
TYPE: Dog Days
LANGUAGE: L
INCIPIT: **Dies caniculares incipiunt**
FACSIMILE: Pulsiano (1994b: 2.2.1)
EDITION: Wormald (1934: 142-53 [11])

London, British Library, Arundel 155
AKA the Eadui Psalter
DATE: overall: 1012-23 (fols 2-135, 171-91); extensive additions and alterations s. xii; calendar: 1012-23; alterations to the calendar, including the addition of the Egyptian Days, s. xii
ORIGIN: Christ Church, Canterbury
CONTENTS: calendar, computus; Roman psalter, changed to Gallican; canticles; prayers; hymns; creeds; prayers
LITERATURE: Wanley (1705: II.292-94); Forshall (1834-40: I.42-43); Wormald (1952: 66 [26]); Ker (1957: 167-71 [135]); Temple (1976: 84-85 [66]); Watson (1979: I.90 [447]); Gneuss (1981: 21 [306]; 2001: 61 [306]); Pulsiano (1994b: 19-37 [175, ASMMF 2.3]); Gameson (1999: 95 [358]); Heslop (1995: 54)

Arundel 155, fols 2r-7v 8.3/11
TYPE: Egyptian Days, twenty-four days
LANGUAGE: L
INCIPIT: ***DIES ĘGYPTIACVS.***
FACSIMILE: Pulsiano (1994b: 2.3.1)
EDITION: Wormald (1934: 170-81 [13])

London, British Library, Cotton Caligula A. xv, fols 120-153, + Egerton 3314, fols 1-78
Caligula A. xv, fols 120-153 formed one manuscript with Egerton 3314, fols 1-78.

---

[30] In Henel as variants to 9.2.3/1 (CCCC 422).

[31] Liuzza referred to the hexameter verses only.

The original volume seems to have been taken apart in the sixteenth century. Original foliation is as follows: Egerton, fols 1-8 (computus notes added s. xii^{ex}); Caligula, fols 120-41 (computus, prognostics, annals); Egerton, fols 9-44, and Caligula, fol. 142 (computus notes, computus, calendar, tables [many additions in hands of s. xiv-xv]); Caligula, fols 143-153 (computus notes, Ælfric's *De temporibus anni*); Egerton, fols 45-78 (computus and astronomy notes from Bede, Isidore, Maurus, additions and scribbles).[32]
DATE: s. xi^2 (*c.* 1073); additions xii-xiv; prognostics: s. xi^2 (*c.* 1073)
ORIGIN: Christ Church, Canterbury
CONTENTS: computus, prognostics, charms; annals of Christ Church, Canterbury; six ages of the world; notes, charms; computus notes; excerpts from Ælfric's *De temporibus anni*
LITERATURE: Wanley (1705: II.233-34); Planta (1802: 45-46); Bond & Thompson (1873-83: III, pl. 145); Förster (1925-26: 74-76); Wormald (1952: 67 [27]); Ker (1957: 173-76 [139]; 1976: 124); Willetts (1966: 26-28); Skeat (1970: I.400-403); Temple (1976: 122 [106]); Watson (1979: I.100 [517]); Gneuss (1981: 28 [411]; 2001: 71 [411]); Hollis & Wright (1992: 259); Gameson (1999: 97 [370]); Liuzza (2001: 215-16 [C])

Caligula A. xv, fol. 125va *2/3*
TYPE: Apuleian Sphere
LANGUAGE: L
INCIPIT: Collige p*er* numeros quicquid cupis esse p*ro*bandu*m*.
FACSIMILE: Cockayne (1864-66: III.150 [diagram only])[33]
EDITION: Förster (1912c: 45-46 [text only]); Pulsiano (1998b: 113, n. 41)
COLLATION: Liuzza (2005: II.39-40 [C; incomplete])[34]
LITERATURE: Förster (1925-26: 75 [1]); Liuzza (2001: 215 [C1])

Caligula A. xv, fols 125vb-126r *9.2.5/3*
TYPE: lunary, specific, illness
LANGUAGE: L/OE (linear gloss)
INCIPIT: **L**un*a* i. qui inciderit / Se þe afealð
EDITION: Cockayne (1864-66: III.150-51 [C] [incomplete])[35]
COLLATION: Förster (1912c: 32-34 [C]); Weißer (1982: 273-77 [*Lo$_{20}$L/E])[36]
LITERATURE: Wanley (1705: II.233-34 [III]); Planta (1802: 45 [29]); Craig (1916: xxxix); Thorndike (1923-58: I.680, n. 2); Förster (1925-26: 75 [2]); Ker (1957: 174 [139.A.a]); Healey & Venezky (1980: 158 [Prog 2.1 (Först), B23.3.2.1]); Quinn & Quinn (1990: 133 [F402]); Hollis & Wright (1992: 257); Voigts & Kurtz (2000: 140.00); Liuzza (2001: 215 [C2])

Caligula A. xv, ff. 129v/27-130r/128.3/12
TYPE: Egyptian Days, twenty-four days
LANGUAGE: L
INCIPIT: **N**on interficias nec sanguis relaxetur.
LITERATURE: Ker (1957: 174 [139.A.h]); Liuzza (2001: 216 [C3])

Caligula A. xv, fol. 130r/13-27 *15/1*
TYPE: unlucky days
LANGUAGE: OE
INCIPIT: **S**yndon twegen dagas on æghwylcum monðe
EDITION: Cockayne (1864-66: III.224);[37] Förster (1929: 262-64 [C])
TRANSLATION: Cockayne (1864-66:

[32] Willetts provided a detailed survey of the construction of the original manuscript. Skeat listed the contents of Egerton 3314. Ker's analysis of Caligula A. xv, fols 120-153, as a two-part composite has been refuted by Willetts.
[33] Reprinted Singer (1961: III.150).
[34] As variants to 2/10 (Bodley 579).
[35] Reprinted Singer (1961: III.150-51).
[36] In Förster as variants to 9.2.5/4 (Tiberius A. iii); in Weißer as variants to Harley 3017, fol. 58v.
[37] Reprinted Singer (1961: III.168).

III.225)[38]
LITERATURE: Wanley (1705: II.234 [VII]); Planta (1802: 45-46 [34]); Thorndike (1923-58: I.695); Förster (1925-26: 75 [6]); Ker (1957: 174 [139.A.e]); Healey & Venezky (1980: 95 [Days 3.1 (Först), B23.2.3.1]); Quinn & Quinn (1990: 132 [F203]); Hollis & Wright (1992: 258); Voigts & Kurtz (2000: 155.00); Liuzza (2001: 216 [C4])

Caligula A. xv, fols 130v/6-131r/4 *8.3/1*
TYPE: Egyptian Days, twenty-four days
LANGUAGE: OE
INCIPIT: **Đ**a ealdan læces gesetton on ledonbocum
EDITION: Cockayne (1864-66: III.152-54);[39] Förster (1929: 266-69 [C])[40]
COLLATION: Henel (1934-35: 336-38 [C])[41]
TRANSLATION: Cockayne (1864-66: III. 153-55);[42] Bonser (1963: 296 [incomplete]); Cameron (1993: 163-64)
LITERATURE: Wanley (1705: II.234 [XII]); Planta (1802: 45-46 [34]); Förster (1925-26: 75 [9]); Ker (1957: 174 [139. A.h]); Bonser (1963: xvii);[43] Healey & Venezky (1980: 95 [Days 3.2 (Först), B23.2.3.2]); Quinn & Quinn (1990: 132 [F203]); Hollis & Wright (1992: 258); Voigts & Kurtz (2000: 156.00); Liuzza (2001: 216 [C5])

Caligula A. xv, fol. 131r/5-11 *3.1.2/2*
TYPE: birth, temporal, 3 miraculous days
LANGUAGE: OE
INCIPIT: **Đ**reo dagas syndon on .xii. monðum mid þrim nihtum
EDITION: Cockayne (1864-66: III.154);[44] Förster (1929: 260 [C])
COLLATION: Henel (1934-35: 346-47 [C])[45]
TRANSLATION: Cockayne (1864-66: III.155)[46]
LITERATURE: Wanley (1705: II.234 [XIII]); Planta (1802: 45-46 [34]); Förster (1925-26: 76 [10]); Ker (1957: 174 [139. A.i]); Bonser (1963: xvii); Healey & Venezky (1980: 95 [Days 3.3 (Först), B23.2. 3.3]); Quinn & Quinn (1990: 132 [F203]); Hollis & Wright (1992: 258); Voigts & Kurtz (2000: 172.00); Liuzza (2001: 216 [C6])

Caligula A. xv, ff. 131v/16-132r/8 *9.2.4/2*
TYPE: lunary, specific, dreams
LANGUAGE: OE
INCIPIT: **O**n anre nihta eald monan swa hwæt swa þe mæteð
EDITION: Cockayne (1864-66: III.154-56);[47] Förster (1925-26: 79-86 [C])
TRANSLATION: Cockayne (1864-66: III. 155-57)[48]
LITERATURE: Wanley (1705: II.234 [XXII]); Planta (1802: 45-46 [34]); Craig (1916: xxxix); Förster (1925-26: 76 [14]); Ker (1957: 175 [139.A.p]); Healey & Venezky (1980: 158 [Prog 2.2 (Först), B23.3.2.2]); Quinn & Quinn (1990: 133 [F402]); Hollis & Wright (1992: 257); Voigts & Kurtz (2000: 112.00); Liuzza (2001: 216 [C7])

Caligula A. xv, fol. 132r/9-35 *9.2.2/2*
TYPE: lunary, specific, birth
LANGUAGE: OE

[38] Reprinted Singer (1961: III.169).
[39] Replicated Cameron (1993: 196); reprinted Singer (1961: III.152-54).
[40] Corrections Henel (1934-35: 336, n. 1).
[41] As variants to 8.3/3 (Harley 3271).
[42] Partly replicated Payne (1904: 19); reprinted Singer (1961: III.153-55).
[43] Bonser erroneously referred to this text as a bloodletting prognostic.
[44] Replicated Förster (1903: 354); reprinted Singer (1961: III.154).
[45] As variants to 3.1.2/3 (Vitellius E. xviii).
[46] Reprinted Singer (1961: III.155).
[47] Partly replicated Förster (1903: 356); reprinted Singer (1961: III.154-56).
[48] Reprinted Singer (1961: III.155-57).

INCIPIT: **G**if mann bið akenned on anre nihte ealne monan.
EDITION: Cockayne (1864-66: III.156-58);[49] Förster (1912c: 21-26 [C]); Mitchell (1995: 273)[50]
TRANSLATION: Cockayne (1864-66: III. 157-59)[51]
LITERATURE: Wanley (1705: II.234 [XXIII]); Planta (1802: 45-46 [34]); Craig (1916: xl); Förster (1925-26: 76 [15]); Ker (1957: 175 [139.A.q]); Healey & Venezky (1980: 158 [Prog 2.3 (Först), B23.3.2.3]); Quinn & Quinn (1990: 133 [F402]); Hollis & Wright (1992: 257); Voigts & Kurtz (2000: 47.00); Liuzza (2001: 216 [C8])

Egerton 3314, fol. 18r/1-25 *8.3/20*
TYPE: Egyptian Days, twenty-four days
LANGUAGE: L
INCIPIT: **Histis mortiferam cognoscite uersib*us* horam.** [title] **D**at prima undenam ianus. pede: septima sextam.
LITERATURE: Skeat (1970: I.402 [6])

Egerton 3314, fols 18v-30r *8.3/21*
TYPE: Egyptian Days, twenty-four days
LANGUAGE: L
INCIPIT: **Iani p*rima* dies. & .vii.^{ma} a fine timetur.**

Egerton 3314, fols 18v-30r *6/18*
TYPE: Dog Days
LANGUAGE: L
INCIPIT: **Dies caniculares.**

[Egerton, 3314, fols 37r/4-38v
TYPE: lunary, collective (added s. xiv^{ex})
LANGUAGE: L
LITERATURE: Skeat (1970: I.402 [11.a])]

Egerton 3314, fol. 50r/3-50v/1 *8.3/22*
TYPE: Egyptian Days, twenty-four days
LANGUAGE: L
INCIPIT: **DE DIEB*VS* EG*YPTIACIS*.** [title] **S**i tenebre ęgyptiis greco sermone uocantur;

London, British Library, Cotton Nero A. ii, fols 3-13

Nero A. ii, fols 3-13, was once part of the prayerbook Galba A. xiv, and was bound by Cotton with a north Italian prayerbook (s. viii-ix), and a series of texts on St. Cuthbert (s. xii).
DATE: s. xi$^{2/4}$
ORIGIN: St. Mary's, Winchester
CONTENTS: calendar, computus; prayers
LITERATURE: Planta (1802: 202); Ker (1957: 198-201 [157]); Gneuss (1981: 23 [342]; 2001: 65 [342]); Muir (1988: ix-xxxiv); Doane (1994: 15-19 [203, ASMMF 1.3])

Nero A. ii, fols 3r-8v *6/11*
TYPE: Dog Days
LANGUAGE: L
INCIPIT: Dies canculares .l.
FACSIMILE: Doane (1994: 1.3.1)
EDITION: Wormald (1934: 30-41 [3]); Muir (1988: 3-14)

London, British Library, Cotton Tiberius A. iii, fols 2-173

Original foliation is: fols 117-73, 2-116.
DATE: s. xi^{med}
ORIGIN: Christ Church, Canterbury
CONTENTS: table of contents; glossed Rule of St. Benedict; injunction to observe the Rule; *Memoriale qualiter*; list of ecclesiastical feast days; Capitula from synod of Aachen in 818 (fols 117-73); post-medieval table of contents; glossed *Regularis concordia*; prognostics; short notes; prayers, directions; Ælfric, glossed *Colloquy*; prognostics; Ælfric's *De temporibus anni*; commonplaces; Life of St. Margaret; Ælfric's homily for Palm Sunday; Sunday letter; homily about a devil captured; homiletic pieces; ordination formula for an archbishop; directions for a confessor; *Monasteriales indicia*; lapidary; warning

[49] Reprinted Singer (1961: III.156-58).
[50] Mitchell confused this text with 9.2.2/3 (Tiberius A. iii).
[51] Reprinted Singer (1961: III.157-59).

against pride; Rule of St. Benedict, ch. 4; Alcuin's *De uirtutibus et uitiis*, ch. 14, 26; cattle charm; Ælfric's *Pastoral Letter* III; horae BVM; prayers, verses (fols 2-116)
LITERATURE: Wanley (1705: II.193-99); Planta (1802: 31-32); Förster (1908c; 1925-26: 66-67; 1944: 41-54); Wormald (1952: 68 [31]); Ker (1957: 241-48 [186]); Bonser (1963: 26); Temple (1976: 118-19 [100]); Gneuss (1981: 25 [363]; 1997; 2001: 67-68 [363]); Hollis & Wright (1992: 259); Liuzza (2001: 216-18 [T]); Wit (2002: 82-83 [9])

Tiberius A. iii, fols 27v/12-32v/16 *7/4*
TYPE: dreambook
LANGUAGE: L/OE
INCIPIT: **De somniorum diuersiitate secundum ordinem abcharii danielis prophete.** / be swefena mistlicnesse æfter endebyrdnessæ abecedes danielis þæt witegan. [title] **A**ues in somnis qui uiderit / fugelas on swefenum se þe gesyhð
EDITION: Cockayne (1864-66: III.198-214 [OE only]);[52] Förster (1910: 47-70); Martin (1977: 186-259 [T]; 1981: 95-168 [T^1,T^2,T^3; Latin only]); Fischer (1982a: 23-161 [L: 2; OE: 2c]); Epe (1995: 110-69 [AA], 172-77 [AB], 180-89 [EA])
COLLATION: Förster (1916: 270-83 [TA])[53]
TRANSLATION: Cockayne (1864-66: III.199-215)
LITERATURE: Wanley (1705: II.194 [II]); Planta (1802: 31 [2]); Förster (1908c: 32 [2]; 1925-26: 66 [2]); Thorndike (1923-58: II.295, n. 3); Ker (1957: 242 [186.7. a]); Bonser (1963: xvii); Healey & Venezky (1980: 160 [ProgGl 1 (Först), C16.1]); Grub (1984: liv [T]); Quinn & Quinn (1990: 153 [H041]); Hollis & Wright (1992: 257); Voigts & Kurtz (2000: 27. 00); Gneuss (2001: 67 [363]); Liuzza (2001: 216 [T1])

Tiberius A. iii, fols 32v/16-35v/14 *9.1/1*
TYPE: lunary, collective
LANGUAGE: L/OE
INCIPIT: **de obseruatione lune & que cauenda sunt** [title] **L**una prima omnibus rebus agendis utilis est. / mona se forma on eallum þingum dondum nytlic ys
EDITION: Cockayne (1864-66: III.184-96 [OE only]); Svenberg (1936: 21, 24-82 [L_2; Latin only]);[54] Förster (1944: 79-129, 165)
COLLATION: Weißer (1982: 380-92 [Lo_2L/E; Latin only])[55]
TRANSLATION: Cockayne (1864-66: III. 185-97)
LITERATURE: Wanley (1705: II.194 [III]); Planta (1802: 31 [3]); Förster (1908c: 32-33 [3]); Craig (1916: xl); Thorndike (1923-58: I.681, n. 1); Förster (1944: 29 [L: 10; OE: 1]); Ker (1957: 242 [186.7.b]); Bonser (1963: xvii);[56] Healey & Venezky (1980: 160 [ProgGl 2 (Först), C16.2]);[57] Hunt (1987: 180, n. 126); Taavitsainen (1988: 39-40); Quinn & Quinn (1990: 153 [H041]); Hollis & Wright (1992: 257); Voigts & Kurtz (2000: 101. 00); Liuzza (2001: 216 [T2]); Wit (2002: 83)

Tiberius A. iii, ff. 35v/15-36r/13 *9.2.4/5*
TYPE: lunary, specific, dreams
LANGUAGE: L/OE
INCIPIT: **L**una prima quicquid uideris / swa wæt swa þu gesihst
EDITION: Förster (1925-26: 67-74 [Tb])

[52] Cockayne's translation is prefaced by the comment "the Saxon glosses some Latin" (1864-66: III.199). Replicated Förster (1908b: 302-05) as variants to 7/2 (also in Tiberius A. iii).

[53] As variants to 7/1 (also in Tiberius A. iii) and 7/3 (Hatton 115).

[54] Corrections Wistrand (1942: 23-35).

[55] As variants to Pal. lat. 235, fols 40r-41r.

[56] Bonser erroneously referred to this text as a bloodletting prognostic.

[57] Formerly Healey and Venezky (1980: 160 [ProgGl 2.1 (Först), C16.2.1]).

LITERATURE: Wanley (1705: II.194 [IV]); Planta (1802: 31 [4]); Förster (1908c: 33 [4]; 1925-26: 66 [4]); Craig (1916: xxxix); Thorndike (1923-58: I. 680, n. 4); Ker (1957: 242 [186.7.c]); Healey & Venezky (1980: 160 [ProgGl 3 (Först), C16.3]); Quinn & Quinn (1990: 153 [H041]); Hollis & Wright (1992: 257); Voigts & Kurtz (2000: 154.00); Liuzza (2001: 216-17 [T3])

Tiberius A. iii, fol. 36r/14-36v/7 *17/4*
TYPE: year prognosis
LANGUAGE: L/OE
INCIPIT: **S**i fuerit kł ianuarius die dominico. / gif bið on dæg drihtenlicu*m*
EDITION: Förster (1908b: 296-97)[58]
TRANSLATION: Thorndike (1923-58: I. 677 [incomplete])
LITERATURE: Wanley (1705: II.194 [V]); Planta (1802: 31 [5]); Hellmann (1896b: 60); Förster (1908b: 298, n. 1; 1908c: 33-34 [5]); Craig (1916: xxxv [3]); Ker (1957: 242 [186.7.d]); Healey & Venezky (1980: 160 [ProgGl 4 (Först), C16.4]); Matter (1982: 387 [7], 390 [1]); Hunt (1987: 180, n. 126); Quinn & Quinn (1990: 153 [H041]); Hollis & Wright (1992: 257); Voigts & Kurtz (2000: 37.00); Liuzza (2001: 217 [T4])

Tiberius A. iii, fol. 36v/8-22 *9.2.2/5*
TYPE: lunary, specific, birth (lacks day 17)
LANGUAGE: L/OE
INCIPIT: **L**una .i. qui natus fuerit. / se þe acenned bið
EDITION: Förster (1912c: 18-21 [T[1]])
LITERATURE: Wanley (1705: II.194 [VI]); Planta (1802: 31 [6]); Förster (1908c: 34 [6]; 1925-26: 66 [6]); Craig (1916: xl); Thorndike (1923-58: I.680, n. 3); Ker (1957: 242 [186.7.e]); Healey & Venezky (1980: 160 [ProgGl 5 (Först), C16.5]); Quinn & Quinn (1990: 153 [H041]); Hollis & Wright (1992: 257); Voigts & Kurtz (2000: 138.00); Liuzza (2001: 217 [T5])

Tiberius A. iii, ff. 36v/23-37r/11 *9.2.5/4*
TYPE: lunary, specific, illness
LANGUAGE: L/OE
INCIPIT: **L**una .i. qui inciderit. / se þe afeallað
EDITION: Förster (1912c: 32-34 [T[1]])
COLLATION: Cockayne (1864-66: III.150-51 [T]);[59] Weißer (1982: 273-77 [*Lo_{19}L/E])[60]
LITERATURE: Wanley (1705: II.194 [VII]); Planta (1802: 31 [7]); Förster (1908c: 34 [7]; 1925-26: 66 [7]); Craig (1916: xxxix); Ker (1957: 242 [186.7.f]); Healey & Venezky (1980: 161 [ProgGl 6 (Först), C16.6]); Quinn & Quinn (1990: 153 [H041]); Hollis & Wright (1992: 257); Voigts & Kurtz (2000: 139.00); Liuzza (2001: 217 [T6])

Tiberius A. iii, f. 37r/12-37v/4 *5.1.2/1*
TYPE: brontology, temporal, hours
LANGUAGE: L/OE
INCIPIT: **S**i tonitruauerit hora uespertina. / gif hit þunrað on tide æfen
EDITION: Förster (1908a: 50-51);[61] Liuzza (2004: 16-17)
TRANSLATION: Liuzza (2004: 17, n. 55)
LITERATURE: Wanley (1705: II.194 [VIII]); Planta (1802: 31 [8]); Förster (1908c: 34-35 [8]); Thorndike (1923-58: I.679, n. 1);[62] Ker (1957: 242 [186.7.g]); Thorndike & Kibre (1963: 1466); Healey & Venezky (1980: 161 [ProgGl 7 (Först), C16.7]); Quinn & Quinn (1990: 153 [H041]); Hollis & Wright (1992: 257); Voigts & Kurtz (2000: 44.00); Liuzza (2001: 217 [T7])

[58] Corrections Förster (1910: 55, n. 5).

[59] As variants to 9.2.5/3 (Caligula A. xv). Reprinted Singer (1961: III.150-51).

[60] As variants to Harley 3017, fol. 58v.

[61] Corrections Förster (1910: 55, n. 5).

[62] Thorndike erroneously referred to this text as a day brontology.

Tiberius A. iii, fols 37v/5-38r/2 *9.2.4/3*
TYPE: lunary, specific dreams (lacks end of day 24 and beginning of 25-26)
LANGUAGE: OE
INCIPIT: **O**n anre nihte ealdne monan swa hwæt swa þe mæteð
EDITION: Förster (1925-26: 79-86 [T])
COLLATION: Cockayne (1864-66: III.154-56)[63]
LITERATURE: Wanley (1705: II.194 [IX, sub 1]); Planta (1802: 31 [9]); Förster (1908c: 35 [9]; 1925-26: 66 [9]); Ker (1957: 242 [186.7.h]); Healey & Venezky (1980: 158 [Prog 3.1 (Först), B23.3.3.1]); Quinn & Quinn (1990: 133-34 [F403]); Hollis & Wright (1992: 257); Voigts & Kurtz (2000: 115.00); Liuzza (2001: 217 [T8])

Tiberius A. iii, fols 38r/2-39v/23 *7/1*
TYPE: dreambook
LANGUAGE: OE
INCIPIT: **G**if mann mæte *þæt* he geseo earn on his heafad ufan.
EDITION: Förster (1916: 270-93 [T/TB]); Epe (1995: 192-211 [EB])
COLLATION: Cockayne (1864-66: III. 168-76 [T])[64]
LITERATURE: Wanley (1705: II.194 [IX, sub 2]); Förster (1908c: 35 [10]; 1925-26: 66 [10]); Ker (1957: 243 [186.7.i]); Healey & Venezky (1980: 158 [Prog 3.2 (Först), B23.3.3.2]); Quinn & Quinn (1990: 133-34 [F403]); Hollis & Wright (1992: 257); Voigts & Kurtz (2000: 48. 00); Liuzza (2001: 217 [T9]); Wit (2002: 83)

Tiberius A. iii, ff. 39v/24-40r/4 *9.2.1/1*
TYPE: lunary, specific, agenda (ends with day 3)
LANGUAGE: OE
INCIPIT: **O**n anre nihte ealdne monan. far þu to cinge.
EDITION: Cockayne (1864-66: III.176 n. 2); Förster (1912c: 43 [T])
LITERATURE: Wanley (1705: II.194 [X]);[65] Planta (1802: 31 [10]); Förster (1908c: 35 [11]; 1925-26: 66 [11]); Craig (1916: xxxix); Ker (1957: 243 [186.7.j]); Healey & Venezky (1980: 159 [Prog 3.3 (Först), B23.3.3.3]); Quinn & Quinn (1990: 133-34 [F403]); Hollis & Wright (1992: 257); Voigts & Kurtz (2000: 113. 00); Liuzza (2001: 217 [T10])

Tiberius A. iii, fol. 40r/5-21 *9.2.5/2*
TYPE: lunary, specific, illness (lacks day 13)
LANGUAGE: OE
INCIPIT: **O**n anre nihte ealdne monan se þe hine adl gestandeð.
EDITION: Cockayne (1864-66: III.182); Förster (1912c: 34-36 [T^2])
TRANSLATION: Cockayne (1864-66: III.183)
LITERATURE: Wanley (1705: II.194 [X]);[66] Förster (1908c: 35 [12]; 1925-26: 66-67 [12]); Craig (1916: xxxix); Thorndike (1923-58: I.679, n. 1); Ker (1957: 243 [186.7.k]); Weißer (1982: 49 [*Lo_{10}E]); Healey & Venezky (1980: 159 [Prog 3.4 (Först), B23.3.3.4]); Quinn & Quinn (1990: 133-34 [F403]); Hollis & Wright (1992: 257); Voigts & Kurtz (2000: 114.00); Liuzza (2001: 217 [T11])

Tiberius A. iii, f. 40r/22-40v/5 *5.1.3/2*
TYPE: brontology, temporal, weekday
LANGUAGE: OE
INCIPIT: **O**n anweardan geare. **G**if se forma þunor cymð on sunnandæge.

---

[63] As variants to 9.2.4/2 (Caligula A. xv). Reprinted Singer (1961: III.154-56).

[64] Collated with 7/3 (Hatton 115). Replicated Förster (1908b: 302-05) as variants to 7/2 (Tiberius A. iii). Partly replicated Griffiths (1996: 221-24).

[65] Wanley was unaware that 9.2.1/1 and 9.2.5/2 are two separate texts; he took the incipit from the former, and the explicit from the latter.

[66] *Ibid.*

EDITION: Cockayne (1864-66: III.180)[67]
TRANSLATION: Cockayne (1864-66: III. 181);[68] Liuzza (2004: 15, n. 50)
LITERATURE: Wanley (1705: II.194 [XI]); Planta (1802: 31 [11]); Förster (1908c: 35-36 [13]); Ker (1957: 243 [186. 7.l]); Healey & Venezky (1980: 159 [Prog 3.6 (Cockayne), B23.3.3.6]); Quinn & Quinn (1990: 133-34 [F403]); Hollis & Wright (1992: 257); Voigts & Kurtz (2000: 117.00); Liuzza (2001: 217 [T12])

Tiberius A. iii, fol. 40v/6-17 *10/1*
TYPE: month prognosis
LANGUAGE: OE
INCIPIT: **Ð**onne se mona bið acenned on sunnandæig.
EDITION: Cockayne (1864-66: III.180-82)
TRANSLATION: Cockayne (1864-66: III. 181-83)
LITERATURE: Wanley (1705: II.194 [XII]); Planta (1802: 31 [12]); Förster (1908c: 36 [14]); Thorndike (1923-58: I. 679); Ker (1957: 243 [186.7.m]); Healey & Venezky (1980: 159 [Prog 3.7 (Cockayne), B23.3.3.7]); Quinn & Quinn (1990: 133-34 [F403]); Hollis & Wright (1992: 257); Voigts & Kurtz (2000: 171. 00); Liuzza (2001: 218 [T13])

Tiberius A. iii, fols 40v/18-41r/11 *3.1.1/1*
TYPE: birth, temporal, development of the foetus
LANGUAGE: OE
INCIPIT: **H**er onginð secgan ymbe mannes gecynde
EDITION: Cockayne (1861: 49-50; 1864-66: III.146);[69] Mitchell (1995: 272); Chardonnens (2000)
TRANSLATION: Cockayne (1864-66: III. 147);[70] Bonser (1963: 265); Deegan (1987: 23); Swanton (1993: 263)
LITERATURE: Wanley (1705: II.194 [XIII]); Planta (1802: 31 [13]); Förster (1908c: 36 [15]); Ker (1957: 243 [186.7. n]); Bonser (1963: xvii, 26); Rubin (1974: 68); Healey & Venezky (1980: 122 [Lch III (Foetus), B21.4]); Quinn & Quinn (1990: 120 [E008]); Hollis & Wright (1992: 270); Voigts & Kurtz (2000: 88. 00); Liuzza (2001: 218 [T14])

Tiberius A. iii, fol. 41r/12-41v/8 *9.2.2/3*
TYPE: lunary, specific, birth
LANGUAGE: OE
INCIPIT: **G**if man biþ acenned on ane nihtne ealdne monan.
EDITION: Förster (1912c: 21-26 [T])
COLLATION: Cockayne (1864-66: III. 156-58)[71]
LITERATURE: Wanley (1705: II.194-95 [XIV]); Planta (1802: 31 [14]); Förster (1908c: 36 [16]; 1925-26: 67 [16]); Craig (1916: xl); Ker (1957: 243 [186.7.o]); Healey & Venezky (1980: 159 [Prog 3.5 (Först), B23.3.3.5]); Quinn & Quinn (1990: 133-34 [F403]); Hollis & Wright (1992: 257); Voigts & Kurtz (2000: 46. 00); Liuzza (2001: 218 [T15])

Tiberius A. iii, fols 41v/8-42r/5 *17/1*
TYPE: year prognosis
LANGUAGE: OE
INCIPIT: **KL** ianuarius gif he byþ on monandæg.
EDITION: Förster (1908b: 297-98)
TRANSLATION: Hampson (1841: I.133-34)
LITERATURE: Wanley (1705: II.195 [XV]); Planta (1802: 31 [15]); Hellmann (1896b: 60); Förster (1908c: 36 [17]); Craig (1916: xxxv [4]); Thorndike (1923-58: I.677-78, n. 3); Ker (1957: 243 [186. 7.p]); Healey & Venezky (1980: 159

[67] Replicated Liuzza (2004: 15).
[68] Replicated Griffiths (1996: 232-33).
[69] Cockayne (1864-66: III.146) replicated in part Cross and Hill (1982: 124), replicated with new errors Deegan (1987: 22-23); reprinted Singer (1961: III.146).
[70] Reprinted Singer (1961: III.147).
[71] As variants to 9.2.2/2 (Caligula A. xv).

[Prog 3.9 (Först), B23.3.3.9]); Matter (1982: 390 [2]); Quinn & Quinn (1990: 133-34 [F403]); Hollis & Wright (1992: 257); Voigts & Kurtz (2000: 41.00); Liuzza (2001: 218 [T16])

Tiberius A. iii, fol. 42r/5-42v/8 *7/2*
TYPE: dreambook
LANGUAGE: OE
INCIPIT: **G**if man mæte *þæt* his mon ehte.
EDITION: Förster (1908b: 302-05);[72] Fischer (1982a: 23-161 [2b]); Epe (1995: 214-17 [EC])
COLLATION: Förster (1916: 270-93 [TC])[73]
TRANSLATION: Griffiths (1996: 226-28)
LITERATURE: Wanley (1705: II.195 [XVI]); Planta (1802: 31 [16]); Förster (1908c: 36-37 [18]); Ker (1957: 243 [186. 7.q]); Fischer (1982a: 13 [2]); Healey & Venezky (1980: 159 [Prog 3.10 (Först), B23.3.3.10]); Quinn & Quinn (1990: 133-34 [F403]); Hollis & Wright (1992: 257); Voigts & Kurtz (2000: 42.00);[74] Liuzza (2001: 218 [T17]); Wit (2002: 83)

Tiberius A. iii, fols 42v/9-43r/2 *3.2/1*
TYPE: birth, non-temporal, gender prediction
LANGUAGE: OE
INCIPIT: **E**ft is oðer wise be þissum þingum *þæt* þu meht witan on bearneacenum wife
EDITION: Cockayne (1864-66: III.144)[75]
TRANSLATION: Cockayne (1864-66: III. 145);[76] Cameron (1993: 183 [incomplete]); Swanton (1993: 263-64)

LITERATURE: Wanley (1705: II.195 [XVII]); Planta (1802: 31 [17]); Hoops (1889: 67); Förster (1908c: 37 [19]); Ker (1957: 243 [186.7.r]); Bonser (1963: xvii, 265); Rubin (1974: 68); Healey & Venezky (1980: 159 [Prog 3.8 (Cockayne), B23. 3.3.8]); Quinn & Quinn (1990: 133-34 [F403]); Hollis & Wright (1992: 257); Voigts & Kurtz (2000: 23.00); Liuzza (2001: 218 [T18])

Tiberius A. iii, fol. 65r/1-11 *9.2.3/3*
TYPE: lunary, specific, bloodletting
LANGUAGE: L
INCIPIT: **L**una .i. tota die bonum est.
EDITION: Förster (1912c: 36-37)
LITERATURE: Wanley (1705: II.196 [XXVIII]); Planta (1802: 31 [25]); Förster (1908c: 39 [29]; 1925-26: 67 [29]); Craig (1916: xxxix); Thorndike (1923-58: I.680, n. 1); Ker (1957: 245 [186.12]); Liuzza (2001: 218 [T19])

Tiberius A. iii, fol. 65r/11-22 *3.1.3/3*
TYPE: birth, temporal, weekday
LANGUAGE: L
INCIPIT: **DE NATIVITATE INFANTVM.** [title] **D**ie dominico. hora diuturna siue nocturna utilissimus erit qui nascetur
COLLATION: Förster (1912b; 301-03 [E_1/Ea])[77]
LITERATURE: Wanley (1705: II.196 [XXIX]); Planta (1802: 32 [26]); Förster (1908c: 39 [30]); Thorndike (1923-58: I. 679); Ker (1957: 245 [186.12]); Liuzza (2001: 218 [T20])

Tiberius A. iii, fol. 65r/22-65v/6 *9.2.2/6*
TYPE: lunary, specific, birth
LANGUAGE: L
INCIPIT: **Incipit Lunaris s*ancti* danielis de natiuitate `inf*antium*´.** [title] **L**una .i. *qui* natus fuerit.
COLLATION: Förster (1912c: 18-21

[72] Corrections Förster (1908c: 37). Replicated Griffiths (1996: 226-28).

[73] As variants to 7/1 (also in Tiberius A. iii) and 7/3 (Hatton 115).

[74] In Voigts and Kurtz filed under the second entry of the dreambook.

[75] Replicated in part Cameron (1993: 183, n. 34); reprinted Singer (1961: III. 144).

[76] Reprinted Singer (1961: III.145).

[77] Collated with 3.1.3/4 (Titus D. xxvi).

[T^{2}])[78]
LITERATURE: Wanley (1705: II.196 [XXX]); Planta (1802: 32 [27]); Förster (1908c: 39-40 [31]); Craig (1916: xl); Thorndike (1923-58: I.680, n. 3); Ker (1957: 245 [186.12]); Liuzza (2001: 218 [T21])

Tiberius A. iii, fol. 65v/7-9 *9.2.5/5*
TYPE: lunary, specific, illness (ends with day 7)
LANGUAGE: L
INCIPIT: Luna .i. qui inciderit
COLLATION: Förster (1912c: 32-34 [T^{3}]); Weißer (1982: 273-77 [*Lo$_{22}$L])[79]
LITERATURE: Wanley (1705: II.196 [XXXI]); Planta (1802: 32 [27]); Förster (1908c: 40 [32]; 1925-26: 67 [32]); Craig (1916: xxxix); Ker (1957: 245 [186.12]); Liuzza (2001: 218 [T22])

London, British Library, Cotton Tiberius C. i, fols 2-42, + Harley 3667

Tiberius C. i, fols 2-42, and Harley 3667 once formed part of one larger volume: the first two quires of Tiberius C. i are marked VI and VII; the quire that makes up Harley 3667 is marked XXI. A number of texts in these manuscripts can also be found in St. John's College 17.
DATE: overall: *c.* 1122; additions to the annals 1135; prognostics: *c.* 1122
ORIGIN: Peterborough
CONTENTS: Tiberius C. i, fols 2-42: computus, astronomy, prognostic; names of the winds; excerpts from Bede, Macrobius, Isidorus, Pliny; Harley 3667: annals of Peterborough Abbey in Easter table, parts of Byrhtferth's computus, astronomy, prognostics; names of the winds
LITERATURE: Wanley (1705: II.220-21); Planta (1802: 37); Nares (1808: III.50); Saxl, Meier & McGurk (1915-66: III.1. 128-34); Van de Vyver (1935: 142); Ker (1957: 259-60 [196]); Kauffmann (1975: 76-77 [37]); Watson (1979: I.107 [559]); Baker & Lapidge (1995: lv-lvii [THa, THb]); Gameson (1999: 102 [404]); Wilcox (2000: 30-45 [231, ASMMF 8.5], 69-71 [275, ASMMF 8.9]); Liuzza (2001: 218-19 [Th])

Tiberius C. i, fol. 7rb/1-15 *8.2/1*
TYPE: Egyptian Days, twelve days
LANGUAGE: L
INCIPIT: **I**sti q*uo*q*ue* dies obseruandi s*unt* in sing*u*lis m*ens*ib*us*.
FACSIMILE: Wilcox (2000: 8.5.1)
LITERATURE: Saxl, Meier & McGurk (1915-66: III.1.130); Wilcox (2000: 34 [231.12]); Liuzza (2001: 219 [Th1])

Tiberius C. i, fol. 7v *2/4*
TYPE: Apuleian Sphere
LANGUAGE: L
INCIPIT: **R**atio sperę pitagori philosophi que*m* apulet*us* scripsit.
FACSIMILE: Murdoch (1984: 310 [detail of fol. 7v]); Wilcox (2000: 8.5.1)
COLLATION: Liuzza (2005: II.40-44 [T; incomplete])[80]
LITERATURE: Saxl, Meier & McGurk (1915-66: III.1.130); Baker & Lapidge (1995: lvi [THa.54], 427 [54]); Wilcox (2000: 34 [231.14]); Liuzza (2001: 219 [Th2])

Harley 3667, fol. 4va, 4vc *2/7*
TYPE: Apuleian Sphere
LANGUAGE: L
INCIPIT: Ratio sp*er*ę pythagori.
FACSIMILE: Wilcox (2000: 8.9.1)
LITERATURE: Kauffmann (1975: 76); Wilcox (2000: 70 [275.3]); Liuzza (2001: 219 [Th3])

Harley 3667, fol. 5r *2/8*
TYPE: Apuleian Sphere

[78] As variants to 9.2.2/5 (also in Tiberius A. iii).

[79] In Förster as variants to 9.2.5/4 (also in Tiberius A. iii); in Weißer as variants to Harley 3017, fol. 58v.

[80] As variants to 2/12 (St. John's College 17).

LANGUAGE: L
INCIPIT: ORGANV*M* PP. De quacú*m*-*que* ré scire uolueris *uel* consulere.
FACSIMILE: Wilcox (2000: 8.9.1)
COLLATION: Liuzza (2005: II.40-44 [Th²; incomplete])[81]
LITERATURE: Wilcox (2000: 70 [275.4]); Liuzza (2001: 219 [Th4])

London, British Library, Cotton Tiberius C. vi
AKA the Tiberius Psalter
DATE: overall: s. xi$^{3/4}$, mid 1060s?; additions s. xii (Latin text on the twenty-four Egyptian Days, and a text on the unlucky days text in Anglo-Norman); prognostics: s. xi$^{3/4}$ (fol. 6v); s. xii (fol. 114r)
ORIGIN: Winchester (Old Minster?)
CONTENTS: computus; illustrations (including Apuleian Sphere); notes, prayers; glossed Gallican psalter with collects; prognostic
LITERATURE: Wanley (1705: II.224); Planta (1802: 38); Bond & Thompson (1873-83: III, pl. 98); Wormald (1952: 68-69 [32]; 1962); Ker (1957: 262 [199]); Temple (1976: 115-17 [98]); Gneuss (1981: 26 [378]; 2001: 69 [378]); Pulsiano (1994b: 38-42 [233, ASMMF 2.4]; 1995: 64 [9]); Gameson (1999: 102 [406])

Tiberius C. vi, fol. 6v *2/5*
TYPE: Apuleian Sphere
LANGUAGE: L
INCIPIT: **COLLIGE PER NVMEROS QVICQVID CVPIS ESSE PROBAND(VM.)**
FACSIMILE: Wormald (1962: pl. 125); Heimann (1966: pl. 9a); Temple (1976: ill. 303); Desham (1977: pl. VIIIa); Jones (1984: 66); Pulsiano (1994b: 2.4.1); Liuzza (2005: II.33, pl. 3)
EDITION: Wanley (1705: II.224 [II; incomplete, verse only])
COLLATION: Liuzza (2005: II.39-40 [Ti; incomplete])[82]
LITERATURE: Planta (1802: 38 [2]); Thorndike (1923-58: I.692); Wormald (1952: 68; 1962: 126, 131 [125]); Bonser (1963: 157, n. 2); Temple (1976: 115); Ohlgren *et al.* (1986: 265-66 [203.7]); Pulsiano (1994b: 39 [233.1])

Tiberius C. vi, fol. 114r/8-18 *8.3/13*
TYPE: Egyptian Days, twenty-four days
LANGUAGE: L
INCIPIT: Non int*er*ficias nec sanguis relaxet*ur*.
FACSIMILE: Pulsiano (1994b: 2.4.4)
LITERATURE: Wormald (1962: 137 [150]); Pulsiano (1994b: 41 [233.2])

[Tiberius C. vi, fol. 114r/19-27
TYPE: unlucky days
LANGUAGE: Anglo-Norman
FACSIMILE: Pulsiano (1994b: 2.4.4)
LITERATURE: Wormald (1962: 137 [150]); Pulsiano (1994b: 41 [233.2])]

London, British Library, Cotton Titus D. xxvi, xxvii
AKA Ælfwine's *Prayerbook*
The two manuscripts originally formed one volume in the order xxvii, xxvi. Ælfwine owned this manuscript as dean of New Minster, Winchester (a. 1032), and the manuscript was probably compiled for him personally. Ælfwine did not write portions of the manuscript himself. One of two main scribes also wrote the calendar and computus of CTC R. 15. 32.
DATE: overall: 1023-31; additions s. xi^{1} (xxvii, fols 55v-56v; xxvi, fols 2r-18r, 76-79v),[83] s. xii (xxvi, fol. 74r); bifolia with

---

[81] As variants to 2/12 and 2/13 (St. John's College 17).

[82] As variants to 2/10 (Bodley 579).

[83] If the last obit, 1023, in the hand of scribe A is indicative of the time of composition, and the manuscript had indeed been completed before 1032, the year in which Ælfwine became abbot, the date for the additions should be 1023-31 (see Günzel 1993: 2, 25-27; Keynes 1996:

miniatures added *c.* 1050 (xxvii, unnumbered leaf + fol. 65, 74-75; xxvi, fols 18-19); prognostics and calendar: 1023-31
ORIGIN: New Minster, Winchester
CONTENTS: xxvii: prognostic, computus, Easter tables with obits in hand A up to 1023, calendar; computus, prognostics, notes, prayer; Ælfric, *De temporibus anni*; notes, computus, prognostic; prayer; miniature of the Crucifixion; devotions to the Holy Cross; prayer; miniature of the Trinity; offices of the Trinity, the Holy Cross, the Virgin Mary; private prayers; xxvi: directions for private devotions; notes, prognostics; prayers; medicinal recipe; decisions at a bishops' synod; miniature of the Apostle Peter; collectar; devotions; litany; private prayers; charm; beginning of St. John's Gospel
LITERATURE: Wanley (1705: II.247-48); Planta (1802: 567); Bond & Thompson (1873-83: III, pl. 60); Wormald (1952: 69 [33]); Ker (1957: 264-66 [202]); Alexander & Kauffman (1973: 32 [11]); Temple (1976: 94-95 [77]); Watson (1979: I.108 [561]); Gneuss (1981: 26 [380]; 2001: 70 [380]); Hollis & Wright (1992: 260); Günzel (1993: 1-78); Corrêa (1995: 50-51); Keynes (1996: 111-23); Liuzza (2001: 219-21 [Æ]); Wit (2002: 84-86 [11])

Titus D. xxvii, fol. 2r *9.2.3/5*
TYPE: lunary, specific, bloodletting
LANGUAGE: L
INCIPIT: **Ad sanguinem minuendam.** [title] **L**una i Tota die bona est.
FACSIMILE: Keynes (1996: pl. X)
EDITION: Birch (1878: 496 [incomplete]);[84] Günzel (1993: 89 [1])
COLLATION: Förster (1912c: 36-37)[85]
LITERATURE: Planta (1802: 567 [XXVII. 1]); Craig (1916: xxxix); Ker (1957: 310 [239.14]); Bonser (1963: xviii); Keynes (1996: 115 [1]); Gneuss (2001: 70 [380]); Liuzza (2001: 219 [Æ1])

Titus D. xxvii, fols 3r-8v *8.3/15*
TYPE: Egyptian Days, twenty-four days
LANGUAGE: L
INCIPIT: ***Dies***
FACSIMILE: Keynes (1996: pl. X-XIII)
EDITION: Wormald (1934: 114-25 [9]); Günzel (1993: 91-102 [4])
LITERATURE: Steele (1919: 121)

Titus D. xxvii, fols 3r-8v *6/13*
TYPE: Dog Days
LANGUAGE: L
INCIPIT: **Dies caniculares incipiunt.**
FACSIMILE: Keynes (1996: pl. X-XIII)
EDITION: Hampson (1841: I.435-46);[86] Wormald (1934: 114-25 [9]); Günzel (1993: 91-102 [4])

Titus D. xxvii, fol. 22r-22v/16 *8.3/16*
TYPE: Egyptian Days, twenty-four days
LANGUAGE: L
INCIPIT: **I**ANI PRIMA DIES. 7 SEPTIMA FINE TIMETVR.- **P**ericulosum est flebotomari in principio mensis ianuarii.
EDITION: Birch (1878: 505 [incomplete]);[87] Günzel (1993: 110-11 [18])
LITERATURE: Planta (1802: 567 [XXVII. 4]); Liuzza (2001: 219 [Æ18a,b])

Titus D. xxvii, fols 22v/16-23r/8 *6/14*
TYPE: Dog Days
LANGUAGE: L
INCIPIT: **E**st etiam istorum temporum obseruanda ratio.
EDITION: Günzel (1993: 111 [18])
COLLATION: Henel (1934-35: 340-41 [T])[88]
LITERATURE: Steele (1919: 121); Liuzza (2001: 219 [Æ18c])

112, 113).

[84] Republished Birch (1892: 269).

[85] As variants to 9.2.3/3 (Tiberius A. iii).

[86] Hampson did not print the entries for the Egyptian Days in this calendar.

[87] Reprinted Birch (1892: 276-77).

[88] Collated with 6/19 and 6/20 (Harley 3271).

Titus D. xxvii, fol. 25r/8-25v/3 *17/6*
TYPE: year prognosis
LANGUAGE: L
INCIPIT: **KL. IAN*VARII*. S**i fuerit in prima feria.
EDITION: Birch (1878: 505 [incomplete]);[89] Günzel (1993: 115 [32])
LITERATURE: Förster (1908b: 298, n. 1); Liuzza (2001: 219 [Æ32])

Titus D. xxvii, fols 27r/8-29v[90] *9.1/2*
TYPE: lunary, collective
LANGUAGE: L
INCIPIT: **ARGVMENTVM LVNARE AD REQVIRENDV*M* QVOMODO *VE*L QVALITER OBSERVETVR.** [title] **L**una .i. hec dies ad omnia agenda. utilis est.
EDITION: Birch (1878: 506 incomplete]);[91] Svenberg (1936: 21, 25-83 [L_1]);[92] Günzel (1993: 117-20 [35])
LITERATURE: Planta (1802: 567 [XXVII. 7]); Thorndike (1923-58: I.681, n. 1); Förster (1944: 29 [6]); Weißer (1982: 48 [Lo_1L]); Liuzza (2001: 219 [Æ35])

Titus D. xxvii, fols 55v-56v/1 *1/1*
TYPE: alphabet prognostic
LANGUAGE: OE
INCIPIT: A. He gangeð 7 biþ his siðfæt gesund.
FACSIMILE: Robinson & Stanley (1991: pl. 29.1-3)
EDITION: Sievers (1877: 189-90);[93] Birch (1878: 508-09);[94] Dobbie (1942: 94 [incomplete, verse ending only]); Günzel (1993: 121-22 [40]); Marsden (2004: 13-15)
TRANSLATION: Griffiths (1996: 218-20)
LITERATURE: Wanley (1705: II.248 [VI]); Planta (1802: 567 [XXVII.9]); Ker (1957: 265 [202.i]); Healey & Venezky (1980: 159 [Prog 4 (Sievers), B23.3.4], 100 [Glor II, Cameron A27]); Quinn & Quinn (1990: 134 [F404]); Hollis & Wright (1992: 258); Voigts & Kurtz (2000: 6.00); Gneuss (2001: 70 [380]); Liuzza (2001: 219-20 [Æ40])

Titus D. xxvi, fols 3v/9-4r/12 *8.1/6*
TYPE: Egyptian Days, three days
LANGUAGE: L
INCIPIT: **hic noctantur dies egiptiaci qui obseruandi sunt per om*n*ia ne quis sanguine*m* audiat in eis minuere** [title] **D**ies enim aegyptiaci in quibus nulliusmodi nec p*er* ulla necessitate
EDITION: Birch (1878: 472-73);[95] Günzel (1993: 144 [56])
COLLATION: Förster (1929: 275 [T])[96]
LITERATURE: Planta (1802: 567 [XXVI. 4]); Steele (1919: 121); Bonser (1963: xviii); Thorndike (1923-58: I.695); Liuzza (2001: 220 [Æ56])

Titus D. xxvi, fol. 4r/13-4v/1 *3.1.2/5*
TYPE: birth, temporal, 3 miraculous days
LANGUAGE: L
INCIPIT: **T**res dies sunt in anno cu*m* totide*m* noctib*us*
EDITION: Birch (1878: 474);[97] Günzel (1993: 145 [57])
COLLATION: Förster (1929: 261 [T])[98]
LITERATURE: Liuzza (2001: 220 [Æ57])

---

[89] Reprinted Birch (1892: 277).

[90] 9.1/2 runs to fol. 29v/9; the rest of the page (a quire end) is empty.

[91] Reprinted Birch (1892: 278).

[92] Corrections Wistrand (1942: 23-35).

[93] Replicated Griffiths (1996: 218-20).

[94] Replicated Skeat (1897: 543); reprinted Birch (1892: 279-80).

[95] Reprinted Birch (1892: 252-53).

[96] Together with Rawlinson C. 814, fol. 60r, as variants to pseudo-Bede *De minutione sanguinis, siue de phlebotomia* (on this text, see pp. 97-98, 278-79).

[97] Birch did not realise that this text is not part of the preceding one (8.1/6). Reprinted Birch (1892: 253).

[98] With pseudo-Bede *De minutione sanguinis, siue de phlebotomia* (see pp. 97-98, 278-79) as variants to Royal 12. C. xii, fol. 87r.

Titus D. xxvi, fol. 4v/2-17 *6/12*
TYPE: Dog Days
LANGUAGE: L
INCIPIT: **Quali tempora ap*er*ienda *sit* uena** [title] **I**ncipiente artucanis. uel arcturi adq*ue* siria stella
EDITION: Birch (1878: 474-475);[99] Günzel (1993: 145 [58])
COLLATION: Henel (1934-35: 332 [T])[100]
LITERATURE: Planta (1802: 567 [XXVI. 5]); Liuzza (2001: 220 [Æ58])

Titus D. xxvi, fol. 5r/1-13 *8.3/14*
TYPE: Egyptian Days, twenty-four days (lacks last four dates)
LANGUAGE: L
INCIPIT: **I**ncipiunt dies aegiptiaci qui in anno obseruandi sunt
EDITION: Birch (1878: 475 [incomplete]);[101] Steele (1919: 110, 111 [incomplete]); Günzel (1993: 145 [59])
LITERATURE: Liuzza (2001: 220 [Æ59])

Titus D. xxvi, fols 5r/14-6r/1 *11/1*
TYPE: colour of the moon
LANGUAGE: L
INCIPIT: **PV**ithagoras u*ero* uir animi sagax
EDITION: Wright & Halliwell (1841-43: I. 15 [incomplete]); Birch (1878: 477);[102] Günzel (1993: 145-46 [60])

Titus D. xxvi, fol. 6r/2-6v/9 *9.2.3/4*
TYPE: lunary, specific, bloodletting
LANGUAGE: L
INCIPIT: **De flebotomatione *u*el de minuendo sanguine** [title] **L**una prima. Tota die bonum est.
EDITION: Birch (1878: 477 [incomplete]);[103] Günzel (1993: 146-47 [61])
COLLATION: Förster (1912c: 36-37)[104]
LITERATURE: Planta (1802: 567 [XXVI. 6]); Craig (1916: xxxix); Liuzza (2001: 220 [Æ61])

Titus D. xxvi, fols 6v/10-7v/1 *3.1.3/4*
TYPE: birth, temporal, weekday
LANGUAGE: L
INCIPIT: **De natiuitate Infantium** [title] **D**ie dominico hora diuturna. **S**iue nocturna uti li erit q*ui* nasc*etur*
EDITION: Birch (1878: 478 [incomplete]);[105] Günzel (1993: 147 [62])
COLLATION: Förster (1912b: 301-03 [E_1/Ed])[106]
LITERATURE: Planta (1802: 567 [XXVI. 7]); Thorndike (1923-58: I.680, n. 3);[107] Liuzza (2001: 220 [Æ62])

Titus D. xxvi, fols 7v/2-8r/13 *9.2.2/7*
TYPE: lunary, specific, birth
LANGUAGE: L
INCIPIT: **incipit lunares S*ancti* danielis de natiuitate.** [title] **L**una .i. qui natus fuerit
EDITION: Birch (1878: 478-79 [incomplete]);[108] Günzel (1993: 147-48 [63])
COLLATION: Förster (1912c: 18-21 [D])[109]
LITERATURE: Planta (1802: 567 [XXVI. 8]); Craig (1916: xl); Thorndike (1923-58: I.680, n. 3); Liuzza (2001: 220 [Æ63])

Titus D. xxvi, fols 8r/14-9r/5 *9.2.5/6*
TYPE: lunary, specific, illness
LANGUAGE: L
INCIPIT: **Incipit lunares de aegris.** [title] **L**una .i. qui inciderit
EDITION: Birch (1878: 479 [incomplete]);[110] Günzel (1993: 148-49 [64])

[99] Reprinted Birch (1892: 253).
[100] As variants to 6/21 (Harley 3271).
[101] Reprinted Birch (1892: 253).
[102] Reprinted Birch (1892: 255).
[103] Reprinted Birch (1892: 255).
[104] As variants to 9.2.3/3 (Tiberius A. iii).
[105] Reprinted Birch (1892: 256).
[106] Collated with 3.1.3/3 (Tiberius A. iii).
[107] Thorndike erroneously referred to this text as a birth lunary.
[108] Reprinted Birch (1892: 256).
[109] As variants to 9.2.2/5 (Tiberius A. iii).
[110] Reprinted Birch (1892: 257).

COLLATION: Förster (1912c: 32-34 [D]); Weißer (1982: 273-77 [*Lo_{21}L])[111]
LITERATURE: Planta (1802: 567 [XXVI. 9]); Craig (1916: xxxix); Thorndike (1923-58: I.680, n. 2); Liuzza (2001: 220 [Æ64])

Titus D. xxvi, fol. 9r/6-9v/13 *9.2.4/7*
TYPE: lunary, specific, dreams
LANGUAGE: L
INCIPIT: **Incipit lunaris de somnis** [title] **L**una .i. quicquid uideri
EDITION: Birch (1878: 479 [incomplete]);[112] Günzel (1993: 149-50 [65])
COLLATION: Förster (1925-26: 67-74 [T])[113]
LITERATURE: Planta (1802: 567 [XXVI. 10]); Craig (1916: xxxix); Thorndike (1923-58: I.680, n. 4); Liuzza (2001: 220 [Æ65])

Titus D. xxvi, fols 9v/14-10v/9 *5.1.2/2*
TYPE: brontology, temporal, hours
LANGUAGE: L
INCIPIT: **De tonitruis dierum uel trium** [title] **S**i notauerit hora uesp*er*tina
EDITION: Birch (1878: 479 [incomplete]);[114] Günzel (1993: 150-51 [66])
COLLATION: Liuzza (2004: 16-17)[115]
LITERATURE: Planta (1802: 567 [XXVI. 11]); Thorndike (1923-58: I.679, n. 1);[116] Liuzza (2001: 221 [Æ66])

Titus D. xxvi, fols 10v/10-11v/6 *17/5*
TYPE: year prognosis
LANGUAGE: L
INCIPIT: **incipiunt signa de temporibus.** [title] **S**i die .i. *feria* fueri`n´t kł ian*u*-*arii*
EDITION: Birch (1878: 480);[117] Günzel (1993: 151 [67])
LITERATURE: Planta (1802: 567 [XXVI. 12]); Förster (1908b: 298, n. 1); Thorndike (1923-58: I.677-78, n. 3); Matter (1982: 387 [3]); Liuzza (2001: 221 [Æ67])

Titus D. xxvi, fols 11v/8-16r *7/5*
TYPE: dreambook
LANGUAGE: L
INCIPIT: **A**ues in somnis uidere. & cu*m* illis pugnare.
EDITION: Birch (1878: 481-83 [incomplete]);[118] Fischer (1982a: 23-161 [3]); Günzel (1993: 151-56 [68])
COLLATION: Förster (1916: 270-93 [Tit]); Martin (1977: 186-259 [J]; 1981: 97-168 [J]); Epe (1995: 110-69, 172-77 [AJ])[119]
LITERATURE: Planta (1802: 567 [XXVI. 13]); Thorndike (1923-58: II.295, n. 3); Grub (1984: liv [J]); Gneuss (2001: 70 [380]); Liuzza (2001: 221 [Æ68]); Wit (2002: 85)

London, British Library, Cotton Vespasian D. xiv, fols 4-169

DATE: overall: s. $xii^{2/4}$, additions in the main hand s. $xii^{2/4}$ (fols 67v, 74v-75v, 102r-103v, 163v-169v), additions s. xii^{ex} (fol. 4r); prognostics: s. $xii^{2/4}$
ORIGIN: Christ Church, Canterbury?[120]

[111] In Förster as variants to 9.2.5/4 (Tiberius A. iii); in Weißer as variants to Harley 3017, fol. 58v.

[112] Reprinted Birch (1892: 257).

[113] As variants to 9.2.4/5 (Tiberius A. iii).

[114] Reprinted Birch (1892: 257).

[115] As variants to 5.1.2/1 (Tiberius A. iii).

[116] Thorndike erroneously referred to this text as a day brontology.

[117] Reprinted Birch (1892: 258).

[118] Reprinted Birch (1892: 258).

[119] In Förster as variants to 7/1 (Tiberius A. iii) and 7/3 (Hatton 115); in Martin (1981) as variants to 7/4 (Tiberius A. iii); In Epe as variants to 7/4 (Tiberius A. iii).

[120] The place of origin is a matter of debate: opinions waver between Christ Church, Canterbury, and Rochester. For a recent discussion of the place of origin, see Irvine (2000: 48-54), who, while emphatically not favouring a Canterbury origin, does inadvertently seem to weaken

CONTENTS: homilies; prognostics
LITERATURE: Wanley (1705: II.202-06); Planta (1802: 476-77); Förster (1920); Ker (1957: 271-77 [209]); Richards (1973); Handley (1974); Hollis & Wright (1992: 259); Treharne (1998: 227-29); Irvine (2000: 48-52); Wilcox (2000: 53-64 [245, ASMMF 8.7]); Liuzza (2001: 221 [V])

Vespasian D. xiv, fol. 75v/3-21 *17/2*
TYPE: year prognosis
LANGUAGE: OE
INCIPIT: Đonne forme gearesdæig byð sunendæig:
FACSIMILE: Wilcox (2000: 8.7.3)
EDITION: Assmann (1889a: 369);[121] Warner (1917: 66 [XXVI])[122]
TRANSLATION: Griffiths (1996: 228-29)
LITERATURE: Wanley (1705: II.204 [XXVIII]); Craig (1916: xxxv [2]); Förster (1920: 52 [25]); Ker (1957: 274 [209. 26]); Healey & Venezky (1980: 159 [Prog 5.1 (Warn), B23.3.5.1]); Matter (1982: 391 [2]); Quinn & Quinn (1990: 134 [F405]); Hollis & Wright (1992: 257); Wilcox (2000: 59 [245.28]); Voigts & Kurtz (2000: 170.00); Liuzza (2001: 221 [V1])

Vespasian D. xiv, fol. 103v/9-25 *5.1.4/1*
TYPE: brontology, temporal, month
LANGUAGE: OE
INCIPIT: **Emb þunre** [title] **O**n Ianuar*ius* monðe gyf hit þunreð:

the case for a Rochester genesis. Christ Church, Canterbury produced many prognostics, while Rochester is not known to have produced any, except possibly those in Vespasian D. xiv. I deem it more likely that the exemplar, if not the place of production for the prognostics, should be Christ Church rather than Rochester.

[121] Partly replicated Förster (1903: 349).

[122] Replicated Griffiths (1996: 228-29), Treharne (1998: 238).

FACSIMILE: Wilcox (2000: 8.7.4)
EDITION: Assmann (1888: 185);[123] Warner (1917: 91 [XXXIV]); Liuzza (2004: 12)
TRANSLATION: Griffiths (1996: 230-32), Liuzza (2004: 12, n. 42)
LITERATURE: Wanley (1705: II.204 [XXXVI]); Förster (1920: 55 [33]); Ker (1957: 274 [209.34]); Healey & Venezky (1980: 159 [Prog 5.2 (Warn), B23.3.5.2]); Quinn & Quinn (1990: 134 [F405]); Braswell (1984: 347); Hollis & Wright (1992: 257); Wilcox (2000: 60 [245. 36]);[124] Voigts & Kurtz (2000: 122.00); Liuzza (2001: 221 [V2])

London, British Library, Cotton Vitellius A. xii, fols 4-77
DATE: s. xi^{ex}
ORIGIN: Salisbury
CONTENTS: *Dialogus Egberti*; computus; notes; Isidore's *De natura rerum*; prognostic; computus; alphabets; calendars
LITERATURE: Wanley (1705: II.239); Planta (1802: 379-80); Van de Vyver (1935: 141, 150); Derolez (1954: 222-26 [8]); Stevens (1979: 194 [V]); Gneuss (1981: 27 [398]; 2001: 72 [398]); Gameson (1999: 104 [419]); Liuzza (2001: 221 [Sa])

Vitellius A. xii, fol. 44r/26-44v/1 *8.1/7*
TYPE: Egyptian Days, three days
LANGUAGE: L
INCIPIT: **DE DIEBVS ĘGYPTIACIS.** [title] **H**os dies maxime obseruare debemus.
LITERATURE: Planta (1802: 380 [5]); Thorndike (1923-58: I.695); Derolez (1954: 224); Liuzza (2001: 221 [Sa1])

Vitellius A. xii, fols 65v-71r *6/15*
TYPE: Dog Days

[123] Partly replicated Förster (1903: 351).

[124] Wilcox (2000: 60) foliated 103v/9-24.

LANGUAGE: L
INCIPIT: **DIES CANICVLARES.**
EDITION: Wormald (1934: 86-97 [7])

Vitellius A. xii, fols 72v-77v *8.3/17*
TYPE: Egyptian Days, twenty-four days
LANGUAGE: L
INCIPIT: **I**ani p*ri*ma dies & septima fine minat*ur*. [verse] Dies eg*yptiacus* [entry]

London, British Library, Cotton Vitellius A. xviii
AKA the Sacramentary of Giso of Wells
DATE: overall: s. xi²; additions to the calendar s. xi/xii-xii¹; calendar: s. xi²; Dog Days original to the calendar; Egyptian Days added s. xi/xii-xii¹
ORIGIN: Wells?
CONTENTS: calendar; sacramentary; prayer, exorcisms, benedictions
LITERATURE: Planta (1802: 381); Warren (1883: 303-07); Watson (1979: I.110 [575]); Gneuss (1981: 27 [400]; 2001: 72 [400]); Gameson (1999: 105 [421])

Vitellius A. xviii, fols 3r-8v *8.3/18*
TYPE: Egyptian Days, twenty-four days
LANGUAGE: L
INCIPIT: *Vicenam* q*uintam iani* p*rimam*q*ue caueto. / Rorat aquarius hanc. manet alt*e*ra sub ca*p*ricorno.* [verse] *Dies eg* [entry]
EDITION: Wormald (1934: 100-111 [8])

Vitellius A. xviii, fols 3r-8v *6/16*
TYPE: Dog Days
LANGUAGE: L
INCIPIT: **Incipiunt d*ies* canicul*ares*.**
EDITION: Wormald (1934: 100-111 [8])

London, British Library, Cotton Vitellius C. viii, fols 22-25
DATE: s. xi¹
ORIGIN: Winchester?[125]
CONTENTS: prayer; prognostic; computus
LITERATURE: Wanley (1705: II.241); Planta (1802: 424); Singer (1917: 110); Ker (1957: 292 [221]; 1959: lxiv); Gneuss (1981: 27 [404]; 2001: 73 [404]); Hollis & Wright (1992: 260); Liuzza (2001: 221-22); Wright & Hollis (2004: 84-95 [255, ASMMF 12.12])

Vitellius C. viii, fol. 22r/12-22v/4 *8.1/2*
TYPE: Egyptian Days, three days
LANGUAGE: OE
INCIPIT: Þry dagas syndon on geare þe we egiptiace hatað
FACSIMILE: Wright & Hollis (2004: 12.12.1)
EDITION: Hampson (1841: II.107); Förster (1929: 271-73 [V2])
TRANSLATION: Hampson (1841: II.107)
LITERATURE: Wanley (1705: II.241 [II]); Planta (1802: 424 [4]); Thorndike (1923-58: I.695); Ker (1957: 292 [221.2]); Healey & Venezky (1980: 95 [Days 4 (Först), B23.2.4]); Quinn & Quinn (1990: 132 [F204]); Hollis & Wright (1992: 258); Voigts & Kurtz (2000: 196.00); Gneuss (2001: 73 [404]); Liuzza (2001: 222 [1]); Wright & Hollis (2004: 89 [255.2.2])

London, British Library, Cotton Vitellius E. xviii
AKA the Vitellius Psalter
The computus of the manuscript shows similarities with the contents of Titus D. xxvi, xxvii. Ælfwine, dean and later abbot of New Minster, Winchester, is mentioned as the writer of the instructions for secret writing in Vitellius E. xviii, but the text is a copy from an older exemplar. The manuscript has sustained severe da-

[125] Ker (1957: 292) noted a strong link between Vitellius C. viii, fols 22-25, and Vitellius E. xviii: the Old English rules for finding Septuagesima and the note on concurrents and epacts in both manuscripts are "closely related to and perhaps the exemplar of no. 224 [i.e. Vitellius E. xviii], arts *e*, *f*". From this I infer that Vitellius C. viii, fols 22-25, will have been in Winchester at some time even if it did not originate there.

mage in the Cottonian Fire. Henel's supposition that one lost leaf preceding the calendar (i.e. *fol. 1**) will have contained a bloodletting lunary is likely in view of the bloodletting lunaries preceding the Winchester calendars in CCCC 422, pp. 27-40, Arundel 60, fols 1r-7v, and Titus D. xxvii, fols 2r-8v.[126]

DATE: overall: 1062;[127] additions s. xii (fols 141r-144r [litany and prayers]) and s. xiii/xiv (fols 9r [list of houses in confraternity], and 17rv [invocations to the Virgin Mary]); calendar and prognostics: 1062

ORIGIN: New Minster, Winchester[128]

CONTENTS: calendar; computus, prognostics, charms, instructions for secret writing; glossed Gallican psalter; prayer; glossed canticles; litany; prayers; lections

LITERATURE: Wanley (1705: II.222-24); Planta (1802: 431); Henel (1934a: 26-28, n. 78); Ker (1957: 298-301 [224]); Rosier (1962: xv-xviii); Bonser (1963: 26); Gneuss (1981: 28 [407]; 2001: 73 [407]); Hollis & Wright (1992: 260); Pulsiano (1994b: 50-56 [258, ASMMF 2.6]; 1995: 64 [10]; 1998a; 1998b); Liuzza (2001: 222 [Vi])

*Vitellius E. xviii, fol. 1*r* *9.2.3/6*

TYPE: lunary, specific, bloodletting (text lost)

LANGUAGE: L

LITERATURE: Henel (1934a: 26, n. 78)

Vitellius E. xviii, fols 2r-7v *8.3/19*

TYPE: Egyptian Days, twenty-four days

LANGUAGE: L

INCIPIT: **Iani prima dies & septima fine timetur.** [verse] ***Dies.*** [entry]

FACSIMILE: Pulsiano (1994b: 2.6.1)

EDITION: Hampson (1841: I.422-33); Wildhagen (1921: 77-94); Wormald (1934: 156-67 [12])

LITERATURE: Liuzza (2001: 222 [Vi1])[129]

Vitellius E. xviii, fols 2r-7v *6/17*

TYPE: Dog Days

LANGUAGE: L

INCIPIT: **Dies kaniculares** *`hic incipiu(nt.)´*

FACSIMILE: Pulsiano (1994b: 2.6.1)

EDITION: Hampson (1841: I.422-33); Wildhagen (1921: 77-94); Wormald (1934: 156-67 [12])

Vitellius E. xviii, fol. 9r/17-26 *15/2*

TYPE: unlucky days

LANGUAGE: OE

INCIPIT: **DE DIEBVS MALIS CVIVSQVE MENSIS:** [title] (T)weigen dagas syndon on æghwilcu*m* monðe.

FACSIMILE: Pulsiano (1994b: 2.6.1)

EDITION: Hampson (1841: II.76); Förster (1929: 262-64 [V])

TRANSLATION: Hampson (1841: II.76)

LITERATURE: Wanley (1705: II.222 [II. 3]); Henel (1934a: 27, n. 78 [fol. 9v]); Ker (1957: 299 [224.d]); Healey & Venezky (1980: 95 [Days 5.1 (Först), B23.2.5.1]); Quinn & Quinn (1990: 132-33 [F205]); Hollis & Wright (1992: 258); Pulsiano (1994b: 51-52 [258.1]; 1998b: 87); Voigts & Kurtz (2000: 204.00); Liuzza (2001: 222 [Vi2])

Vitellius E. xviii, fol. 13r/27-37 *6/1*

TYPE: Dog Days

LANGUAGE: OE

INCIPIT: **E**ahtatina nihtu*m* ær hlafmæssan gangeð se styrra up

FACSIMILE: Pulsiano (1994b: 2.6.1)

EDITION: Henel (1934-35: 331)

[126] Henel (1934a: 26, n. 78).

[127] Pulsiano (1998a; 1998b: 99-103), in a captivating analysis, assigned the composition of the psalter to 1062. Other scholars have assigned the manuscript to *c.* 1060.

[128] Ker (1957: 301) suggested Old Minster, though he mentioned that the calendar may have been produced in New Minster.

[129] Liuzza referred to the hexameter verses only.

LITERATURE: Wanley (1705: II.223 [II. 11]); Henel (1934a: 27, n. 78 [fol. 15r]); Ker (1957: 299 [224.g]); Healey & Venezky (1980: 161 [Prohib, B23.4]); Quinn & Quinn (1990: 134 [F407]); Hollis & Wright (1992: 258); Pulsiano (1994b: 52 [258.1]; 1998b: 88); Voigts & Kurtz (2000: 21.00); Liuzza (2001: 222 [Vi3])

Vitellius E. xviii, fol. 14v 2/6
TYPE: Apuleian Sphere
LANGUAGE: L
INCIPIT: (**SP**)**ERE:**– [title] (Ratio spere pythagori ph)ilosophi qua*m* appollogius descripsit
FACSIMILE: Pulsiano (1994b: 2.6.1)
COLLATION: Liuzza (2005: II.44-45 [Vi; incomplete])[130]
LITERATURE: Wanley (1705: II.223 [III]); Henel (1934a: 28, n. 78 [fol. 14v]); Pulsiano (1994b: 52 [258.1]; 1998b: 88); Liuzza (2001: 222 [Vi4])

Vitellius E. xviii, fol. 15r/1-5 3.1.2/3
TYPE: birth, temporal, 3 miraculous days
LANGUAGE: OE
INCIPIT: (Ð)ry dagas syndon on twelf monðum mid þrim ni(ht)um
FACSIMILE: Pulsiano (1994b: 2.6.1)
EDITION: Henel (1934-35: 346-47); Pulsiano (1998a: 6-7)[131]
LITERATURE: Henel (1934a: 27, n. 78 [fol. 13r]); Ker (1957: 300 [224.h]); Healey & Venezky (1980: 95 [Days 5.4 (Henel), B23.2.5.4]); Quinn & Quinn (1990: 132-33 [F205]); Hollis & Wright (1992: 258); Pulsiano (1994b: 52 [258.1]); Voigts & Kurtz (2000: 198.00); Liuzza (2001: 222 [Vi5])

Vitellius E. xviii, fol. 15r/6-15 8.1/3
TYPE: Egyptian Days, three days
LANGUAGE: OE
INCIPIT: **F**ind eft þry dagas on twelf monðum. þa syndon swiðe unhalwende
FACSIMILE: Pulsiano (1994b: 2.6.1)

[130] Collated with 2/9 (Sloane 475).

[131] Reprinted Pulsiano (1998b: 101).

EDITION: Förster (1929: 273-74 [W]);[132] Pulsiano (1998a: 7)[133]
LITERATURE: Henel (1934a: 27, n. 78 [fol. 13r]); Ker (1957: 300 [224.i]); Healey & Venezky (1980: 95 [Days 5.2 (Först), B23.2.5.2]); Quinn & Quinn (1990: 132-33 [F205]); Hollis & Wright (1992: 258); Pulsiano (1994b: 52 [258.1]); Voigts & Kurtz (2000: 25.00);[134] Liuzza (2001: 222 [Vi6])

Vitellius E. xviii, fol. 15r/16-15v/6 8.3/2
TYPE: Egyptian Days, twenty-four days
LANGUAGE: OE
INCIPIT: **Þ**a ealdan læcas gesettan on ledenbocum.
FACSIMILE: Pulsiano (1994b: 2.6.1)
EDITION: Hampson (1841: II.76 [incomplete]); Förster (1929: 266-69 [V])[135]
COLLATION: Henel (1934-35: 336-38 [V])[136]
TRANSLATION: Hampson (1841: II.77)
LITERATURE: Henel (1934a: 27-28, n. 78 [fol. 13rv]); Ker (1957: 300 [224.j]); Healey & Venezky (1980: 95 [Days 5.3 (Först), B23.2.5.3]); Quinn & Quinn (1990: 132-33 [F205]); Hollis & Wright (1992: 258); Pulsiano (1994b: 52 [258.1]; 1998b: 89); Voigts & Kurtz (2000: 176.00); Liuzza (2001: 222 [Vi7])

Vitellius E. xviii, fol. 16r/9-39 2/1
TYPE: Apuleian Sphere
LANGUAGE: L/OE
INCIPIT: **VITA VEL DE MORTE:**– [title] **S**pera apulei platonici de uita uel de morte
FACSIMILE: Pulsiano (1994b: 2.6.1); Pul-

[132] Corrections Henel (1934-35: 336, n. 1).

[133] Reprinted Pulsiano (1998b: 88-89, 101-02).

[134] Filed under the manuscript reading "Find eft" (incipit).

[135] Corrections Henel (1934-35: 336, n. 1).

[136] As variants to 8.3/3 (Harley 3271).

siano & Treharne (1998: pl. 11)
EDITION: Förster (1912c: 46-47 [text only]); Pulsiano (1998b: 90, 96)[137]
COLLATION: Liuzza (2005: II.39-40 [Vi; incomplete])[138]
LITERATURE: Wanley (1705: II.223 [IV]); Henel (1934a: 28, n. 78 [fol. 16r]); Ker (1957: 300 [224.r]); Healey & Venezky (1980: 148 [OccGl 37 (Först), C37]); Quinn & Quinn (1990: 163-64 [H232]); Pulsiano (1994b: 53 [258.1]); Liuzza (2001: 222 [Vi8])

London, British Library, Harley 585
DATE: overall: s. xi$^{1/10}$; additions s. xii-xiv;[139] prognostic: s. xi$^{1/10}$
ORIGIN: England[140]
CONTENTS: *Herbarium pseudo-Apulei*; *Medicina de quadrupedibus*; table of contents for *Herbarium* (booklet 1); *Lacnunga* and *Lorica* of Gildas (booklet 2)[141]
LITERATURE: Wanley (1705: II.304-05); Nares (1808: I.353-55); Grattan & Singer (1952: 206-08); Beccaria (1956: 249-50 [75]); Ker (1957: 305-306 [231]); Bonser (1963: 25); Talbot (1967: 21-23); Rubin (1974: 62-65); Gneuss (1981: 28 [421]; 2001: 75 [421]); Meaney (1984a: 245, 255-64); Vriend (1984: xxiii-xxviii [H]); Hollis & Wright (1992: 219); Cameron (1993: 31, 45-47); Doane (1994: 26-36 [265, ASMMF 1.5]); Liuzza (2001: 222-23)

Harley 585, fol. 190r/7-190v/16 *8.1/4*
TYPE: Egyptian Days, three days
LANGUAGE: OE
INCIPIT: Þry dagas syndon on geare þe we egiptiaci hatað
FACSIMILE: Doane (1994: 1.5.4)
EDITION: Cockayne (1864-66: III.76 [117-118]);[142] Leonhardi (1905: 152-53 [CXVII-CXVIII], 156); Förster (1929: 271-73 [H]); Grattan & Singer (1952: 198 [clxxxix])[143]
TRANSLATION: Cockayne (1864-66: III.77);[144] Grattan & Singer (1952: 199); Bonser (1963: 299 [incomplete]); Cameron (1993: 165)
LITERATURE: Nares (1808: I.355 [123]); Beccaria (1956: 250 [75.6]); Ker (1957: 306 [231.2]); Rubin (1974: 64); Healey & Venezky (1980: 140 [Med 3 (Grattan-Singer), B21.3]); Quinn & Quinn (1990: 120 [E007]); Hollis & Wright (1992: 219); Doane (1994: 35 [265.4]); Voigts & Kurtz (2000: 197.00); Gneuss (2001: 75 [421]); Liuzza (2001: 223 [1])

London, British Library, Harley 863
AKA the Leofric Psalter
The psalter was commissioned by Leofric, bishop of Exeter, 1046-72, and was probably given to Exeter cathedral. The calendar was added later.
DATE: overall: s. xi$^{3/4}$; calendar added s. xii^{ex}; calendar: s. xii^{ex}
ORIGIN: Exeter

[137] Pulsiano (1998b: 90, 96) numbered fol. 16r/8-18: he did not count the lines for the letter values and the diagram.

[138] As variants to 2/10 (Bodley 579).

[139] Ker dated fols 1-114 to s. x/xi, the table of contents on fols 115-129, and part of the *Lacnunga* on fols 179/11-193, to s. xi^1. Doane (1994: 26), however, dated the manuscript overall to s. xi$^{1/10}$, and mentioned that "despite Ker's dating of the two hands, probably no great interval separates them; the change of hands on fol. 179r seems to be a continuation of the same campaign of writing, following the same exemplar".

[140] Doane (1994: 26) suggested western England.

[141] On the booklets of Harley 585, see Robinson (1978: 234-35).

[142] Replicated Förster (1903: 353); reprinted Singer (1961: III.76).

[143] Replicated Cameron (1993: 165, n.13).

[144] Replicated Payne (1904: 19); reprinted Singer (1961: III.77).

CONTENTS: notes; calendar, Gallican psalter; canticles; litany; prayers; office
LITERATURE: Nares (1808: I.462-63); Ker (1957: 306-07 [232]); Watson (1979: I.120 [638]); Gneuss (1981: 28 [425]; 2001: 75 [425]); Pulsiano (1996: 37-43 [266, ASMMF 4.4])

Harley 863, fols 1r-6v *8.3/23*
TYPE: Egyptian Days, twenty-four days
LANGUAGE: L
INCIPIT: **Iani *pri*ma dies & septima fine timet*ur*.** [verse] **DIES MALA.** [entry]
FACSIMILE: Watson (1979: II, pl. 102 [detail of fol. 1r]); Pulsiano (1996: 4.4.1)
EDITION: Hampson (1841: I.449-60)[145]

London, British Library, Harley 3271
DATE: s. xi[1] (1032?)
ORIGIN: New Minster, Winchester?[146]
CONTENTS: grammatical texts; Tribal Hidage; notes on nations; Ælfric's *Grammar*; encyclopedic notes, prognostics and computus notes; *Beatus quid est*; prognostic; Office for the Invention of St. Stephen; Abbo of st. Germain's *Bella Parisiacae uribs* book 3 (with OE glosses and poetic version); prognostics and mass; Ælfric's sermon on the Seven Gifts of the Holy Spirit; excerpts from his *Letter to Sigeweard*; six ages of the world
LITERATURE: Nares (1808: III.13); Beccaria (1956: 250-51 [76]); Ker (1957: 309-12 [239]); Watson (1979: I.134 [743]); Gneuss (1981: 29 [435]; 2001: 77 [435]); Hollis & Wright (1992: 260); Liuzza (2001: 224-25 [G]); Chardonnens (2007b)

Harley 3271, fols 90v/20-91r/24 *8.3/3*
TYPE: Egyptian Days: twenty-four days (parts iii-vi (fols 90v/18-91r/4) precede i-ii (fol. 91r/5-24))
LANGUAGE: OE
INCIPIT: **DE DIEBVS MALIS.** [title] Þa ealdan læcas gesettan on ledenbocun:
EDITION: Henel (1934-35: 336-37)[147]
TRANSLATION: Griffiths (1996: 233-35)
LITERATURE: Nares (1808: III.13 [5]); Henel (1934a: 28, n. 78 [fol. 13rv]); Ker (1957: 310 [239.8-9]); Healey & Venezky (1980: 95 [Days 6 (Henel), B23.2.6]); Quinn & Quinn (1990: 133 [F206]); Hollis & Wright (1992: 258); Voigts & Kurtz (2000: 177.00); Liuzza (2001: 224 [G1,2]); Chardonnens (2007b: 29 [8])

Harley 3271, fol. 102v/1-16 *9.2.3/7*
TYPE: lunary, specific, bloodletting
LANGUAGE: L
INCIPIT: **DE SANGVINE MINVERE:–** [title] **L**VNA **i.** **T**ota die bona est.
LITERATURE: Beccaria (1956: 251 [76. 1]); Ker (1957: 310 [239.14]); Bayless (1993: 98); Liuzza (2001: 224 [G3]); Chardonnens (2007b: 32 [22])

Harley 3271, fol. 120v/1-20 *8.3/24*
TYPE: Egyptian Days, twenty-four days (the text is an extremely sloppy copy and has been repeated on fol. 122rv)
LANGUAGE: L (with one Old English gloss: dies primus lunę / se forma monandæg)
INCIPIT: \`IAN*VARIVS*´ \`Ia*ni* prima dies & septima fine timetur´ In principio mensis Ianuarii. dies primus.
COLLATION: Henel (1934-35: 339-40 [Ha])[148]

[145] The calendar contains a set of hexameter verses not printed by Hampson (1841: I.449-60). The verses he did append to the calendar are not from Harley 863 as he clearly indicated (1841: I.448), but Steele (1919: 119) replicated these as belonging to the calendar of Harley 863.

[146] The place of origin is unknown, but Winchester is a likely candidate (see Chardonnens 2007b).

[147] Replicated Griffiths (1996: 233-35).

[148] The goose prohibition is collated with that of 8.3/25 (Harley 3271). The Egyptian Days are taken from 8.3/25.

LITERATURE: Beccaria (1956: 251 [76. 4]); Ker (1957: 311 [239.19]); Healey & Venezky (1980: 151 [OccGl 67 (Henel-Ker), C67]); Quinn & Quinn (1990: 171 [H285]); Liuzza (2001: 224 [G4]); Chardonnens (2007b: 32 [27])

Harley 3271, fols 120v/20-121r/4 *6/19*
TYPE: Dog Days (a line in the right margin indicates that 8.1/8 should have followed 6/19; they are now separated by a mass of seventeen lines)[149]
LANGUAGE: L
INCIPIT: Est etiam istor*um* temporu*m* obseruanda ratio.
COLLATION: Henel (1934-35: 340-41 [Ha])[150]
LITERATURE: Beccaria (1956: 251 [76. 4]); Ker (1957: 311 [239.19]); Liuzza (2001: 224 [G4]); Chardonnens (2007b: 33 [28])

Harley 3271, fol. 121r/21-30 *8.1/8*
TYPE: Egyptian Days, three days (on the link with 6/19, see above)
LANGUAGE: L
INCIPIT: P*ost* viii kł april*is*. illa diȩ lunȩ
LITERATURE: Beccaria (1956: 251 [76. 4]); Ker (1957: 311 [239.19]); Liuzza (2001: 224 [G5]); Chardonnens (2007b: 33 [30])

Harley 3271, fol. 122r-122v/7 *8.3/25*
TYPE: Egyptian Days, twenty-four days
LANGUAGE: L
INCIPIT: VERSVS AD DIES AEGYPTIACOS. INVENI`A´NDAS. [title] **I**ANI PRIMA DIES ET SEPTIMA. FINE TIMETVR. **IANVAR*IVS*.** **I**n principio m*en*sis ianuarii dies prim*us*.
EDITION: Henel (1934-35: 339-40 [Hb])[151]
LITERATURE: Nares (1808: III.13 [10]); Beccaria (1956: 251 [76.2]); Ker (1957: 311 [239.19]); Thorndike (1923-58: I. 695); Thorndike & Kibre (1963: 651); Liuzza (2001: 224 [G6]); Chardonnens (2007b: 33 [32])

Harley 3271, fol. 122v/7-19 *6/20*
TYPE: Dog Days
LANGUAGE: L
INCIPIT: DE DIEB*VS* CANICVLARIBVS. [title] **E**st etia*m* istorum te*m*poru*m* obseruanda ratio:
COLLATION: Henel (1934-35: 339-41 [Hb])[152]
LITERATURE: Beccaria (1956: 251 [76. 3]); Ker (1957: 311 [239.19]); Thorndike & Kibre (1963: 508); Liuzza (2001: 224 [G7]); Chardonnens (2007b: 33 [33])

Harley 3271, fol. 122v/19-28 *8.1/9*
TYPE: Egyptian Days, three days
LANGUAGE: L
INCIPIT: DE TRIBVS DIEBVS AEGYPTIAC*IS*. [title] P*ost* viii. kł apr*ilis* illa die lunȩ.
LITERATURE: Beccaria (1956: 251 [76. 4]); Ker (1957: 311 [239.19]); Liuzza (2001: 224 [G8]); Chardonnens (2007b: 33 [34])

Harley 3271, fols 122v/29-123v/25 *12/1*
TYPE: regimen
LANGUAGE: L (with one Old English gloss: cataplasma / cliþa)[153]
INCIPIT: MEDICINA YPOGRATIS. QVID VSITARE DEBEATVR. PER SINGVLOS MENSES. [title] DE IAN-

[149] Ker (1957: 311) wrote "a Missa pro sacerdote occupies fol. 121/4-30". The mass, however, is on ll. 4-20.

[150] Collated with 6/14 (Titus D. xxvii) and 6/20 (also in Harley 3271).

[151] In Henel the text of the Egyptian Days is based on 8.3/25, but the goose prohibition is collated with that of 8.3/24 (also in Harley 3271)

[152] Collated with 6/14 (Titus D. xxvii) and 6/19 (also in Harley 3271).

[153] This gloss is not incorporated in the *Complete Corpus of Old English* (Healey and Venezky 2000).

VARIO. **M**ense ian*uario* non minuare sanguine*m*.
LITERATURE: Nares (1808: III.13 [11]); Beccaria (1956: 251 [76.5]); Ker (1957: 311 [239.19]); Thorndike & Kibre (1963: 868); Quinn & Quinn (1990: 171 [H285]); Liuzza (2001: 224 [G9]); Chardonnens (2007b: 33 [35])

Harley 3271, fols 123v/25-124r/9 *6/21*
TYPE: Dog Days
LANGUAGE: L (with one Old English gloss: catarticu*m* / spiwdrenc)
INCIPIT: DE FLEBOTOMAT`I´TIONE. MENSIS. AGVSTI. [title] Incipiente ortu canis u*e*l ar`c´turi atq*ue* siri stellæ.
EDITION: Henel (1934-35: 332 [H])[154]
LITERATURE: Beccaria (1956: 251 [76.6-7]); Ker (1957: 311 [239.19]); Thorndike & Kibre (1963: 726 [Dog Days], 1157 [moonbook]); Healey & Venezky (1980: 151 [OccGl 67 (Henel-Ker), C67]); Quinn & Quinn (1990: 171 [H285]); Liuzza (2001: 225 [G10,11]; Chardonnens (2007b: 34 [36])

London, British Library, Harley 3667
See Tiberius C. i, fols 2-42, + Harley 3667

London, British Library, Harley 6258B
DATE: s. xii$^{4/4}$; additions by the original scribe
ORIGIN: England
CONTENTS: OE *Herbarium*; *Medicina de quadrupedibus*; herb cures; *Peri didaxeon*
LITERATURE: Nares (1808: III.347); Löweneck (1896: v-viii); Ker (1957: xix); Bonser (1963: 25); Rubin (1974: 65-67); Meaney (1984a: 241-43); Vriend (194: xxviii-xxxviii [O]); Hollis & Wright (1992: 327-28); Cameron (1993: 33); Doane (1994: 44-48 [278, ASMMF 1.7]); Glaze (2007); Maion (2007)

Harley 6258B, fol. 51v/25-52v/9 *6/2*
TYPE: Dog Days (in medical tract)
LANGUAGE: OE
INCIPIT: **Incipit lib*er* qui dicit*ur* pe*ri* didaxeon.** [title] er onginþ seo boc p*er*i didax`e´on.
FACSIMILE: Doane (1994: 1.7.2-3)
EDITION: Cockayne (184-66: III.82-84); Löweneck (1896: 3-5)
TRANSLATION: Cockayne (1864-66: III.83-85)
LITERATURE: Healey & Venezky (2000: [PeriD, Cameron B21.6]);[155] Hollis & Wright (1992: 327); Doane (1994: 48 [278.5]); Voigts & Kurtz (2000: 89.00)

London, British Library, Royal 2. B. v
AKA the Regius Psalter
DATE: overall: s. x^{med} (psalter, canticles), additions s. x^{ex}-xi^{2}; prognostic: s. x^{ex}
ORIGIN: overall: Winchester (s. x-xi, fols 1-7 also from Winchester (St. Mary's?), transferred to Christ Church, Canterbury (s. xi and later [whence some of the additions and alterations originate]);[156] prognostic: Winchester
CONTENTS: office of the Virgin Mary; glossed maxims and proverbs; glossed Roman psalter with commentary; glossed canticles with scholia; encyclopedic notes, and prognostic; prayers; notes
LITERATURE: Wanley (1705: II.182); Warner & Gilson (1921: I.40-41); Ker (1957: 318-20 [249]); Gneuss (1981: 30 [451]; 2001: 79 [451]); Pulsiano (1994b: 57-64 [284, ASMMF 2.7]; 1995: 65 [14]); Liuzza (2001: 225 [R])

[154] Henel did not print the moonbook.

[155] Not in Healey and Venezky (1980). Pertains to *Peri didaxeon* in its entirety.

[156] Gneuss (1981: 30) suggested Worcester?, Winchester?, Christ Church Canterbury (see Pulsiano 1995: 65), which is probably based on the fact that the companion volume to Royal 2. B. v, Royal 4. A. xiv, resided in Worcester (see Sisam and Sisam 1959: 52-56).

Royal 2. B. v, fol. 190r/10-190v/7 5.1.4/2
TYPE: brontology, temporal, month (lacks entry for December)
LANGUAGE: L
INCIPIT: Si tonitruu*m* fuerit *in* m*en*se ianuario
FACSIMILE: Pulsiano (1994b: 2.7.7)
EDITION: Liuzza (2004: 8)
TRANSLATION: Liuzza (2004: 8, n. 28)
LITERATURE: Warner & Gilson (1921: I. 41 [8f]); Pulsiano (1994b: 63 [284.8]);[157] Gneuss (2001: 79); Liuzza (2001: 225 [R1])

London, British Library, Royal 12. D. xvii
AKA Bald's *Leechbook*
DATE: s. x^{med}
ORIGIN: Old Minster, Winchester
CONTENTS: Bald's *Leechbook* (fols 1r-58v [book I], fols 58v-108v [book II]); *Leechbook III* (fols 109r-127v)
LITERATURE: Wanley (1705: II.176-80); Payne (1904: 39-62); Warner & Gilson (1921: II.48); Wright & Quirk (1955: 11-30); Beccaria (1956: 263-64 [82]); Ker (1957: 332-33 [264]); Bonser (1963: 24-25); Talbot (1967: 18-20); Rubin (1974: 55-61); Gneuss (1981: 31 [479]; 2001: 83 [479]); Meaney (1984a: 236); Hollis & Wright (1992: 213); Cameron (1993: 30-32, 35-45); Doane (1994: 60-64 [298, ASMMF 1.10]); Getz (1998: 47-48); Nokes (2004)

Royal 12. D. xvii, fols 5v/20-6r/13 [in table of contents] 54v/19-55v/19 [text] 6/3
TYPE: Dog Days (in medical tract)
LANGUAGE: OE
INCIPIT: .lxxii **L**æcedomas on hwilce tid blod sie to forganne on hwilce to forlætenne [toc] .LXXII. On hwilce tid blod sie to forganne *on* hwilce to lætenne. [text]
FACSIMILE: Wright (1955: pl. 5b-6a (toc),54b-55b (text)); Doane (1994: 1.10.1 (toc), 1.10.2 (text))
EDITION: Cockayne (1864-66: II.14-16 (toc) II.146-48 (text) [I.lxxii]);[158] Leonhardi (1905: 5 (toc) 44-45 (text) [I.LXXII]); Mitchell (1995: 236 (text) [incomplete])
TRANSLATION: Cockayne (1864-66: II. 15-17 (toc) II.147-49 (text));[159] Bonser (1963: 296-97 [incomplete]); Cameron (1993: 161-62 (text)); Swanton (1993: 259-60 (text)); Mitchell (1995: 236 (text) [incomplete])
LITERATURE: Wanley (1705: 177 [LXXII]); Ker (1957: 332 [264.1]); Rubin (1974: 142); Healey & Venezky (1980: 121 [Lch II (1 Head) (toc) Lch II (1) (text), B21.2.1.1.1 (toc) B21.2.1.1.2 (text)]); Quinn & Quinn (1990: 119 [E003]); Hollis & Wright (1992: 211); Doane (1994: 61 [298.1a (toc) 298.1b (text)]); Voigts & Kurtz (2000: 102.00); Nokes (2004: 59-60, 63, 65)

London, British Library, Sloane 475, fols 125-231
Fols 125-231 of this composite volume are in various English hands.
DATE: s. xi^{ex} or xi/xii (fols 125-231); additions on fol. 209v-210v s. xiv
ORIGIN: England?[160]
CONTENTS: excerpts of Isidore's *Etymologiae*; Galen's *De febribus*; recipes, charms, prognostic; medical glossary; tract on urine; gynaecological tract; prognostics; medical recipes
LITERATURE: Thorndike (1923-58: I. 723-26); Beccaria (1956: 255-59 [78]);

[157] Pulsiano noted that this prognostic covers the months January, March, July and August whereas the text lists entries for all months except December.

[158] Replicated Cameron (1993: 195); reprinted Singer (1961: II.14-16, 146-48).

[159] Reprinted Singer (1961: II.15-17, 147-49).

[160] The place of origin of fols 125-231 is now taken to be England (Beccaria 1956: 255-59; Gneuss 2001: 85; Liuzza 2001: 225), but the redactions of the prognostics are continental (see pp. 42-3).

Cameron (1983: 144); Gameson (1999: 121 [567]); Gneuss (2001: 85 [498.1]); Liuzza (2001: 225-27 [S]); Wit (2002: 81 [7])

[Sloane 475, fols 4v/24-6r/1
TYPE: Egyptian Days, twenty-four days (in regimen)
LANGUAGE: L
LITERATURE: Beccaria (1956: 255 [78. 2]); Thorndike & Kibre (193: 632); Liuzza (2001: 226 [S1])]

[Sloane 475, fol. 6r/1-7
TYPE: Dog Days
LANGUAGE: L
LITERATURE: Liuzza (2001: 226 [S2])]

[Sloane 475, fol. 6r/7-13
TYPE: Egyptian Days, three days
LANGUAGE: L
LITERATURE: Liuzza (2001: 226 [S2])]

[Sloane 475, fols 7v/12-8r/16
TYPE: Dog Days (in medical tract)
LANGUAGE: L
LITERATURE: Beccaria (1956: 255 [78. 5])]

[Sloane 475, fol. 8r/16-24
TYPE: Egyptian Days, twenty-four days
LANGUAGE: L
EDITION: Steele (1919: 110 [lists dates only])
LITERATURE: Beccaria (1956: 255 [78. 6]); Gameson (1999: 121 [566]); Liuzza (2001: 226 [S3])]

[Sloane 475, fols 35r/18-36r/6
TYPE: regimen
LANGUAGE: L
LITERATURE: Beccaria (1956: 256 [78. 12]); Thorndike & Kibre (1963: 1033)]

[Sloane 475, fol. 37r/4-22
TYPE: lunary, specific, bloodletting
LANGUAGE: L
LITERATURE: Beccaria (1956: 256 [78. 14]); Liuzza (2001: 226 [S4])]

[Sloane 475, fols 58v/25-60r/17
TYPE: regimen
LANGUAGE: L
LITERATURE: Beccaria (1956: 257 [78. 15])]

[Sloane 475, fols 81r-82r/13
TYPE: lunary, specific, illness
LANGUAGE: L
EDITION: Weißer (1982: 365-73 [*Lo_{18}L])
LITERATURE: Beccaria (1956: 257 [78. 18]); Thorndike & Kibre (1963: 838); Liuzza (2001: 226 [S5])]

[Sloane 475, fol. 82r/13-25
TYPE: regimen
LANGUAGE: L
LITERATURE: Beccaria (1956: 257 [78. 19])]

[Sloane 475, fol. 82v/1-15
TYPE: regimen
LANGUAGE: L
LITERATURE: Beccaria (1956: 257 [78. 19])]

Sloane 475, fols 132v-133v/11 2/9
TYPE: Apuleian Sphere (opening lines and diagram lacking; dry-point circle on fol. 132v indicates that a diagram was to have appeared on this page)
LANGUAGE: L
INCIPIT: & partíris in trigintas **.xxx.** partes & quicquit remanserit in spera res pisties.
COLLATION: Liuzza (2005: II.44-45 [S; incomplete])[161]
LITERATURE: Thorndike (1923-58: I. 679);[162] Beccaria (1956: 258 [78.24a]);

[161] Collated with 2/6 (Vitellius E. xviii).

[162] Thorndike (1923-58: I.679) called this a weekday and name prognostic. The values for the weekdays and the letters in a name are part of the Apuleian Sphere, and it is likely that Thorndike was thinking along the wrong lines because of the absence of part of the explanatory texts and the diagram.

Liuzza (2001: 226 [S6])

Sloane 475, fol. 135v/4-13 *4/1*
TYPE: bloodletting, weekday
LANGUAGE: L
INCIPIT: **Incipiunt** ora se quod. sanguinem minuare debes.[title] in primis die dominico
LITERATURE: Thorndike (1923-58: I. 679); Liuzza (2001: 226 [S7])

Sloane 475, fols 211r-16v/4 *9.1/3*
TYPE: lunary, collective
LANGUAGE: L
INCIPIT: æc dies utilis est omib*us* reb*us* agendis.
EDITION: Svenberg (1936: 25-83 [L_3])[163]
LITERATURE: Craig (1916: xl); Thorndike (1923-58: I.681, n. 1); Förster (1944: 29 [12]); Beccaria (1956: 258 [78.28]); Martin (1981: 39 [17]]); Weißer (1982: 48 [Lo_3L]); Cameron (1983: 144 [7]); Gameson (1999: 121 [567]); Gneuss (2001: 85 [498.1]); Liuzza (2001: 226 [S8])

Sloane 475, fols 216v/4-217r/6 *8.3/26*
TYPE: Egyptian Days, twenty-four days
LANGUAGE: L
INCIPIT: Si ténębrę ęgýptus grecoa sermóne uocántur.
LITERATURE: Thorndike (1923-58: I. 695); Svenberg (1936: 14 [6]); Beccaria (1956: 258 [78.29]); Thorndike & Kibre (1963: 1466); Cameron (1983: 144 [8]); Gameson (1999: 121 [567]); Gneuss (2001: 85 [498.1]); Liuzza (2001: 226 [S9])

Sloane 475, fol. 217r/7-217v/12 *17/7*
TYPE: year prognosis
LANGUAGE: L
INCIPIT: Natalis d*omi*ni p*ri*ma dies si acciderit dominica
LITERATURE: Craig (1916: xxxiv); Thorndike (1923-58: I.678); Beccaria (1956: 259 [78.29]); Martin (1981: 39 [17]); Matter (1982: 389 [1]); Cameron (1983: 144 [9]); Liuzza (2001: 226 [S10])

Sloane 475, fols 217v/13-218r/19 *7/6*
TYPE: dreambook
LANGUAGE: L
INCIPIT: **A**ues in somnis uidere cu*m* ipsis pugnarę
COLLATION: Martin (1977: 186-259 [S]; 1981: 95-168 [S]); Epe (1995: 110-69 [AS])[164]
LITERATURE: Beccaria (1956: 259 [78. 29]); Thorndike (1923-58: II.295, n. 3); Thorndike & Kibre (1963: 170); Grub (1984: liv [S]); Hunt (1987: 180, n. 127); Gameson (1999: 121 [567]); Gneuss (2001: 85 [498.1]); Liuzza (2001: 227 [S11]); Wit (2002: 81)

London, Lambeth Palace Library, MS 427, fols 1-202

AKA the Lambeth Psalter

This composite manuscript originally contained the psalter prefaces, the psalter and canticles; fols 3-4 (prognostics) and the leaves after fol. 202 were added at a later date.
DATE: overall: s. xi[1] (fols 1-2, 5-202); additions s. xi-xv; prognostics: s. xii[1/4]
ORIGIN: Winchester?, transferred to Lanthony secunda[165]
CONTENTS: psalter prefaces; prognostics, computus; psalter preface; glossed Gallican psalter; glossed prayer; glossed form

[163] Corrections Svenberg (1939: 78-80; 1963: 16), Wistrand (1942: 23-35).

[164] In Martin (1981) as variants to 7/4 (Tiberius A. iii); in Epe as variants to the first series of entries in 7/4.

[165] O'Neill rejected Ker's suggestion that the manuscript originated from the priory of Lanthony. It is assumed that O'Neill referred to the psalter in its original state, so without fols 3-4 and the material added on fols 203-209, whereas the ascription "R. Lanthonie" is on fol. 209v, which, therefore, need not conflict with O'Neill's findings.

of confession; alliterative verse; glossed canticles
LITERATURE: Wanley (1705: II.268-69 [4° 188]); Lindelöf (1909-14: II.1-15); James & Jenkins (1930-32: IV.588-90); Ker (1957: 342-43 [280]); Gneuss (1981: 33 [517]; 2001: 87 [517]); O'Neill (1991); Pulsiano (1995: 65-66 [16])

Lambeth Palace 427, fol. 3ra *9.2.3/8*
TYPE: lunary, specific, bloodletting
LANGUAGE: L
INCIPIT: **L**una i Tota die bonu*m est*
LITERATURE: Wanley (1705: II.268]); Lindelöf (1909-14: II.1); James & Jenkins (1930-32: IV.588 [1]); O'Neill (1991: 144 [2])

Lambeth Palace 427, fol. 3rb *9.2.4/8*
TYPE: lunary, specific, dreams
LANGUAGE: L
INCIPIT: i *Q*uicqu*i*d uid*e*ris
LITERATURE: Wanley (1705: II.268]); Lindelöf (1909-14: II.1); James & Jenkins (1930-32: IV.588 [1]); O'Neill (1991: 144 [2])

Oxford, Bodleian Library, Bodley 579, fols 38-59 (2675)
AKA the *Leofric Missal*
Leofric, bishop of Crediton (1046-50) and Exeter (1050-72), gave the manuscript to Exeter Cathedral (s. xi^med^).[166] The manuscript consists of three units. Orchard has argued that Leofric A was the sacramentary of Archbishop Plegmund of Canterbury (devised *c.* 860-920); B are the changes and expansions to A made for Dunstan at Canterbury (s. x^2/4^, x^3/4^, 979-87); C are the changes and expansions made at Exeter (s. xi^med^)
DATE: Leofric B, fols. 38-59: 979-87 (fols 38-59); calendar and prognostics: 979-87
ORIGIN: section B: Christ Church, Canterbury, transferred to Exeter; calendar and prognostics: Christ Church, Canterbury (on the basis of a Glastonbury calendar)
CONTENTS: Section A: Gregorian sacramentary; Section B: computus, calendar, prognostics; Section C: manumissions, notes, masses, benedictions, exorcisms
LITERATURE: Warren (1883: xix-lxvi); Madan, Craster & Denholm-Young (1922-53: II.1.487-89 [2675]); Myres (1952: 14 [3]); Wormald (1952: 75-76 [49]); Ker (1957: 378-79 [315]); Pächt & Alexander (1966-73: I.33 [422], III.3 [20], III.4 [25]); Temple (1976: 44-45 [17]); Desham (1977); Gneuss (1981: 37 [585]; 2001: 95 [585]); Watson (1984: I.19 [103]); Nelson & Pfaff (1995: 93-94); Pfaff (1995a: 11-14); Liuzza (2001: 227 [L]); Orchard (2002)

Bodley 579, fols 39r-44v *6/22*
TYPE: Dog Days
LANGUAGE: L
INCIPIT: **DIES CANICVLARES.**
FACSIMILE: http://image.ox.ac.uk/show?collection=bodleian&manuscript=msbodl579
EDITION: Wormald (1934: 44-55 [4]); Orchard (2002: II.)

Bodley 579, fols 49v-50r *2/10*
TYPE: Apuleian Sphere
LANGUAGE: L
INCIPIT: **COLLIGE PER NVMERVM QVICQVID CVPIS ESSE PROBANDVM.**
FACSIMILE: Warren (1883: 44-45);[167] Heimann (1966: pl. 7a, 7c); Pächt & Alexander (1966-73: III, pl. III [25] [of fol. 49v]); Temple (1976: ill. 55-56); Desham (1977: 149; pl. II, VIIIb); Jordan (1986: 291, pl. 7, 294, pl. 9]); Orchard

[166] The date, origin and construction of Bodley 579 are extremely complicated matters, for which see Orchard's lucid analysis (2002: I).

[167] Replicated Singer (1928: 146, fig. 55), Grattan and Singer (1952: 40, 41, fig. 19-20), Jordan (1986: 292, pl. 8).

(2002: II.78-79 [287, 288; pl. 2, 3]); Liuzza (2005: II.31, pl. 1 [of fol. 50r]); http://image.ox.ac.uk/show?collection=bod leian& manuscript=msbodl579
EDITION: Voigts (1986: 298 [verse only]); Liuzza (2005: II.39-40 [L; incomplete])
TRANSLATION: Voigts (1986: 301, 305, n. 30 [verse only])
LITERATURE: Madan, Craster & Denholm-Young (1922-53: II.1.488 [2675. B]); Wormald (1952: 75-76); Temple (1976: 45); Ohlgren *et al.* (1986: 79 [95.3-4]); Liuzza (2001: 227 [L1]); Orchard (2002: I.189 [14, 15])

Bodley 579, fol. 56r/6-20 *9.2.3/9*
TYPE: lunary, specific, bloodletting
LANGUAGE: L
INCIPIT: **L**VNA PRIMA BONA EST
FACSIMILE: http://image.ox.ac.uk/show?collection=bodleian&manuscript=msbodl579
EDITION: Warren (1883: 54); Orchard (2002: II.94 [315])
LITERATURE: Liuzza (2001: 227 [L2]); Orchard (2002: I.192 [26k])

Oxford, Bodleian Library, Digby 63 (1664)
Digby 63 is written by the Frankish scribe Rægenbold, who brought the opening pages of the manuscript with him to England.
DATE: overall: 867-92; additions s. ix/x(?) (fols 9r, 25r, 41r [scribbles]), s. xi-xii (additions to the calendar); prognostic and calendar: 867-92
ORIGIN: Francia (fols 1-39), Northumbria (remainder). Kept at Old Minster, Winchester by *c.* 1000?
CONTENTS: computus
LITERATURE: Bond & Thompson (1873-83: II, pl. 168); Madan, Craster & Denholm-Young (1922-53: II.1.71-72 [1664]); Ker (1957: 381 [319]); Pächt & Alexander (1966-73: III.2 [16]); Gneuss (1981: 38 [611]; 2001: 98 [611]); Watson (1984: I.67 [419]), Stevens (1992: 134-36); Liuzza (2001: 227 [Di])

[Digby 63, fol. 36r/8-20
TYPE: Egyptian Days, twenty-four days
LANGUAGE: L
LITERATURE: Thorndike (1923-58: I. 686, 695); Liuzza (2001: 227 [Di1])]

[Digby 63, fol. 36r/21-36v/11
TYPE: Egyptian Days, three days
LANGUAGE: L
LITERATURE: Thorndike (1923-58: I. 685-86, 695); Liuzza 2001: 227 [Di1])]

Digby 63, fols 40r-45v *8.3/27*
TYPE: Egyptian Days, twenty-four days
LANGUAGE: L
INCIPIT: dies mala.
EDITION: Wormald (1934: 2-13 [1])
LITERATURE: Thorndike (1923-58: I. 686)[168]

Oxford, Bodleian Library, Douce 296 (21870)
DATE: s. $xi^{2/4}$
ORIGIN: Crowland
CONTENTS: calendar and computus; Gallican psalter; canticles; creeds; litany; prayers; office
LITERATURE: Madan, Craster & Denholm-Young (1922-53: IV.584 [21870]); Pächt & Alexander (1966-73: III.6 [43]); Temple (1976: 96-97 [79]); Gneuss (1981: 39 [617]; 2001: 98 [617]); Watson (1984: I.76 [471]); Keynes (1985)

Douce 296, fols 1r-6v *8.3/28*
TYPE: Egyptian Days, twenty-four days
LANGUAGE: L
INCIPIT: **IANI PRIMA DIES ET SEPTIMA FÍNE TIMETVR.** [verse] **Dies aegypti** [entry]
EDITION: Wormald (1934: 254-65 [20])

Douce 296, fols 1r-6v *6/23*
TYPE: Dog Days
LANGUAGE: L
INCIPIT: **Dies canicul*ares* incipiunt.**

[168] Thorndike remarked that 3 March and 3 July are the only dates listed, but more were entered into the calendar.

EDITION: Wormald (1934: 254-65 [20])

Oxford, Bodleian Library, Hatton 113 (5210)
Formerly Junius 99
AKA *St. Wulstan's Homiliary*, part 1
Hatton 113 and 114 formed one manuscript up to *c.* 1200, and were intended as a continuation of Oxford, Bodleian Library, Junius 121. The original manuscript was copied for use by Wulfstan II, bishop of Worcester (1062-95).
DATE: overall: s. $xi^{3/4}$ (fols ii verso-xi verso between 1064-83; fols ii recto, 1-144 between 1062-70), additions by Coleman (1080-1100), alterations to text and glosses (nearly contemporary with composition of the manuscript), marginalia added s. xii and xii/xiii, several layers of glosses in the Tremulous Worcester hand s. xiii^{1}; calendar: 1064-83
ORIGIN: Worcester
CONTENTS: letter to Wulfstan; prayers; calendar; computus; table of contents; homilies (Wulfstan, pseudo-Wulfstan, Ælfric)
LITERATURE: Wanley (1705: II.26-30); Turner (1916: lvi [3]); Bannister (1916); Madan, Craster & Denholm-Young (1922-53: II.2.967-68 [5134, 5210]); Ker (1957: 391-99 [331]); Gneuss (1981: 40 [637]; 2001: 100 [637]); Watson (1984: I. 85 [520]); Franzen (1991: 30-34 [MS C]; 1998: 26-34 [384a, ASMMF 6.6]); Gameson (1999: 138 [727])

Hatton 113, fols iii recto-viii verso *8.3/29*
TYPE: Egyptian Days, twenty-four days
LANGUAGE: L
INCIPIT: **D**ies mala.
FACSIMILE: Atkins (1928: 241-42, pl. xxxvi and xxxvii [of fols iv verso-v recto); Watson (1984: II, pl. 25a [detail of fol. viii verso); Franzen (1998: 6.6.1)
EDITION: Atkins (1928: 241-52); Wormald (1934: 198-209 [16])

Hatton 113, fols iii recto-viii verso *6/24*
TYPE: Dog Days
LANGUAGE: L
INCIPIT: **DIES CANICVLARES INCIPIVNT.**
FACSIMILE: Franzen (1998: 6.6.1)
EDITION: Atkins (1928: 241-52); Wormald (1934: 198-209 [16])

Oxford, Bodleian Library, Hatton 115 (5135)
Formerly Junius 23
With Lawrence, University of Kansas, Kenneth Spencer Research Library, Pryce C 2:2. The manuscript consist of five booklets with additions, which were bound together after 1200 but probably before the second layer of glosses by the Tremulous Worcester hand (s. xiii^{1}).[169]
DATE: table of contents: *c.* 1200 (fol. v

[169] Franzen (1998: 45) assigned the union of the five booklets into what is now known as Hatton 115 to s. xii at the earliest (though she did mention that booklets 1-3 may still have been separate from booklets 4 and 5 in s. xiii^{1}). Although this date stands to reason as booklet 5 was written in s. xii^{med}, it is problematic because the table of contents on fol. v recto lists rubricated items from booklets 1-3 only and dates to *c.* 1200. Moreover, the first layer of glosses in the Tremulous hand is in booklets 1-3 only, whereas the second layer covers 1-4 (Franzen 1991: 41-44; 1998: 46-47). It seems likely, therefore, that booklets 1-3 were originally bound together, and that the manuscript as it is now was put together in s. xiii^{1} (after the composition of the table of contents and after the first layer of glosses, but before the second layer of glosses in the Tremulous hand). A text fragment and two glosses by the Tremulous hand on fol. 154 (i.e. the fly-leaf of booklet 5), are of later date than the two layers of glosses. This, together with the absence of glosses on fols 148-153, makes one wonder (a) whether there was an intermediary stage in which Hatton 115 consisted of booklets 1-4 only.

recto[170]); booklet 1: 1060-80 (fols 1-64); additional material: 1080-1100 (fol. 65); additional material and booklets 2 and 3: 1060-80 (fols 66-67 [add.], 68-94 [2], 95-139 [3]); booklet 4: s. xi (fols 140-47); booklet 5: s. xii^{med} (fols 148-55); additions s. xii^{ex} (fol. 155r), s. xiii^{1} (fol. 154r [Tremulous hand]); first layer of glosses and additions in the table of contents by the Tremulous hand (on fols 1-139a), second layer of glosses in the Tremulous hand (on fols 1-147), text fragment[171] and two glosses in the Tremulous hand (fol. 154), s. xiii^{1};[172] prognostics: s. xii^{med} (booklet 5)
ORIGIN: booklets 1-3: England. Booklets 1-3 were in Worcester by *c.* 1200, when a table of contents was added, and the shelf mark "XXII" on fol. 1r in a hand of s. xii/xiii (cf. "Sermones anglice XX" (retouched) on the spine of Hatton 113 and "Sermones anglici XXI" in Hatton 114, fol. 1r). Around this time, therefore, booklets 1-3 must have been a unit, but Hatton 115 as it is now did not yet exist; booklet 4: England. Booklet 4 was originally not bound with 1-3 as the table of contents does not cover the items in booklet 4. Ker commented that booklet 4 "has long been bound with the rest [i.e. 1-3], but was not originally so, since 2 out of 7 wormholes on fol. 139 do not reappear on fol. 140: fols 140 and 147, the outer pages of the quire [=booklet 4], show signs of exposure";[173] booklet 5: Christ Church, Canterbury?[174] It is certain that booklets 4 and 5 were in Worcester s. xiii^{1}, when they were bound with booklets 1-3. prognostics: Christ Church, Canterbury? (s. xii^{med}), transferred to Worcester (before or in s. xiii^{1})
CONTENTS: table of contents; homilies, short pieces (1); homily, two short pieces (additions); homilies (2); homilies, Old Testament pieces (3); Vercelli homily IX (4); prognostics, two notes on fasting (5)
LITERATURE: Wanley (1705: II.36-40); Förster (1912a: 55, n. 1); Turner (1916: lvi [4]); Madan, Craster & Denholm-Young (1922-53: II.2.968-69 [5135]); Ker (1957: 399-403 [332]; 1976: 124-25); Collins (1976: 50-51 [7]); Gneuss (1981: 40 [639]; 2001: 101 [639]); Franzen (1991: 38-44 [MS E]; 1998: 44-54 [385, ASMMF 6.8]); Hollis & Wright (1992: 259); Treharne (1998: 235-39); Gameson (1999: 138 [729]); Liuzza (2001: 227-28 [H])

Hatton 115, fol. 148r *9.2.4/4*
TYPE: lunary, specific, dreams (lacks day 11)
LANGUAGE: OE

[170] The table of contents lists items of booklets 1-3, which implies that 4-5 were not part of the manuscript at this time. Moreover, material added between booklets 1 and 2 may not have been positioned where it is now (Ker 1957: 402; Franzen 1991: 43; 1998: 45). The Tremulous hand added entries to the table of contents for non-rubricated items on fols 58-67, from booklet 1 and the added material (Franzen (1991: 43).

[171] A prognostic copied in the same state of the Tremulous hand is in CCCC 391, p. 721 (Franzen 1991: 14-15, 69).

[172] For a description of the work of the Tremulous hand in Hatton 115, see Franzen (1991: 41-44, 84-102).

[173] Ker (1957: 399); see also Robinson (1978: 235-36).

[174] The date and origin of booklet 5 are disputed (see Ker 1957: 403; Franzen 1991: 40; 1998: 44-45). I have adopted the date advanced by Treharne (1998: 235-39). She placed the origin of booklet 5 in the south, possibly Kent, on the basis of script, language and content. Similarities with prognostics in Tiberius A. iii (Christ Church, Canterbury) and Vespasian D. xiv (Christ Church, Canterbury?) would posit an exemplar, if not the origin of booklet 5, in Christ Church.

INCIPIT: **Ð**Ære æresten nyhte þonne niwe mone byð ecymen.
FACSIMILE: Franzen (1998: 6.8.5)
EDITION: Cockayne (1864-66: III.158-60); Förster (1925-26: 90-92)[175]
TRANSLATION: Cockayne (1864-66: III. 159-61); Griffiths (1996: 224-26)
LITERATURE: Wanley (1705: II.40 [33]); Craig (1916: xxxix); Ker (1957: 402 [332. 35.a]); Healey & Venezky (1980: 159 [Prog 6.1 (Först), B23.3.6.1]); Quinn & Quinn (1990: 134 [F406]); Hollis & Wright (1992: 258); Franzen (1998: 51 [385.35.a]); Voigts & Kurtz (2000: 178. 00); Liuzza (2001: 227-28 [H1])

Hatton 115, fol. 148v/1-18 *9.2.2/4*
TYPE: lunary, specific, birth (ends with day 14)
LANGUAGE: OE
INCIPIT: **SE** ðe bið acenned on annihtne mona.
FACSIMILE: Franzen (1998: 6.8.5); Pulsiano & Treharne (1998: pl. 18)
EDITION: Cockayne (1864-66: III.160-62); Förster (1912c: 21-24 [H])
TRANSLATION: Cockayne (1864-66: III. 161-63)
LITERATURE: Wanley (1705: II.40 [34]); Craig (1916: xl); Ker (1957: 402 [332.35. b]); Healey & Venezky (1980: 159 [Prog 6.2 (Först), B23.3.6.2]); Quinn & Quinn (1990: 134 [F406]); Hollis & Wright (1992: 258); Franzen (1998: 51 [385.35. b]); Voigts & Kurtz (2000: 141.00); Liuzza (2001: 228 [H2])

Hatton 115, ff. 148v/19-149r/11 *3.1.3/2*
TYPE: birth, temporal, weekday
LANGUAGE: OE
INCIPIT: **SWA** hwilc man swa on sunnandæg. oððe on niht acenned bið.
FACSIMILE: Franzen (1998: 6.8.5); Pulsiano & Treharne (1998: pl. 18-19)[176]
EDITION: Cockayne (1864-66: III. 162);[177] Förster (1912b: 297-300)[178]
TRANSLATION: Cockayne (1864-66: III. 163)
LITERATURE: Wanley (1705: II.40 [35]); Ker (1957: 402 [332.35.c]); Healey & Venezky (1980: 160 [Prog 6.3 (Först), B23.3.6.3]); Quinn & Quinn (1990: 134 [F406]); Hollis & Wright (1992: 258); Franzen (1998: 51 [385.35.c]); Voigts & Kurtz (2000: 153.00); Liuzza (2001: 228 [H3])

Hatton 115, fol. 149r/12-149v/7 *17/3*
TYPE: year prognosis
LANGUAGE: OE
INCIPIT: **G**if middeswintres messedeg b`i´ð on sunnandeg.
FACSIMILE: Franzen (1998: 6.8.5); Pulsiano & Treharne (1998: pl. 19 [of fol. 149r (not 149v!)])
EDITION: Cockayne (1864-66: III.162-64)[179]
TRANSLATION: Cockayne (1864-66: III. 163-65)
LITERATURE: Wanley (1705: II.40 [36]); Hellmann (1896b: 58, 61); Craig (1916: xxxv [1]); Ker (1957: 402 [332.35.d]); Healey & Venezky (1980: 160 [Prog 6.4 (Cockayne), B23.3.6.4]); Matter (1982: 391 [1]); Quinn & Quinn (1990: 134 [F406]); Hollis & Wright (1992: 258); Franzen (1998: 51 [385.35.d]); Voigts & Kurtz (2000: 52.00); Liuzza (2001: 228 [H4])

Hatton 115, fol. 149v/8-23 *16/1*
TYPE: wind prognostic
LANGUAGE: OE
INCIPIT: **HER** segh ymb drihtnes gebyrd. ymb þa .xii. niht hs tide. [title] Gyf se

[175] Replicated Griffiths (1996: 224-26).
[176] The caption for pl. 19 in Pulsiano and Treharne refers to fol. 149v.
[177] Partly replicated Förster (1903: 355).
[178] Corrections Förster (1912c: 49).
[179] Partly replicated Förster (1903: 349; 1908b: 299); adapted Treharne (1998: 237-38).

wind byoð on þa forma niht.
FACSIMILE: Franzen (1998: 6.8.5)
EDITION: Cockayne (1864-66: III.164); Förster (1912a: 56-58)
TRANSLATION: Cockayne (1864-66: III. 165)
LITERATURE: Hellmann (1896b: 58, 65); Ker (1957: 402 [332.35.e]); Healey & Venezky (1980: 160 [Prog 6.5 (Först), B23.3.6.5]); Quinn & Quinn (1990: 134 [F406]); Hollis & Wright (1992: 258); Franzen (1998: 52 [385.35.e]); Voigts & Kurtz (2000: 78.00); Liuzza (2001: 228 [H5])

Hatton 115, fols 149v/24-150r/17 *14/2*
TYPE: sunshine prognostic
LANGUAGE: OE
INCIPIT: **Þ**y forma dæg drihtnes gebyrde. gyf sunne scyneð.
FACSIMILE: Franzen (1998: 6.8.5)
EDITION: Cockayne (1864-66: III.164-66); Förster (1912a: 65 [H])[180]
TRANSLATION: Cockayne (1864-66: III. 165-67)
LITERATURE: Hellmann (1896b: 58, 65); Ker (1957: 402 [332.35.f]); Healey & Venezky (1980: 160 [Prog 6.6 (Först), B23.3.6.6]); Quinn & Quinn (1990: 134 [F406]); Hollis & Wright (1992: 258); Franzen (1998: 52 [385.35.f]); Voigts & Kurtz (2000: 200.00); Liuzza (2001: 228 [H6])

Hatton 115, fol. 150v/1-9 *5.1.3/3*
TYPE: brontology, temporal, weekday
LANGUAGE: OE
INCIPIT: **O**N anwardne ger gyf hyt þunrie on sunandæg.
FACSIMILE: Franzen (1998: 6.8.5)
EDITION: Cockayne (1864-66: III.166-68); Liuzza (2004: 15)
TRANSLATION: Cockayne (1864-66: III. 167-69)
LITERATURE: Wanley (1705: II.40 [37]); Ker (1957: 402 [332.35.i]); Healey & Venezky (1980: 160 [Prog 6.7 (Cockayne), B23.3.6.7]); Quinn & Quinn (1990: 134 [F406]); Hollis & Wright (1992: 258); Franzen (1998: 52 [385.35. i]); Voigts & Kurtz (2000: 116.00); Liuzza (2001: 228 [H8])

Hatton 115, fols 150v/10-152v/3 *7/3*
TYPE: dreambook
LANGUAGE: OE
INCIPIT: **G**yf mon meteð *þæt* he geseo earn on his heafod unfan ge settan.
FACSIMILE: Franzen (1998: 6.8.5)
EDITION: Förster (1916: 270-93 [H])
COLLATION: Cockayne (1864-66: III. 168-76 [J]);[181] Epe (1995: 192-211 [EH])[182]
TRANSLATION: Cockayne (1864-66: III. 169-77)[183]
LITERATURE: Wanley (1705: II.40 [38]); Ker (1957: 402 [332.35.j]); Healey & Venezky (1980: 160 [Prog 6.8 (Först), B23.3.6.8]); Quinn & Quinn (1990: 134 [F406]); Hollis & Wright (1992: 258); Franzen (1998: 52 [385.35.j]); Voigts & Kurtz (2000: 55.00); Liuzza (2001: 228 [H10])

Hatton 115, fols 152v/4-153v/16 *9.2.1/2*
TYPE: lunary, specific, agenda (deliberately ends with day 17)[184]
LANGUAGE: OE
INCIPIT: **O**N annihte monan fær to cy-

[180] Förster designated the manuscript variously as Hatton 115 and 116. He used the first three entries to complete 14/1 (CCCC 391), the remainder as variants to 14/1.

[181] Collated with 7/1 (Tiberius A. iii). Replicated Förster (1908b: 302-05) as variants to 7/2 (Tiberius A. iii). Partly replicated Griffiths (1996: 221-24).

[182] As variants to 7/1 (Tiberius A. iii).

[183] Replicated Griffiths (1996: 221-24).

[184] Strong punctuation after day 17 indicates the end of copying. The term 'strong punctuation' is borrowed from Ker (1957: 247 [186.29]).

ninge.
FACSIMILE: Franzen (1998: 6.8.5)
EDITION: Cockayne (1864-66: III.176-80); Förster (1912c: 43-45 [C])
TRANSLATION: Cockayne (1864-66: III. 177-81)
LITERATURE: Wanley (1705: II.40 [39]); Craig (1916: xxxix); Ker (1957: 402 [332. 35.k]); Healey & Venezky (1980: 160 [Prog 6.9 (Först), B23.3.6.9]); Quinn & Quinn (1990: 134 [F406]); Hollis & Wright (1992: 258); Franzen (1998: 52 [385.35.k]); Voigts & Kurtz (2000: 110. 00); Liuzza (2001: 228 [H11])

Oxford, St. John's College, MS 17
AKA the *Ramsey Computus*
A medical section precedes and follows the computus on fols 1-2, 175-77. Nero C. vii, fols 80-84, originally belonged to St. John's College 17. This manuscript is a copy of an autograph by Byrhtferth of Ramsey which was used in the making of Byrhtferth's *Enchiridion*. Some prognostics in St. John's College 17 are also in Tiberius C. i, fols 2-42, + Harley 3667.
DATE: 1110-11, additions s. xiii^{ex} [185]
ORIGIN: Thorney Abbey[186]
CONTENTS: medicine; science, runes, computus, prognostics; Byrhtferth's computus, calendar; excerpts from Bede's *De temporum ratione*, *De natura rerum*; excerpts from Helperic's *De computo ecclesiastico*; Thorney annals; grammar, science, computus
LITERATURE: Coxe (1852: II.5-8); Singer (1917: 117-27); Haskins (1924: 83-84); Van de Vyver (1935: 144-45, 147); Derolez (1954: 26-34 [3]); Ker (1957: 435 [360]); Hart (1970); Rubin (1974: 67-68); Kauffmann (1975: 56-57 [9]); Lapidge (1980: 21-22 [IV.5]); Gneuss (1981: 43 [683]); Baker (1982: 124-27); Cameron (1983: 150; 1993: 33, 54-58); Watson (1984: I.146 [867]); Alexander & Temple (1985: 3 [5]); Wallis (1985: I; 1995: 122-27); Baker & Lapidge (1995: liii-lv [J]); Gameson (1999: 144 [794]); Liuzza (2001: 229-30 [J])

St. John's College 17, f. 1va-1vb/16 *6/25*
TYPE: Dog Days (in medical tract)
LANGUAGE: L
INCIPIT: Hi q*ua*ttuor humores d*omi*nant*ur* in suis locis.
EDITION: Singer (1917: 130-33 [3])
TRANSLATION: Singer (1917: 152 [incomplete])
LITERATURE: Coxe (1852: II.5 [1]); Derolez (1954: 27); Cameron (1983: 153 [3]); Wallis (1985: I.167-68 [A1b]; 1995: 122 [2a]); Hanna (2002: 27-28 [1])

St. John's College 17, f. 1vb/17-32[187] *6/26*
TYPE: Dog Days (in medical tract)
LANGUAGE: L
INCIPIT: DE FLEBOTOMIA. [title] Si necessitas fuer*it* o*mn*i t*em*p*or*e
EDITION: Singer (1917: 130-33 [3])
TRANSLATION: Singer (1917: 152 [incomplete])
LITERATURE: Coxe (1852: II.5 [1]); Bonser (1963: xix); Cameron (1983: 153 [3]); Wallis (1985: I.168-70 [A2)]; 1995: 122 [2b]); Hanna (2002: 27-28 [1])

St. John's College 17, f. 3va/29-35 *8.1/10*
TYPE: Egyptian Days, three days
LANGUAGE: L
INCIPIT: Hi tres dies pl*us* *sun*t obseruandi.
LITERATURE: Singer (1917: 118); Thorndike & Kibre (1963: 613); Wallis (1985: I. 192-94 [B3a]; 1995: 122 [3c]); Hanna

[185] The date of this manuscript is uncertain, and, according to some scholars, depends heavily on the annals in the computistical part of the manuscript.

[186] The place of origin is uncertain; the latest opinion is that it was copied in Thorney Abbey.

[187] Foliation refers to that part of the text pertaining to the Dog Days. The entire tract occupies fols 1vb/17-2rb/44, 2va/27-33.

(2002: 28 [3]);[188] Liuzza (2001: 229 [J1])

St. John's College 17, f. 3va/36-41 3.1.2/6
TYPE: birth, temporal, 3 miraculous days
LANGUAGE: L
INCIPIT: Tres dies *sunt* in *quoque* anno cu*m* t*ri*b*us* noctib*us*
LITERATURE: Singer (1917: 118); Wallis (1985: I.194-95 [B3b]; 1995: 122 [3c]); Hanna (2002: 28 [3]);[189] Liuzza 92001: 229 [J2])

St. John's College 17, f. 4ra/1-30 9.2.3/10
TYPE: lunary, specific, bloodletting (text has undergone extensive revision)
LANGUAGE: L
INCIPIT: **Luna .i. T**ota die bona *est.*
LITERATURE: Coxe (1852: II.5 [8]); Thorndike (1923-58: I.680, n. 1); Derolez (1954: 27); Weißer (1982: 57 [5]); Wallis (1985: I.202-04 [B6]; 1995: 122 [3f]); Hanna (2002: 28 [3]);[190] Liuzza (2001: 229 [J3])

St. John's College 17, f. 4ra/31-45 3.1.3/5
TYPE: birth, temporal, weekday
LANGUAGE: L
INCIPIT: **D**ie d*omi*nico hora diut*ur*na siue noct*ur*na q*ui* nascent*ur*
LITERATURE: Wallis (1985: I.204-10 [B7]; 1995: 123 [3g]); Hanna (2002: 28 [3]);[191] Liuzza (2001: 229 [J4])

St. John's College 17, f. 4rb/1-30 9.2.2/8
TYPE: lunary, specific, birth
LANGUAGE: L
INCIPIT: **Luna i** Q*ui* nat*us* fuerit
LITERATURE: Weißer (1982: 57 [4]); Wallis (1985: I.202-04 [B6]; 1995: 122 [3f]); Hanna (2002: 28 [3]);[192] Liuzza (2001: 229 [J5])

St. John's College 17, fol. 4rb/31-4rc/16 9.2.5/7
TYPE: lunary, specific, illness
LANGUAGE: L
INCIPIT: **Luna i** Q*ui* cecid*er*it
COLLATION: Weißer (1982: 273-77 [*Ox_2L])[193]
LITERATURE: Wallis (1985: I.202-04 [B6]; 1995: 122 [3f]); Hanna (2002: 28 [3]);[194] Liuzza (2001: 229 [J6])

St. John's College 17, f. 4rc/17-46 9.2.4/9
TYPE: lunary, specific, dreams
LANGUAGE: L
INCIPIT: **Lun*a* i** Q*ui*cq*ui*d uid*er*is
LITERATURE: Weißer (1982: 57 [6]); Wallis (1985: I.202-04 [B6]; 1995: 122 [3f]); Hanna (2002: 28 [3]);[195] Liuzza (2001: 229 [J7])

St. John's College 17, fol. 8rb 2/11
TYPE: Apuleian Sphere (consists of diagram only; contains coded writing)
LANGUAGE: L
EDITION: Derolez (1954: 29 [coded writing only])
FACSIMILE: Singer (1917: 121, fig. 1; 1928: 167, fig. 65[196])
LITERATURE: Coxe (1852: II.6 [16]); Derolez (1954: 29); Bonser (1963: 157, n. 4); Wallis (1985: I.248-50 [C2]; 1995: 123 [4b]); Hanna (2002: 32 [7]); Liuzza (2001: 229 [J8])[197]

St. John's College 17, ff. 16r-21v 8.3/30
TYPE: Egyptian Days, twenty-four days
LANGUAGE: L
INCIPIT: **IANI PRIMA DIES ET SEP-**

[188] Hanna did not distinguish the individual prognostics on fols 3v-4r.

[189] *Ibid.*

[190] *Ibid.*

[191] *Ibid.*

[192] *Ibid.*

[193] As variants to Harley 3017, fol. 58v.

[194] Hanna did not distinguish the individual prognostics on fols 3v-4r.

[195] *Ibid.*

[196] Replicated Grattan and Singer (1952: 48, fig. 23), Singer (1961: I.xxv, fig. 3).

[197] Wallis and Liuzza erroneously referred to fol. 8v.

TIMA FINE TIMETVR. [verse] ***Dies* mala.** [entry]
EDITION: Steele (1919: 113);[198] Baker & Lapidge (1995: 391-416 [15])
LITERATURE: Wallis (1985: I.306-23 [D1]; 1995: 123 [5]); Hanna (2002: 28-29 [10]); Liuzza (2001: 229 [J9])[199]

St. John's College 17, f. 40va/18-39 8.2/2
TYPE: Egyptian Days, twelve days
LANGUAGE: L
INCIPIT: Isti dies obseruandi s*un*t in singu*lis* m*en*sib*us*.
LITERATURE: Wallis (1985: I.456-57 [G1]; 1995: 123 [8]); Liuzza (2001: 229 [J10a])

St. John's College 17, f. 40vb/18-31 15/3
TYPE: unlucky days
LANGUAGE: L
INCIPIT: S*un*t in unoq*uoque* m*en*se duo dies. q*uo*d cu*m* in eis incipit*ur*. n*on* finit*ur* u*n*q*uam*.
LITERATURE: Wallis (1985: I.457 [G2]; 1995: 123 [8]); Liuzza (2001: 229 [J10b])

St. John's College 17, fol. 40vb/32-49 8.3/31
TYPE: Egyptian Days, twenty-four days
LANGUAGE: L
INCIPIT: De dieb*us* ęgyptiacis q*ui* maledicti s*un*t in anno. [title] His dieb*us* n*on* debent ho*min*es se flebotomare.
LITERATURE: Wallis (1985: I.457-58 [G3]; 1995: 123 [8]); Liuzza (2001: 229 [J10c])

St. John's College 17, fol. 41ra 2/12
TYPE: Apuleian Sphere
LANGUAGE: L
INCIPIT: Ratio sperę phytagori phylosophi que*m* apulei*us* descripsit.
EDITION: Liuzza (2005: II.40-44 [J; incomplete])
LITERATURE: Wallis (1985: I.458-59 [G4]; 1995: 123 [8]); Baker & Lapidge (1995: liv [J.c], 427 [54]); Hanna (2002: 32 [11]); Liuzza (2001: 229-30 [J11])

St. John's College 17, fol. 41rb 2/13
TYPE: Apuleian Sphere (diagram has been excised)[200]
LANGUAGE: L
INCIPIT: **D**e quacumq*ue* re scire uolueris *ue*l consulere.
COLLATION: Liuzza (2005: II.40-44 [J[2]; incomplete])[201]
LITERATURE: Wallis (1985: I.459-60 [G5]; 1995: 123 [8]); Baker & Lapidge (1995: liv [J.c], 427 [54]); Hanna (2002: 32 [11]); Liuzza (2001: 229-30 [J11])

St. John's College 17, fols 157vb/9-158va/8 13/1
TYPE: *Sortes Sanctorum* (lacks entry ii.ii.ii; ends with a prayer)
INCIPIT: **.c.c.c.** Animu*m* tuu*m* si dubitante*m* sentis crede p*rimo* modu*m* d*e*o adiuuante i*m*petrabis q*u*ę uis;
LANGUAGE: L
LITERATURE: Coxe (1852: II.7 [49]); Thorndike (1923-58: I.680, n. 1); Derolez (1954: 28); Wallis (1985: I.574-76 [L4]; 1995: 124 [13.b]); Hanna (2002: 31 [25]); Liuzza (2001: 230 [J12])

St. John's College 17, f. 159rb/5-38 17/8
TYPE: year prognosis
LANGUAGE: L
INCIPIT: **Si** p*ri*ma feria kł ian*uarii* fuerit.

[198] Steele printed the hexameter verse for February only.

[199] Liuzza referred to the hexameter verses only.

[200] Exactly when the diagram was excised is not known, but it must have happened in the sixteenth century or after, because the sixteenth(?)-century writer who, in the margins, added comments upon the medieval texts, also added a description in the top margin of fol. 41v. This description is now incomplete since the opening part was lost when the diagram on its reverse side was excised.

[201] Partly as variants to 2/12 (also in St. John's College 17).

LITERATURE: Wallis (1985: I.580-81 [L8]); Hanna (2002: 31 [28]); Liuzza (2001: 230 [J13])

Rome, Vatican City, Bibliotheca Apostolica Vaticana, Reg. lat. 12
AKA the Bury St. Edmunds Psalter
DATE: s. $xi^{2/4}$
ORIGIN: Christ Church, Canterbury?[202]
CONTENTS: penitential prayers; calendar, computus; Gallican psalter; canticles; paternoster, creeds; litany; prayers
LITERATURE: Thompson et al. (1913-30: X, XI, pl. 166-68); Wilmart (1937-45: I. 30-35); Temple (1976: 100-02 [84]); Gneuss (1981: 58 [912]; 2001: 140 [912]); Ohlgren (1992: 2-3 [3])

Reg. lat. 12, fols 7r-12v *8.3/32*
TYPE: Egyptian Days, twenty-four days
LANGUAGE: L
INCIPIT: **Dies mala.**
FACSIMILE: Thompson et al. (1913-30: X, XI, pl. 168a [of fol. 11v])
EDITION: Wormald (1934: 240-51 [19])

Reg. lat. 12, fols 7r-12v *6/27*
TYPE: Dog Days
LANGUAGE: L
INCIPIT: **Dies caniculares.**
EDITION: Wormald (1934: 240-51 [19])

Rouen, Bibliothèque municipale, MS 274 (Y. 6)
AKA the *Missal of Robert of Jumièges*
The calendar antedates the rest of the manuscript. The manuscript was donated to Jumièges by Robert of Jumièges, bishop of London (1044-50), archbishop of Canterbury (1050-52), during his appointment in London.
DATE: overall: s. xi^1; calendar: 1000-06
ORIGIN: Christ Church, Canterbury?
CONTENTS: computus, calendar; sacramentary
LITERATURE: Warren (1883: 275-93); Omont (1886-88: I.53); Wilson (1896: xix-lxx); Atkins (1928); Ker (1957: 449 [377]); Temple (1976: 89-91 [72]); Gneuss (1981: 58 [921]; 141 [921])

Rouen 274, fols 6r-11v *6/28*
TYPE: Dog Days
LANGUAGE: L
INCIPIT: Dies caniculares.
EDITION: Wilson (1896: 9-20); Atkins (1928: 241-52)

Salisbury, Cathedral Library, MS 150
DATE: overall: 969-78; glosses added s. xi/xii; additions s. xii; calendar: 969-78
ORIGIN: overall: Shaftesbury?, transferred to Salisbury (s. xi^2);[203] calendar: Shaftesbury?
CONTENTS: calendar, computus; glossed Gallican psalter; prayer; glossed canticles; litanies
LITERATURE: Bond & Thompson (1873-83: II, pl. 188-89); Ker (1957: 449-51 [379]); Sisam & Sisam (1959: 1-47); Temple (1976: 45-46 [18]); Stroud (1979); Gneuss (1981: 46 [740]; 2001: 111 [740]); Gameson (1999: 152 [875])

Salisbury 150, fols 3r-8v *8.3/33*
TYPE: Egyptian Days, twenty-four days
LANGUAGE: L
INCIPIT: **DIES EGYP*TIACVS***
FACSIMILE: Bond & Thompson (1873-83: II, pl. 188 [of fol. 5r]); Temple (1976: ill. 60-61 [of fols 3r, 5r])
EDITION: Wormald (1934: 16-27 [2])

---

[202] Wormald opted for Bury St. Edmunds, and Gneuss noted a pre-eleventh-century Bury St. Edmunds provenance. The whole manuscript probably originated from Christ Church, Canterbury, and was intended for use at Bury St. Edmunds.

[203] The place of origin is a matter of debate. Places suggested are the west country, Salisbury, Shaftesbury, Sherborne and a transfer to Salisbury, and Wilton.

SUPPLEMENT

NB The existence of a large number of manuscripts after 1100 containing Egyptian Days and/or Dog Days in the calendar is acknowledged (see Wormald 1939-46). References to these manuscripts are not included in this supplement.

Cambridge, Pembroke College, MS 103
DATE: s. xii^{ex}
ORIGIN: Reading Abbey?
CONTENTS: sacramentary; religious writings; proverbs; prognostics
LITERATURE: James and Minnis (1915: 97-100); Wit (2002: 89-90 [17])

CPC 103, fols 75r-77v
TYPE: dreambook
LANGUAGE: L
LITERATURE: James and Minnis (1915: 99 [7]); Thorndike and Kibre (1963: 735); Martin (1977: 81-82 [C]; 1981: 17-18 [C]); Grub (1984: liv [C]); Wit (2002: 89)

CPC 103, fols 77v-79v
TYPE: lunary, collective[204]
COLLATION: Weißer (1982: 307-14 [Ca_2L])[205]
LANGUAGE: L
LITERATURE: James and Minnis (1915: 99 [8]); Thorndike and Kibre (1963: 837)

CPC 103, fols 77v-79v
TYPE: brontology, temporal, hours?[206]
LANGUAGE: L
LITERATURE: James and Minnis (1915: 99 [8])

Cambridge, Trinity College, B. 11. 2 (241)
DATE: overall: 930s or s. x^{med}, additions s. xi; prognostic: s. xi$^{3/4}$
ORIGIN: overall: St. Augustine's, Canterbury, transferred to and expanded in Exeter; prognostic: Exeter
CONTENTS: Amalarius' *Liber officialis*; antiphon; prognostic; excerpts from Amalarius
LITERATURE: James (1900-04: I.327-28 [241]); Temple (1976: 48 [21]); Gneuss (1981: 14 [174]; 2001: 44 [174])

CTC B. 11. 2
TYPE: Egyptian Days, twenty-four days
LANGUAGE: L
EDITION: James (1900-04: I.328)
LITERATURE: Gneuss (2001: 44 [144])

Cambridge, University Library, Gg. 5. 35
AKA the *Cambridge Songs Manuscript*, the *Canterbury Classbook*
DATE: s. xi^{med}; additions on fols 425v-431v and 444v-446v, *c.* 1100
ORIGIN: St. Augustine's, Canterbury
CONTENTS: miscellany of curriculum texts, riddles and poems; medical treatises; *Cambridge Songs*, *Meters of Boethius*, medical treatises
LITERATURE: Hardwick et al. (1856-67: III.201-205 [1567]); Sigerist (1923: 160-67); Beccaria (1956: 237-39 [70]); Ker (1957: 21-22 [16]); Gneuss (1981: 6 [12]; 2001: 27-28 [12]); Cameron (1983: 150-51; 1993: 48-53); Doane & Grade (2001: 1-31 [96, ASMMF 9.1])

CUL Gg. 5. 35, fols 425v-427v
TYPE: series of medical tracts containing moonbooks, Dog Days, regimens and Egyptian Days
LANGUAGE: L
EDITION: Cameron (1993: 51, 52, n. 11, 13, 14 [incomplete])
TRANSLATION: Cameron (1993: 51, 52

---

[204] James and Minnis 1915: 99) wrote: "Prognostics of weather etc. and divinations such as are often attributed to Esdras 'Luna prima hec est utilis omnibus augmentis... Si hora nona (tonitrus fuerit) habundantia et pax significat'". Esdras would suggest a year prognosis, but the incipit pertains to an agenda or collective lunary, the explicit to an hour brontology.

[205] As variants to Harley 978, fols 16r-18r.

[206] see note 204.

[incomplete])
FACSIMILE: Doane & Grade (2001: 9.1. 14)
LITERATURE: Beccaria (1956: 238 [70.2-6]); Cameron (1983: 154 [4-10]; 1993: 50-53); Doane & Grade (2001: 24-25 [96.45])

Exeter, Cathedral Library, MS 3507
DATE: s. x^2
ORIGIN: Christ Church, Canterbury, or Sherborne?
CONTENTS: computus; notes; Isidore's *De natura rerum*
LITERATURE: Derolez (1954: 219-22 [7]); Ker (1957: 153-54 [116*]); Ker & Piper (1969-92: II.813-14); Stevens (1979: 191 [E]; 1992: 136-37); Gneuss (1981: 19 [258]; 2001: 54 [258])

Exeter 3507, fol. 63v
TYPE: Egyptian Days, twenty-four days?
LANGUAGE: L
LITERATURE: Derolez (1954: 221); Ker & Piper (1969-92: II.813 [3c])

Exeter 3507, fols 63v-64r
TYPE: Egyptian Days, three days
LANGUAGE: L
LITERATURE: Derolez (1954: 221); Ker & Piper (1969-92: II.813 [3d])

London, British Library, Egerton 821
Formerly Cambridge, Trinity College, O. 7. 36 (1364); Halliwell 60
DATE: s. xii
ORIGIN: England
CONTENTS: astrological, medical and computistical miscellany
LITERATURE: Madden (1843: 1840.16); James (1900-04: III.372-73 [1364]); Thorndike (1923-58: I.726-30)

Egerton 821, fol. 1r-1v/17
TYPE: year prognosis
LANGUAGE: L
LITERATURE: James (1900-04: III.372); Thorndike (1923-28: I.678, n. 1); Svenberg (1963: 13 [6]); Matter (1982: 387 [9])

Egerton 821, fols 1v/17-2v/26
TYPE: zodiacal year prognosis
LANGUAGE: L

Egerton 821, fols 2v/26-5r/3
TYPE: zodiacal brontology
LANGUAGE: L
LITERATURE: James (1900-04: III.372); Svenberg (1963: 13 [6])

Egerton 821, fol. 7r/22-7v/22
TYPE: term of imprisonment, zodiacal
LANGUAGE: L
LITERATURE: James (1900-04: III.372)

Egerton 821, fols 7v/23-8r/25
TYPE: zodiacal lunary, agenda
LANGUAGE: L
EDITION: Förster (1944: 20)

Egerton 821, fols 8r/25-12r/14
TYPE: zodiacal lunary, collective
LANGUAGE: L
EDITION: Weißer (1982: 244-52 [Lo_5L])
LITERATURE: Thorndike (1923-58: I. 681, n. 2); Förster (1944: 19)

Egerton 821, fols 12r/15-14v/21
TYPE: dreambook
LANGUAGE: L
LITERATURE: James (1900-04: III.373)

Egerton 821, fol. 15r/13-15v
TYPE: Apuleian Sphere
LANGUAGE: L
LITERATURE: James (1900-04: III.373)

Egerton 821, fols 17v/1-24r/2
TYPE: zodiacal mansions
LANGUAGE: L
EDITION: Svenberg (1963: 45-59 [H])

Egerton 821, fol. 32r/15-32v/11
TYPE: lunary, specific, illness
LANGUAGE: L
EDITION: Weißer (1982: 272-73 [*Lo_8L])
LITERATURE: Thorndike (1923-58: I. 680, n. 2)

Egerton 821, fols 55r/12-56r/12
TYPE: *Sortes Sanctorum*[207]
LANGUAGE: L
LITERATURE: Thorndike (1923-58: I. 727); Svenberg (1963: 13 [6])

(London, British Library, Royal 13. A. xi
DATE: s. xi/xii or xii^in
ORIGIN: Normandy or NW France, not yet in England by 1100
CONTENTS: computus, Bede's *De natura rerum*; computus; cosmology; horoscope; notes on eclipses; astronomy; computus
LITERATURE: Warner & Gilson (1921: II. 80-81); Van de Vyver (1935: 145); Gneuss (1981: 31 [483]; 2001: 83 [483]); Gameson (1999: 119 [548])

Royal 13. A. xi, fols 12v/11-13r/3
TYPE: Egyptian Days, twenty-four days
LANGUAGE: L
LITERATURE: Warner & Gilson (1921: II. 80 [2]); Gameson (1999: 119 [548]); Gneuss (2001: 83 [483])

Royal 13. A. xi, fol. 13r/3-7
TYPE: Egyptian Days, three days
LANGUAGE: L

Royal 13. A. xi, fols 28r/13-28v/20, 29v
TYPE: Apuleian Sphere
LANGUAGE: L
LITERATURE: Warner & Gilson (1921: II. 80 [5]); Gameson (1999: 119 [548])

Royal 13. A. xi, fol. 29v
TYPE: Apuleian Sphere
LANGUAGE: L
COLLATION: Liuzza (2005: II.40-44 [R; incomplete])[208]
LITERATURE: Warner & Gilson (1921: II. 80 [5])

London, British Library, Sloane 2839
DATE: *c.* 1100
ORIGIN: England(?)
CONTENTS: medicine
LITERATURE: Thorndike (1923-58: I. 723); Beccaria (1956: 261-63 [81]); Kauffmann (1975: 58-59 [12]); Gameson (1999: 122 [578]); Gneuss (2001: 85 [498.9]); Glaze (2007)

Sloane 2839, fols 107r-110v
TYPE: medical tract containing Dog Days, regimen, twenty-four Egyptian Days, moonbook, three Egyptian Days
LANGUAGE: L
LITERATURE: Beccaria (1956: 262-63 [81.7-12]); Gameson (1999: 122 [578])

Los Angeles, Getty Museum, Ludwig XII. 5
Formerly Cologne, Schnütgen-Museum Ludwig XII. 5
DATE: s. xii¹ (fols 2-141); additions s. xiii¹ (142-151), xiv-xvi (152-219)
ORIGIN: England
CONTENTS: compendium of the quadrivium containing notes on philosophy, history, medicine, geography, ecclesiastical history, arithmetic, music, prognostics, calendar and computus, astronomy, architecture and agriculture
LITERATURE: Euw & Plotzek (1979-85: III.158-69)

Ludwig XII. 5, fols 9v-11v
TYPE: solar prognostic
LANGUAGE: L
LITERATURE: Euw & Plotzek (1979-85: III.159 [25])

Ludwig XII. 5, fol. 46r
TYPE: Apuleian Sphere
LANGUAGE: L
FACSIMILE: Euw & Plotzek (1979-85: III pl. 82)
LITERATURE: Euw & Plotzek (1979-85: III.160 [43-44])

Ludwig XII. 5, fols 46r-47r
TYPE: Apuleian Sphere
LANGUAGE: L

[207] Svenberg (1963: 13) called these *Sortes Sangallenses*.
[208] As variants to 2/12 (St. John's College 17).

FACSIMILE: Euw & Plotzek (1979-85: III pl. 82-83 [of fols 46r, 47r])
LITERATURE: Thorndike & Kibre (1963: 1039); Euw & Plotzek (1979-85: III.160 [45-47])

Ludwig XII. 5, fol. 47rv
TYPE: Apuleian Sphere
LANGUAGE: L
FACSIMILE: Euw & Plotzek (1979-85: III pl. 83-84)
COLLATION: Liuzza (2005: II.40-44 [Gl; incomplete])[209]
LITERATURE: Euw & Plotzek (1979-85: III.160 [48-49])

Ludwig XII. 5, fols 48r-49v
TYPE: *Sortes Sanctorum*
LANGUAGE: L
LITERATURE: Euw & Plotzek (1979-85: III.160 [50])

Ludwig XII. 5, fol. 49v
TYPE: weekday prognostic
LANGUAGE: L
LITERATURE: Euw & Plotzek (1979-85: III.160 [51])

Ludwig XII. 5, fols 51r-55v
TYPE: Egyptian Days, twenty-four days
LANGUAGE: L
LITERATURE: Euw & Plotzek (1979-85: III.161 [55])

(Oxford, Bodleian Library, Barlow 35 (6467)
DATE: s. x; additions s. xi^{in}
ORIGIN: continent, in England by s. xi^{in}
CONTENTS: computus; Alcuin's *Interrogationes Sigewulfi*; glossary; charm; pseudo-Cicero's *Synonyma*; glossaries
LITERATURE: Madan, Craster & Denholm-Young (1922-53: II.2.1058 [6467]); Gneuss (1981: 35 [541]; 2001: 91 [541])

Barlow 35, fol. 5r/16-32
TYPE: year prognosis
LANGUAGE: L
LITERATURE: Madan, Craster & Denholm-Young (1922-53: II.2.1058 [A])

[209] As variants to 2/12 (St. John's College 17).

APPENDIX TWO

REFERENCE LIST

Below, I provide a list of the Anglo-Saxon prognostics and the manuscripts in which they are found. This is a condensed version of the information provided in chapters two and three, and appendix one.[1]

MS	date	orig	pages	type	sq	num	lang	ctxt
CCCC 9	s. xi^2	Wo	3-14	Dog Days		6/5	L	cal
CCCC 391	1064-9	Wo	*712†*-3	sunshine prognostic		14/1	OE	ps
			713-4	brontology, weekday		5.1.3/1		
			714	brontology, night hour		5.1.1.1/1		
			714	brontology, compass		5.2/1		
			714-5	brontology, day hour		5.1.1.2/1		
			715	birth, weekday	α	3.1.3/1		
			716	lunary, birth		9.2.2/1		
			717-8	lunary, illness		9.2.5/1		
			718	birth, 3 days	γ	3.1.2/1		
				Egyptian Days, 3		8.1/1		
			718-20	lunary, dreams		9.2.4/6	L	
			720-1	lunary, dreams	α	9.2.4/1	OE	
	s. xiii^1		(721	Egyptian Days, 3		—	ME	gst)
CCCC 422 part B	*c.* 1061	NM[2]	27	lunary, bloodletting		9.2.3/1	L/OE	com
			29-40	Egyptian Days, 24		8.3/4	L	cal
				Dog Days		6/4	L/OE	
	s. xii	Sher	49	Egyptian Days, 3	γ	8.1/5	L	gst
				birth, 3 days		3.1.2/4		

[1] Abbreviations: Header row: ctxt=context, lang=language, num=number, orig=place of origin, sq=sequence; Place of origin: Ca=Canterbury, CC=Christ Church, Canterbury, Col=Colchester, Cr=Crowland, E=England, Ex=Exeter, Fr=Francia, NM=New Minster, Winchester, Nth=Northumbria, OM=Old Minster, Winchester, Pe=Peterborough, Sal=Salisbury, Sha=Shaftesbury, Sher=Sherborne, StA=St. Augustine's, Canterbury, StM=St. Mary's, Winchester, Th=Thorney, We=Wells, Wi=Winchester, Wo=Worcester; Language: AN=Anglo-Norman, L=Latin, L/OE=Latin with running glosses in Old English, ME=Middle English, OE=Old English; Context: cal=calendar, com=computus, gst=guest text, med=medicine, ps=prognostic section.

[2] Transferred to, and expanded in Sherborne.

MS	date	orig	pages	type	sq	num	lang	ctxt
CTC O. 7. 41	after 1112	Col	1r	Apuleian Sphere		2/2	L	com
			1v-7r	Egyptian Days, 24 Dog Days		8.3/5 6/6		cal
CTC R. 15. 32	s. xi^{ex} [3]	StA	15-26	Egyptian Days, 24		8.3/6	L	cal
	1035-6	NM[4]		Dog Days		6/7		
	s. xi^{in}		37	Egyptian Days, 24		8.3/7		com
CUL Kk. 5. 32 ff. 49-60	1021-2	StA	50r-5v	Egyptian Days, 24 Dog Days		8.3/8 6/8	L	cal
Add. 37517	s. x/xi	Ca (StA?)	2r-3r	Egyptian Days, 24 Dog Days		8.3/9 6/9	L	cal
Arundel 60	1073?	NM	1r	lunary, bloodletting		9.2.3/2	L	com
			2r-7v	Egyptian Days, 24 Dog Days		8.3/10 6/10		cal
Arundel 155	s. xii [5]	CC	2r-7v	Egyptian Days, 24		8.3/11	L	cal
Caligula A. xv ff. 120-53 + Egerton 3314 ff. 1-78	s. xi^{2} (*c.* 1073)	CC	125va 125vb-6r 129v-30r	Apuleian Sphere lunary, illness Egyptian Days, 24		2/3 9.2.5/3 8.3/12	L L/OE L	com
			130r 130v-1r 131r	unlucky days Egyptian Days, 24 birth, 3 days		15/1 8.3/1 3.1.2/2	OE	
			131v-2r 132r	lunary, dreams lunary, birth	α	9.2.4/2 9.2.2/2		
Caligula A. xv + **Egerton 3314**			18r	Egyptian Days, 24		8.3/20	L	
			18v-30r	Egyptian Days, 24 Dog Days		8.3/21 6/18		cal
			50rv	Egyptian Days, 24		8.3/22		com
Nero A. ii ff. 3-13	s. xi$^{2/4}$	StM	3r-8v	Dog Days		6/11	L	cal
Tiberius A. iii ff. 2-173 (see next page)	s. xi^{med}	CC	27v-32v 32v-5v 35v-6r 36rv 36v 36v-7r 37rv	dreambook lunary, collective lunary, dreams year prognosis lunary, birth lunary, illness brontology, hour		7/4 9.1/1 9.2.4/5 17/4 9.2.2/5 9.2.5/4 5.1.2/1	L/OE	ps

[3] Additions to a Winchester calendar from 1035-36.
[4] Transferred to, and expanded in St. Augustine's, Canterbury.
[5] Additions to a calendar from 1012-23.

MS	date	orig	pages	type	sq	num	lang	ctxt
Tiberius A. iii, ff. 2-173 (continued)	s. xi^{med}	CC	37v-8r	lunary, dreams		9.2.4/3	OE	ps
			38r-9v	dreambook		7/1		
			39v-40r	lunary, agenda		9.2.1/1		
			40r	lunary, illness		9.2.5/2		
			40rv	brontology, weekday		5.1.3/2		
			40v	month prognosis		10/1		
			40v-1r	birth, foetus		3.1.1/1		
			41rv	lunary, birth		9.2.2/3		
			41v-2r	year prognosis		17/1		
			42rv	dreambook		7/2		
			42v-3r	birth, gender		3.2/1		
			65r	lunary, bloodletting	α	9.2.3/3	L	ps
			65r	birth, weekday		3.1.3/3		
			65rv	lunary, birth		9.2.2/6		
			65v	lunary, illness		9.2.5/5		
Tiberius C. i ff. 2-42 + Harley 3667	*c.* 1122	Pe	7rb	Egyptian Days, 12		8.2/1	L	com
			7v	Apuleian Sphere		2/4		
Tiberius C. i + **Harley 3667**			4va, 4vc	Apuleian Sphere		2/7		
			5r	Apuleian Sphere		2/8		
Tiberius C. vi	s. xi$^{3/4}$	Wi (OM?)	6v	Apuleian Sphere		2/5	L	com
	s. xii		114r	Egyptian Days, 24 (unlucky days)		8.3/13 —	AN)	gst
Titus D. xxvi, **xxvii**	1023-31	NM	2r	lunary, bloodletting		9.2.3/5	L	com
			3r-8v	Egyptian Days, 24		8.3/15		cal
				Dog Days		6/13		
			22rv	Egyptian Days, 24	β	8.3/16		com
			22v-3r	Dog Days		6/14		
			25rv	year prognosis		17/6		
			27r-9v	lunary, collective		9.1/2		
			55v-6v	alphabet prognostic		1/1	OE	gst
Titus D. **xxvi**, xxvii (see next page)			3v-4r	Egyptian Days, 3	γ	8.1/6	L	ps
			4rv	birth, 3 days		3.1.2/5		
			4v	Dog Days		6/12		
			5r	Egyptian Days, 24		8.3/14		
			5r-6r	moon, colour		11/1		
			6rv	lunary, bloodletting	α	9.2.3/4		
			6v-7v	birth, weekday		3.1.3/4		
			7v-8r	lunary, birth		9.2.2/7		
			8r-9r	lunary, illness		9.2.5/6		
			9rv	lunary, dreams		9.2.4/7		

MS	date	orig	pages	type	sq	num	lang	ctxt
Titus D. **xxvi**, xxvii (continued)	1023-31	NM	9v-10v 10v-1v 11v-6r	brontology, hour year prognosis dreambook		5.1.2/2 17/5 7/5	L	ps
Vespasian D. xiv ff. 4-169	s. xii$^{2/4}$	CC?	75v 103v	year prognosis brontology, month		17/2 5.1.4/1	OE	gst
Vitellius A. xii ff. 4-77	s xi^{ex}	Sal	44rv	Egyptian Days, 3		8.1/7	L	com
			65v-71r	Dog Days		6/15		cal
			72v-7v	Egyptian Days, 24		8.3/17		cal
Vitellius A. xviii	s. xi/xii-xii^{1} [6]	We?	3r-8v	Egyptian Days, 24		8.3/18	L	cal
	s. xi^{2}			Dog Days		6/16		
Vitellius C. viii ff. 22-25	s. xi^{1}	Wi?	22rv	Egyptian Days, 3		8.1/2	OE	com
Vitellius E. xviii	1062	NM	*1*r*	lunary, bloodletting		9.2.3/6	L	com
			2r-7v	Egyptian Days, 24 Dog Days		8.3/19 6/17	L	cal
			9r 13r	unlucky days Dog Days		15/2 6/1	OE	com
			14v	Apuleian Sphere		2/6	L	com
			15r	birth, 3 days Egyptian Days, 3	γ	3.1.2/3 8.1/3	OE	com
			15rv	Egyptian Days, 24		8.3/2	OE	com
			16r	Apuleian Sphere		2/1	L/OE	com
Egerton 3314, see Caligula A. xv, ff. 120-53 + Egerton 3314, ff. 1-78								
Harley 585	s. xi$^{1/10}$	E	190rv	Egyptian Days, 3		8.1/4	OE	med
Harley 863	s. xii^{ex}	Ex	1r-6v	Egyptian Days, 24		8.3/23	L	cal
Harley 3271	s. xi^{1} (1032?)	Wi?	90v-1r	Egyptian Days, 24		8.3/3	OE	com
			102v	lunary, bloodletting		9.2.3/7	L	gst
			120v 120v-1r 121r	Egyptian Days, 24 Dog Days Egyptian Days, 3	β	8.3/24 6/19 8.1/8	L	ps
			122rv 122v 122v	Egyptian Days, 24 Dog Days Egyptian Days, 3	β	8.3/25 6/20 8.1/9	L	ps
			122v-3v 123v-4r	regimen Dog Days		12/1 6/21	L	ps

[6] Additions to a calendar from s. xi^{2}.

MS	date	orig	pages	type	sq	num	lang	ctxt
Harley 3667, see Tiberius C. i, ff. 2-42 + Harley 3667								
Harley 6258B	s. xii$^{4/4}$	E	51v-2v	Dog Days in med tract		6/2	OE	med
Royal 2.B.v	s. x^{ex}	Wi	190rv	brontology, month		5.1.4/2	L	gst
Royal 12. D.xvii	s. x^{med}	OM	54v-5v	Dog Days in med tract		6/3	OE	med
Sloane 475 ff. 125-231	s. xi^{ex} or xi/xii	E(?)	132v-3v 135v 211r-6v 216v-7r 217rv 217v-8r	Apuleian Sphere bloodletting, weekday lunary, collective Egyptian Days, 24 year prognosis dreambook		2/9 4/1 9.1/3 8.3/26 17/7 7/6	L	med
Lambeth Palace 427 ff. 1-202	s. xii$^{1/4}$	Wi?	3r	lunary, bloodletting lunary, dreams	α	9.2.3/8 9.2.4/8	L	com
Bodley 579, fols 38-59	979-87	CC	39r-44v	Dog Days		6/22	L	cal
			49v-50r 56r	Apuleian Sphere lunary, bloodletting		2/10 9.2.3/9		com
Digby 63	867-92	(Fr	36r 36rv	Egyptian Days, 24 Egyptian Days, 3		— —	L	com)
		Nth	40r-5v	Egyptian Days, 24		8.3/27		cal
Douce 296	s. xi$^{2/4}$	Cr	1r-6v	Egyptian Days, 24 Dog Days		8.3/28 6/23	L	cal
Hatton 113	1064-83	Wo	iii r-viii v	Egyptian Days, 24 Dog Days		8.3/29 6/24	L	cal
Hatton 115	s. xii^{med}	CC?[7]	148r 148v 148v-9r	lunary, dreams lunary, birth birth, weekday	α	9.2.4/4 9.2.2/4 3.1.3/2	OE	ps
			149rv 149v 149v-50r 150v 150v-2v 152v-3v	year prognosis wind prognostic sunshine prognostic brontology, weekday dreambook lunary, agenda		17/3 16/1 14/2 5.1.3/3 7/3 9.2.1/2		
St. John's College 17 (see next page)	1110-1	Th	1vab 1vb	Dog Days in med tract Dog Days in med tract		6/25 6/26	L	med
			3va	Egyptian Days, 3 birth, 3 days	γ	8.1/10 3.1.2/6		com

[7] Transferred to Worcester.

MS	date	orig	pages	type	sq	num	lang	ctxt
St. John's College 17 (continued)	1110-1	Th	4ra	lunary, bloodletting	α	9.2.3/10	L	com
			4ra	birth, weekday		3.1.3/5		
			4rb	lunary, birth		9.2.2/8		
			4rbc	lunary, illness		9.2.5/7		
			4rc	lunary, dreams		9.2.4/9		
			8rb	Apuleian Sphere		2/11		
			16r-21v	Egyptian Days, 24		8.3/30		cal
			40va	Egyptian Days, 12		8.2/2		com
			40vb	unlucky days		15/3		
			40vb	Egyptian Days, 24		8.3/31		
			41ra	Apuleian Sphere		2/12		
			41rb	Apuleian Sphere		2/13		
			157vb-8va	*Sortes Sanctorum*		13/1		
			159rb	year prognosis		17/8		
Reg. lat. 12	s. $xi^{2/4}$	CC?	7r-12v	Egyptian Days, 24 Dog Days		8.3/32 6/27	L	cal
Rouen 274	1000-6	CC?	6r-11v	Dog Days		6/28	L	cal
Salisbury 150	969-78	Sha?	3r-8v	Egyptian Days, 24		8.3/33	L	cal

APPENDIX THREE

CONCORDANCE TO ANGLO-SAXON PROGNOSTICS

The following is a concordance to the indexation of prognostics in some of the major catalogues, manuals and bibliographies of Old English. The first column represents the numbers I have assigned to the prognostics.[1] The other columns contain references to Ker's *Catalogue of Manuscripts*; the Cameron number and short title for the *Dictionary of Old English* [*DOE*]; Quinn and Quinn's *A Manual of Old English Prose* [Q&Q]; Voigts and Kurtz's *Scientific and Medical Writings in Old and Middle English* [V&K]; and, finally, the series *Anglo-Saxon Manuscripts in Microfiche Facsimile* [ASMMF][2] The Old English prognostics have also been listed in Hollis and Wright's *Old English Prose of Secular Learning*.[3]

	Ker	Cameron	short title (*DOE*)	Q&Q	V&K	ASMMF
1/1	202.i	B23.3.4 A27	Prog 4 (Sievers) Glor II	F404	6	
2/1	224.r	C37	OccGl 37 (Först)	H232		258.1
2/4						231.14
2/5						233.1
2/6						258.1
2/7						275.3
2/8						275.4
3.1.1/1	186.7.n	B21.4	Lch III (Foetus)	E008	88	
3.1.2/1	67.d.vi	B23.2.1.1	Days 1.1 (Först)	F201	173	
3.1.2/2	139.A.i	B23.2.3.3	Days 3.3 (Först)	F203	172	
3.1.2/3	224.h	B23.2.5.4	Days 5.4 (Henel)	F205	198	258.1
3.1.2/4						60.11
3.1.3/1	67.d.iii	B23.3.1.3	Prog 1.3 (Först)	F401	53	
3.1.3/2	332.35.c	B23.3.6.3	Prog 6.3 (Först)	F406	153	385.35.c
3.1.3/3	186.12					
3.2/1	186.7.r	B23.3.3.8	Prog 3.8 (Cockayne)	F403	23	

[1] See the introductions to the genres in the text edition.

[2] Ker (1957), Healey and Venezky (1980, 2000), Quinn and Quinn (1990), Voigts and Kurtz (2000), Pulsiano and Doane (1994-), respectively.

[3] Hollis and Wright (1992).

	Ker	Cameron	short title (*DOE*)	Q&Q	V&K	ASMMF
5.1.1.1/1	67.d.ii	B23.3.1.2	Prog 1.2 (Först)	F401	118	
5.1.1.2/1	67.d.ii	B23.3.1.2	Prog 1.2 (Först)	F401	118	
5.1.2/1	186.7.g	C16.7	ProgGl 7 (Först)	H041	44	
5.1.3/1	67.d.ii	B23.3.1.2	Prog 1.2 (Först)	F401	118	
5.1.3/2	186.7.l	B23.3.3.6	Prog 3.6 (Cockayne)	F403	117	
5.1.3/3	332.35.i	B23.3.6.7	Prog 6.7 (Cockayne)	F406	116	385.35.i
5.1.4/1	209.34	B23.3.5.2	Prog 5.2 (Warn)	F405	122	245.36
5.1.4/2						284.8
5.2/1	67.d.ii	B23.3.1.2	Prog 1.2 (Först)	F401	118	
6/1	224.g	B23.4	Prohib	F407	21	258.1
6/2[4]	page xix	B21.6	PeriD		89	278.5
6/3[5]	264.1	B21.2.1.1.1 B21.2.1.1.2	Lch II (1 Head) Lch II (1)	E003	102	298.1a 298.1b
6/4	70.B.c	C88	OccGl 88 (Meritt)	H320	148	
6/19	239.19					
6/20	239.19					
6/21	239.19	C67	OccGl 67 (Henel-Ker)	H285		
7/1	186.7.i	B23.3.3.2	Prog 3.2 (Först)	F403	48	
7/2	186.7.q	B23.3.3.10	Prog 3.10 (Först)	F403	42	
7/3	332.35.j	B23.3.6.8	Prog 6.8 (Först)	F406	55	385.35.j
7/4	186.7.a	C16.1	ProgGl 1 (Först)	H041	27	
8.1/1[6]	67.d.vii	B23.2.1.2	Days 1.2 (Först)	F201	174	
8.1/2	221.2	B23.2.4	Days 4 (Först)	F204	196	255.2.2
8.1/3	224.i	B23.2.5.2	Days 5.2 (Först)	F205	25	258.1
8.1/4[7]	231.2	B21.3	Med 3 (Grattan-Singer)	E007	197	265.4
8.1/5						60.11
8.1/8	239.19					
8.1/9	239.19					
8.2/1						231.12
8.3/1	139.A.h	B23.2.3.2	Days 3.2 (Först)	F203	156	

[4] References pertain to the medical work in its entirety, not just to the prognostic.

[5] *Ibid.*

[6] The fragmentary text on the three Egyptian Days copied by the Tremulous Worcester hand in CCCC 391, p. 721 and probably based on 8.1/1 is sometimes included in reference works as well: Ker 67, Cameron B23.2.1.3, *DOE* Days 1.3 (Först), Q&Q F201, V&K 195.

[7] References pertain to the medical work in its entirety, not just to the prognostic.

	Ker	Cameron	short title (*DOE*)	Q&Q	V&K	ASMMF
8.3/2	224.j	B23.2.5.3	Days 5.3 (Förster)	F205	176	258.1
8.3/3	239.8-9	B23.2.6	Days 6 (Henel)	F206	177	
8.3/6						84.6.e
8.3/7						84.6.n
8.3/13						233.2
8.3/24	239.19	C67	OccGl 67 (Henel-Ker)	H285		
8.3/25	239.19					
9.1/1	186.7.b	C16.2	ProgGl 2 (Förster)	H041	101	
9.2.1/1	186.7.j	B23.3.3.3	Prog 3.3 (Förster)	F403	113	
9.2.1/2	332.35.k	B23.3.6.9	Prog 6.9 (Förster)	F406	110	385.35.k
9.2.2/1	67.d.iv	B23.3.1.4	Prog 1.4 (Förster)	F401	132	
9.2.2/2	139.A.q	B23.3.2.3	Prog 2.3 (Förster)	F402	47	
9.2.2/3	186.7.o	B23.3.3.5	Prog 3.5 (Förster)	F403	46	
9.2.2/4	332.35.b	B23.3.6.2	Prog 6.2 (Förster)	F406	141	385.35.b
9.2.2/5	186.7.e	C16.5	ProgGl 5 (Förster)	H041	138	
9.2.2/6	186.12					
9.2.3/1	70.B.a	B23.2.2	Days 2 (Henel)	F202	84	60
9.2.3/2						174.1
9.2.3/3	186.12					
9.2.3/7	239.14					
9.2.4/1	67.d.viii	B23.3.1.6	Prog 1.6 (Förster)	F401	192	
9.2.4/2	139.A.p	B23.3.2.2	Prog 2.2 (Förster)	F402	112	
9.2.4/3	186.7.h	B23.3.3.1	Prog 3.1 (Förster)	F403	115	
9.2.4/4	332.35.a	B23.3.6.1	Prog 6.1 (Förster)	F406	178	385.35.a
9.2.4/5	186.7.c	C16.3	ProgGl 3 (Förster)	H041	154	
9.2.4/6	67.d.viii					
9.2.5/1	67.d.v	B23.3.1.5	Prog 1.5 (Förster)	F401	142	
9.2.5/2	186.7.k	B23.3.3.4	Prog 3.4 (Förster)	F403	114	
9.2.5/3	139.A.a	B23.3.2.1	Prog 2.1 (Förster)	F402	140	
9.2.5/4	186.7.f	C16.6	ProgGl 6 (Förster)	H041	139	
9.2.5/5	186.12					
10/1	186.7.m	B23.3.3.7	Prog 3.7 (Cockayne)	F403	171	
12/1	239.19			H285		
14/1	67.d.i	B23.3.1.1	Prog 1.1 (Förster)	F401	4	
14/2	332.35.f	B23.3.6.6	Prog 6.6 (Förster)	F406	200	385.35.f
15/1	139.A.e	B23.2.3.1	Days 3.1 (Förster)	F203	155	

	Ker	Cameron	short title (*DOE*)	Q&Q	V&K	ASMMF
15/2	224.d	B23.2.5.1	Days 5.1 (Först)	F205	204	258.1
16/1	332.35.e	B23.3.6.5	Prog 6.5 (Först)	F406	78	385.35.e
17/1	186.7.p	B23.3.3.9	Prog 3.9 (Först)	F403	41	
17/2	209.26	B23.3.5.1	Prog 5.1 (Warn)	F405	170	245.28
17/3	332.35.d	B23.3.6.4	Prog 6.4 (Cockayne)	F406	52	385.35.d
17/4	186.7.d	C16.4	ProgGl 4 (Först)	H041	37	

APPENDIX FOUR

VALUES, DATES, COMPOSITION

The following are tables of reference for easy comparison of the values, dates and manner of composition of Apuleian Spheres, Dog Days, moonbooks, Egyptian Days, collective lunaries and unlucky days.

Apuleian Spheres

	letter values	weekday values	lunar values	diagram
1	to left of diagram	under diagram	absent	regular circular (1rc)
2	in rings of diagram	absent	absent	regular circular (1rc)
3	in central circle of diagram	under diagram	absent	compartmentalised circular (3cc)
4	2 around diagrams (4aI, 4aII)	around first diagram	absent	2 regular circular (4dIrc, 4dIIrc)
5	2 to left & right of diagrams (5aI, 5aII)	absent	absent	uita/mors (5um)
6	2 in rings of diagram (6aI, 6aII)	above diagram	absent	regular circular (6rc)
7	to left of diagrams	absent	to right of diagrams	regular circular, uita/mors (7dIrc, 7dIIum)
8,13	unnecessary	absent	absent	rhomboid (8r)
9	absent	under diagram	absent	absent
10	2 to left & right of uita/mors (10aI, 10aII)	around figure mors	around rhomboid	uita/mors & rhomboid (10dIum, 10dIIr)
11	absent	absent	absent	compartmentalised circular (11cc)
12	2 in rings of diagrams (12aI, 12aII)	under diagram	absent	2 regular circular (12dIrc, 12dIIrc)

table 26: Apuleian Spheres, components[1]

[1] **2/2** weekday values added at a later date | **2/8, 2/13** fixed letter values of Greek alphabet employed | this type of Apuleian Sphere (Petosiris I) uses numerical values for the days of the moon, but list is not supplied in 2/8 | diagram of 2/13 excised; in view of relatedness to 2/8, it will have been rhomboid | **2/9** leaf that should have contained diagram was never written upon; dry-point markings show outline of circle.

	incipit	number in intro	number in example
Apuleian	Spera apulei platonici de uita et de morte uel de omnibus negotiis & quicquid inquirere uolueris	30	not applicable
Pythagorean	Ratio spere phytagori phylosophi quem apuleius descripsit ut de quacumque re scire uolueris uel consulere	30	not applicable
Petosiris I	De quacumque re scire uolueris uel consulere	30	29
Petosiris II	Ratio spere phytagori phylosophi quem apuleius descripsit ut de quacumque re scire uolueris uel consulere	29	29

table 27: Apuleian Spheres, textual variants of explanatory texts in prose

	1, 3, 6, 9, 10	4, 12
Sunday	**xiii**	**xiii**
Monday	**xviii**	**xviii**
Tuesday	**xv**	**xv**
Wednesday	**xxv**	**xxv**
Thursday	**xi**	**xi**
Friday	**xv**	**xv**
Saturday	**xxvi**	*xvii*

table 28: Apuleian Spheres, values for the weekdays[2]

	7	10		7	10		10
1	**īclxxxix**	*mlxxxix*	11	**īcc`cc´lxv**	*mdcxciiii*	21	mclxxxvi
2	**īcvi**	**mcvi**	12	**īcclxxvi**	*mcccxliii*	22	mdxvi
3	**īxviii**	*mxix*	13	**īcclxxxi**	*mcclxxxiiii*	23	mccccxix
4	**īlxxxv**	**mlxxxv**	14	**īccx**	*mcclxxxii*	24	mccclxv
5	**īlxv**	*mxv*	15	**dxxxii**	*mccx*	25	mcclxiiii
6	**īliiii**	**mliiii**	16	**dcccxcii**	*dxxxii*	26	mciiii
7	**īc`c´cxxxix**	*mccccxxxix*	17		dcccxciii	27	dccclxxx
8	**īcc`cc´lv**	*mccccłvi*	18		mdcxciiii	28	mcvi
9	**īdcxxxi**	*mccclxv*	19		dclxxxviii	29	mcv
10	**īdcxciii**	*mdccxxix*	20		dccli	30	mcxliiii

table 29: Apuleian Spheres, values for the days of the moon

[2] **2/1** value of Sunday emended from xii to xiii, of Monday from xvii to xviii, of Thursday from x to xi | value of Saturday lacking through fire damage.

	small numbers							large numbers
	1: 1, 3	2: 2	3: 4aI, 12aI	4: 4aII, 6aII, 12aII	5: 5aI, 10aI	6: 6aI	7: 7	5aII, 10aII
A	**iii**	**iii**	**iii**	**iii**	**iii**	**iii**	**iii**	dcccc
B	**iii**	**iii**	**iii**	**iii**	**iii**	**iii**	**iii**	ccc
C	**xxii**	**xxii**	*xxviii*	*xxviii*	*xxviii*	**xxii**	**xxii**	c
D	**xxiiii**	*xxiii*	**xxiiii**	**xxiiii**	**xxiiii**	*xxiii*	**xxiiii**	d
E	**xv**	**xv**	**xv**	**xv**	*xxv*	**xv**	**xv**	ccl
F	**iii**	**iii**	**iii**	**iii**	**iii**	**iii**	**iii**	xl
G	**vii**	**vii**	**vii**	**vii**	**vii**	**vii**	**vii**	cccc
H	**vi**	**vi**	**vi**	**vi**	**vi**	**vi**	**vi**	cc
I	**xv**	**xv**	**xv**	**xv**	**xv**	**xv**	**xv**	ī
K	**xv**	**xv**	*vi*	**xv**	xvi	xvi	*vi*	c
L	**xxi**	**xxi**	**xxi**	**xxi**	**xxi**		**xxi**	l
M	**xxiii**	*xxvi*	*xxvi*	**xxiii**	**xxiii**		*xxvi*	ī
N	**xv**	**xv**	**xv**	**xv**	**xv**		**xv**	xc
O	**viii**	*ix*	**viii**	*ix*	*ix*		**viii**	xl
P	**xiiii**	**xiiii**	**xiiii**	**xiiii**	**xiiii**		**xiiii**	cccc
Q	**xxi**	**xxi**	**xxi**	**xxi**	**xxi**		**xxi**	d
R	**xiii**	**xiii**	**xiii**	*xii*	*xii*		**xiii**	lxxx
S	**ix**	**ix**	**ix**	**ix**	**ix**		**ix**	lx
T	**viii**	**viii**	**viii**	*ix*	*ix*		**viii**	clx
V	**v**	**v**	**v**	*vi*	xvi		**v**	v̄
X	**vi**	**vi**	*x*	xvi	*x*	**vi**	*x*	x̄
Y	**iii**	**iii**	**iii**	*vi*	*vi*	**iii**	**iii**	cl
Z	**iii**	**iii**	**iii**	**iii**	**iii**	**iii**	**ii⟨i⟩**	ī

table 30: Apuleian Spheres, values for the letters of the alphabet[3]

[3] On aI and aII, see table 28 | **2/1** values for 'x', 'y' and 'z' lacking through fire damage | **2/2** value of 'c' emended from xxv to xxii, of 'h' from v to vi, of 'l' from xx to xxi | **2/3** value of 'c' emended from xxiii to xxii, of 'n' from xii to xv | **2/4aI** value of 't' emended from vii to viii | **2/5aI** value of 'd' emended from xxviiii to xxiiii | **2/6aII** value of 'c' emended from xxvii to xxviii, of 'x' from vi to xvi (but Apuleian Sphere in Harley 3017 also reads vi for this letter) | **2/12aII** value of 'o' emended from viii to ix.

	rc + um				cc	r	
	1: 1rc, 4dIIrc, 6rc, 12dIIrc	2: 2rc	3: 4dIrc, 7dIrc, 7dIIum, 12dIrc	4: 5um, 10dIum	3cc, 11cc	1: 8r	2: 10dIIr
i	**u**	*m*	**u**	**u**	zmi	**mom**	*mou*
ii	**u**	**u**	**u**	**u**	zmi	**mou**	**mou**
iii	**u**	**u**	**u**	**u**	zmi	**mou**	**mou**
iiii	**u**	*m*	**u**	**u**	zmi	**mom**	*mou*
v	**m**	**m**	**m**	**m**	tme	**mom**	**mom**
vi	**m**	**m**	**m**	**m**	tme	**mom**	**mom**
vii	**u**	**u**	**u**	**u**	zmi	**mou**	**mou**
viii	**m**	**m**	**m**	**m**	tme		**mom**
ix	**u**	**u**	**u**	**u**	zmi	**mom**	*mou*
x	**u**	**u**	**u**	**u**	zme	**mau**	*meu*
xi	**u**	**u**	**u**	**u**	ype	**meu**	**meu**
xii	**m**	**m**	**m**	**m**	tme	**mom**	**mom**
xiii	**u**	**u**	**u**	**u**	ype	**meu**	**meu**
xiiii	**u**	**u**	**u**	**u**	ype	**meu**	**meu**
xv	**m**	**m**	**m**	**m**	ypo	**mom**	**mom**
xvi	**u**	**u**	*m*	**u**	ype	**meu**	**meu**
xvii	**u**	**u**	**u**	**u**	ype	**meu**	**meu**
xviii	**m**	**m**	**m**	**m**	ypo	**meu**/ *mou*	mom
xix	**u**	**u**	**u**	**u**	ype	**mom**/ *mau*	*mau*
xx	**u**	**u**	**u**	**u**	zme	**meu**	*mau*
xxi	**m**	**m**	*u*/**m**	**m**	ypo	**mou**/ *mom*	mam
xxii	**u**	**u**	*m*	**u**	zme		**mau**
xxiii	**u**	**u**	**u**/*m*	**u**	zme	**mau**	**mau**
xxiiii	**m**	**m**	*u*/**m**	*u*	ypo		**mau**
xxv	**m**	**m**		**m**	tmi	**mam**	**mam**
xxvi	**u**	**u**	**u**	*m*	zme	**mau**	*mam*
xxvii	**u**	*m*	*m*	**u**	zme	**mam**/ *mau*	*mau*
xxviii	**m**	*u*	**m**	**m**	tmi	**mam**/ *mom*	**mam**
xxix	**m**	**m**	*u*	**m**	tmi		**mam**

	rc + um				cc	r	
	1: 1rc, 4dIIrc, 6rc, 12dIIrc	2: 2rc	3: 4dIrc, 7dIrc, 7dIIum, 12dIrc	4: 5um, 10dIum	3cc, 11cc	1: 8r	2: 10dIIr
XXX	**m**			**m**	tmi	**mam**	**mam**

table 31: Apuleian Spheres, values for the diagrams[4]

	text	letter values	weekday values	lunar values	values for outcome
1	Apuleian	small 1	redaction 1	not applicable	rc/um 1
2	Petosiris II	small 2	absent	not applicable	rc/um 2
3	verse + Apuleian	small 1	redaction 1	not applicable	cc
4,12	Pythagorean	small 3 + 4	redaction 2	not applicable	rc/um 3 + 1
5	verse	small 5 + large	absent	absent	rc/um 4
6	Pythagorean	small 6 + 4	redaction 1	not applicable	rc/um 1
7	absent	small 7	absent	redaction 1	rc/um 3 (2*)
8,13	Petosiris I	not applicable	absent	not applicable	r 1
9	verse + Pythagorean	lost	redaction 1	not applicable	absent
10	verse + Apuleian	small 5 + large	redaction 1	redaction 2	rc/um 4 + r 2
11	absent	absent	absent	not applicable	cc

table 32: Apuleian Spheres, composition[5]

[4] Abbreviations: cc=compartmentalised circular, m=mors, mam=magna mors, mau =magna uita, mc=mors cita, meu=media uita, mom=modica mors, mou=modica uita, r=rhomboid, rc=regular circular, tme=thanatos megas (glossed by "mors cita" in 2/3 and 2/11), tmi=thanatos mikros (glossed by "mors longa" in 2/3, and "mors hominis" in 2/11), u=uita, um=uita/mors, ype=ypergeion (glossed by "super terram" in 2/3), ypo=ypogeion (glossed by "subterior" in 2/3), zme=zoe megale (glossed by "uita longa" in 2/3, and "uita cita" in 2/11), zmi=zoe mikra (glossed by 'uita minor' in 2/3, and "uita hominis" in 2/11). On dI, dII, see table 26 | **2/4dIrc** values xvi, xvii and xx listed under uita and mors | value xviii emended from mors xvii | value xxiiii emended from mors xx, introducing an ambiguity already present in 2/7dIrc, 2/7dIIum and 2/12dIrc | value xix lacking | **2/4dIIrc** value xvi listed twice under uita | value xxvii emended from xvi | value xxviii emended from xxvii | **2/6rc** values v, vi, viii, xii, xxi, xxiiii lacking through fire damage | **2/7dIrc, 2/7dIIum, 2/12dIrc** value xii listed under uita and mors | value xiii emended from uita xii | **2/11cc** values xi, xiii, xiiii, xv, xvi, xvii, xviii, xix, xxi and xxiiii lacking.

[5] **2/2** letter values should have been absent because Petosiris II employs Greek alphabet | weekday values added at a later date and therefore not taken into consideration | **2/9** dry-point circle present but diagram not drawn; regular circular like other Pythagorean redactions? | **2/13** diagram excised; in view of relatedness to 2/8, redaction will have been r 1.

Dog Days

	1s, 6c, 7c, 10c, 11c, 17c, 28c	3m, 13c	4c	5c, 18c	23c	8c	9c, 15c, 22c	12s, 14s, 19s, 20s, 21s, 26m	16c	24c	27c
start	14/7	17/7	14/7	14/7	14/7	14/7	14/7		18/7	14/7	11/7
star			17/7			19/7	17/7	18/7		18/7	
end	5/9	5/9	5/9		4/9	5/9		5/9	5/9		5/9

table 33: Dog Days, dates[6]

Moonbooks

	bad days of the moon	good days
6/3,12,26	5, 10, 15, 20, 25, 30	
6/14,19,20	4, 5, 10, 15, 20, 25, 30	
6/21	5, 10, 15, 20, 25, 30	4, 14, 24
8.3/1,2,3	4, 5	

table 34: moonbooks, days of the moon

Egyptian Days

	first Monday	second Monday	third Monday
1, 3	end of April	beginning of August	end of December
2, 4	end of April	beginning of August	beginning of December
5-10	25 March	1 August	end of December

table 35: three Egyptian Days, Mondays[7]

	Jan	Feb	Mar	Apr	May	June	July	Aug	Sept	Oct	Nov	Dec
1, 2	3	2	7	5	8	7	5	13	9	2	9	13

table 36: twelve Egyptian Days, dates

[6] Abbreviations: c=calendar; m=embedded in medical tract; s=stand-alone text | **6/2, 6/25** dates for Dog Days not given but phenomenon of Dog Days discussed in connection with periods of activity of the humours..

[7] The three Egyptian Days fall on Mondays around the times mentioned | **8.1/5** dates mentioned, but not that the Egyptian Days fall on a Monday.

	2s, 3s, 5v, 6c, 8c, 10cv, 15c, 16s, 17cv, 18cv, 19cv, 21v, 22v, 23v, 24s, 25s, 26v, 28cv, 29c, 30cv, 32c	1s, 5c, 11c, 12s, 13t, 20v, 23c, 31s	4c	7v	9c	14s	27c	33c
Jan	**1,25**	**1,25**	**25**	**1,25**	**1,25**	2,24		2,**25**
Feb	**4,26**	**4,26**		5,18	**4,26**	8,24	2	6
Mar	**1,28**	**1,28**	12,23	**1,28**	10,21	3,27	3	
Apr	**10,20**	**10,20**	3,21	**10,20**	3,24	3,23		4,11
May	**3,25**	**3,25**	23	**3,25**	**3,25**	6,17		4,**25**
June	**10,16**	**10,16**	7	**10,16**	**10**,26	9,**16**	7	20
July	**13,22**	**13,22**	14,**22**	**13,22**	**13,22**	7,**22**	3	6,**13**
Aug	**1,30**	**1,30**	**30**	**1,30**	**30**	7,20		
Sept	**3,21**	**3,21**	7	**3,21**	13,20	2,25	2	
Oct	**3,22**	**3,22**		**3,22**	**3,22**	**3**,26	**3**	4
Nov	**5,28**	**5,28**	24	**5,28**	**5,28**			24
Dec	**12,15**	7,22	11,27	**12,15**	**12,15**		13	**12**

table 37: twenty-four Egyptian Days, dates[8]

Unlucky days

Jan	Feb	Mar	Apr	May	June	July	Aug	Sept	Oct	Nov	Dec
3, 4	5, 7	6, 7	5, 8	8, 9	5, 27	3, 13	8, 13	5, 9	5, 15	7, 9	3, 13

table 38: unlucky days, days of the moon[9]

[8] Abbreviations: c=calendar; s=stand-alone text; v=verse | **8.3/5c** second date of March emended from 29 to 28 | **8.3/8c** dates present for January, March, April, and first date of February only | three dates listed for March: 1, 27 and 28. The entry for 27 March is probably an error which was not corrected | **8.3/10c** second dates of February and October missing | **8.3/11c** second date of June missing | **8.3/15c** three dates listed for December: 12, 15 and 25. It is unlikely that the third entry was intended seriously | **8.3/17c** second date of February only | **8.3/17v** verse for December missing | **8.3/18c** three dates listed for December: 7, 12 and 15. The entry for 12 December was erased | **8.3/19c** dates missing for July, February, September, first date of March and second date of January | second date of October emended from 24 to 22 | **8.3/23c** second date of April emended from 19 to 20 | **8.3/23v** no verses after April | **8.3/28c** first dates of June and July only | **8.3/28v** first date of December emended from 6 to 7 | **8.3/29c** second date of October emended from 23 to 22 | **8.3/30c** dates present for January and first date of March only | **8.3/32c** dates missing for January, December, second date of July and first date of September.

[9] **15/1** 17 instead of 27 June | 12 instead of 13 December.

Collective Lunaries

	1	3	2		1	3	2
1	$+d_1d_{2m}efg$	$+d_1d_2ef$	+efd	16	$-abd_{1m}d_{2m}efg$	$-abd_1d_2ef$	fed
2	$+ad_1d_2efg$	$+acd_1d_2ef$	+acefd	17	ad_1d_2efg	ad_1d_2ef	fed
3	$aced_1d_2fg$	$aced_1d_2f$	-acfed	18	$+d_{1m}d_{2m}efg$	$+ad_1d_2ef$	fed
4	$abed_1d_2fg$	$+abed_1d_2f$	+abefd	19	$+d_{1m}d_2efg$	$+ad_1d_2ef$	fed
5	$abcd_1d_2efg$	$abcd_1d_2ef$	abcefd	20	$-d_1d_2efg$	$-ad_1d_2ef$	fed
6	$ced_{1m}d_2fg$	$acebd_1d_2f$	acefd	21	$-acd_1d_{2m}efg$	$-acd_1d_2ef$	fed
7	$abcd_{1m}d_{2m}efg$	$abcd_1d_2ef$	abefd	22	ad_1d_2egf	ad_1d_2ef	fed
8	$acd_{1m}d_{2m}feg$	acd_1d_2ef	aefd	23	$+d_1d_2efg$	$+d_1d_2ef$	fed
9	$+abed_{1m}d_{2m}fg$	$abed_1d_2f$	+fd	24	$+d_1d_2efg$	$+d_1d_2ef$	fed
10	$+ad_1d_2efg$	$+ad_{1m}d_2ef$	+fed	25	ad_1d_2efg	ad_1d_2ef	fed
11	$ad_1d_{2m}efg$	ad_1d_2ef	afd	26	d_1d_2efg	d_1ef	fed
12	$+ad_{1m}d_{2m}efg$	$+ad_1d_2ef$	+fed	27	d_1d_2efg	d_1d_2ef	fed
13	$-abd_{1m}d_{2m}efg$	abd_1d_2ef	-fed	28	d_1d_2efg	d_1d_2ef	fed
14	$+ad_{1m}d_{2m}efg$		+f	29	d_1d_2fg	d_1d_2f	fed
15	$ad_{1m}d_2efg$	ad_1d_2ef	-afd	30	d_1d_2efg	d_1d_2ef	fed

table 39: collective lunaries, components[10]

[10] Abbreviations: +/-=general quality of the day; a=agenda; b=fugitive; c=property; d=birth (gender unspecified, otherwise $_1$=male; $_2$=female; $_m$=birthmark); e=illness; f= dream; g=bloodletting. Classifications of the components of collective lunaries show a large degree of uniformity in Wistrand (1942: 11-12), Förster (1944: 6-7, 32-33), Weißer (1982: 15-20), Taavitsainen (1988: 98-101). I have adopted Weißer's classification makes a distinction between the overall quality of a day and the agenda component and indicates the presence or absence of birthmarks (the structure of the birth component is used by some scholars as a means of grouping collective lunaries together, cf. Svenberg (1936: 17-18) | **9.1/1** day 5 $abcd_1d_2fg$ in Weißer (1981: 64) | day 7 $gabcd_{1m}d_{2m}efg$ in Weißer (1981: 64), but the first bloodletting instruction is part of the agenda component and does not form a bloodletting component on its own | day 8 $acd_{1m}d_{2m}efg$ in Weißer (1981: 64).

BIBLIOGRAPHY

Manuscripts

Cambridge, Corpus Christi College, MS 9; MS 391; MS 422, part B
—, Trinity College, O. 7. 41; R. 15. 32
—, University Library, Kk. 5. 32, fols 49-60
London, British Library, Additional 37517; Arundel 60; Arundel 155; Cotton Caligula A. xv, fols 120-153; Cotton Nero A. ii, fols 3-13; Cotton Tiberius A. iii, fols 2-173; Cotton Tiberius C. i, fols 2-42; Cotton Tiberius C. vi; Cotton Titus D. xxvi; Cotton Titus D. xxvii; Cotton Vespasian D. xiv, fols 4-169; Cotton Vitellius A. xii, fols 4-77; Cotton Vitellius A. xviii; Cotton Vitellius C. viii, fols 22-25; Cotton Vitellius E. xviii; Egerton 3314, fols 1-78; Harley 585; Harley 863; Harley 3271; Harley 3667; Harley 6258B; Royal 2. B. v; Royal 12. D. xvii; Sloane 475, fols 125-231
—, Lambeth Palace, MS 427
Oxford, Bodleian Library, Bodley 579; Digby 63; Douce 296; Hatton 113; Hatton 115
—, St. John's College, MS 17
Rome, Vatican City, Bibliotheca Apostolica Vaticana, Reg. lat. 12
Rouen, Bibliothèque municipale, MS 274
Salisbury, Cathedral Library, MS 150

Printed Primary Sources and Studies

Adamson, M.W. (1995). *Medieval Dietetics. Food and Drink in Regimen sanitatis Literature from 800 to 1400*. German Studies in Canada 5. Frankfurt am Main: Lang.

Alauzier, L. d' (1970-71). "Des jours néfastes au moyen âge", *Bulletin de la société achéologique du Tarn-et-Garonne* 96, 79-80.

Alexander, J.J.G., and C.M. Kauffmann (1973). *English Illuminated Manuscripts 700-1500*. Brussels: Bibliotheque Royale Albert Ier.

Alexander, J.J.G., and E. Temple (1985). *Illuminated Manuscripts in Oxford College Libraries, The University Archives and the Taylor Institution*. Oxford: OUP.

Artemidori Daldiani et Achmetis Sereimi F. oneirocritica, Astrampsychi et Nicephori versus etiam oneirocritici (1603). Paris: Marcus Orry.

Assmann, B., ed. (1888). "Eine Regel über den Donner", *Anglia* 10, 185.

—, ed. (1889a). "Prophezeiung aus dem 1. Januar für das Jahr", *Anglia* 11, 369.

—, ed. (1889b). *Angelsächsische Homilien und Heiligenleben*. Bibliothek der angelsächsischen Prosa 3. Kassel: Wigand.

Atkins, I. (1928). "An Investigation of Two Anglo-Saxon Kalendars (Missal of Robert of Jumièges and St. Wulfstan's Homiliary)", *Archeologia* 78 (2nd ser. 28), 219-54.

Auty, R., *et al.* (1980-99). *Lexikon des Mittelalters*. 10 vols. Munich, Zürich: Artemis Verlag, LexMA Verlag.

Baader, G., and G. Keil, ed. (1982). *Medizin im mittelalterlichen Abendland*. Wege der Forschung 363. Darmstadt: Wissenschaftliche Buchgesellschaft.

Baker, P.S. (1980). "The Old English Canon of Byrhtferth of Ramsey", *Speculum* 55, 22-37.

— (1982). "Byrthferth's *Enchiridion* and the Computus in Oxford, St John's College 17", *ASE* 10, 123-42.

—, and M. Lapidge, ed. (1995). *Byrhtferth's Enchiridion*. EETS, ss 15. London: OUP.

Bannister, H.M. (1916). "Note on Hatton 113", in Turner (1916), lx-lxii.

Barlow, C.W. (1950). *Martini Episcopi Bracarensis Opera omnia*. Papers and Monographs of the American Academy in Rome 12. New Haven: Yale UP.

Bartholomaeus Anglicus (1485). *Liber de proprietatibus rerum*. Strasbourg.

Bayless, M. (1993). "*Beatus quid est* and the Study of Grammar in Late Anglo-Saxon England", *Historiographia Linguistica* 20, 67-110.

Beccaria, A. (1956). *I codici di medicina del periodo presalernitano (secoli IX, X e XI)*. Rome: Storia e letteratura.

Berriot, F., ed. (1989). *Exposicions et significacions des songes et les songes Daniel (manuscrits français de la Bibliothèque nationale de Paris et de la Staatsbibliothek de Berlin, XIVe, XVe et XVIe siècles)*. Travaux d'humanisme et renaissance 234. Geneva: Droz.

Best, R.I., ed. (1940), "An Irish Version of the 'Somniale Danielis'", in Ryan (1940), 3-22.

Betz, H.D., transl. (1986). *The Greek Magical Papyri in Translation, Including the Demotic Spells*. Chicago and London: Univ. of Chicago Press.

Bezold, C., and F. Boll (1911). *Reflexe astrologischer Keilinschriften bei griechischen Schriftstellern*. Sitzungsberichte der Heidelberger Akademie der Wissenschaften, philosophisch-historische Klasse 2.7.

Birch, W. de G. (1878). "On Two Anglo-Saxon Manuscripts in the British Museum", *Transactions of the Royal Society of Literature*, 2nd ser. 11, 463-512.

— (1892). *Liber Vitae. Register and Martyrology of New Minster and Hyde Abbey, Winchester*. Hampshire Record Society. London and Winchester: Simpkin and Warren.

Blum, C. (1943). "Some Observations on Artemon Miletos and his Dreambook", *Eranos. Acta Philologica Suecana* 41, 28-32.

Boissonade, J.F., ed. and transl. (1814). Marinus: *Vita Procli*. Leipzig.

Boll, F., C. Bezold, and W. Gundel (1966). *Sternglaube und Sterndeutung. Die Geschichte und das Wesen der Astrologie*. 5th rev. edn. Darmstadt: Wissenschaftliche Buchgesellschaft.

Bolte, J., ed. (1901-06). *Georg Wickrams Werke*. 8 vols. Bibliothek des litterarischen Vereins in Stuttgart 222, 223, 229, 230, 232, 236, 237, 241. Tübingen: Litterarischen Verein in Stuttgart.

Bond, E.A., and E.M. Thompson (1873-83). *Facsimiles of Manuscripts and Inscriptions*. 1st ser. 3 vols. The Palaeographical Society. London: William Clowes and Sons.

Bonser, W. (1963). *The Medical Background of Anglo-Saxon England. A Study in History, Psychology, and Folklore*, Publications of the Wellcome Historical Medical Library, ns 3. London: Wellcome Historical Medical Library.

Borst, A. (1993). *The Ordering of Time, From the Ancient Computus to the Modern Computer*. Cambridge: Polity Press. Translated from *Computus. Zeit und Zahl in der Geschichte Europas*.

Bosworth, J., and T.N. Toller, ed. (1882-98). See Bosworth and Toller (1882-1972).

—, ed. (1882-1972). *An Anglo-Saxon Dictionary*. Oxford: OUP. 3 vols. Vol. 1: *An Anglo-Saxon Dictionary* (Bosworth and Toller 1882-98); vol. 2: *Supplement* (Toller 1908-21); vol. 3: *Enlarged Addenda and Corrigenda to the Supplement* (Campbell 1972).

Bottéro, J. (1974). "Symptômes, signe, écritures en Mésopotamie ancienne", in

Vernant *et al.* (1974), 70-197.
Bradley, H., ed. (1897). "An Anglo-Saxon Enigma", *Athenaeum* 1897:I, 682-83.
Braekman, W.L. (1981). *Fortune-Telling by the Casting of Dice.* Scripta 4. Brussels: OMIREL.
—— (1988). *Studies on Alchemy, Diet, Medecine [sic] and Prognostication in Middle English.* Scripta 22. Brussels: OMIREL. [year of publication on title page 1986]
Brand, J. (1849-55). *Observations on the Popular Antiquities of Great Britain, Chiefly Illustrating the Origin of Our Vulgar and Provincial Customs, Ceremonies, and Superstitions.* 3 vols. rev. and expanded Sir Henry Ellis. London: Bohn.
Brandin, L., ed. (1914). "Traduction française en vers des *sortes apostolorum*", *Romania* 43, 481-94.
Braswell, L. (1978). "Popular Lunar Astrology in the Late Middle Ages", in *University of Ottawa Quarterly* 48, 187-94.
—— (1984). "Utilitarian and Scientific Prose", in Edwards (1984), 337-87.
Bremmer, R.H. Jr, ed. (1998). *Franciscus Junius F. F. and His Circle.* Amsterdam and Atlanta (GA): Rodopi.
——, and L.S. Chardonnens (2001). "Old English Prognostics: between the Moon and the Monstrous", in Olsen and Houwen (2001), 153-66.
——, and K. Dekker (2006). See Pulsiano and Doane (1994-).
——, and K. Dekker, ed. (2007). *The Transfer of Encyclopaedic Knowledge in the Early Middle Ages. The Foundations of Learning.* Mediaevalia Groningana. Leuven, Paris and Dudley (MA): Peeters. [forthcoming]
Brodersen, K. (2006). Astrampsychos *Das Pythagoras-Orakel und Über magische Steine, Über Traumdeutung, Liebesbindezauber.* Texte zur Forschung 88. Darmstadt: Wissenschaftliche Buchgesellschaft.
Brown, A.K. (1978). "The English Compass Points", *Medium Ævum* 47, 221-46.
Brown, T.J., F. Wormald, A.S.C. Ross, and E.G. Stanley (1969). *The Durham Ritual. A Southern English Collectar of the Tenth Century With Northumbrian Additions. Durham Cathedral Library A. IV. 19.* EEMF 16. Copenhagen: Rosenkilde and Bagger.
Browne, G. M. (1976). "The Origin and Date of the *Sortes Astrampsychi*", *Illinois Classical Studies* 1, 53-55.
——, and R. Stewart, ed. (1983-2001). *Sortes Astrampsychi.* 2 vols. Bibliotheca scriptorum graecorum et romanorum teubneriana. Leipzig: Teubner.
Büchsenschütz, B. (1868). *Traum und Traumdeutung im Alterthume.* Berlin: Calvary.
Budge, E.A.W. (1899). *Egyptian Magic.* London: Kegan Paul, Trench, Trübner.
—— (1913). *Syrian Pathology and Therapeutics, or "The Book of Medicines".* 2 vols. Oxford: OUP.
Budny, M. (1997). *Insular, Anglo-Saxon, and Early Anglo-Norman Manuscript Art at Corpus Christi College, Cambridge, An Illustrated Catalogue.* 2 vols. Kalamazoo, Michigan: Medieval Institute Publications.
Bühler, C.F. (1962). "Two Middle English Texts of the *Somnia Danielis*", *Anglia* 80, 264-73.
Burnett, C. (1997). *The Introduction of Arabic Learning into England.* The Panizzi Lectures 1996. London: The British Library.
——, and N. Mann, ed. (2005). *Britannia Latina. Latin in the Culture of Great Britain from the Middle Ages to the Twentieth Century.* Warburg Institute Colloquia 8. London, Turin: The Warburg Institute, Nino Aragno Editore.

Cameron, A.F. (1973). "A List of Old English Texts", in Frank and Cameron (1973), 25-306.

—— *et al.*, ed. (1980-). *Dictionary of Old English*. Toronto: Pontifical Institute of Mediaeval Studies.

Cameron, M.L. (1983). "The Sources of Medical Knowledge in Anglo-Saxon England", *ASE* 11, 135-55.

—— (1993). *Anglo-Saxon Medicine*. CSASE 7. Cambridge: CUP.

Campbell, A. (1968). *Old English Grammar*. rev. edn. Oxford: OUP.

——, ed. (1972). See Bosworth and Toller (1882-1972).

Camus, J. (1891). "Notices et extraits des manuscrits français de Modène antérieurs au xvie siècle", *Revue des langues romanes* 35, 169-262.

Cappelli, A. (1990, rpt. 1995). *Lexicon abbreviaturarum*. 6th edn. Milan: Ulrico Hoepli.

Chabaneau, C. (1880a). "Les sorts des apotres", *Revue des langues romanes*, 3rd ser. 4, 157-78.

—— (1880b). "Les sorts des apotres", *Revue des langues romanes*, 3rd ser. 4, 264-74.

Chabas, F. (1865). *Le calendrier des jours fastes et néfastes de l'année égyptienne. Traduction complète du Papyrus Sallier IV*. Paris: Dejussieu.

Chardonnens, L.S. (1999). "The Anglo-Saxon Prognostic Calendar", in Lemmen (1999), 1-19.

——, ed. (2000). "A New Edition of the Old English 'Formation of the Foetus'", *Notes and Queries*, ns 47, 10-11.

—— (2006). *Anglo-Saxon Prognostics. A Study of the Genre with a Text Edition*. Unpublished Ph.D. Thesis Leiden Univ.

—— (2007a). "Cijferen met middeleeuwse kopiisten en moderne filologen", *Madoc* 21:1. [forthcoming]

—— (2007b). "London, British Library, Harley 3271: the Composition and Structure of an Eleventh-Century Anglo-Saxon Miscellany", in Lendinara, Lazzari and D'Aronco (2007). [forthcoming]

—— (2007c). "Context, Language, Date and Origin of Anglo-Saxon Prognostics", in Bremmer and Dekker (2007). [forthcoming]

Cilliers, L (2004). "Vindicianus' *Gynaecia* and Theories on Generation and Embryology from the Babylonians up to Graeco-Roman Times", in Horstmanshoff and Stol, 343-67.

—— (2005). "Vindicianus's *Gynaecia*: Text and Translation of the Codex Monacensis (Clm 4622)", *The Journal of Medieval Latin* 15, 153-236.

Clayton, M. (1990). *The Cult of the Virgin Mary in Anglo-Saxon England*. CSASE 2. Cambridge: CUP.

——, and H. Magennis (1994). *The Old English Lives of St Margaret*. CSASE 9. Cambridge: CUP.

Clemoes, P., ed. (1959). *The Anglo-Saxons. Studies in Some Aspects of Their History and Culture, Presented to Bruce Dickins*. London: Bowes & Bowes.

—— (1997). *Ælfric's Catholic Homilies, The First Series, Text*. EETS, ss 17. London: OUP.

——, and K. Hughes, ed. (1971). *England Before the Conquest. Studies in Primary Sources Presented to Dorothy Whitelock*. Cambridge: CUP.

Cockayne, T.O., ed. (1861). *Narratiunculæ anglice conscriptæ*. London: J. R. Smith.

—— (1864-66). *Leechdoms, Wortcunning, and Starcraft of Early England. Being a Collection of Documents, for the Most Part Never before Printed, Illustrating the History of Science in this Country before the Norman Conquest*. 3 vols. Rolls Series 35. London: Longmans, Green,

Reader, and Dyer. rev. edn C.W. Singer (1961), London: The Holland Press.

Colgrave, B., and R.A.B. Mynors, ed. and transl. (1991). *Bede's Ecclesiastical History of the English People*. rev. edn. Oxford: OUP.

Collins, R.L. (1976). *Anglo-Saxon Vernacular Manuscripts in America*. New York: The Scheide Library, The Pierpont Morgan Library.

Cordoñer, C. (2003). "Un manuscrito escolar del siglo IX: Royal 15.B.XIX", *Segno e Testo* 1, 229-45.

Corrêa, A. (1995). "Daily Office Books. Collectars and Breviaries", in Pfaff (1995b), 45-60.

Coxe, H.O. (1852). *Catalogus codicum MSS. qui in collegiis aulisque Oxoniensibus hodie adservantur*. 2 vols. Oxford: OUP.

Craig, H. (1916). *The Works of John Metham, Including the Romance of Amoryus and Cleopes*. EETS, os 132. London: Kegan Paul.

Crawford, S.J., ed. (1922). *The Old English Version of the Heptateuch, Ælfric's Treatise on the Old and New Testament and His Preface to Genesis*. EETS, os 160. London: OUP.

Cross, J.E. and T.H. Hill, ed. and transl. (1982). *The* Prose Solomon and Saturn *and* Adrian and Ritheus. McMaster Old English Studies and Texts 1. Toronto, Buffalo, London: Univ. of Toronto Press.

Cuissard, C. (1882). *Étude sur les jours égyptiens des calendriers*. LmASC 5. Orléans: E. Colas.

Damico, H., D. Fennema and K. Lenz, ed. (1998). *Medieval Scholarship. Biographical Studies on the Formation of a Discipline*. Vol 2: *Literature and Philology*. New York and London: Garland.

D'Aronco, M.A. (2005). "How 'English' is Anglo-Saxon Medicine? The Latin Sources for Anglo-Saxon medical Texts", in Burnett and Mann (2005), 27-41.

— (2007). "The Transmission of Medical Knowledge in Anglo-Saxon England: the Voices of the Manuscripts", in Lendinara, Lazzari and D'Aronco (2007). [forthcoming]

Daunou, P.C.F. (1842-48). *Cours d'études historiques*. 19 vols. Paris.

Davril, A., T.M. Thidobeau and B.-G. Guyot, ed. (1995-2000). *William Durandus' Rationale diuinorum officiorum*. 3 vols. Corpus Christianorum, Continuatio Mediaevalis CXL, CXLA, CXLB. Turnhout: Brepols.

Dawson, W.R. (1926). "Some Observations on the Egyptian Calendars of Lucky and Unlucky Days", *Journal of Egyptian Archaeology* 12, 260-64.

Deegan, M. (1987). "Pregnancy and Childbirth in Anglo-Saxon Medical Texts. A Preliminary Survey", in Deegan and Scragg (1987), 17-26.

—, and D.C. Scragg, ed. (1987). *Medicine in Early Medieval England, Four Studies*. Manchester: Manchester Centre for Anglo-Saxon Studies, Univ. of Manchester.

Dekker, C (2007). "Anglo-Saxon Encyclopaedic Notes: Tradition and Function", in Bremmer and Dekker (2007). [forthcoming]

Derolez, R. (1954). *Runica Manuscripta. The English Tradition*. Rijksuniversiteit te Gent, Werken uitgegeven door de faculteit van de wijsbegeerte en letteren 118. Bruges: De Tempel.

— (1971). "The Orientation System in the Old English *Orosius*", in Clemoes and Hughes (1971), 253-68.

Derow, J.P. (1993). "Jorg Immendorff's 'Café Deutschland Gut': Consolidation with Klucel G and the Engelbrecht Radiant Heat Source", *The Book and Paper Group Annual* 12, 8-11.

Desham, R. (1977). "The Leofric Missal and Tenth-Century English Art", *ASE* 6, 145-73.

Diepgen, P. (1912). *Traum und Traumdeutung als medizinisch-naturwissenschaftliches Problem im Mittelalter*. Berlin: Springer.

Dieterich, A. (1901). "ABC-Denkmäler", in *Rheinisches Museum für Philologie*, neue Folge 56, 77-105.

DiTommaso, L. (2005). *The Book of Daniel and the Apocryphal Daniel Literature*. Studia in Veteris Testamenti Pseudepigrapha 20. Leiden, Boston: Brill.

—— (2006). "Pseudepigrapha Notes I: 1. *Lunationes Danielis*; 2. Biblical Figures outside the Bible", *Journal for the Study of the Pseudepigrapha* 15:2, 119-44.

Divjak, J., ed. (1971). *Aurelius Augustinus. Epistolae ad Galatas expositionis liber unus*. Sancti Aurelii Augustini Opera IV.1, 53-141. Corpus Scriptorum Ecclesiasticorum Latinorum 84. Vienna: Hoelder, Pichler, Tempsky.

Doane, A.N. (1994). See Pulsiano and Doane (1994-)

——, and T.J. Grade (2001). See Pulsiano and Doane (1994-).

Dobbie, E.V.K., ed. (1942). *The Anglo-Saxon Minor Poems*. Anglo-Saxon Poetic Records 6. London and New York: Routledge and Kegan Paul.

Dobschütz, E. von (1912). *Das Decretum Gelasianum de libris recipiendis et non recipiendis*. Texte und Untersuchungen zur Geschichte der altchristlichen Literatur, 3rd ser., vol. 8.4. Leipzig: J. C. Hinrichs'sche Buchhandlung.

Dold, A. (1948). *Die Orakelsprüche im St. Galler Palimpsestcodex 908 (die sogenannten "sortes Sangallenses")*. Österreichische Akademie der Wissenschaften, philosophisch-historische Klasse, Sitzungsberichte 225:4. Vienna: Rudolf M. Rohrer.

Drexl, F. (1921). "Das anonyme Traumbuch des Cod. Paris. gr. 2511", *Laographia* 8, 347-75.

—— (1922). "Das Traumbuch des Patriarchen Nikephoros", in Koeniger (1922), 94-118.

—— (1923). "Das Traumbuch des Patriarchen Germanos", *Laographia* 7, 433-48.

—— (1925). *Achmetis Oneirocriticon*. Bibliotheca scriptorum graecorum et romanorum Teubneriana. Leipzig: Teubner.

—— (1926). "Das Traumbuch des Propheten Daniel nach dem Cod. Vatic. Palat. gr. 319", *Byzantinische Zeitschrift* 26, 290-314.

Ducange, C. du Fresne, *et al.* (1937-38). *Glossarium mediae et infimae latinitatis*. 10 vols. new edn. Paris.

Eales, R., and R. Sharpe, ed. (1995). *Canterbury and the Norman Conquest. Churches, Saints and Scholars 1066-1109*. London and Rio Grande: The Hambledon Press.

Edwards, A.S.G., ed. (1984, rpt. 1986). *Middle English Prose, A Critical Guide to Major Authors and Genres*. New Brunswick: Rutgers UP.

——, ed. (2004). *A Companion to Middle English Prose*. Cambridge: D. S. Brewer.

Einarsson, S. (1937). "Old and Middle English Notes", *Journal of English and Germanic Philology* 36, 183-87.

Elliott, R.W.V. (1989). *Runes. An Introduction*. 2nd edn. Manchester, New York: Manchester UP, St. Martin's Press.

Elsakkers, M. (2004). "Her anda neylar: an Intriguing Criterion for Abortion in Old Frisian Law", *Scientiarum Historia* 30, 107-54.

Epe, A., ed. (1995). *Wissensliteratur im angelsächsischen England. Das Fachschrifttum der vergessenen artes mechanicae und artes magicae. Mit besonderer Berücksichtigung des Somniale Danielis. Edition der (lateinisch-)altenglischen Fassungen*. Münster: Verlag Tebbert.

Eriksson, S. (1956). *Wochentagsgötter, Mond und Tierkreis. Laienastrologie in der römischen Kaiserzeit.* Studia Graeca et Latina Gothoburgensia 3. Stockholm: Almqvist and Wiksell.
Euw, A. von, and J.M. Plotzek (1979-85). *Die Handschriften der Sammlung Ludwig.* 4 vols. Cologne: Schnütgen-Museum.
Evans, E. ed. (1969). *Aurelius Augustinus. Enchiridion ad Laurentium de fide et spe et caritate.* Sancti Aurelii Augustini Opera XIII.2, 21-114. CCSL 46. Turnhout: Brepols.
Ferckel, C. (1914). "Ein deutscher anatomischer Vindiciantext", *Sudhoff* 7, 306-18.
Fischer, S.R., ed. (1982a). *The Complete Medieval Dreambook. A Multilingual, Alphabetical Somniale Danielis Collation.* Bern, Frankfurt am Main: Peter Lang.
—— (1982b). "Ein deutsches 'Somniale Danielis'-Fragment aus dem späten Mittelalters", *ZfdA* 110, 145-51.
—— (1983). "Dreambooks and the Interpretation of Medieval Literary Dreams", *Archiv für Kulturgeschichte* 65, 1-20.
—— (1989). *Das Somniarium. Ein mittelalterliches Traumbuch.* Bern: Peter Lang.
Flint, V.I.J. (1991). *The Rise of Magic in Early Medieval Europe.* Princeton: Princeton UP.
Forshall, J. (1834-40). *Catalogue of Manuscripts in the British Museum.* ns I. 3 vols. London: British Museum.
Fowler, R., ed. (1972). *Wulfstan's Canons of Edgar.* EETS, os 266. London: OUP.
Förster, M. (1903). "Die Kleinliteratur des Aberglaubens im altenglischen", *Archiv* 110, 346-58.
—— (1906). "Zur altenglischen Mirabilien-Version", *Archiv* 117, 367-70.
—— (1908a). "Beiträge zur mittelalterlichen Volkskunde I", *Archiv* 120, 43-52.
—— (1908b). "Beiträge zur mittelalterlichen Volkskunde II", *Archiv* 120, 296-305.
—— (1908c). "Beiträge zur mittelalterlichen Volkskunde III", *Archiv* 121, 30-46.
—— (1910). "Beiträge zur mittelalterlichen Volkskunde IV", *Archiv* 125, 39-70.
—— (1911). "Beiträge zur mittelalterlichen Volkskunde V", *Archiv* 127, 31-84.
—— (1912a). "Beiträge zur mittelalterlichen Volkskunde VI", *Archiv* 128, 55-71.
—— (1912b). "Beiträge zur mittelalterlichen Volkskunde VII", *Archiv* 128, 285-308.
—— (1912c). "Beiträge zur mittelalterlichen Volkskunde VIII", *Archiv* 129, 16-49.
—— (1916). "Beiträge zur mittelalterlichen Volkskunde IX", *Archiv* 134, 264-93.
—— (1920). "Der Inhalt der altenglischen Handschrift Vespasianus D. XIV.", *Englische Studien* 54, 46-68.
—— (1921). "Das älteste kymrische Traumbuch (um 1350)", *Zeitschrift für celtische Philologie* 13, 55-92.
—— (1925). "Die Weltzeitalter bei den Angelsachsen", in *Neusprachliche Studien. Festgabe Karl Luick zu seinem sechzigsten Geburtstag. Die neueren Sprachen* 33, Beiheft 6, 183-203.
—— (1925-26). "Die altenglischen Traumlunare", *Englische Studien* 60, 58-93.
—— (1929). "Die altenglischen Verzeichnisse von Glücks- und Unglückstagen", in Malone and Ruud (1929), 258-77.
—— (1936). "Zwei kymrische Orakelalphabete für Psalterwahrsagung", *Zeitschrift für celtische Philologie* 20, 228-43.
—— (1944). "Vom Fortleben antiker Sammellunare im englischen und in anderen Volkssprachen", *Anglia* 67/68, 1-171.
Frank, R., and A.F. Cameron, ed. (1973). *A Plan for the Dictionary of Old English.* Toronto and Buffalo: Univ. of Toronto Press.
Frantzen, A.J. (1983a). *The Literature of Penance in Anglo-Saxon England.* New Brunswick (NJ): Rutgers UP.

—— (1983b). "The Tradition of Penitentials in Anglo-Saxon England", *ASE* 11, 23-56.

Franzen, C. (1991). *The Tremulous Hand of Worcester. A Study of Old English in the Thirteenth Century*. Oxford: OUP.

—— (1998). See Pulsiano and Doane (1994-).

Frings, T. (1933). "Eduard Sievers, geboren zu Lippoldsberg a. d. Weser am 25. November 1850 gestorben zu Leipzig am 30. März 1932", *Berichte über die Verhandlungen der sächsischen Akademie der Wissenschaften zu Leipzig, philologisch-historische Klasse* 85:1.

Gameson, R. (1999). *The Manuscripts of Early Norman England (c. 1066-1130)*. Oxford: OUP.

Ganz, P. (1978). "Eduard Sievers", *Beiträge zur Geschichte der deutschen Sprache und Literatur* 100, 40-85.

Gardiner, A.H., ed. (1935). *Chester Beatty Gift*. 2 vols. HPBM, 3rd ser. London: British Museum.

Gasquet, A., and E. Bishop (1908). *The Bosworth Psalter. An Account of a Manuscript Formerly Belonging to O. Turville-Petre Esq. of Bosworth Hall now Addit. MS. 37517 at the British Museum*. London: George Bell and Sons.

Gaster, M. (1891). *Chrestomatie Română. Texte tipă rite şi manuscrise [sec. xvi-xix], dialectale şi populare*. 2 vols. Leipzig, Bucharest: F. A. Brockhaus, Socecŭ & Co.

Gebelin, A.C. de, ed. (1773-82). *Monde primitif, analysé et comparé avec le monde moderne*. 9 vols. Paris: Nicolas Ruault.

Getz, F. (1998). *Medicine in the English Middle Ages*. Princeton: Princeton UP.

Gilson, J.P. (1912). *Catalogue of Additions to the Manuscripts in the British Museum in the Years MDCCCCVI-MDCCCCX*. London: British Museum.

Gittos, H. (2005) "Is there any Evidence for the Liturgy of Parish Churches in Late Anglo-Saxon England? The Red Book of Darley and the Status of Old English", in Tinti (2005), 63-82.

Glaze, F. E. (2007). "Master-Student Medical Dialogues: the Evidence of London, British Library, Sloane 2839", in Lendinara, Lazzari and D'Aronco. [forthcoming]

Gneuss, H. (1964). "Englands Bibliotheken im Mittelalter und ihr Untergang", in Gneuss (1996a), I.91-121.

—— (1981). "A Preliminary List of Manuscripts Written or Owned in England up to 1100", *ASE* 9, 1-60.

—— (1986). "Anglo-Saxon Libraries from the Conversion to the Benedictine Reform", in Gneuss (1996a), II.643-688.

—— (1992). "Bücher und Leser in England im zehnten Jahrhundert", in Gneuss (1996a), IV.104-30.

—— (1994). "Guide to the Editing and Preparation of Texts for the *Dictionary of Old English*", in Scragg and Szarmach (1994), 7-26.

—— (1996a). *Books and Libraries in Early England*. Variorum Collected Studies Series 558. Aldershot: Ashgate.

—— (1996b). *English Language Scholarship. A Survey and Bibliography from the Beginnings to the End of the Nineteenth Century*. Medieval and Renaissance Texts and Studies 125. Binghampton (NY): Center for Medieval and Early Renaissance Studies.

—— (1997). "Origin and Provenance of Anglo-Saxon Manuscripts. The Case of Cotton Tiberius A. III", in Robinson and Zim (1997), 13-48.

—— (2001). *Handlist of Anglo-Saxon Manuscripts. A List of Manuscripts and Manuscript Fragments Written or Owned in England up to 1100*. Medieval and Renaissance Texts and Studies 241. Tempe (AZ): Arizona Center for Medieval and Renaissance Studies.

—— (2003). "Addenda and Corrigenda to the *Handlist of Anglo-Saxon Manuscripts*. *ASE* 32, 293-305.

Godden, M. (1977). "Old English", in Rigg (1977), 9-33.

—— (1979). *Ælfric's Catholic Homilies, The Second Series, Text*. EETS, ss 5. London: OUP.

—— (1992). "New Year's Day in Late Anglo-Saxon England", *Notes and Queries* 237, ns 39, 148-50.

—— (2000). *Ælfric's Catholic Homilies, Introduction, Commentary and Glossary*. EETS, ss 18. London: OUP.

——, and M. Lapidge, ed. (1991). *The Cambridge Companion to Old English Literature*. Cambridge: CUP.

Gorman, M. (1996). "The Glosses on Bede's *De temporum ratione* Attributed to Byrhtferth of Ramsey", *ASE* 25, 209-32.

Graffunder, P. (1906). "Daniels Traumdeutungen. Ein mitterlaterliches Traumbuch in deutschen Versen", *ZfdA* 48, 507-31.

Graham, T. (2001). "Anglo-Saxon Studies. Sixteenth to Eighteenth Centuries", in Pulsiano and Treharne (2001), 415-433.

—— *et al.* (2003). See Pulsiano and Doane (1994-).

Granlund, J., *et al.* (1956-82). *Kulturhistorisk leksikon for nordisk middelalder fra vikingetid til reformationstid*. 22 vols. Copenhagen: Rosenkilde and Bagger.

Grattan, J.H.G., and C.W. Singer (1952). *Anglo-Saxon Magic and Medicine, Illustrated Specially from the Semi-Pagan Text* Lacnunga. Publications of the Wellcome Historical Medical Museum, ns 3. London: OUP.

Greenfield, S.B., and F.C. Robinson (1980). *A Bibliography of Publications on Old English to the End of 1972*. Manchester: Manchester UP.

Gretsch, M. (1999). *The Intellectual Foundations of the English Benedictine Reform*. CSASE 25. Cambridge: CUP.

—— (2001). "Winchester Vocabulary and Standard Old English: the Vernacular in Late Anglo-Saxon England", *Bulletin of the John Rylands University Library of Manchester* 83:1, 41-88.

—— (2004), "The Taunton Fragment: a New Text from Anglo-Saxon England", *ASE* 33, 145-93.

Griffiths, B. (1996). *Aspects of Anglo-Saxon Magic*. Hockwold-cum-Wilton: Anglo-Saxon Books.

Grub, J. (1984). *Das lateinische Traumbuch im Codex Upsaliensis C 664 (9. Jh.). Eine frühmittelalterliche Fassung der lateinischen Somniale Danielis-Tradition*. Lateinische Sprache und Literatur des Mittelalters 19. Frankfurt am Main, Bern and New York: Peter Lang.

Gumbert, J.P. (2004). "Codicological Units: towards a Terminology for the Stratigraphy of the Non-Homogeneous Codex", *Segno e Testo* 2, 17-42.

Gundel, W. (1907). *De stellarum appellatione et religione Romana*. Religionsgeschichtliche Versuche und Vorarbeiten 3:2, 93-252.

—— (1927). "Individualschicksal, Menschentypen und Berufe in der antiken Astrologie", *Jahrbuch der Charakterologie* 4, 133-93.

——, and H.G. Gundel (1959). *Sternglaube, Sternreligion und Sternorakel. Aus der Geschichte der Astrologie*. 2nd edn. Heidelberg: Quelle & Meyer.

——, and H.G. Gundel (1966). *Astrologumena. Die astrologische Literatur in der Antike und ihre Geschichte. Sudhoff*, Beiheft 6. Wiesbaden: Franz Steiner Verlag.

Günzel, B. (1993). *Ælfwine's Prayerbook (London, British Library, Cotton Titus D. xxvi + xxvii)*. HBS 108. London: Boydell Press.

Haag, G. (2003). *Traum und Traumdeutung in mittelhochdeutscher Literatur. Theoretische Grundlagen und Fallstudien*. Germanistik. Stuttgart: Hirzel.

Hahn, I. (1992). *Traumdeutung und gesellschaftliche Wirklichkeit. Artemidorus Daldianus als sozialgeschichtliche Quelle*. Exnia 27. Konstanz: Universitätsverlag Konstanz.

Hall, J.R. (2001). "Anglo-Saxon Studies in the Nineteenth Century. England, Denmark, America", in Pulsiano and Treharne (2001), 434-54.

Hampson, R.T. (1841). *Medii aevi kalendarium. Dates, Charters, and Customs of the Middle Ages, with Kalendars from the Tenth to the Fifteenth Century, and an Alphabetical Digest of Obsolete Names of Days, Forming a Glossary of the Dates of the Middle Ages with Tables and other Aids for Ascertaining Dates*. 2 vols. London: Causton.

Handley, R. (1974). "British Museum MS. Cotton Vespasian D. xiv", *Notes and Queries*, ns 21, 243-50.

Hanna, R. (2002). *A Descriptive Catalogue of the Western Medieval Manuscripts of St. John's College Oxford*. Oxford: OUP.

Hanson, A.E. (2004), "*Aphorismi* 5.28-63 and the Gynaecological Texts of the *Corpus Hippocratum*", in Horstmanshoff and Stol (2004), 277-304.

Hardwick, C., *et al.* (1856-67, rpt. 1980). *A Catalogue of the Manuscripts Preserved in the Library of the University of Cambridge*. 5 vols. Cambridge: CUP.

Harmening, D. (1979). *Superstitio. Überlieferungs- und theoriegeschichtliche Untersuchungen zur kirchlich-theologischen Aberglaubensliteratur des Mittelalters*. Berlin: Erich Schmidt.

Harris, J.R. (1888). "The 'sortes sanctorum' in the St. Germain Codex (g^1)", *American Journal of Philology* 9, 58-63.

—— (1901). *The Annotators of the Codex Bezae (With some Notes on Sortes sanctorum)*, London: CUP.

Harrison, K. (1973). "The Beginning of the Year in England, *c*. 500-900", *ASE* 2, 51-70.

— (1978). "Easter Cycles and the Equinox in the British Isles", *ASE* 7, 1-8.

Hart, C. (1970). "The Ramsey *Computus*", *English Historical Review* 85, 29-44.

Hartel, W. von (1886). "Bibliotheca patrum latinorum Hispaniensis V", Sitzungsberichte der philosophisch-historische Klasse der kaiserlichen Akademie der Wissenschaften 113, 215-84.

Hartung, A.E., gen. ed. (1998). *A Manual of the Writings in Middle English, 1050-1500. Vol 10: Science and Information*. New Haven: Connecticut Academy of Arts and Sciences.

Haskins, C.H. (1915). "The Reception of Arabic Science in England", *English Historical Review* 30, 56-69.

—— (1924). *Studies in the History of Mediaeval Science*. Cambridge: Harvard UP.

Healey, A. diP., and R.L. Venezky (1980). *A Microfiche Concordance to Old English*, Toronto, Buffalo, London: Pontifical Institute of Mediaeval Studies.

—— (2000). *The Complete Corpus of Old English in Electronic Form*. <http://ets.umdl.umich.edu/o/oec/index.html [accessed 14 April 2005]>.

Heimann, A. (1966). "Three Illustrations from the Bury St. Edmunds Psalter and Their Prototypes. Notes on the Iconography of Some Anglo-Saxon Drawings", *Journal of the Warburg and Courtauld Institutes* 29, 39-59.

Heinevetter, F. (1912). *Würfel- und Buchstabenorakel in Griechenland und Kleinasien*. Breslau: Graß, Barth & Comp.

Hélin, M. (1925). *La clef des songes*. Documents scientifiques du XVe siècle 2. Paris.

Hellmann, G. (1896a) "Über der chaldaïschen Ursprung modernen Gewitteraberglaubens", *Meteorologische Zeitschrift* 13, 236-38.

—— (1896b). *Die Bauern-Praktik 1508*. Neudrucke von Schriften und Karten über Meteorologie und Erdmagnetismus 5. Berlin: A. Asher & Co.

Henel, H. (1934a). *Studien zum altenglischen Computus*. Beiträge zur englischen Philologie 26. Leipzig: Tauchnitz.

—— (1934b). "Planetenglaube in Ælfrics Zeit", *Anglia* 58, 292-317.

—— (1934-35). "Altenglischer Mönchsaberglaube", *Englische Studien* 69, 329-49.

—— (1942). *Ælfric's De temporibus anni*. EETS , os 213. London: OUP.

Hercher, R. (1863). *Astrampsychi oraculorum decades CIII*. Jahresbericht über das königliche Joachimsthalsche Gymnasium. Berlin: Unger.

Hermes, L. (1996). *Traum und Traumdeutung in der Antike*. Antike Aktuell. Zurich: Artemis & Winkler.

Hervagius, J. (1563). *Opera Bedae Venerabilis presbyteri Anglosaxonis*. 4 vols. Basel: Hervagius.

Heslop, T.A. (1995). "The Canterbury Calendars and the Norman Conquest", in Eales and Sharpe (1995), 53-85.

Hessels, J.H., ed. (1890). *An Eighth-Century Latin-Anglo-Saxon Glossary Preserved in the Library of Corpus Christi College, Cambridge (MS. No. 144)*. Cambridge: CUP.

Hickes, G., and H. Wanley (1705). *Antiquæ literaturæ septentrionalis*. 2 vols. Oxford: Sheldon.

Hill, B.H. (1961-63). "Frisian Law and the Foetus", *Janus. Archives internationales pour l'histoire de la médecine et la géographie médicale* 50, 55-59.

Hill, J. (2001). "The Benedictine Reform and Beyond", in Pulsiano and Treharne (2001), 151-69.

Hirsh, J.C. (1997). "Fate, Faith and Paradox. Medieval Unlucky Days as a Context for 'Wytte hath Wondyr'", *Medium Ævum* 66, 288-92.

Hoffmann-Krayer, E., H. Bächtold-Stäubli, *et al.* (1927-42). *Handwörterbuch des deutschen Aberglaubens*. 10 vols. Berlin: De Gruyter.

Hohler, C.E. (1972). "The Red Book of Darley", *Nordiskt Kollokvium i Latinsk Liturgiforskning* 2, 39-47.

Hollis, S. (2001). "Scientific and Medical Writings", in Pulsiano and Treharne (2001), 188-208.

——, and M. Wright (1992). *Old English Prose of Secular Learning*. Annotated Bibliographies of Old and Middle English Literature 4. Cambridge: D. S. Brewer.

Holowchack, M.A. (2002). *Ancient Science and Dreams. Oneirology in Greco-Roman Antiquity*. Lanham: UP of America.

Holthausen, F. (1908). "Ein altschwedische Donnerregel", *Archiv* 121, 129.

Hoops, J. (1889). *Über die altenglischen Pflanzennamen*. Freiburg i. B.: Chr. Lehmann.

Horstmanshoff, H.F.J, and M. Stol, ed. (2004). *Magic and Rationality in Ancient Near Eastern and Graeco-Roman Medicine*. Studies in Ancient Medicine 27. Leiden, Boston: Brill.

Hughes, A., ed. (1958-60). *The Portiforium of Saint Wulstan (Corpus Christi College, Cambridge, MS. 391)*. 2 vols. HBS 89-90. Leighton Buzzard: Faith Press.

Hugonnard-Roche, H. (1996). "The Influence of Arabic Astronomy in the Medieval West", in Rashed (1996), I.284-305.

Hunt, T. (1987). "*Deliciae Clericorum*. Intellectual and Scientific Pursuits in Two Dorset Monasteries", *Medium Ævum* 56, 159-82.

——, ed. (1994-97). *Anglo-Norman Medicine*. 2 vols. Cambridge: D.S. Brewer.

Iconclass (2002). <http://www.iconclass.nl [accessed 14 April 2005]>.

Irvine, S. (2000). "The Compilation and Use of Manuscripts Containing Old English in the Twelfth Century", in Swan and Treharne (2000), 41-61.

Jahoda, G. (1969, rpt. 1971). *The Psychology of Superstition*. Harmondsworth: Penguin Books.

James, M.R. (1900-04). *The Western Manuscripts in the Library of Trinity College, Cambridge, A Descriptive Catalogue*. 4 vols. Cambridge: CUP.

— (1912). *A Descriptive Catalogue of the Manuscripts in the Library of Corpus Christi College Cambridge*. 2 vols. Cambridge: CUP.

—, and C. Jenkins (1930-32). *A Descriptive Catalogue of the Manuscripts in the Library of Lambeth Palace*. 5 vols. Cambridge: CUP.

—, and E.H. Minnis (1915). *A Descriptive Catalogue of the Manuscripts in the Library of Pembroke College, Cambridge, With a Handlist of the Printed Books to the Year 1500*. Cambridge: CUP.

Jastrow, M. (1905-12). *Die Religion Babyloniens und Assyriens*. 2 vols. Giessen: Alfred Töpelmann.

Jenkinson, F.J.H., ed. (1908). *The Hisperica Famina*. Cambridge: CUP.

Joannes de Sacrobosco (1566). *Libellus de anni ratione, seu, ut vocatur vulgo, computus ecclesiasticus*. Antwerp: Jean Richard.

John, E. (1963). "The Beginning of the Benedictine Reform in England", *Revue Bénédictine* 73, 73-87.

Jones, C.W. (1938). "The Byrhtferth Glosses", *Medium Ævum* 7, 81-97.

— (1939). *Bedae Pseudepigrapha. Scientific Writings Falsely Attributed to Bede*. Ithaca and London: Cornell UP, OUP.

— (1943). *Bedae Opera de temporibus*. Cambridge (Mass.): The Mediaeval Academy of America.

—, ed. (1975-80). *Bedae Venerabilis Opera*. Part VI. *Opera didascalia*. 3 vols. CCSL 123A-C. Turnhout: Brepols.

Jones, P.M. (1984). *Medieval Medical Miniatures*. London: The British Library and the Wellcome Institute for the History of Medicine.

Jones, W.H.S., ed. and transl. (1931, rpt. 1979). *Hippocrates*. Vol. IV. Cambridge (MS): Harvard UP.

Jordan, L. (1986). "Demonic Elements in Anglo-Saxon Iconography", in Szarmach and Oggins (1986), 283-317.

Kaiser, M., and F.S. Krauss (1965). Artemis von Daldis *Traumbuch*. 2nd edn. Basel: Schwabe.

Kauffmann, C.M. (1975). *Romanesque Manuscripts 1066~1190*. Survey of Manuscripts Illuminated in the British Isles 3. London: Harvey Miller.

Keil, G. (1957). "Die verworfenen Tage", *Sudhoff* 41, 27-58.

— (1960). "Eine lateinsiche Fassung von Meister Alexanders Monatsregeln. Bairische Gesundheitsregeln aus dem Ende des 14. Jahrhunderts", in Baader and Keil (1982), 228-59.

Keiser, G. (1998). "Scientific and Practical Writings", in Hartung (1998).

— (2004). "Scientific, Medical, and Utilitarian Prose", in Edwards (2004), 231-47.

Ker, N.R. (1957). *Catalogue of Manuscripts Containing Anglo-Saxon*. Oxford: OUP.

— (1959). "Three Old English Texts in a Salisbury Pontifical, Cotton Tiberius C I", in Clemoes (1959), 262-79.

— (1976). "A Supplement to *Catalogue of Manuscripts Containing Anglo-Saxon*", *ASE* 5, 121-31.

——, and A.J. Piper (1969-92). *Medieval Manuscripts in British Libraries*. 4 vols. Oxford: OUP.

Keskiaho, J. (2004). "Eighth-Century Anglo-Latin Ecclesiastical Attitudes to Dreams and Visions", *Ennen ja nyt* 2004:4. <http://www.ennenjanyt.net/4-04/referee/keskiaho.html [accessed 1 March 2007]>.

Keynes, S. (1985). "The Crowland Psalter and the Sons of King Edmund Ironside", *Bodleian Library Record* 11:6, 359-70.

—— (1996). *The Liber vitae of the New Minster and Hyde Abbey Winchester*. EEMF 26. Copenhagen: Rosenkilde and Bagger.

Kieckhefer, R. (1989). *Magic in the Middle Ages*. Cambridge Medieval Textbooks. Cambridge: CUP.

Killy, W., and R. Vierhaus, ed. (1995-2000). *Deutsche biographische Enzyklopädie*. 11 vols. München: K. G. Saur.

Kitson, P. (1990). "On Old English Nouns of More than One Gender", *English Studies* 71, 185-221.

Klingshirn, W.E. (2002). "Defining the *Sortes Sanctorum*. Gibbon, Du Cange, and Early Christian Lot Divination", *Journal of Early Christian Studies* 10, 77-130.

Klopfer, H., and M. Lackner (1989). *Das arabische Traumbuch des Ibn-Sirin*. Diederichs' gelbe Reihe: 80. Munich: Diederichs.

Knowles, D. (1949). *The Monastic Order in England. A History of its Development from the Times of St Dunstan to the Fourth Lateran Council 943-1216*. corrected edn. Cambridge: CUP.

—— (1951). *Decreta Lanfranci, Monachis Cantuariensibus transmissa. The Monastic Constitutions of Lanfranc*. London: Thomas Nelson and Sons.

Koeniger, A.M. (1922). *Beiträge zur Geschichte des christlichen Altertums und der byzantinischen Literatur. Festgabe Albert Ehrhard zum 60. Geburtstag (14. März 1922)*. Bonn, Leipzig: Schroeder.

Kooper, E., ed. (2003). *Current Research in Dutch Universities and Polytechnics on Old English, Middle English, and Historical Linguistics. Papers Read at the Twenty-Fourth Research Symposium Held in Utrecht on 13 December 2002*. Utrecht.

Korhammer, P.M. (1973). "The Origin of the Bosworth Psalter", *ASE* 2, 173-87.

—— (1985). "The Orientation System in the Old English Orosius: Shifted or not?", in Lapidge and Gneuss (1985), 251-69.

Körntgen, L. (1993). *Studien zu den Quellen der frühmittelalterlichen Bußbücher*. Quellen und Forschungen zum Recht im Mittelalter 7. Sigmaringen: Jan Thorbecke Verlag.

Kottje, R. (1980). *Die Bussbücher Halitgars von Cambrai und des Hrabanus Maurus. Ihre Überlieferung und ihre Quellen*. Beiträge zur Geschichte und Quellenkunde des Mittelalters 8. Berlin, New York: Walter de Gruyter.

Kotzor, G. (1981). *Das altenglische Martyrologium*. 2 vols. Bayerische Akademie der Wissenschaften, Abhandlungen, philosophisch-historische Klasse, neue Folge 88/1-2. Munich: Verlag der Bayerischen Akademie der Wissenschaften.

Kruger, S.F. (1992). *Dreaming in the Middle Ages*. Cambridge Studies in Medieval Literature 14. Cambridge: CUP.

Kurland, M.L. (1972). "Oneiromancy: An Historic Review of Dream Interpretation", *American Journal of Psychotherapy* 26, 408-16.

Lapidge, M. (1980). "The Revival of Latin Learning in Late Anglo-Saxon England", in Mare and Barker-Benfield (1980), 18-22.

—— (2006). *The Anglo-Saxon Library*. Oxford: OUP.

—, and H. Gneuss, ed. (1985). *Learning and Literature in Anglo-Saxon England. Studies Presented to Peter Clemoes on the Occasion of his Sixty-Fifth Birthday*. Cambridge: CUP.

Leemans, C., ed. and transl. (1843-85). *Papyri graeci musei antiquarii publici Lugduni Batavi regis Augustissimi jussu*. 2 vols. Leiden: Brill.

Lehmann, P. (1914). "Apuleiusfragmente", *Hermes. Zeitschrift für klassische Philologie* 49, 612-20.

Lemmen, H., ed. (1999). *Current Research in Dutch Universities and Polytechnics on Old English, Middle English, and Historical Linguistics. Papers Read at the Twentieth Research Symposium, Utrecht, 11 December 1998*. Utrecht.

Lendinara, P. (1991). "The World of Anglo-Saxon Learning", in Godden and Lapidge (1991), 264-81.

— (1999). *Anglo-Saxon Glosses and Glossaries*. Variorum Collected Studies Series 622. Aldershot: Ashgate.

—, L. Lazzari, and M.A. D'Aronco, ed. (2007). *Form and Content of Instruction in Anglo-Saxon England in the Light of Contemporary Manuscript Evidence. Papers Presented at the International Conference Udine, April 6th-8th 2006*. Fédération Internationale des Instituts d'Études Médiévales. Textes et Études du Moyen Âge 39. Turnhout: Brepols. [forthcoming]

Lenker, U. (2000). "The Monasteries of the Benedictine Reform and the 'Winchester School'. Model Cases of Social Networks in Anglo-Saxon England?", *European Journal of English Studies* 4:3, 225-38.

Leonhardi, G., ed. (1905). *Kleinere angelsächsische Denkmäler*. Vol. 1. Bibliothek der angelsächsischen Prosa 6. Hamburg: Henri Grand.

Lewis, N. (1976, rpt. 1996). *The Interpretation of Dreams and Portents in Antiquity*. Wauconda: Bolchazy-Carducci Publishers.

Liebermann, F., ed. and transl. (1903-16). *Die Gesetze der Angelsachsen*. 3 vols. Halle: Niemeyer.

Lindelöf, U., ed. (1909-14). *Der Lambeth Psalter. Eine altenglische Interlinearversion des Psalters in der Hs. 427 der erzbischöflichen Lambeth Palace Library*. 2 vols. Acta Societatis Scientiarum Fennicæ 35:1, 43:3. Helsingfors: Duckerei der finnischen Litteraturgesellschaft.

Lindsay, W.M. ed (1911). *Isidore of Seville's Etymologiarum sive originum*. 2 vols. Oxford: OUP.

Liuzza, R.M. (2001). "Anglo-Saxon Prognostics in Context. A Survey and Handlist of Manuscripts", *ASE* 30, 181-230.

— (2004). "What the Thunder Said. Anglo-Saxon Brontologies and the Problem of Sources", *The Review of English Studies*, ns 55, 1-23.

— (2005). "The Sphere of Life and Death: Time, Medicine, and the Visual Imagination", in O'Brien O'Keeffe and Orchard (2005), II.28-52.

Logeman, H. (1889). "Anglo-Saxonica Minora", *Anglia* 11, 97-120.

Loiseleur, J. (1872). "Les jours égyptiens. Leurs variations dans les calendriers du moyen-âge", *Mémoires de la société nationale des antiquaires de France* 33, 4th ser. 3, 198-253.

Löweneck, M. (1896). *Peri didaxeon. Einer Sammlung von Rezepten in englischer Sprache aus dem 11./12. Jahrhundert*. Erlanger Beiträge zur englischen Philologie und vergleichenden Litteraturgeschichte 12. Erlangen: Fr. Junge.

Madan, F., H.H.E. Craster, and N. Denholm-Young (1922-53, rpt. 1980). *A Summary Catalogue of Western Manuscripts in the Bodleian Library at Oxford*. 7 vols. Oxford: OUP.

Madden, F. (1843). *List of Additions to the Manuscripts in the British Museum in the Years*

MDCCCXXXVI-MDCCCXL. London: Trustees of the British Museum.
Magnusson, M., and H. Pálsson, ed. and transl. (1965). *The Vinland Sagas. The Norse Discovery of America*. Harmondsworth: Penguin Books.
Maion, D. (2007). "The Fortune of the so-called *Practica Petrocelli Salernitani* in England: New Evidence and some Considerations", in Lendinara, Lazzari and D'Aronco (2007). [forthcoming]
Malone, K., and M.B. Ruud, ed. (1929). *Studies in English Philology. A Miscellany in Honor of Frederick Klaeber*. Minneapolis: Univ. of Minnesota Press.
Mare, A. C. de la, and B. C. Barker-Benfield, ed. (1980). *Manuscripts at Oxford. An Exhibition in Memory of Richard William Hunt (1908-1979), Keeper of Western Manuscripts at the Bodleian Library Oxford, 1945-1975*. Oxford: Bodleian Library.
Marsden, R., ed. (2004). *The Cambridge Old English Reader*. Cambridge: CUP.
Martin, E. (1867). "Mittelrheinische und niederländische Gedichte in einer Berliner HS.", *ZfdA* 13, 348-77.
Martin, L.T. (1977). *The Somniale Danielis. An Edition of a Medieval Latin Dream Interpretation Handbook*. Unpublished Ph.D. Thesis Univ. of Wisconsin.
— (1979). "The Earliest Versions of the Latin *Somniale Danielis*", *Manuscripta* 23, 131-41.
— (1981). *Somniale Danielis. An Edition of a Medieval Latin Dream Interpretation Handbook*. Lateinische Sprache und Literatur des Mittelalters 10. Frankfurt am Main, Bern and Cirencester: Peter D. Lang.
Matheson, L.M., ed. (1994). *Popular and Practical Science of Medieval England*. Medieval Texts and Studies 11. East Lansing: Colleagues.
Masullo, R., ed. and transl. (1985). *Marinus. Vita di Procli*. Napels: M. d'Auria Editore.
Matter, E.A. (1982). "The 'Revelatio Esdrae' in English and Latin Traditions", *Revue Bénédictine* 92, 376-92.
Mavroudi, M. (2002). *A Byzantine Book on Dream Interpretation. The Oneirocriticon of Achmet and its Arabis Sources*. The Medieval Mediterranean 36. Leiden, Boston: Brill.
McCarren, V.P., and D. Moffat, ed. (1998). *A Guide to Editing Middle English*. Ann Arbor: Univ. of Michigan Press.
McGowan, J.P. (2001a). "An Introduction to the Corpus of Anglo-Latin Literature", in Pulsiano and Treharne (2001), 11-49.
— (2001b). "Anglo-Latin Prose", in Pulsiano and Treharne (2001), 296-323.
McGurk, P., D.N. Dumville, M.R. Godden, and A. Knock (1983). *An Eleventh-Century Anglo-Saxon Illustrated Miscellany. British Library Cotton Tiberius B. V, Part I, Together With Leaves From Cotton Nero D. II*. EEMF 21. Copenhagen: Rosenkilde and Bagger.
McLachlan, L. (1929). "St Wulstan's Prayer Book", *Journal of Theological Studies* 30, 174-77.
McNeill, J.T., and H.M. Gamer (1938, rpt. 1965). *Medieval Handbooks of Penance. A Translation of the Principal Libri poenitentiales and Selections from Related Documents*. Records of Civilization, Sources and Studies 29. New York: Octagon Press.
Meaney, A.L. (1984a). "Variant Versions of Old English Medical Remedies and the Compilation of Bald's *Leechbook*", *ASE* 13, 235-68.
— (1984b). "Ælfric and Idolatry", *Journal of Religious History* 13, 199-35.
— (1985). "Ælfric's Use of His Sources in His Homily on Auguries", *English Studies* 66, 477-95.

Means, L. (1992). "Electionary, Lunary, Destinary, and Questionary. Toward Defining Categories of Middle English Prognostic Material", *Studies in Philology* 89, 367-403.

— (1993). *Medieval Lunar Astrology, A Collection of Representative Middle English Texts*. Lewiston, Queenston, Lampeter: Edwin Mellen.

— (1994). "A Translation of Martin of Spain's *De geomancia*", in Matheson (1994), 61-121.

Meens, R. (1994). *Het tripartite boeteboek. Overlevering en betekenis van vroegmiddeleeuwse biechtvoorschriften*. Middeleeuwse Studies en Bronnen 41. Hilversum: Verloren.

Meister, R. (1951). *Die Orakelsprüche im St. Galler Palimpsestcodex 908 (die sogenannten "sortes Sangallenses")*. Österreichische Akademie der Wissenschaften, philosophisch-historische Klasse, Sitzungsberichte 225:5. Vienna: Rudolf M. Rohrer.

Mercati, S.G. (1932). "Onirocritico lunare secondo i codici Vaticano Greco 342 e Berlinese Greco 168", *Byzantinische Zeitschrift* 32, 263-66.

Meritt, H.D. (1945). *Old English Glosses (A Collection)*. The Modern Language Association of America 16. London, New York: OUP, The Modern Language Association of America.

— (1954). *Fact and Lore About Old English Words*. Standford University Publications, Language and Literature 13. Stanford: Stanford UP.

Meyer, C. (1884). *Der Aberglaube des Mittelalters und der nächstfolgenden Jahrhunderte*. Basel: Felix Schneider.

Meyer, P. (1881). "Notice du MS. A 454 de la Bibliothèque de Rouen", *Bulletin de la Société des anciens textes français* 7, 76-111.

Migne, J.-P., ed. (1861-1904). *Venerabilis Bedae, Anglo-Saxonis Presbyteri Opera omnia*. 6 vols. Patrologiæ cursus completus, ser. latina 90-95. Paris.

Miles, D., R. Jayatilaka, and M. Godden (2002). *Fontes Anglo-Saxonici. A Register of Written Sources Used by Anglo-Saxon Authors*. Oxford: Fontes Anglo-Saxonici Project. CD-ROM Version 1.1.

Miller, G.H. (1909, rpt. 1994). *Dictionary of Dreams*. Ware: Wordsworth Reference.

Miller, P.C. (1994). *Dreams in Late Antiquity. Studies in the Imagination of a Culture*. Princeton: Princeton UP.

Mitchell, B. (1980). "The Dangers of Disguise. Old English Texts in Modern Punctuation", *The Review of English Studies*, ns 31, 385-413.

— (1998). *An Invitation to Old English and Anglo-Saxon England*. rev. edn. Oxford, UK, Cambridge, US: Blackwell.

Mommsen, T., ed. (1863). *Inscriptiones Latinae antiquissimae. Ad. C. Caesaris mortem*. Corpus Inscriptionum Latinarum 1. Berlin: Reimer.

Mooij-Valk, S. (2003). Artemidoros van Daldis *Droomboek*. 's-Hertogenbosch: Voltaire.

Mooney, L.R. (1994). "Diet and Bloodletting. A Monthly Regimen", in Matheson (1994), 245-61.

— (1998). "Editing Astrological and Prognostic Texts", in McCarren and Moffat (1998), 123-32.

Muir, B.J., ed. (1988). *A Pre-Conquest Prayer-Book (BL MSS Cotton Galba A.xiv and Nero A.ii (ff.3-13))*. HBS 103. Woodbridge: The Boydell Press.

Muratori, L.A., ed. (1723-58). *Rerum Italicarum scriptores ab anno aerae Christianae quingentesimo ad millesiumquingentesimum, quorum potissima pars nunc primum in lucem prodit ex Ambrosianae, Estensis, aliarumque insignum bibliothecarum codicibus*. 25 vols. Milan: Societas Palatina.

Murdoch, J.E. (1984). *Album of Science, Antiquity and the Middle Ages*. New York: Charles Scribner's Sons.

Myres, J.N.L. (1952). *Latin Liturgical Manuscripts and Printed Books*. Oxford: Bodleian Library.

Näf, B. (2004). *Traum und Traumdeutung im Altertum*. Darmstadt: Wissenschaftliche Buchgesellschaft.

Napier, A.S., ed. (1883). *Wulfstan. Sammlung der ihm zugeschriebenen Homilien nebst Untersuchungen über ihre Echtheit*. Sammlung englischer Denkmäler in kritischen Ausgaben 4. Berlin: Weidmannsche Buchhandlung.

Nares, R. (1808). *A Catalogue of the Harleian Manuscripts in the British Museum*. 3 vols. London: British Museum.

Nelson, J.L., and R.W. Pfaff (1995). "Pontificals and Benedictionals", in Pfaff (1995), 87-98.

Nokes, R. S. (2004). "The Several Compilers of Bald's *Leechbook*", *ASE* 33, 51-76.

North, J.D. (1986a) "Celestial Influence—the Major Premiss of Astrology", in Zambelli (1986), 45-100.

—— (1986b). *Horoscopes and History*. Warburg Institute Surveys and Texts 13. London: The Warburg Institute, University of London.

Oberhelman, S.M. (1981). *The Oneirocritic Literature of the Late Roman and Byzantine Eras of Greece. Manuscript Studies, Translations and Commentaries to the Dream-Books of Greece during the First Millennium A.D., with Greek and English Catalogues of the Dream-Symbols and with a Discussion of Greek Oneiromancy from Homer to Manuel the Palaeologian*. 2 vols. Unpublished Ph.D. Thesis Minneapolis, Univ. of Minnesota.

—— (1986). "The Interpretation of Dream-Symbols in Byzantine Oneirocritic Literature", *Byzantinoslavica: Revue internationale des études byzantines* 47, 8-24.

—— (1991). *The Oneirocriticon of Achmet. A Medieval Greek and Arabic Treatise on the Interpretation of Dreams*. Lubbock: Texas Tech UP.

O'Brien O'Keeffe, K., and A. Orchard, ed. (2005). *Latin Learning and English Lore. Studies in Anglo-Saxon Literature for Michael Lapidge*. 2 vols. Toronto, Buffalo, London: Univ. of Toronto Press.

Oess, G., ed. (1910). *Der altenglische Arundel-Psalter. Eine Interlinearversion in der Handschrift Arundel 60 des Britischen Museums*. Anglistische Forschungen 30. Heidelberg: Carl Winter.

Ohlgren, T.H. (1992). *Anglo-Saxon Textual Illustration. Photographs of Sixteen Manuscripts*. Kalamazoo: Medieval Institute Publications.

—— *et al.* (1986). *Insular and Anglo-Saxon Illuminated Manuscripts. An Iconographic Catalogue c. A.D. 625 to 1100*. New York and London: Garland.

Oliphant, R.T. (1966). *The Harley Latin-Old English Glossary, Edited from British Museum MS Harley 3376*. Janua Linguarum, ser. practica 20. The Hague and Paris: Mouton & co.

Olsen, K.E., and L.A.J.R. Houwen, ed. (2001). *Monsters and the Monstrous in Medieval Northwest Europe*. Leuven, Paris and Stirling (VA): Peeters.

Omont, H. (1886-88). *Catalogue général des manuscrits des bibliothèques publiques de France, Départements, Rouen*. 2 vols. Paris: Plon.

O'Neill, P. (1991). "Latin Learning at Winchester in the Early Eleventh Century. The Evidence of the Lambeth Psalter", *ASE* 20, 143-66.

Önnerfors, A. (1960). "Zur Überlieferungsgeschichte des sogenannten Somniale Danielis", *Eranos. Acta Philologica Suecana* 58, 142-58.

—— (1977). *Mediaevalia. Abhandlungen und Aufsätze*. Lateinische Sprache und Literatur des Mittelalters 6. Frankfurt am Main, Bern, Las Vegas: Peter Lang.

Oppenheim, A.L. (1956). *The Interpretation of Dreams in the Ancient Near-East, With a Translation of an Assyrian Dream-Book*. Transactions of the American Philosophical Society, ns 46:3. Philadelphia: The American Philosophical Society.

Orchard, A. (1995). *Pride and Prodigies. Studies in the Monsters of the* Beowulf-*Manuscript*. Woodbridge: D. S. Brewer.

Orchard, N. (1995). "The Bosworth Psalter and the St. Augustine's Missal", in Eales and Sharpe (1995), 87-94.

—— (2002). *The Leofric Missal*. 2 vols. HBS 113, 114. Woodbridge: The Boydell Press.

Orrick, A.H., ed. (1968). *Nordica et Anglica. Studies in Honor of Stefán Einarsson*. Janua Linguarum, ser. major 22. The Hague: Mouton.

Pächt, O., and J.J.G. Alexander (1966-73). *Illuminated Manuscripts in the Bodleian Library Oxford*. 3 vols. Oxford: OUP.

Pack, R.A. (1963). *Artemidori Daldiani Onirocriticon libri V*. Bibliotheca scriptorum graecorum et romanorum Teubneriana. Leipzig: Teubner.

Payne, J.F. (1904). *English Medicine in the Anglo-Saxon Times*. Oxford: OUP.

Penot, D. (1998). *L'interprétation des rêves. Manuel d'oniromancie arabe*. La Chapelle-Villars: Alif éditions.

Perry, G.G., ed. (1914). *Religious Pieces in Prose and Verse. Edited from Robert Thornton's MS. (Cir. 1440) in the Lincoln Cathedral Library*. rev. edn. EETS, os 26. London: OUP.

Peter Comestor (1474). *Historia scholastica*. Strasbourg.

Pfaff, R.W. (1995a). "Massbooks, Sacramentaries and Missals", in Pfaff (1995b), 7-34.

—— (1995b). *The Liturgical Books of Anglo-Saxon England*. *Old English Newsletter*, Subsidia 23.

Philippson, E.A. (1929). *Germanisches Heidentum bei den Angelsachsen*. Kölner anglistische Arbeiten 4. Leipzig: Bernhard Tauchnitz.

Pick, D, and L. Roper, ed. (2004). *Dreams and History. The Interpretation of Dreams from Ancient Greece to Modern Psychoanalysis*.London: Routledge.

Piper, F. (1862). *Die Kalendarien und Martyrologien der Angelsachsen, so wie das Martyrologium und der Computus der Herrad von Landsperg nebst Annalen der Jahre 1859 und 1860*. Berlin: Königlichen Geheimen ober-Hofbuchdruckerei.

Pithou, F., and P. Pithou (1687). *Codex canonum uetus ecclesiæ Romanæ*. Paris: Imprimerie Royale.

Planta, J. (1802). *A Catalogue of the Manuscripts in the Cottonian Library, Deposited in the British Museum*. London: British Museum.

Pongracz, M., and I. Santner (1963). *Das Königreich der Träume, 4000 Jahre moderne Traumdeutung*. Wien, Hamburg: Paul Zsolnay Verlag.

Pope, J.C., ed. (1967-68). *Homilies of Ælfric. A Supplementary Collection, Being Twenty-One Full Homilies of His Middle and Later Career for the Most Part not Previously Edited, with Some Short Pieces Added to the Second and Third Series*. 2 vols. EETS, os 259, 260. London: OUP.

—— (1998). "Eduard Sievers (1850-1932)", in Damico, Fennema and Lenz (1998), 177-99.

Pradel, F. (1907). *Griechische und süditalienische Gebete, Beschwörungen und Rezepte des Mittelalters*. Religionsgeschichtliche Versuche und Vorarbeiten 3:3. Giessen: Alfred Töpelmann.

Preisendanz, K., *et al.*, ed. and transl. (1928-31). *Papyri graecae magicae. Die griechischen Zauberpapyri*. 2 vols. Leipzig and Berlin: Teubner.

Pulsiano, P. (1994a). "Additional Evidence for an Old English 'Canterbury Vocabulary'", *Neuphilologische Mitteilungen* 95, 257-65.

—— (1994b). See Pulsiano and Doane (1994-).

—— (1995). "Psalters", in Pfaff (1995b), 61-85.

—— (1996). See Pulsiano and Doane (1994-).

—— (1998a). "Abbot Ælfwine and the Date of the Vitellius Psalter", *American Notes and Queries*, ns 11, 3-12.

—— (1998b). "The Prefatory Matter of London, British Library, Cotton Vitellius E. xviii", in Pulsiano and Treharne (1998), 85-116.

——, and A.N. Doane, gen. ed. (1994-). *Anglo-Saxon Manuscripts in Microfiche Facsimile.* Binghampton (NY), Tempe (Arizona): Center for Medieval and Renaissance Texts and Studies, Arizona Center for Medieval and Renaissance Studies. Vol. 1: *Books of Prayers and Healing* (Doane 1994); vol. 2: *Psalters 1* (Pulsiano 1994b); vol. 4: *Glossed Texts, Aldhelmia, Psalms* (Pulsiano 1996); vol. 6: *Worcester Manuscripts* (Franzen 1998); vol. 8: *Wulfstan Texts and Other Homiletic Materials* (Wilcox 2000); vol. 9: *Deluxe and Illustrated Manuscripts containing Technical and Literary Texts* (Doane and Grade 2001); vol. 11: *Corpus Christi College, Cambridge I: MSS 41, 57, 191, 302, 303, 367, 383, 422* (Graham *et al.* 2003); vol. 12: *Manuscripts of Trinity College, Cambridge* (Wright and Hollis 2004); vol. 13: *Manuscripts in the Low Countries* (Bremmer and Dekker 2006).

——, and E.M. Treharne, ed. (1998). *Anglo-Saxon Manuscripts and their Heritage.* Aldershot: Ashgate.

——, and E.M. Treharne, ed. (2001). *A Companion to Anglo-Saxon Literature.* Oxford: Blackwell.

Quinn, K.J., and K.P. Quinn (1990). *A Manual of Old English Prose.* New York, London: Garland Publishing.

Raith, J., ed. (1964). *Die altenglische Version des Halitgar'schen Bussbuches (sog. Poenitentiale Pseudo-Ecgberti).* 2nd edn. Bibliothek der angelsächsischen Prosa 13. Darmstadt: Wissenschaftliche Buchgesellschaft.

Rashed, R., ed. (1996). *Encyclopedia of the History of Arabic Science.* 3 vols. London, New York: Routledge.

Reiche, R. (1973). "Einige lateinische Monatsdiätetiken aus Wiener und St. Galler Handschriften, *Sudhoff* 57, 113-41.

Reiner, E. (1995). *Astral Magic in Babylonia.* Transactions of the American Philosophical Society, ns 85:4. Philadelphia: The American Philosophical Society.

Renzi, S. de (1852-59). *Collectio Salernitana ossia documenti inediti, e trattati di medicina appartenenti alla scuolo medica Salernitana.* 5 vols. Naples: Sebezio.

Rhodes, E.W., ed. (1889). *Defensor's* Liber Scintillarum, *With an Interlinear Anglo-Saxon Version Made Early in the Eleventh Century.* EETS, os 93. London: OUP.

Richards, M.P. (1973). "On the Date and Provenance of MS Cotton Vespasian D. XIV ff. 4-169", *Manuscripta* 17, 30-35.

—— ed. (1994). *Anglo-Saxon Manuscripts.* Basic Readings in Anglo-Saxon England 2. New York and London: Garland.

Riché, P (2004). *Abbon de Fleury. Un moine savant et combatif (vers 950-1004).* Turnhout: Brepols.

Richter, A.E., and E. Friedberg, ed. (1879-81). *Corpus iuris canonici.* 2nd edn. 2 vols. Leipzig: Tauchnitz.

Riess, E. (1891-93). "Nechepsonis et Petosiridis, fragmenta magica", *Philologus*, Suppl. 6, 325-94.

Rigg, A.G., ed. (1977). *Editing Medieval Texts English, French, and Latin Written in England. Papers Given at the Twelfth Annual Conference on Editorial Problems, University of Toronto, 5-6 November 1976.* New York, London: Garland Publishing.

Roberts, J., C. Kay and L. Grundy (2000). *A Thesaurus of Old English.* Second impression. 2 vols. Amsterdam, Atlanta: Rodopi.

Robinson, F.C., and E.G. Stanley (1991). *Old English Verse Texts from Many Sources. A Comprehensive Collection.* EEMF 23. Copenhagen: Rosenkilde and Bagger.

Robinson, P.R. (1978). "Self-Contained Units in Composite Manuscripts in Anglo-Saxon England", *ASE* 7, 231-38.

— (1988). *Catalogue of Dated and Datable Manuscripts c. 737-1600 in Cambridge Libraries.* 2 vols. Cambridge: D. S. Brewer.

—, and R. Zim, ed. (1997). *Of the Making of Books. Medieval Manuscripts, Their Scribes and Readers, Essays Presented to M. B. Parkes.* Aldershot: Scolar Press.

Rocquain, F. (1880). "Les sorts des saints ou des apotres", *Bibliothèque de l'école des Chartes* 41, 457-74.

Rohde, E.S. (1922). "The Folk-Lore of Herbals", *Folklore* 33, 243-64.

Rose, V., ed. (1894). *Theodori Prisciani Euporiston libri III, cum physicorum fragmento et additamentis Pseudo-Theodoreis.* Leipzig: Teubner.

Rosier, J.L., ed. (1962). *The Vitellius Psalter, Edited from British Museum MS Cotton Vitellius E. xviii.* Ithaca (NY): Cornell UP.

Rubin, S. (1974). *Medieval English Medicine.* New York: Barnes & Noble.

Ryan, J., ed. (1940). *Essays and Studies Presented to Professor Eoin Macneill on the Occasion of His Seventieth Birthday May 15th, 1938.* Dublin: At the Sign of the Three Candles.

Salmasius, C. (1648). *De annis climactericis et antiqua astrologia diatribae.* Leiden: Elsevier.

Salvioni, C., J. Subak, and H. Schneegans (1909). "Zu Sizilianische Gebete, Beschwörungen und Rezepte in griechischer Umschrift", *Zeitschrift für romanische Philologie* 33, 323-38.

Salzman, M.R. (1990). *On Roman Time. The Codex-Calendar of 354 and the Rhythm of Urban Life in Late Antiquity.* Berkeley: Univ. of California Press.

Sammons, J.L., and E. Schürer, ed. (1970). *Lebendige Form. Interpretationen zur Deutschen Literatur. Festschrift für Heinrich E. K. Henel.* Munich: Wilhelm Fink.

Sauer, H. (1998). "Max Förster (1869-1954)", in Damico, Fennema and Lenz (1998), 339-49.

— (2001). "Anglo-Saxon Studies in the Nineteenth Century. Germany, Austria, Switzerland, in Pulsiano and Treharne (2001), 455-71.

Savage, E.A. (1911). *Old English Libraries. The Making, Collection, and Use of Books during the Middle Ages.* London: Methuen.

Saxl, F., H. Meier, and P. McGurk (1915-66). *Verzeichnis astrologischer und mythologischer illustrierter Handschriften des lateinischen Mittelalters. Catalogue of Astrological and Mythological Illuminated Manuscripts of the Latin Middle Ages.* 4 vols. Heidelberg and London: Carl Winter and Univ. of London.

Schindler, H.B. (1858). *Der Aberglaube des Mittelalters. Ein Beitrag zur Culturgeschichte.* Wiesbaden: Dr. Martin Sändig.

Schleissner, M.R., ed. (1995). *Manuscript Sources of Medieval Medicine. A Book of Essays.* New York and London: Garland.

Schmitt, W. (1965). "Ein deutsches Traumbüchleins aus dem späten Mittelalter, *Studia Neophilologica* 37, 96-111.

— (1966). "Das Traumbuch des Hans Lobenzweig", *Archiv für Kulturgeschichte* 48, 181-

218.
Schmitz, H.J. (1883). *Die Bussbücher und die Bussdisciplin der Kirche.* Mainz: Franz Kirchheim.
Schmitz, W. (1877). *Beiträge zur lateinischen Sprach- und Literaturkunde.* Leipzig: Teubner.
Schneegans, H. (1908). "Sizilianische Gebete, Beschwörungen und Rezepte in griechischer Umschrift", *Zeitschrift für romanische Philologie* 32, 571-94.
Schönbach, A. (1875). "Zu ZS. 17, 84", *ZfdA* 18, 81-82.
—— (1890). "Bedeutung der Buchstaben", *ZfdA* 34, 1-6.
Scragg, D.G. (2001). "Secular Prose", in Pulsiano and Treharne (2001), 268-80.
——, and P.E. Szarmach, ed. (1994). *The Editing of Old English. Papers from the 1990 Manchester Conference.* Cambridge: D. S. Brewer.
Seidlin, O. (1981). "In Memoriam. Heinrich Henel (18.4.1905-7.3.1981)", *Monatshefte für deutschen Unterricht, deutsche Sprache und Literatur* 73, 289-90.
Serjeantson, Mary S. (1936). "The Vocabulary of Folklore in Old and Middle English", *Folklore* 47, 42-73.
Seymour, M.C., ed. (1975). *John Trevisa. On the Properties of Things. John Trevisa's Translation of Bartholomaeus Anglicus* De proprietatibus rerum. 2 vols. Oxford: OUP.
Sievers, E. (1875). "Bedeutung der Buchstaben", *ZfdA* 18, 297.
—— (1877). "Bedeutung der Buchstaben", *ZfdA* 21, 189-90.
Sigerist, H.E. (1923, rpt. 1977). *Studien und Texte zur frühmittelalterlichen Rezeptliteratur.* Studien zur Geschichte der Medizin 13. Vaduz: Topos Verlag.
—— (1942). "The *Sphere of Life and Death* in Early Mediaeval Manuscripts", *Bulletin of the History of Medicine* 11, 292-303.
Simpson, J.A., and E.S.C. Weiner, ed. (1992). *The Oxford English Dictionary on CD-ROM.* 2nd edn. CD-ROM Version 1.01. Oxford: OUP.
Singer, C.W. (1917). "A Review of the Medical Literature of the Dark Ages, with a New Text of about 1110", *Proceedings of the Royal Society of Medicine* 10:II, Section of the History of Medicine, 107-60.
—— (1928, rpt. 1958). *From Magic to Science. Essays on the Scientific Twilight.* New York: Dover.
—— (1961). See Cockayne (1864-66).
Sisam, C., and K. Sisam, ed. (1959). *The Salisbury Psalter, Edited from Salisbury Cathedral MS. 150.* EETS, os 242. London: OUP.
Skeat, T.C. (1970). *The British Museum Catalogue of Additions to the Manuscripts 1936-1945.* 2 vols. London: The Trustees of the British Museum.
Skeat, W.W. (1888). "Notes on English Etymology". *Transactions of the Philological Society* 1888-90, 1-22.
——, ed. and transl. (1881-1900). *Ælfric's Lives of Saints, Being a Set of Sermons on Saints' Days Formerly Observed by the English Church.* 2 vols. EETS, os 76, 82, 94, 114. London: OUP.
—— (1897). "An Anglo-Saxon Enigma", *Athenæum* 1897:I, 543.
Smith, F. (1919-33, rpt. 1976). *The Early History of Veterinary Literature and its British Development.* 4 vols. London: Allen.
Södergård, Ö. (1954). "Note sur les jours périlleux de l'année", *Neuphilologische Mitteilungen* 55, 267-71.
Soldt, W.H. van (1995). *Solar Omens of Enuma Anu Enlil. Tablets 23 (24) - 29 (30).* Uitgaven van het Nederlands historisch-archaeologisch instituut te Istanbul 73. Leiden: Nederlands historisch-archaeologisch instituut te Istanbul.

Spindler, R. (1934). *Das altenglische Bussbuch (sog. Confessionale Pseudo-Egberti). Ein Beitrag zu den kirchlichen gesetzen der Angelsachsen*. Leipzig: Bernhard Tauchnitz.
Stafford, P.A. (1978). "Church and Society in the Age of Ælfric", in Szarmach and Huppé (1978), 11-42.
Stanley, E.G. (1975). *The Search for Anglo-Saxon Paganism*. Cambridge: D.S. Brewer.
— (1998). "The Sources of Junius's Learning as Revealed in the Junius Manuscripts in the Bodleian Library", in Bremmer (1998), 159-76.
Stanton, R (2002). *The Culture of Translation in Anglo-Saxon England*. Cambridge: D.S. Brewer.
Steele, R. (1919). "Dies Aegyptiaci", *Proceedings of the Royal Society of Medicine* 12, Section of the History of Medicine, Supplement, 108-121.
Steinmeyer (1874). "Bedeutung der Buchstaben", *ZfdA* 17, 84.
Steinschneider, M. (1863). "Das Traumbuch Daniels und die oneirokritische Litteratur des Mittelalters. Eine bibliographische Studie". *Serapeum* 24, 193-216.
Stenton, F. (1971). *Anglo-Saxon England*. 3rd edn. Oxford: OUP.
Stephen, L., and S. Lee (1885-1900). *Dictionary of National Biography*. 63 vols. London: Smith, Elder & Co.
Stevens, W.M. (1979). "Introduction to Hrabani *De computo liber*", in Stevens (1995), VIII.165-96.
— (1981). "Scientific Instruction in Early Insular Schools", in Stevens (1995), IV.83-111.
— (1985, rev. 1995). "Bede's Scientific Achievement", in Stevens (1995), II.1-58.
— (1992). "Sidereal Time in Anglo-Saxon England", in Stevens (1995), V.125-52.
— (1993). "Cycles of Time. Calendrical and Astronomical Reckonings in Early Science", in Stevens (1995), I.27-51.
— (1995). *Cycles of Time and Scientific Learning in Medieval Europe*. Variorum Collected Studies Series 482. Aldershot: Ashgate.
Stevenson, J., ed. and transl. (1995). *The "Laterculus Malalianus" and the School of Archbishop Theodore*. CSASE 14. Cambridge: CUP.
Stewart, R. (1995). "The Textual Transmission of the *Sortes Astrampsychi*", *Illinois Classical Studies* 20, 135-47.
Stolberg-Wernigerode, O., Graf zu (1953-). *Neue deutsche Biographie*. Berlin: Duncker and Humblot.
Stoop, E. de (1909). "Onirocriticon du prophète Daniel dédié au roi Nabuchodonosor", *Revue de philologie, de littérature et d'histoire anciennes*, ns 33, 93-111.
Stroud, D.I. (1979). "The Provenance of the Salisbury Psalter", *The Library*, 6th ser. 1, 225-35.
Stuart, H. (1979). "A Ninth-Century Account of Diets and *Dies Aegyptiaci*", *Scriptorium* 33, 237-44.
Suchier, W. (1957). "Altfranzösische Traumbücher", *Zeitschrift für französische Sprache und Literatur* 67, 129-67.
Sudhoff, K. (1908). "Monatsregeln für den Aderlaß aus Cod. monac. lat. 13076 vom Jahre 1356", *Sudhoff* 1, 447-48.
— (1909a). "Medizinische Monatsregeln für Aderlaß, Schröpfen, Baden, Arzneigebrauch und Auswahl der Speisen und Getränke aus einer Pariser Handschrift des 14. Jahrhunderts", *Sudhoff* 2, 136-39.
— (1909b). "Nachtrag zu den 'medizinischen Monatsregeln'", *Sudhoff* 2, 384.
— (1909c). "Ein Monats-Regimen", *Sudhoff* 2, 434-36.

—— (1916). "Todes- und Lebensprobe, ägyptische Tage", *Sudhoff* 9, 308.
Svenberg, E., ed. (1936). *De Latinska Lunaria. Text och Studier*. Göteborg: Elanders Boktryckeri Aktiebolag.
—— (1939). "Nya kollektivlunaria", *Eranos. Acta Philologica Suecana* 37, 75-83.
—— ed. (1963). *Lunaria et Zodiologia Latina*. Studia Graeca et Latina Gothoburgensia 16. Göteborg: Elanders Boktryckeri Aktiebolag.
Swan, M. (2001). "Authorship and Anonymity", in Pulsiano and Treharne (2001), 71-83.
——, and E.M. Treharne, ed. (2000). *Rewriting Old English in the Twelfth Century*. CSASE 30.
Swanton, M., transl. (1993). *Anglo-Saxon Prose*. London: Dent.
Symons, T., ed. and transl. (1953). *Regularis Concordia, Anglicae nationis monachorum sanctimonialiumque. The Monastic Agreement of the Monks and Nuns of the English Nation*. London: Thomas Nelson and Sons.
Szarmach, P.E., and B.F. Huppé, ed. (1978). *The Old English Homily and its Backgrounds*. Albany (NY): State Univ. of New York Press.
Szarmach, P.E., and V.D. Oggins, ed. (1986). *Sources of Anglo-Saxon Culture*. Studies in Medieval Culture 20. Kalamazoo (MI): Medieval Institute Publications.
Taavitsainen, I. (1987). "The Identification of Middle English Lunaries", *Neuphilologische Mitteilungen* 88, 18-26.
—— (1988). *Middle English Lunaries. A Study of the Genre*. Mémoires de la société néophilologique de Helsinki 47. Helsinki: Société Néophilologique.
—— (1994). "A Zodiacal Lunary for Medical Professionals", in Matheson (1994), 283-300.
——, and Päivi Pahta, ed. (2004). *Medical and Scientific Writing in Late Medieval England*. Studies in English Language. Cambridge: CUP.
Talbot, C.H. (1967). *Medicine in Medieval England*. London: Oldbourne.
Temple, E. (1976). *Anglo-Saxon Manuscripts 900~1066*. Survey of Manuscripts Illuminated in the British Isles 2. London: Harvey Miller.
Thompson, E.M., *et al.* (1903-12). *Facsimiles of Ancient Manuscripts*. 1st ser. 10 vols. The New Palaeographical Society. London: OUP.
—— (1913-30). *Facsimiles of Ancient Manuscripts*. 2nd ser. 13 vols. The New Palaeographical Society. London: OUP.
Thompson, V. (2005). "The Pastoral Contract in Late Anglo-Saxon England: Priest and Parishioner in Oxford, Bodleian Library, MS Laud Miscellaneous 482", in Tinti (2005), 106-20.
Thomson, R.M., and M. Gullick (2001). *A Descriptive Catalogue of the Medieval Manuscripts in Worcester Cathedral Library*. Cambridge: D. S. Brewer.
Thorndike, L.(1923-58). *A History of Magic and Experimental Science during the First Thirteen Centuries of our Era*. 8 vols. New York: Columbia UP.
——, and P. Kibre (1963). *A Catalogue of Incipits of Mediaeval Scientific Writings in Latin*. rev. edn. The Mediaeval Academy of America 29. London: The Mediaeval Academy of America.
Thorpe, B., ed. (1840). *Ancient Laws and Institutes of England; Comprising Laws Enacted under the Anglo-Saxon Kings from Æthelbirht to Cnut, with an English Translation of the Saxon; the Laws Called Edward the Confessor's; the Laws of William the Conqueror and Those Ascribed to Henry the First; also, Monumenta Ecclesiastica Anglicana from the Seventh to the Tenth Century; and the Ancient Latin Version of the Anglo-Saxon Laws*. 2 vols. London.

— ed. (1844-46). *The Homilies of the Anglo-Saxon Church in the Original Anglo-Saxon, with an English Version*. 2 vols. London.

Tinti, F., ed. (2005). *Pastoral Care in Late Anglo-Saxon England*. Anglo-Saxon Studies 6. Woodbridge: The Boydell Press.

Tobler, A. (1883). *Die altvenezianische Übersetzung der Sprüche des Dionysius Cato*. Abhandlungen der königlichen Akademie der Wissenschaften zu Berlin, philosophisch-historische Classe, Abhandlung 1. Berlin: Verlag der königlichen Akademie der Wissenschaften.

Toller, T.N. ed. (1908-21). See Bosworth and Toller (1882-1972).

Tolles, T.G. (1983). "The Somniale Danielis. Visions of an Early Latin Manuscript Tradition", *Manuscripta* 27, 181-82.

Treharne, E.M. (1998). "The Dates and Origins of Three Twelfth-Century Old English Manuscripts", in Pulsiano and Treharne (1998), 227-53.

— (2000). "The Production and Script of Manuscripts Containing English Religious Texts in the First Half of the Twelfth Century", in Swan and Treharne (2000), 11-40.

— (2001). "English in the Post-Conquest Period", in Pulsiano and Treharne (2001), 403-14.

— (2003). "English 1050-1200. Dispelling the Myths", in Kooper (2003), 55-69.

—, and P. Pulsiano (2001). "An Introduction to the Corpus of Anglo-Saxon Vernacular Literature", in Pulsiano and Treharne (2001), 3-10.

—, and M. Swan (2000). "Introduction", in Swan and Treharne (2000), 1-10.

Tschann, J., and M.B. Parkes (1996). *Facsimile of Oxford, Bodleian Library, MS Digby 86*. EETS, ss 16. Oxford: OUP.

Turner, C.H. (1916). *Early Worcester Manuscripts. Fragments of Four Books and a Charter of the Eighth Century Belonging to Worcester Cathedral*. Oxford: OUP.

Turville-Petre, E.O.G. (1968). "An Icelandic Version of the *Somniale Danielis*", in Orrick (1968), 19-36.

Vernant, J.P. *et al.* (1974). *Divination et rationalité*. Paris: Éditions du Seuil.

Viré, G., ed. (1992). *Hyginus. De astronomia*. Stuttgart and Leipzig: Teubner.

Voigts, L.E. (1984). "Medical Prose", in Edwards (1984), 315-35.

— (1986). "The Latin Verse and Middle English Prose Texts on the Sphere of Life and Death in Harley 3719", *Chaucer Review* 21, 291-305.

— (1994). "The Golden Table of Pythagoras", in Matheson (1994), 123-39.

— (1995). "Multitudes of Middle English Medical Manuscripts, or the Englishing of Science and Medicine", in Schleissner (1995), 183-95.

—, and P.D. Kurtz (2000). *Scientific and Medical Writings in Old and Middle English. An Electronic Reference*. Ann Arbor (MI): Univ. of Michigan Press. [CD-ROM]

Vriend, H.J. de (1984). *The Old English Herbarium and Medicina de quadrupedibus*. EETS, os 286. London: OUP.

Vyver, A. van de (1935). "Les œuvres inédites d'Abbon de Fleury", *Revue Bénédictine* 47, 125-69.

— (1936). "Les plus anciennes traductions latines médiévales (X[e]-XIe siècles) de traités d'astronomie et d'astrologie", *Osiris* 1, 658-91.

Waitz, G. (1879). "Handschriften in englischen und scottischen Bibliotheken (Fortsetzung)", *Neues Archiv der Gesellschaft für ältere deutsche Geschichtskunde* 4, 583-625.

Wallace-Hadrill, J.M. (1988). *Bede's Ecclesiastical History of the English People, A Historical Commentary*. Oxford: OUP.

Wallis, F. (1985). *MS Oxford St John's College 17. A Mediaeval Manuscript in its Context.* 2 vols. Unpublished Ph.D. Thesis Univ. of Toronto.

— (1995). "Medicine in Medieval Calendar Manuscripts", in Schleissner (1995), 105-43.

—, ed. and transl. (1999). *Bede. The Reckoning of Time.* Liverpool: Liverpool UP.

Wanley, H. (1705). See Hickes and Wanley (1705: II).

Warner, G.F., and J.P. Gilson (1921). *Catalogue of Western Manuscripts in the Old Royal and King's Collections in the British Museum.* 4 vols. London: British Museum, OUP.

Warner, R. D.-N., ed. (1917, rpt. 1971). *Early English Homilies from the Twelfth-Century Manuscript Vesp. D. XIV.* EETS, os 152. London: OUP.

Warren, F.E., ed. (1883). *The Leofric Missal as Used in the Cathedral of Exeter during the Episcopate of its First Bishop A.D. 1050-1072, together with some Account of the Red Book of Derby, the Missal of Robert of Jumièges, and a Few Other Early Manuscript Service Books of the English Church.* Oxford: OUP.

Wasserschleben, F.W.H. (1851). *Die Bussordnungen der abendländischen Kirche nebst einer rechtsgeschichtlichen Einleitung.* Halle: Ch. Graeger.

Watson, A.G. (1979). *Catalogue of Dated and Datable Manuscripts c. 700-1600 in the Department of Manuscripts, the British Library.* 2 vols. London: British Library.

— (1984). *Catalogue of Dated and Datable Manuscripts c. 435-1600 in Oxford Libraries.* 2 vols. Oxford: OUP.

Wedel, T.O. (1920, rpt. 1968). *The Mediæval Attitude toward Astrology, Particularly in England.* Yale Studies in English 60. New Haven: Yale UP.

Weinstock, S. (1949). "Lunar Mansions and Early Calendars", *Journal of Hellenic Studies* 69, 48-69.

Weißer, C. (1976). "Zur Quellenfrage des spätmittelhochdeutschen Krankheits-Speziallunars", *Studia Neophilologica* 48, 325-29.

— (1981). "Das Krankheitslunar aus medizinhistorischer Sicht. Ein Beitrag zur iatromathematisch-astrologischen Fachliteratur des Mittelalters", *Sudhoff* 65, 390-400.

— (1982). *Studien zum mittelalterlichen Krankheitslunar. Ein Beitrag zur Geschichte laienastrologischer Fachprosa.* Würzburger medizinhistorische Forschungen 21. Hannover: Horst Wellm.

Who was Who, 1916-1928 (1947). London: Adam and Charles Black.

Wickersheimer, E. (1914). "Figures médico-astrologiques des IXe, Xe, et XIe siècles", *Janus. Archives internationales pour l'histoire de la médecine et la géographie médicale* 19, 157-77.

— (1966). *Les manuscrits latins de médecine du haut moyen âge dans les bibliothèques de France.* Documents, études et répertoires publiés par l'institut de recherche et d'histoire des textes 11. Paris: Centre national de la recherche scientifique.

Wilcox, J. (1994). *Ælfric's Prefaces.* Durham Medieval Texts 9. Durham: Durham Medieval Texts, Department of English Studies.

— (2000). See Pulsiano and Doane (1994-).

— (2001). "Transmission of Literature and Learning. Anglo-Saxon Scribal Culture", in Pulsiano and Treharne (2001), 50-70.

Wildhagen, K., ed. (1921). *Das Kalendarium der Handschrift Vitellius E XVIII (Brit. Mus.). Ein Beitrag zur Chronologie und Hagiologie Altenglands.* Halle: Max Niemeyer.

Wilhelm, F. (1914-18). *Denkmäler deutscher Proza des 11. und 12. Jahrhunderts.* 2 vols. Münchener Texte 8. Munich: Callway.

Willets, P.J. (1966). "A Reconstructed Astronomical Manuscript from Christ Church Library Canterbury", *British Museum Quarterly* 30, 22-30.

Wilmart, A. (1937-45). *Bibliotheca Apostolicae Vaticanae, Codices Reginenses Latini.* 2 vols. Rome: Bibliotheca Vaticana.

Wilson, H.A., ed. (1896). *The Missal of Robert of Jumièges.* HBS 11. London: Harrison and Sons.

— ed. (1918). *The Calendar of St. Willibrord from MS. Paris. Lat. 10837.* HBS 55. London: Harrison and Sons.

Winnefeld, H. (1887). *Sortes Sangallenses.* Bonn: Max. Cohen.

Wissowa, G., *et al.*, ed. (1894-1978). *Paulys Real-Encyclopädie der classischen Altertumswissenschaft.* 1st ser. 24 vols [1st]; 2nd ser. 10 vols [2nd]; supplement 15 vols [suppl.]. Stuttgart: Metzler.

Wistrand, E. (1942). *Lunariastudien.* Göteborgs Högskolas Årsskrift 48:4. Göteborg: Elanders Boktryckeri Aktiebolag.

Wit, M. de (2002). *Codices legere bonum significat. De Somniale Danielis (een middeleeuws droomboek) in handschriften en maatschappij der Middeleeuwen (met handschriftenbijlage, speciaalstudie en edities van Vaticaanse Somnialia).* Unpublished MA thesis Univ. of Utrecht.

Worm, O. (1626). *Fasti Danici. Universam tempora computandi rationem antiquitus in Dania et vicinis regionibus libris tribus exhibentes.* Copenhagen: Salomon Sartorius.

Wormald, F., ed. (1934, rpt. 1988). *English Kalendars before A.D. 1100.* HBS 72. Woodbridge: The Boydell Press.

— (1939-46). *English Benedictine Kalendars after A.D. 1100.* 2 vols. HBS 77, 81. London: Harrison and Sons.

— (1952). *English Drawings of the Tenth and Eleventh Centuries.* London: Faber and Faber.

— (1962). "An Eleventh-Century Psalter with Pictures, British Library, Cotton MS Tiberius C. VI", in Wormald (1984-88), vol. I, 123-37.

— (1984-88). *Collected Writings*, ed. J.J.G. Alexander, T.J. Brown and J. Gibbs. 2 vols. Oxford: OUP.

Wright, C.E., and R.C. Quirk, ed. (1955). *Bald's Leechbook, British Museum Royal Manuscript 12 D. XVII.* EEMF 5. Copenhagen: Rosenkilde and Bagger.

Wright, M., and S. Hollis (2004). See Pulsiano and Doane (1994-).

Wright, T., and J.O. Halliwell, ed. (1841-43, rpt. 1966). *Reliquiæ antiquæ. Scraps from Ancient Manuscripts, Illustrating Chiefly Early English Literature and the English Language.* 2 vols. New York: AMS Press.

Wright, T., and R.P. Wülcker, ed. (1884). *Anglo-Saxon and Old English Vocabularies.* 2 vols. 2nd edn. London: Trübner.

Yampolsky, P. (1950). "The Origin of the Twenty-Eight Lunar Mansions", *Osiris* 9, 62-83.

Zambelli, P., ed. (1986). *Astrologi hallucinati. Starts and the End of the World in Luther's Time.* Berlin: Walter de Gruyter.

Zelzer, M., ed. (1982). *St. Ambrosius. Epistulae extra collectionem.* Sancti Ambrosi Opera X.3, 141-311. Corpus Scriptorum Ecclesiasticorum Latinorum 82. Vienna: Hoelder, Pichler, Tempsky.

Zupitza, J., ed. (1880). *Ælfrics Grammatik und Glossar.* Sammlung englischer Denkmäler in kritischen Ausgaben 1. Berlin: Weidmann.

INDEX OF NAMES

The Index of Names and the Index of Subjects do not cover the footnotes, the critical apparatus of the text edition, and the appendices, with the exception of the entry on manuscripts in the Index of Subjects.

INDEX OF SUBJECTS

Brill's Studies in Intellectual History

Series Editor: A.J. Vanderjagt

Brill's Texts and Sources in Intellectual History

Subseries Editor: Han van Ruler

Recent volumes in the series:

114. Pott, S., M. Mulsow & L. Danneberg (eds.). *The Berlin Refuge 1680-1780*. Learning and Science in European Context. 2003. ISBN 978 90 04 12561 2
115. Gersh, S. & B. Roest (eds.). *Medieval and Renaissance Humanism*. Rhetoric, Representation and Reform. 2003. ISBN 978 90 04 13274 0
116. Lennon, T.M. (ed.). *Cartesian Views*. Papers presented to Richard A. Watson. 2003. ISBN 978 90 04 13299 3
117. Von Martels, Z. & A. Vanderjagt (eds.). *Pius II – 'El Più Expeditivo Pontefice'*. Selected Studies on Aeneas Silvius Piccolomini (1405-1464). 2003. ISBN 978 90 04 13190 3
118/1. Gosman, M., A. Macdonald & A. Vanderjagt (eds.). *Princes and Princely Culture 1450-1650*. Volume One. 2003. ISBN 978 90 04 13572 7
118/2. Gosman, M., A. Macdonald & A. Vanderjagt (eds.). *Princes and Princely Culture 1450-1650*. Volume Two. 2005. ISBN 978 90 04 13690 8
119. Lehrich, C.I. *The Language of Demons and Angels*. Cornelius Agrippa's Occult Philosophy. 2003. ISBN 978 90 04 13574 1
120. Bunge, W. van (ed.). *The Early Enlightenment in the Dutch Republic, 1650–1750*. Selected Papers of a Conference held at the Herzog August Bibliothek, Wolfenbüttel 22–23 March 2001. 2003. ISBN 978 90 04 13587 1
121. Romburgh, S. van, *"For My Worthy Freind Mr Franciscus Junius."* An Edition of the Correspondence of Francis Junius F.F. (1591-1677). 2004. ISBN 978 90 04 12880 4
122. Mulsow, M. & R.H. Popkin (eds.). *Secret Conversions to Judaism in Early Modern Europe*. 2004. ISBN 978 90 04 12883 5
123. Goudriaan, K., J. van Moolenbroek & A. Tervoort (eds.). *Educa-tion and Learning in the Netherlands, 1400-1600*. 2004. ISBN 978 90 04 13644 1
124. Petrina, A. *Cultural Politics in Fifteenth-Century England: The Case of Humphrey, Duke of Gloucester*. 2004. ISBN 978 90 04 13713 4
125. Schuurman, P. *Ideas, Mental Faculties and Method*. The Logic of Ideas of Descartes and Locke and Its Reception in the Dutch Republic, 1630–1750. 2004. ISBN 978 90 04 13716 5
126. Bocken, I. *Conflict and Reconciliation: Perspectives on Nicholas of Cusa*. 2004. ISBN 978 90 04 13826 1
127. Otten, W. *From Paradise to Paradigm*. A Study of Twelfth-Century Humanism. 2004. ISBN 978 90 04 14061 5
128. Visser, A.S.Q. *Joannes Sambucus and the Learned Image*. The Use of the Emblem in Late-Renaissance Humanism. 2005. ISBN 978 90 04 13866 7
129. Mooij, J.J.A. *Time and Mind*. History of a Philosophical Problem. 2005. ISBN 978 90 04 14152 0
130. Bejczy, I.P. & R.G. Newhauser (eds.). *Virtue and Ethics in the Twelfth Century*. 2005. ISBN 978 90 04 14327 2
131. Fisher, S. *Pierre Gassendi's Philosophy and Science*. Atomism for Empiricists. 2005. ISBN 978 90 04 11996 3

132. Wilson, S.A. *Virtue Reformed.* Rereading Jonathan Edwards's Ethics. 2005. ISBN 978 90 04 14300 5
133. Kircher, T. *The Poet's Wisdom.* The Humanists, the Church, and the Formation of Philosophy in the Early Renaissance. 2005. ISBN 978 90 04 14637 2
134. Mulsow, M. & J. Rohls (eds.). *Socinianism and Arminianism.* Antitrinitarians, Calvinists and Cultural Exchange in Seventeenth-Century Europe. 2005. ISBN 978 90 04 14715 7
135. Rietbergen, P. *Power and Religion in Baroque Rome.* Barberini Cultural Policies. 2006. ISBN 978 90 04 14893 2
136. Celenza, C. & K. Gouwens (eds.). *Humanism and Creativity in the Renaissance.* Essays in Honor of Ronald G. Witt. 2006. ISBN 978 90 04 14907 6
137. Akkerman, F. & P. Steenbakkers (eds.). *Spinoza to the Letter.* Studies in Words, Texts and Books. 2005. ISBN 978 90 04 14946 5
138. Finkelstein, A. *The Grammar of Profit: The Price Revolution in Intellectual Context.* 2006. ISBN 978 90 04 14958 8
139. Ittersum, M.J. van. *Profit and Principle.* Hugo Grotius, Natural Rights Theories and the Rise of Dutch Power in the East Indies, 1595-1615. 2006. ISBN 978 90 04 14979 3
140. Klaver, J.M.I. *The Apostle of the Flesh: A Critical Life of Charles Kingsley.* 2006. ISBN 978 90 04 15128 4
141. Hirvonen, V., T.J. Holopainen & M. Tuominen (eds.). *Mind and Modality.* Studies in the History of Philosophy in Honour of Simo Knuuttila. 2006. ISBN 978 90 04 15144 4
142. Davenport, A.A. *Descartes's Theory of Action.* 2006. ISBN 978 90 04 15205 2
143. Mazzocco, A. *Interpretations of Renaissance Humanism.* 2006. ISBN 978 90 04 15244 1
144. Verbaal, W., Y. Maes & J. Papy (eds.). *Latinitas Perennis, Volume I: The Continuity of Latin Literature.* 2007. ISBN 978 90 04 15327 1
145. Boulton, D'Arcy J.D. & J.R. Veenstra (eds.). *The Ideology of Burgundy.* The Promotion of National Consciousness, 1364-1565. 2006. ISBN 978 90 04 15359 2
146. Ruler, H. van, A. Uhlmann & M. Wilson (eds.). *Arnold Geulincx* Ethics. With Samuel Beckett's Notes. Translated by M. Wilson. 2006. ISBN 978 90 04 15467 4 (Published as Vol. 1 in the subseries *Brill's Texts and Sources in Intellectual History*)
147. Radding, C.M. & A. Ciaralli (eds.). *The* Corpus Iuris Civilis *in the Middle Ages.* Manuscripts and Transmission from the Sixth Century to the Juristic Revival. 2007. ISBN 978 90 04 15499 5
148. Birkedal Bruun, M. *Parables: Bernard of Clairvaux's Mapping of Spiritual Topography.* 2007. ISBN 978 90 04 15503 9
149. Lehner, U. *Kants Vorsehungskonzept auf dem Hintergrund der deutschen Schulphilosophie und -theologie.* 2007. ISBN 978 90 04 15607 4
150. Warnar, G. *Ruusbroec.* Literature and Mysticism in the Fourteenth Century. Translated by D. Webb. 2007. ISBN 978 90 04 15869 6
151. Treschow, M., Otten, W. & W. Hannam (eds.). *Divine Creation in Ancient, Medieval, and Early Modern Thought.* Essays Presented to the Rev'd Dr Robert D. Crouse. 2007. ISBN 978 90 04 15619 7
152. Juste, D. *Les* Alchandreana *primitifs.* Étude sur les plus anciens traités astrologiques latins d'origine arabe (Xe siècle). 2007. ISBN 978 90 04 15827 6 (Published as Vol. 2 in the subseries *Brill's Texts and Sources in Intellectual History*)
153. Chardonnens, L.S. *Anglo-Saxon Prognostics, 900-1100.* Study and Texts. 2007. ISBN 978 90 04 15829 0 (Published as Vol. 3 in the subseries *Brill's Texts and Sources in Intellectual History*)
154. Melve, L. *The Medieval Public Sphere.* Continuity and Innovation in the Polemical Literature of the Investiture Contest. 2007. ISBN 978 90 04 15884 9
155. Velema, W. *Republicans.* Essays on Eighteenth-Century Dutch Political Thought. 2007. ISBN 978 90 04 16191 7
156. Boone, R.A. *War, Domination, and the* Monarchy of France. Claude de Seyssel and the Language of Politics in the Renaissance. 2007. ISBN 978 90 04 16214 3